Drug Interactions
in Anesthesia

Drug Interactions in Anesthesia

N. TY SMITH, M.D.
Department of Anesthesiology
Veterans Administration Medical Center
Professor of Anesthesiology
University of California
San Diego, California

ALDO N. CORBASCIO, M.D., D.Sc.
Professor of Pharmacology
University of the Pacific
San Francisco, California

Second Edition

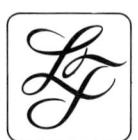

Lea & Febiger
Philadelphia
1986

Lea & Febiger
600 Washington Square
Philadelphia, PA 19106-4198
U.S.A.
(215) 922-1330

First Edition, 1981
  Reprinted, 1982
Second Edition, 1986

Library of Congress Cataloging-in-Publication Data

Main entry under title:

Drug interactions in anesthesia.

  Includes bibliographies and index.
  1. Drug interactions. 2. Anesthesiology. I. Smith,
N. Ty (Norman Ty), 1932–   . II. Corbascio, Aldo N.,
1928–   . [DNLM: 1. Anesthesia. 2. Anesthetics.
3. Drug Interactions. QV 38 D79325]
RD82.7.D78D78   1986   615'.781   85–18236
ISBN 0-8121-0998-8

Copyright © 1986 by Lea & Febiger. Copyright under the International Copyright Union. All rights reserved. This book is protected by copyright. *No part of it may be reproduced in any manner or by any means without written permission from the publishers.*

Printed in the United States of America

Print No. 4 3 2 1

"To Penelope and Caterina:

The beacons which light our way."

FOREWORD

Modern man accepts drug therapy as a necessary means to attain and maintain good health. If an adverse drug interaction occurs as a consequence of multiple drug therapy, however, modern man does not accept it as an act of God, but rather as a fault for which someone must be held responsible. It is mandatory, therefore, for all anesthesiologists, indeed all physicians, to be fully knowledgeable about drug interactions. That drug interactions do not lead more frequently to problems in everyday living is remarkable, considering the enormous quantity and variety of pills that people ingest. Perhaps interactions are much more common than we appreciate. Patients coming to the operating room are subjected to an intense pharmacologic siege brought about by the drugs introduced by the anesthetist on a body that has already been exposed to other drugs in the preanesthetic period. The possibilities for drug interactions are innumerable. All anesthesiologists must address themselves to and understand this reality.

Anesthesia is the sum of amnesia, analgesia, sedation, hypnosis, relaxation, and attenuation of noxious reflexes.[1,2] As a result of this definition, many anesthetists have concluded that the optimal way to produce the anesthetic state is to use the smallest amount of a variety of drugs, each of which contribute to one of the previously mentioned states. Thus, a common sequence is the frequent use of two or three premedicants before delivery to the operating suite followed by the intravenous administration of atropine or an atropine-like drug. Next comes a small dose of a nondepolarizing muscle relaxant (to minimize fasciculations and muscle pain secondary to succinylcholine), an analgesic, a sedative/hypnotic, the succinylcholine, and then one, two, or three inhalation and/or intravenous agents. The resultant pharmacologic stew produced in the short interval of anesthetic induction is one that our anesthetic ancestors never dreamed about and would probably condemn, being fully aware of the dangers of poly-pharmacy and the difficulty of extricating one drug response from another.

Thus, the anesthesiologist contributes to the plethora of potential drug interactions now associated with anesthesia and surgery. Is this desirable? Is this something that we should be seeking in the future development of anesthetic agents and adjuvants? I doubt it. Yet the idea of developing a perfect, single-agent anesthetic is not popular at this time, and therefore, anesthetic-induced drug interaction will continue to be a daily reality. For this reason, a text dealing with anesthetic drug interactions is not only relevant but extremely important. The possibility that an understanding of potential drug interactions may allow the more rational development of new anesthetics should not be discounted. The importance of drugs administered hours, perhaps days, after the use of anesthetic agents and adjuvants in the operating or recovery rooms is still another area of concern. There is little doubt that there will be further anesthetic drug development in the foreseeable future. Hopefully, those who direct or influence our specialty may seriously consider single compounds that can produce the same effects as three others and demand that they be used instead of the multiple-agent approach. Whether this tree will ever bear fruit is difficult to say. It is clear that, for the moment, we must not ignore the complexities of potential and real drug interactions, and that we must try to understand the fundamentals and mechanisms of the subject. Thus, it is important to know and understand the types and mechanisms, as well as the physical and chemical bases, of these interactions. In addition, such seemingly unrelated concepts as competition at the plasma protein level and at receptor binding sites, effects of altered drug excretion, accelerated and/or inhibited drug metabolism, and the importance of physiologic changes and homeostatic alterations to these changes must be fully mastered. It is with a text designed to explore these complex and often difficult-to-comprehend subjects that mastery begins.

> Theodore H. Stanley, M.D.
> Professor of Anesthesiology/Surgery
> University of Utah
> Salt Lake City, Utah

REFERENCES

1. Gray, T.C., and Rees, G.J.: The role of apnea in anesthesia for major surgery. Brit Med J 2:891, 1952.
2. Woodbridge, P.D.: Changing concepts concerning depth of anesthesia. Anesthesiology 18:536, 1957.

PREFACE

We need not justify the necessity for another edition of a book on drug interactions. Change in this field has occurred at least as rapidly as in other areas of medicine. This swift change is reflected in this second edition by five additional chapters on subjects that either warranted a separate treatment in the first edition or that have matured considerably.

The least change that might be expected during the interval between editions is the detection of new interactions among existing pairs of agents, the combination of suspected interactions, the formulation of new principles, or the application of old principles applied to allow a better understanding of interactions.

All of this has indeed happened, particularly in the application of old principles. During the past several decades, pharmacokinetics has contributed enormously to the intelligent use of the inhaled anesthetic agents. Its contribution to our understanding of the behavior of intravenous agents has until recently been much more modest. Lately, however, pharmacokinetics has contributed increasingly not only to our understanding of individual drugs, but to interactions among them. In fact, it has allowed us to predict specific interactions that have in turn been searched for and uncovered. To recognize the importance of these endeavors, we have added a new chapter on pharmacokinetics, one that complements the information contained in the chapter on mechanisms.

But more exciting information has appeared since the first edition. New drugs and new classes of drugs, as well as new receptor sites and theories, have been investigated and implemented in clinical practice. These new drugs and new classes interact not only with each other, but also with existing agents. The most prominent addition to drugs has been the calcium-channel blockers. This group of drugs has been rapidly introduced into therapy with considerable advantages to the patients but at an increased cost in terms of interactions. We are just beginning to uncover and to explain some of these interactions.

In addition to the chapter on calcium-channel blockers, other headings have been included in the second edition: "Antibronchospastic Drugs," "Antihistaminics," "Antiepileptic Agents," and "Inorganic Cations." This last chapter represents a unique class of drugs, one that has been around since the beginning of medicine, but one that is still poorly understood.

The identification of receptor sites invariably leads to a proliferation of antagonists and agonists/antagonists. Conversely, the development of a pure antagonist agent is essential to help to complete the understanding of the receptor sites and of *endogenous* ligands, that is, the body's "drugs" that react with the receptor sites. Thus, successively, neuromuscular blocking agents, adrenergic agents, opiates, and benzodiazepines have followed the same pattern of inquiry and development. The benzodiazepine receptor sites are emphasized in a greatly expanded chapter on "Sedatives and Hypnotics," while opiates receive extensive treatment in a carefully crafted revision of "Narcotics and Narcotic Antagonists." Similarly, the chapter entitled "Neuromuscular Blocking Agents" has been revised to reflect the addition of two new agents to the clinical toolbox.

Several other chapters have received careful and extensive revision for the second edition, including chapters 1, 3, 7, 9, 11, 12, 14, 17, 19, 23, 25, 26, and 27. All in all, the second edition contains a considerable amount of new information.

Concerns have been raised about two features in the first edition, one relating to too little information, the other relating to too much. It has been observed that, on the one hand, the emphasis was placed on drugs used in the United States to the apparent exclusion of those used in Europe, for example. On the other hand, it has been perceived that much of the information contained in the first edition was "unnecessary" for practice in the operating room.

In regard to the first point, the contributors must be ultimately selective in the information they present because the number of drugs accessible to the clinician is overwhelming. The contributors to this book have collected information where it is available on drug interactions; frequently, of course, a drug is omitted simply because no interaction information is available. Recently, a phenomenon has occurred that makes a general, comprehensive compendium of drugs difficult to achieve. Many countries have set up their own equivalent to the U.S. Food and Drug Administration. Each of these organizations requires a long, involved process for approval of a new drug. For this reason, few drugs are available in every country; many are available in only a few. Thus, it would be wasteful to try to describe every drug in detail. Fortunately, general principles of drug interactions *usually* apply to classes of drugs, and knowledge of these principles can make possible the prediction of interaction in individual drugs. For example, although individual calcium-channel blocking agents differ in their interactions, major drug interactions should be relatively easy to predict if one is aware of a few guiding principles, as well as the characteristics of each drug of interest.

In regard to the point that the first edition presented information not strictly pertinent to the anesthesiologist, we feel strongly that anesthesiologists must be informed in areas beyond the narrow bounds of the operating room. For example, they must also be aware of drug interactions that occur in the surgical intensive care unit, the medical intensive care unit, the coronary care unit, the emergency room, and the delivery room. The knowledge that ethanol and insulin taken together can lead to profound coma, or of the availability of agents that can quickly reverse benzodiazepine-induced coma, is useful to any anesthetist trained to help in the therapy of comatose patients. In addition, the anesthetist should know not only about the potential interactions among preoperative drugs and anesthetic agents, but also about interactions among those strictly given by the internists because many of these interactions affect the perianesthetic and perisurgical care of the patient. Finally, although the title of the book does refer to anesthesia, the book is also intended as a reference source for those working outside the field of anesthesia.

The first edition was found clinically useful. In particular, the case-report format has received wide approval. With this encouragement, we have continued this approach in the second edition. We have also adhered to the original chapter arrangement: an initial section on general principles; followed by chapters on the pharmacology and interactions of groups of drugs, chapters complete in themselves, so that the reader will not be forced to peruse several sources for the required information; and a clinical orientation exemplified by abundant case reports.

Finally, we must extend our thanks to Robin A. Brien, Administrative Assistant to Dr. Smith, for her invaluable help in coordinating the editorial phases of this publication.

We hope that you enjoy reading this book, and that we may hear from you concerning its usefulness, whatever your area of interest.

San Diego, California   N. Ty Smith
San Francisco, California Aldo N. Corbascio

CONTRIBUTORS

Milton H. Alper, M.D.
  Professor of Anesthesia
  Harvard Medical School
  Anesthesiologist-in-Chief
  The Children's Hospital
  Boston, MA

Aaron H. Anton, Ph.D.
  Professor of Anesthesiology and
    Pharmacology
  Case Western Reserve School of Medicine
  Cleveland, OH

John L. Atlee, III, M.D.
  Associate Professor of Anesthesiology
  University of Wisconsin Medical School
  Madison, WI

R. Dennis Bastron, M.D.
  Professor of Anesthesia
  Department of Anesthesia
  Arizona Health Sciences Center
  Tucson, AZ

Burnell R. Brown, Jr., M.D., Ph.D.
  Professor and Head, Anesthesiology
  Professor, Pharmacology and Toxicology
  University of Arizona Health Sciences
    Center
  Clinical Head, Department of
    Anesthesiology
  University of Arizona Medical Center
  Tucson, AZ

Helmut F. Cascorbi, M.D., Ph.D.
  Professor and Chairman, Dept. of
    Anesthesiology
  Case Western Reserve University
  School of Medicine
  Cleveland, OH

Henry Casson, M.D.
  Associate Professor of Anesthesiology
  Oregon Health Sciences University
  School of Medicine
  Portland, OR

Aldo N. Corbascio, M.D., D.Sc.
  Professor of Pharmacology
  University of the Pacific
  San Francisco, CA

David J. Cullen, M.D.
  Associate Professor, Anesthesiology
  Harvard Medical School
  Director of Recovery Room—Acute Care
    Area
  Massachusetts General Hospital
  Boston, MA

Sanjay Datta, M.D.
  Associate Professor of Anesthesia
  Harvard Medical School
  Senior Staff Anesthesiologist
  Director of Obstetric Anesthesia
  Brigham and Women's Hospital
  Boston, MA

Hall Downes, M.D., Ph.D.
  Professor of Pharmacology and
    Anesthesiology
  Oregon Health Sciences University
  Portland, OR

Joel D. Everett, M.D.
  Visiting Clinical Anesthetist
  University of Utah
  School of Medicine
  Salt Lake City, UT

Joan W. Flacke, M.D.
  Professor of Anesthesiology
  University of California, Los Angeles
  School of Medicine
  Los Angeles, CA

Werner E. Flacke, M.D.
  Professor of Anesthesiology and
    Pharmacology
  University of California, Los Angeles
  School of Medicine
  Los Angeles, CA

CONTRIBUTORS

Pierre Foëx, M.D., D. Phil.
Clinical Reader (Clinical Physiology)
University of Oxford
Honorary Consultant (Clinical Physiology)
Oxford Hospitals
Oxford, England

J.S. Gravenstein, M.D.
Graduate Research Professor of
Anesthesiology
University of Florida
College of Medicine
Gainesville, FL

Carol A. Hirschman, M.D.
Professor of Anesthesiology and
Pharmacology
Oregon Health Sciences University
Portland, OR

Carl C. Hug, Jr., M.D., Ph.D.
Professor of Anesthesiology and
Pharmacology
Emory School of Medicine
Director of Cardiothoracic Anesthesia
Emory Clinic
Atlanta, GA

David C. Janowsky, M.D.
Professor, Department of Psychiatry
University of California, San Diego
La Jolla, CA

Esther C. Janowsky, M.D.
Associate Clinical Professor
Department of Anesthesiology
University of California, San Diego
San Diego, CA

Robert M. Julien, M.D., Ph.D.
Staff Anesthesiologist
St. Vincent Hospital and Medical Center
Portland, OR

Patricia A. Kapur, M.D.
Assistant Professor of Anesthesiology
University of California, Los Angeles
School of Medicine
Los Angeles, CA

Harry G.G. Kingston
Associate Professor of Anesthesiology
Oregon Health Sciences University
Portland, OR

Igor Kissin, M.D., Ph.D.
Professor of Anesthesia
Director of Basic Research
Department of Anesthesiology
University of Alabama Medical Center
Birmingham, AL

David E. Longnecker, M.D.
Distinguished Professor of Anesthesiology
University of Virginia
Charlottesville, VA

Edward Lowenstein, M.D.
Professor of Anesthesia
Harvard Medical School
Anesthetist
Massachusetts General Hospital
Boston, MA

George E. McLain, Jr., M.D.
Research Associate
Department of Anesthesiology
Arizona Health Sciences Center
College of Medicine
Tucson, AZ

Robert G. Merin, M.D.
Professor of Anesthesiology
University of Texas Medical School
Staff Anesthesiologist
Hermann Hospital
Houston, TX

Ronald D. Miller, M.D.
Professor and Chairman of Anesthesiology
Professor of Pharmacology
University of California
School of Medicine
San Francisco, CA

Edwin S. Munson, M.D.
Professor and Chairman of Anesthesiology
University of Kentucky
College of Medicine
Attending Anesthesiologist
University of Kentucky Hospital
Staff Physician, Anesthesiology Service
Veterans Administration Medical Center
Lexington, KY

John L. Neigh, M.D.
Associate Professor of Anesthesia
University of Pennsylvania
Director, Department of Anesthesia
Presbyterian-University of Pennsylvania
Medical Center
Philadelphia, PA

J.G. Reves, M.D.
  Professor of Anesthesiology
  Director, Division of Cardiothoracic
    Anesthesia
  Duke University Medical Center
  Durham, NC

M. Frances Rhoton, Ph.D.
  Associate Professor of Anesthesiology
  Case Western Reserve University
  School of Medicine
  Cleveland, OH

S. Craig Risch, M.D.
  Associate Professor, Department of
    Psychiatry
  University of California, San Diego
  La Jolla, CA

Ben F. Rusy, M.D.
  Professor of Anesthesiology
  University of Wisconsin Medical School
  Madison, WI

N. Ty Smith, M.D.
  Professor of Anesthesiology
  University of California, San Diego
  Staff Anesthesiologist
  VA Medical Center
  San Diego, CA

Theodore H. Stanley, M.D.
  Professor of Anesthesiology/Surgery
  University of Utah
  Salt Lake City, UT

Robert K. Stoelting, M.D.
  Professor and Chairman
  Department of Anesthesia
  Indiana University
  School of Medicine
  Indianapolis, IN

K.C. Wong, M.D., Ph.D.
  Professor of Anesthesiology and
    Pharmacology
  Chairman, Department of Anesthesiology
  University of Utah
  School of Medicine
  Salt Lake City, UT

CONTENTS

Foreword vii
Theodore H. Stanley, M.D.

1. Dangers and Opportunities 1
   N. Ty Smith, M.D.

2. The Preoperative Visit 12
   J.S. Gravenstein, M.D.
   M.F. Rhoton, M.D.
   Helmut F. Cascorbi, M.D., Ph.D.

3. Mechanisms: General Principles .. 16
   Werner E. Flacke, M.D.
   Joan W. Flacke, M.D.

4. Pharmacokinetics and Drug Interactions 39
   Aldo N. Corbascio, M.D., D.Sc.

5. The Effect of pH 51
   J.S. Gravenstein, M.D.
   A.H. Anton, Ph.D.

6. The Role of the Liver 63
   Burnell R. Brown, Jr., M.D., Ph.D.
   George E. McLain, Jr., M.D.

7. Sympathomimetic Drugs 71
   K.C. Wong, M.D., Ph.D.
   Joel D. Everett, M.D.

8. Antibronchospastic Drugs 100
   Harry G.G. Kingston, M.B., B.Ch., F.F.A.R.C.S.
   Hall Downes, M.D., Ph.D.
   Carol A. Hirschman, M.D.

9. Beta-Adrenergic Blockers 114
   Edward Lowenstein, M.D.
   Pierre Foëx, M.D.

10. Calcium-Channel Blockers and Other Vasodilating Antianginal Agents 135
    Patricia A. Kapur, M.D.

11. Antihypertensives and Alpha Blockers 147
    Robert K. Stoelting, M.D.

12. Cholinergic and Anticholinergic Agents 160
    Werner E. Flacke, M.D.
    Joan W. Flacke, M.D.

13. Histamine H_2 Blockers 176
    Henry Casson, M.D.

14. Digitalis 179
    John L. Atlee, III, M.D.
    Ben F. Rusy, M.D.

15. Inorganic Cations 196
    Aldo N. Corbascio, M.D., D.Sc.
    N. Ty Smith, M.D.

16. Diuretics 206
    Robert G. Merin, M.D.
    R. Dennis Bastron, M.D.

17. Antidysrhythmic Agents 225
    John L. Atlee, III, M.D.

18. Antiepileptic Agents 245
    Robert M. Julien, M.D., Ph.D.

19. Psychotropic Agents 261
    Esther C. Janowsky, M.D.
    S. Craig Risch, M.D.
    David S. Janowsky, M.D.

20. Sedatives and Hypnotics 282
    N. Ty Smith, M.D.

21.	Intravenous Anesthetic Agents J.G. Reves, M.D. Igor Kissin, M.D., Ph.D.	308	25.	Local Anesthetics Edwin S. Munson, M.D.	391
22.	Narcotics and Narcotic Antagonists Carl C. Hug, Jr., M.D., Ph.D. David E. Longnecker, M.D.	321	26.	Drugs and Anesthetic Depth David J. Cullen, M.D.	407
23.	Inhalation Anesthetic Agents John L. Neigh, M.D.	340	27.	Agents in Obstetrics: Mother, Fetus, and Newborn Milton H. Alper, M.D. Sanjay Datta, M.D.	427
24.	Neuromuscular Blocking Agents Ronald D. Miller, M.D. N. Ty Smith, M.D.	363		Index	439

1

DANGERS AND OPPORTUNITIES

N. TY SMITH

The first known anesthetic death could have been prevented by knowledge in a specific area of drug interactions. Mortality and morbidity continue to arise from our understandable ignorance of many facets of this subject. On the other hand, drug interactions have helped to transform the course of anesthetic management, which currently relies on the skilled administration of several drugs to the same patient. Certainly, combination therapy and drug interactions are the basis of "balanced" anesthesia. Hence the art lies in the avoidance of hazardous interactions and in the expert application of useful ones. This introductory chapter examines the role of drug interactions in the practice of anesthesia. The emphasis is on the practical side of the subject, including the contributions of research to the clinical understanding of drug interactions.

CASE REPORT

In 1848, 16-year-old Hannah Greener came under the care of Dr. Meggison, a country practitioner near Newcastle, England, for the removal of a great toenail. She was terrified of the impending procedure, and accepted gratefully the offer of the new anesthetic agent, chloroform. This only partially calmed her, and she approached the operation with fear. The story of her sudden death during the first few whiffs of chloroform and of the futile attempts to resuscitate her with brandy is too well known to repeat here. There is now little doubt that her death was a direct result of the interaction between chloroform and the excess epinephrine discharged from her adrenals. Had Dr. Meggison chosen ether, her life probably would have been spared. The clarification of the cause of Hannah's mysterious death had to wait over half a century for the classic studies of Goodman Levy, who demonstrated unequivocally that chloroform sensitizes the myocardium to the dysrhythmic actions of epinephrine.[1,2]

Even today, physicians often wait until an interaction has occurred and then ascertain the cause, rather than anticipate an interaction on theoretical grounds. The major difference is that, because of an expanded pool of pharmacologic knowledge, the time scale of this sequence has been compressed—from over 60 years in the case of chloroform, to a few hours or days.

A Useful Drug Interaction

Drug interactions have exerted a profound effect on the development of modern anesthesia. Neuromuscular blocking agents are an example. Previously, adequate muscle relaxation could be obtained only with the primary anesthetic agent, usually ether. This relaxation was achieved at the risk of profound central nervous, circulatory, and occasionally respiratory depression. The introduction of muscle relaxants allowed the use of lower concentrations of potent inhaled agents, or even their abandonment in favor of the intravenous agents. The latter led to the implementation of the concept of "balanced" anesthesia, which meant balancing the dosage of drugs with different actions to provide adequate amnesia, muscle relaxation, analgesia, and attenuation of reflexes.

The safe use of curare was certainly an essential feature of this revolution in anesthetic practice. The changes brought about by curare, however, were not the consequence of the introduction of a single drug, but were due to the skillful exploitation of the interactions among three drugs: curare, neostigmine, and atropine. It is not an overstatement to claim that the rapid expansion of modern surgery is closely connected with the purposeful application of drug interactions.

Dangers and Opportunities

The guiding principles, then, of the succeeding chapters are avoiding or at least attenuating undesirable and dangerous drug interactions, using desirable and useful interactions to maximum advantage, and converting ostensibly undesirable interactions into useful ones.

One example should suffice for the last principle. About 25 years ago, the combination of ether and curare was banned in our training program because of a well-known study by Beecher and Todd,[3] who had demonstrated that the mortality following the combination was 1 in 50. Thus my teacher's suggestion to use ether and curare for a case met with my resistance. He explained that the basis of the ether-curare combination was marked synergism, and the solution was simply to use less of each drug, particularly curare. Today we should take this principle for granted—when there is synergism or addition between two agents, less of one, or preferably of both, should be used. However, one still sees, for example, nondepolarizing blocking agents administered on a fixed schedule, irrespective of the anesthetic used. The result can be troublesome, particularly with halothane, enflurane, or isoflurane. Small increments of the neuromuscular blocking agent and low concentrations of the inhaled agent will suffice, with adjustment of muscle relaxation according to the concentration of the inhaled agent. This approach takes advantage of a drug interaction, rather than being controlled or hindered by it.

The "Ideal" Opiate Antagonist

The evolution of opiate anesthesia and the opiate antagonists illustrates a useful drug interaction, as well as the search for the "ideal" drug interaction. Ideally, an antagonist should (1) have no effect of its own, (2) reverse only the "undesirable" effects of the agonist, and (3) last longer than the agonist. The first is easily attained. The third, a long duration of action, is nebulous, since the opiates vary considerably in this respect. If the antagonist administered in the recovery room lasts too long, pain relief may be delayed. The second criterion (selective antagonism) is even less well defined. The definition of desirability depends upon the circumstances. For example, the amphetamines have hypertensive, anorectic, and cortical stimulating properties. Each of these properties may be desirable if the agent is used to elevate blood pressure, decrease the appetite, or elevate the mood; the other two automatically become side-effects. The opiates, with their protean effects, are no exception. Physicians often employ the usually undesirable effect of ventilatory depression in patients who are resisting the ventilator, and the somnolence produced by some opiates is considered desirable in patients on long-term ventilation. It is currently an open question whether specificity of action should be built into the agonists themselves, or into the antagonists.

An Interaction Gone Astray

Occasionally, a useful drug combination goes beyond its original intent. The addition of epinephrine to a local anesthetic is an example. Its usefulness in decreasing the toxicity and prolonging the duration of the local anesthetic is well documented. In the presence, however, of certain inhaled agents, particularly halothane, an additional and undesirable interaction may occur: a decrease in the dysrhythmic threshold to epinephrine. We now know that enflurane and isoflurane are better agents to use in the presence of exogenously administered epinephrine, halothane permits limited use, and cyclopropane is unacceptable. Interestingly enough, the presence of lidocaine increases the threshold to epinephrine-induced dysrhythmias.[8]

Still another unanticipated interaction is the advance warning that epinephrine may provide against local anesthetic toxicity. If rapid intravascular absorption following injection of the test dose occurs, it may be difficult to detect any effects of the anesthetic, whereas those of epinephrine are usually obvious—tachycardia, palpitations, and headache. If these manifestations are present, one should assume that significant amounts of the local anesthetic have also been absorbed and that central nervous system toxicity may occur on further injection.

On the other hand, if the epinephrine is absorbed slowly during a peridural anesthetic, as is appropriate, still another type of interaction occurs. Blood pressure and systemic vascular resistance may actually *decrease* more when epinephrine is in the anesthetic solution than when it is not.[4] Why should this happen when the original drug interaction depended on the vasoconstrictive properties of epinephrine? In high concentrations, as present in the epidural space, epinephrine does have an *alpha*-adrenergic (vasoconstrictive) action. In low concentrations—diluted in the bloodstream—it acts as a *beta*-adrenergic substance. Presumably this vasodilating action adds to the vasodepressant effects of lidocaine—both direct and indirect from the sympathetic block—to produce noticeably greater hypotension. Thus a drug interaction that began as straightforward has become complex.

RESEARCH INTO DRUG INTERACTIONS

The rest of this chapter will deal with the state of research into drug interactions, and with the impact of this research on daily practice. Research is defined here as any concerted effort that increases our knowledge and allows the useful transfer of that knowledge to the practicing physician.

The Problem of Definitions

The terminology used to describe drug interactions is in a sad state. The lack of standard definitions has created a problem in this book, since we must use terms as other authors have used them, and their definitions either vary or are nonexistent. For accuracy, I shall outline below some of the definitions that have been proposed. For the sake of standardization, I shall give my own preferences.

The commonly used terms are *addition, antagonism, synergism,* and *potentiation*. Before synergism or antagonism can be defined, there must be some agreement on the definition of *addition*, or the mode of summation of drug effects. Two definitions of addition are generally used: (1) *dose addition*, when one-half the dose of drug A plus one-half an equi-effective dose of drug B evokes the same effect as the entire dose of drug A or drug B alone; (2) *effect addition*, when the intensity of the combined effect equals the sum of the intensities of the effect that each drug evokes when administered alone. Effect addition is certainly additive behavior as it may be expected from a superficial examination; each drug simply brings its own effect into the partnership. I prefer the dose-addition definition, although with dose-addition, the combined drug effect is not so obvious. It is more easily understood by considering a simple experiment. Equipotent amounts of drug A and drug B can be established. If upon administration of one-half of each of these amounts, the same effect is achieved as from either drug alone in its full amount, dose addition exists. The same is true if we use one-third of drug A and two-thirds of drug B, one-quarter of drug A and three-quarters of drug B, one-fifth of drug A and four-fifths of drug B, etc. Thus the one moiety of the combined drug does not add its own effect to that of the other moiety, but complements the effect of the latter exactly to the intensity that would be achieved by the sum of the fractional doses if both were fractions of either A or B.

Synergism has been defined as a type of interaction in which the effect of a combination of drugs is greater than the effect of (1) any drug given singly, (2) the combined effects of the drugs, or (3) the effect of the sum of the drugs, i.e., greater than addition as defined in the previous paragraph. The third definition might be called *dose synergism*, and in keeping with our acceptance of the dose addition concept, I prefer this definition.

The first definition of synergism is the one most widely used or implied in case and clinical reports. The rationale given is that synergism literally means "working together," and any combination that gives a greater effect than either drug alone is synergistic. However, it would seem that if the effect of the combination of two drugs is less than the sum of the effects of the drugs, the drugs are actually working against each other. For example, if two lumberjacks can saw down trees at the rate of ten trees each per day, and if together they can saw down only 12 trees, it would seem that somehow they were working against each other, perhaps by getting in each other's way; the relationship is in fact antagonism.

Potentiation has had several definitions, most of them the same as the definitions given for synergism above. I prefer the following definition: the enhancement of action of one drug by a second drug that has no detectable action of its own. Thus, although cocaine has no sympathomimetic action of its own, it potentiates the action of epinephrine.

In its simplest form, the definition of *antagonism* is the opposing action of one drug toward another. When drugs exert opposite physiologic actions, as do nitroprusside and methoxamine, or when an inactive drug diminishes the effect of an active drug (naloxone and a narcotic) the understanding of the concept of antagonism, physiologic or pharmacologic, is straightforward. However, when two drugs produce a similar effect, they may still antagonize each other if the combined effect is less than that of the sum of the drugs, as defined by dose addition.

We can thus summarize the aforementioned definitions: additive interaction may be represented by 2 + 2 = 4; synergism by 2 + 2 = 5; potentiation by 0 + 2 = 3; and antagonism by 0 + 2 < 2; 1 + 2 < 3; or 2 + 2 < 4.

The Present State of Drug Interaction Research

Quantifying Drug Interactions. The quantification of drug interactions is an interesting part of pharmacology in which one goes beyond the stage of saying that, for example, synergism is present, and tries to determine how much. This area, however, is replete with complex notions, large numbers of curves placed together on the same graph, and difficult mathematic calculations. Research is usually done *in vitro*, or in animals, at best. It is therefore beyond the scope of this book. Suffice it to say that research into the quantification of drug interaction is still in a rudimentary state, and is rarely useful to the clinician.

The extent of knowledge of interactions among more than two drugs is even more discouraging. Few studies even semiquantitatively examine the interaction among three agents, and none has attempted more than three. The experiments are long, the data involve four dimensions, and the display of data requires a three-dimensional plot. That the simplest technique involves one dimension for each drug[5] plus one additional dimension has discouraged most investigators.

Even the qualitative description of multiple-drug interactions can be overwhelming. Thus we were unable to find an author willing to write a chapter on this subject. The problem must be faced, however; the large number of drugs used by anesthesiologists and other physicians mandates it. It is not unusual for the anesthetist to use six to ten drugs per patient, including preanesthetic medication. Preoperatively, a patient may be receiving more than 40 medications concurrently, many of which are multicomponent preparations![6]

This information on multiple-drug interaction should be important. For example, one would intuitively expect that the interaction among quinidine, a nondepolarizing neuromuscular blocking agent, and an antibiotic would be more severe than that between any two of these agents.

The Incidence of Drug Interactions. Another difficulty in drug-interaction research has been in estimating the incidence of drug interactions in all hospitalized patients and not just in those patients undergoing anesthesia and surgical procedures. Some attempts have been made,[6,10] but the results vary considerably. Problems arise from variations in the strictness of criteria for the incidence and the clinical relevance of a drug interaction, from whether a study was prospective or retrospective, from the attitude of physicians toward filling out "yet another form," and from whether an interaction or a potential interaction was reported. (A potential interaction means that two or more drugs that *might* cause an interaction are administered to the same patient.)

One attempt to estimate the incidence of drug interactions has been to establish the relationship between the number of drug *reactions* and the total number of drugs given. It is assumed that this relationship should be linear; that is, twice as many

Table 1–1

Number of Drugs Given	Reaction Rate (%)
0–5	4.2
6–10	7.4
11–15	24.2
16–20	40.0
21+	45.0

(From Smith, J.W., Seidl, L.G., and Cluff, L.E.: Studies on the epidemiology of adverse drug reactions. V. Clinical factors influencing susceptibility. Ann. Intern. Med., 65:629, 1966.)

drugs should produce twice the incidence of reactions. Thus any greater increase in drug reactions would be partly due to drug interactions. According to Table 1–1, the number of drug reactions does increase out of proportion to the increase in the number of drugs consumed. One could argue, however, that a larger number of drugs taken indicates a more severely ill patient, and that reactions are determined partly by the condition of the patient.

Bringing Information to the Physician. Of more interest to the practicing physician than the methodology and the rigidity of assessing drug interactions is the accumulation and maintenance of an accurate mass of information about well-documented drug interactions, and a method for disseminating this information in a clinically useful way. This is even more difficult than it sounds. The widespread circulation of inaccurate, poorly documented, or clinically irrelevant information has retarded the general acceptance of the medical significance of drug interactions. Although certain examples of enhancement of toxicity or antagonism of beneficial effects resulting from the use of specific drug combinations are widely recognized by physicians, in general the substantial number of potential drug interactions and the pharmacologic complexities involved in many of these interactions have made it impractical for most anesthesiologists to have adequate drug-interaction information available when therapy is prescribed, when the patient is evaluated, or when anesthesia is administered.

There are a few reliable sources of information on drug interactions. None of them emphasizes the interactions of interest to the anesthesiologist, although some do provide information for those wishing to explore the problem further. Hansten has written a book that summarizes a large number of interactions in a convenient and easy-to-read format.[11] This useful book is now in its 4th edition. The American Pharmaceutical and Medical Associations have sponsored a book that goes into more detail.[12] It includes short treatises on groups of drugs and the interactions within these groups, as well as a number of succinct monographs dealing with individual drug-drug interactions. The National Institutes of Health have published three enormous volumes, which cover all of the drug interactions reported or investigated between 1967 and 1974.[13] These volumes have been a valuable resource for the serious student of drug interactions, but they are impossible to carry around on preanesthetic rounds. In contrast to these large books is a small drug interaction "wheel" (Medisc, Excerpta Medica Services). Whereas this pocket-sized device is probably of more interest to internists than to those whose primary interests lie in the operating room, and whereas it gives no other information than the possibility of an interaction, it may alert the physician as to when to seek more information.

Other books continue to be published and republished. *Drug Interactions Index*[14] summarizes many interactions important to the family practitioner. It briefly states each interaction and outlines suggestions on how to prevent or deal with the interactions. The index itself is extensively cross referenced, although it is moderately clumsy to use, and no references are cited. *Drug Interactions Indexed*[15] is a much smaller volume. It tabulates interactions in the following form: "When a person is on this drug . . . , And this drug is added . . . , This interaction may occur." Again, no references are cited. *Drug Interactions Handbook*[16] is intended for the layman. Its principal utility to the physician is its extensive listings of trade/generic names, not only for single-drug prescription items, but also for over-the-counter and multicomponent items.

The field of drug interactions is changing so rapidly, partly because of the continual addition of new drugs, that several attempts have been made to help the physician keep up via the newsletter format. *Drug Interactions Newsletter*[17] is specifically oriented in this direction, while *The Medical Letter*[18] gives occasional information on drug interactions. A good compromise between reasonably detailed information and fairly rapid updating is *United States Pharmacopeia Dispensing Information,*[19] which is revised annually, with updates bimonthly. Its major drawback is the lack of citations, but the information appears to be carefully screened. The currently best all-around source is the *MEDIPHOR Drug Interaction Facts,* discussed below.

With few exceptions, little information directly applicable to operating room practice is contained in these volumes. And much of the information that does exist shows a lack of understanding about this area. The following example, relating to the interaction between sulfonamides and thiopental, should demonstrate this point. "Increase in thiopental levels, possibly leading to toxicity. Respiratory depression can result. Pay particular attention to respiratory inadequacy when using thiopental in patients taking sulfonamides."

It would not be surprising, however, if the physician were wary of books or schemes that claim to specify drug interactions, since the history of drug interaction recounts many false alarms. In the case of the antihypertensive agents, we have successively believed that reserpine, guanethidine, *alpha*-methyldopa, and propranolol are all dangerous drugs to the anesthetized patient, and that they should be discontinued before operation if at all possible. We have repeatedly conveyed this information to our colleagues. It is no won-der if surgeons mistrust drug-interaction information from anesthesiologists. In fact, many patients have been denied timely operations because of this belief. The attitude toward various antihypertensive agents has changed several times over the past few years, but gradually some fundamental guidelines have emerged. (1) We now believe that many of the initially reported problems were due not to the drugs but to the disease and the resulting propensity to labile arterial pressures. (2) Current opinion suggests that to withdraw some antihypertensive agents (clonidine or propranolol) can be dangerous or even lethal. (3) Perhaps therapy *should be initiated before anesthesia* in patients with uncontrolled hypertension. (4) Finally some have gone so far as to suggest that a *beta*-adrenergic blocking agent should be given prophylactically before induction of anesthesia in any patient in whom it is desirable to avoid hypertensive episodes.

Another consideration in transmitting drug-interaction information properly to the physician is the classification of drug interactions in a way that can provide guidelines for dealing with the interaction effectively. Although drug interactions are often thought of in absolute terms, they represent only one of many factors influencing the clinical response to drugs. Moreover, most interacting drug combinations *can* be given concurrently if the interacting potential is kept in mind by the physician and proper adjustments in dosage or route of administration are made.

The Stanford MEDIPHOR system was the first to take advantage of the power of the computer to store, manipulate, and retrieve large data bases related to drug interactions. It and the report class-designation were developed by Cohen et al. beginning in 1969.[6] It provides in a convenient manner both necessary information and useful guidelines.

Each prescription for a hospitalized patient is entered at a terminal at the hospital pharmacy, and a computer-stored record is created and maintained for each patient. The record is updated by entries of relevant information about all medication changes, and newly prescribed drugs are checked for potential interactions with drugs already included in the patient drug profile. When an interaction is found by the search programs, the computer generates a report (Fig. 1–1), which is printed at a terminal located in the hospital pharmacy and sent to the nursing unit along with the medication. A sample of the report is shown below. A brief description of the report class-designation follows. In general, Class 1 contains interactions having clinically significant effects that would be expected to occur relatively quickly after administering the drug combination. The patient's physician is informed about the potential interaction, its implication, and some suggestions on how to deal with it before the first dose of the interacting drug is administered. For example, the interaction between monoamine oxidase inhibitors and certain sympathomimetic amines is included in this class.

Class 2 interactions have consequences that may be less immediate, but nonetheless serious. In this case, the first dose of the interacting drug may be administered, but the physician is contacted before the drug combination is continued as prescribed. The interference with the hypotensive effects of guanethidine when a tricyclic antidepressant is given concurrently is an example of a Class 2 interaction.

Class 3 is assigned to interactions that have well-documented clinical significance, but do not ordinarily lead to clinically apparent consequences until the interacting drug combination has been administered repeatedly. Information about such an interaction is placed conspicuously in the patient's chart, but the drugs are administered as prescribed unless the physician changes his order. The interaction between phenobarbital and coumarin anticoagulants is included in this class.

```
                    Sample of a drug interaction report produced on the pharmacy report printer
        STANFORD UNIVERSITY MEDICAL CENTER. DIVISION OF CLINICAL PHARMACOLOGY. DRUG INTERACTION REPORT
                                            REPORT #0

        T D                                      0002001   E1A
        (Patient name)                           (Account no.)                    (Med rec no.)

        12/31/74    IF THE CONSEQUENCES OF THIS INTERACTION OCCUR, THEY MAY NOT BE EVIDENT UNTIL THIS
                    DRUG COMBINATION HAS BEEN ADMINISTERED FOR A VARIABLE PERIOD OF TIME, BUT THEY MAY
                    POTENTIALLY LEAD TO SYMPTOMS OF TOXICITY OR LOSS OF THERAPEUTIC EFFICACY OF ONE OR
                    BOTH OF THE DRUGS LISTED IN THIS REPORT.

        DIURIL(CHLOROTHIAZIDE) WITH DIABINESE(CHLORPROPAMIDE)

        OLD DRUG: DIURIL(CHLORPROPAMIDE)
            MEMBER OF CLASS: SULFONYLUREAS
            DRUG STARTED ON 12/31/74

        NEW DRUG: DIURIL(XHLOEORHIAZIDE)
            MEMBER OF CLASS: THIAZIDE DIURETICS

        PHARMACOLOGICAL EFFECTS: PHARMACOLOGICAL EFFECTS OF DIABINESE DECREASED.

        MECHANISMS: ANTAGONISTIC PHARMACOLOGICAL ACTIVITIES.

        CLINICAL FINDINGS: IMPAIRED THERAPEUTIC EFFECTIVENESS OF DIABINESE.
            HYPERGLYCEMIA.

        CLINICAL MANAGEMENT SUGGESTIONS: MAY NEED HIGHER DOSE OF DIABINESE

        REFERENCES:
            RUNYAN, J.W., JR.: NEJM, 267: 541(1962)
            SHAPIRO, A.P., ET AL.: NEJM, 265: 1028(1961)
            SAMAAN, N., ET AL.: LANCET, 2: 1244(DEC 14, 1963)
            BASABE, J., ET AL.: EXCERPTA MED INT CONG SERIES, 231:476(1971)

        COMMENTS:
            THIAZIDES CAUSE INCREASED BLOOD GLUCOSE IN 15 TO 25% OF PATIENTS AFTER SEVERAL MONTHS OF
            THERAPY. THE FREQUENCY IS HIGHER IN DIABETICS. THE INHIBITION OF INSULIN RELEASE FROM
            PANCREAS.

                The drug interaction report is based on information available to the hospital pharmacy.
            The report may involve drugs that have been discontinued if prescription changes have not been
            forwarded promptly to the pharmacy or if the drug's interactive potential persists for a period
            after it has been stopped.
                Please request clinical pharmacology consultation if additional information about the
            interaction is desired.  This report is provided for informational purposes only.  While the
            information is believed to be correct, neither Stanford University nor the Stanford University
            Hospital is responsible for the accuracy or validity of this report nor for the clinical
            consequences of administering or not administering any of the drugs herein mentioned.
                                                                                       WARD COPY
        (Tatro DS, Briggs RL, Chavez-Pardo R, Feinberg LS, Hannigan JF, Moore TN, Cohen SN:  Online
        drug interaction surveillance, in Computer Concepts: Gouveia WA (Ed) Am J Hosp Pharm 32:417-
        420,1975.)
```

Fig. 1–1. A report from the Stanford MEDIPHOR system.

Class 4 contains interactions that are not sufficiently well documented to warrant distributing reports to physicians, and are used for investigational purposes only.

In general, the MEDIPHOR system* has been useful.[20] The two major problems encountered with the system were undue repetition of the issuance of the reports, and the legal implications. Given today's legal climate, the latter is a justifiable concern. One would hope, however, that the availability of information would not increase the liability of the user of the information. Such an atmosphere would be counterproductive, of course.

Since the first edition of this book, the MEDIPHOR system has evolved in three ways. First, the system currently used at Stanford has been expanded in several areas. For example, laboratory test data and other information are included with the pharmacologic information. Second, the MEDIPHOR system has been licensed by Stanford as a commercial product and is available for use in hospitals.

Third, the MEDIPHOR data base is partially available in printed form: *Drug Interaction Facts*.[21] This publication is in loose-leaf format, so that it can be readily updated. New material is distributed quarterly. As a matter of fact, a new revision was mailed in July, 1984. The publication is not only well referenced, but the citations are carefully screened by an outstanding panel. The format is such that it is easy to estimate the rapidity of onset, severity of the interaction, and validity of the doc-

---

*Medication Services, Inc., San Raphael, California.

umentation. Again, however, relatively little information is available for use in the operating room.

Perhaps the MEDIPHOR system could be modified for use in anesthesia. The reader can, however, appreciate the magnitude of the task. Would it require the services of a computer? Certainly. The drug file used in the Stanford reporting system contains more than 4,000 pharmaceutical preparations.[6] In the case of multicomponent preparations, entries identify each generic component of the preparation, as well as its interaction class. Thus the computer can search for interactions of drugs included in various brand-name compounds and in other multicomponent preparations. The interaction search, which occurs following entry of a new prescription to the patient's medication record, often requires a substantial amount of computing time (occasionally as long as 1 to 2 minutes) when the patient is receiving many other drugs. The computer must search every new prescription for possible interactions with the components of *each* of the previous medications. The task would be more complex for an anesthesia-drug interaction search system, since the computer would have to search for possible interactions among the patient's present medications and the proposed anesthesia or ancillary agents each time the anesthesiologist contemplated using a new agent during the anesthetic course. The system would require interactive information terminals both on the wards for preanesthetic rounds and in the operating rooms.

What to Do Until the Computer Comes. Once information on a potential drug interaction has been received by the anesthesiologist, the problem is only partially solved. The physician must then know how to minimize the occurrence of drug interactions. There are many ways to accomplish this, some obvious, others not. In the case of the Stanford computerized system, the task is simplified by an educational printout that accompanies each drug-interaction warning (Fig. 1–1). Until such a service is generally available for anesthesiologists, we must adhere to the old rules, however.

1. Obtain a careful history from each patient. When inquiring about the drug history, whether prescribed or self-administered, use understandable terms, for example, pain, fever, or flu reliever for aspirin, or blood pressure tablets for antihypertensive drugs. Do not neglect useful information that can be obtained from a history of experiences with drugs.
2. Restrict the number of drugs to the essential minimum. This advice is easier for the anesthesiologist to give than to take. I am aware that multiple-drug use is part of the practice of many anesthesiologists and, as outlined above, that drug interactions can be made useful, rather than harmful, if carefully controlled. On the other hand, the concept that fewer drugs are associated with fewer drug interactions has considerable merit.
3. If multiple-drug therapy is required, avoid those drugs that are likely to cause serious interactions or make control of therapy difficult. Some drug combinations are best avoided. Certainly, drugs (for example, monoamine oxidase inhibitors) that can cause serious reactions should be avoided wherever possible. Substitute drugs that can be more safely given. For example, with oral coumarin anticoagulants, consider indomethacin for phenylbutazone, paracetamol (acetaminophen) for aspirin, diazepam for a barbiturate sedative, flurazepam or nitrazepam for a barbiturate hypnotic. When muscle relaxants or potent inhaled agents are used, consider vancomycin or oleandomycin for neomycin, streptomy-

cin, or any one of the many antibiotics that can increase the neuromuscular blocking properties of our agents (see Chap. 24). If fixed combination drugs must be used, the components must be known.
4. Always keep in mind genetic factors and associated diseases or pathophysiologic conditions that may enhance an interaction. Pseudocholinesterase deficiency comes to mind immediately. The combination of this condition plus succinylcholine plus peritoneal lavage with certain antibiotics could be disastrous. As outlined in Chapters 16 and 24, the presence of renal pathology can accentuate many drug interactions.
5. Changes of drug therapy should be kept to a minimum. Again this advice may seem gratuitous to the anesthesiologist, who must by definition change the patient's drug regimen many times in order to administer an anesthetic. However, one must also consider the role of the anesthesiologist outside the operating room in the long-term care of the patient, for example in the intensive-care unit. If changes are necessary and involve known interactions, some change in dose can be anticipated, but the time, course, and extent of interaction vary with the drugs and the individual patient. Any dose adjustment should only be made on the basis of results derived from close observation of therapy over a period of time after the change. This is particularly important with oral coumarin anticoagulants.
6. Pay special attention to problem drugs. These include oral coumarin anticoagulants, oral sulfonylurea, hypoglycemics, digitalis, anticonvulsants, antihypertensive drugs, CNS-depressant or antipsychotic drugs, or neuromuscular blocking agents.
7. Educate the patient and the patient's attending physician. This implies that the anesthesiologist must be educated first. Warn them of the possible dangers that may arise with changes, cessations, or alterations in medication, whether prescribed or self-administered.

The Future of Drug-Interaction Research

What are the future needs of research into drug interactions, as well as the clinical understanding of their complexities? (1) We need better methods for quantifying drug interactions. These methods should be clinically relevant, and the results should be understandable and made available to clinicians, and not just to an elite few. (2) The complexities of interactions among more than two drugs must be solved. The solutions may require new mathematic and statistical methods, or they may be based on available methods, as we attempted to do in our early work.[5] (3) A system must be developed for recording and evaluating drug interactions on a prospective basis. A multihospital cooperative study may be necessary, as is done so well in the Veterans Administration Hospitals. (4) Current information should be available to the physician immediately. Thus any drug-interaction warning system, such as that developed at Stanford, should include a mechanism for a continual updating of the information in its files—with all the complexities that this implies. The Stanford system, as well as MEDIPHOR, has just such capabilities. (5) One set of information could give the probability of a clinically important interaction if two or more drugs are given. The physician, after all, considers various probabilities when making diagnostic and therapeutic decisions.

What is the clinician's responsibility in this problem? The anesthesiologist not only must be well informed about drug interactions, but also must be alert for them, both on preanesthetic rounds and each time a drug is administered in the operating or recovery room. This is not possible unless the proper information is supplied. The research scientist can determine whether the information is clinically useful only by observing and by receiving feedback from the clinician on how it is used, the ease with which it is used, and its comprehensibility.

In summary, we have presented a philosophy of drug interactions as seen from the anesthesiologist's viewpoint. We have shown that some drug interactions can be very hazardous, some can be useful, and others can be useful only if manipulated properly. To avoid troublesome interactions and to take advantage of useful ones requires extensive knowledge. Unfortunately, the progress of research into drug interactions and the rate of transfer of knowledge to the clinician is still slow. We need more help in discriminating between relevant and irrelevant interactions, and in gaining access to already accumulated knowledge. Computerized systems for detection of drug interactions are needed for the anesthesiologist similar to the one available for internists. Finally, a system for the continual education of the physician must be set up.

REFERENCES

1. Levy, A.G.: Sudden death under light chloroform anaesthesia. J. Physiol., 42:III, 1911.
2. Levy, A.G.: Chloroform Anaesthesia. London, John Bole & Sons & Danielsson, 1922.
3. Beecher, H.K., and Todd, D.P.: A Study of Deaths Associated with Anesthesia and Surgery. Springfield, Ill., Charles C Thomas, 1954.
4. Bonica, J.J., et al.: Circulatory effects of peridural block: II. Effects of epinephrine. Anesthesiology, 34:514, 1971.
5. Gershwin, M.E., and Smith, N. Ty: Interaction between drugs using three-dimensional isobolographic interpretation. Arch. Int. Pharmacodyn. Ther., 201:154, 1973.
6. Cohen, S.N., et al.: A computer-based system for the study and control of drug interactions in hospitalized patients. In Drug Interactions. Edited by P.L. Morselli, S. Garattini, and S.N. Cohen. New York, Raven Press Brooks, Ltd., 1974.
7. Borda, L.T., Slone, D., and Jick, H.: Assessment of adverse reactions within a drug surveillance program. J.A.M.A., 205:645, 1968.
8. Ogilvie, R.I., and Ruedy, J.: Adverse reactions during hospitalization. Can. Med. Assoc. J., 97:1445, 1967.
9. Seidl, L.G., et al.: Studies on the epidemiology of adverse drug reactions. Bull. Johns Hopkins Hosp., 119:299, 1966.
10. Stewart, R.B., and Cluff, L.E.: Studies on the epidemiology of adverse drug reactions VI: Utilization and interactions of prescription and nonprescription drugs in outpatients. Johns Hopkins Med. J., 129:319, 1971.
11. Hansten, P.D.: Drug Interactions. Third Edition. Philadelphia, Lea & Febiger, 1975.
12. Ascione, F.J.: Evaluations of Drug Interactions. Second Edition. Washington, D.C., American Pharmaceutical Association, 1976.
13. Drug Interactions: an annotated bibliography with selected excerpts, 1967–1970. Vol. 1, 1972, HEW publication no. (NIH) 73–322; Vol. 2, 1974, (NIH) 75–322; Vol. 3, 1975, (NIH) 76–3004.
14. Lerman, F., and Weibert, R.T.: Drug Interactions Index. Oradell, NJ, Medical Economics Co., Inc., 1983.
15. Litton Industries: Drug Interactions Indexed. Oradell, NJ, Medical Economics Co., 1975.
16. Harkness, R.: Drug Interactions Handbook. Englewood Cliffs, NJ, Prentice-Hall, 1984.
17. Hansten, P.D.: Drug Interactions Newsletter. San Francisco, CA, Applied Therapeutics, Inc., 1980.
18. Abramowicz, M. (Ed.): The Medical Letter. New Rochelle, NY, The Medical Letter, Inc., 1984.
19. United States Pharmacopeia Dispensing Information. U.S. Pharmacopeial Convention, Inc., 20th Ed., 1980.
20. Tatro, D.S., et al.: Online drug interaction surveillance. In Computer Concepts. Edited by W.A. Gouveia. Am. J. Hosp. Pharm., 32:417, 1975.

|2|

THE PREOPERATIVE VISIT

J.S. GRAVENSTEIN, M.F. RHOTON, and HELMUT F. CASCORBI

Recently, in consultation with an internist, we performed a careful preoperative assessment and developed a special plan for anesthesia for a patient with sickle cell anemia. This extra effort was questioned by the internist on the grounds that our obligations were the same for all patients regardless of concomitant diseases and that good anesthetic management is supposed to prevent hypoxia, acidosis, stasis, and cooling.

We were unable to counter these arguments satisfactorily. Our colleague was right. All patients deserve the same meticulous anesthesia care, with avoidance of hypoxia and acidosis, as do patients with sickle cell disease. Theoretically, therefore, an extra effort in detecting preoperative problems should not be necessary since, again theoretically, everybody should receive the best possible anesthetic management.

In reality, however, not all patients do receive the best possible anesthetic care. Hypotension, bouts of hypoxemia, and acidosis do occur occasionally and special efforts to prevent such occurrences are in order for patients who cannot tolerate even small deviations from normal. A good preoperative screen is therefore necessary to detect the patients who require these special efforts. Such careful preoperative analysis, unfortunately, is not universal, and thousands of patients each year receive anesthesia and undergo operations without the benefits of a thorough and complete preoperative evaluation. These patients receive little more than a rapid review of the record before induction, because of the time constraints of anesthetic practice. Nonetheless, this perfunctory procedure does identify the occasional patient with a family history of unusual problems (for example, malignant hyperpyrexia) that might have eluded the examination of family physician, internist, or surgeon. Moreover, when combined with good anesthetic management, a brief preinduction assessment does seem to lower morbidity and mortality levels.

In light of these arguments, why do we insist on a complete preoperative workup? First, we believe that the encounter with the anesthesiologist before an operation is psychologically beneficial to the patient. Here the anesthesiologist has an opportunity to answer questions, allay unfounded fears, provide support, and instill confidence.

Second, there is a small group of patients (in our hospital, probably less than 1%) for whom a complete anesthetic history and an examination of the drug regimen for potential drug-interaction problems requires postponement of the anesthesia and the operation. For these selected patients, a complete anesthetic evaluation is lifesaving. Since they cannot be identified in advance, it is mandatory to screen *all* patients for the benefit of these few. Hence the routine preoperative workup is an obligation we cannot escape.

What happens during a preanesthetic visit? The physician meets the patient, seeks to establish rapport and inspire confidence, in short, develops the elements of a patient-physician relationship. Simultaneously, the anesthesiologist seeks the special information (history of disease, drug intake, previous anesthetics) that will influence his choice of anesthesia for this particular patient. We find that the experienced clinician seems to employ intuition, which is difficult to define and impossible to teach. Analysis of "intuition," however, reveals a structure that can be identified and taught. We call this the *key-words* structure. At first glance, many key words might appear to be common, informational medical terms. Indeed, these words only become special when the anesthesiologist recognizes them as signals to be translated into a *category*. These categories then invite a clear exposition of the therapeutic issues under the heading *problems*, which makes it easier to outline options or *actions*. Given the *key word* "crush injury" we think of the *category* "muscle damage." The *problem* is potassium release with succinylcholine and the logical *action* is avoidance of depolarizing drugs.

Let us take a more complex but common anesthetic problem.

CASE REPORT

Mrs. S., a 40-year-old white housewife, was plump, but not grossly overweight. She was seeing a surgeon because of repeated attacks of biliary colic. Scheduled for elective cholecystectomy, she was examined preoperatively by the anesthesiologist. During the interview, the patient related nothing unusual except a history of asthma. The patient also revealed that she was taking steroids, phenobarbital, and that she used an isoproterenol inhaler whenever she felt tightness in the chest. The last serious attack of asthma had occurred fifteen months before.

Some experienced anesthesiologists might have decided to premedicate her with 20 mg of diazepam intramuscularly 1 hour before anesthesia, to add intravenous atropine prior to induction of anesthesia with thiopental, and to maintain anesthesia with halothane, 60% N_2O, and oxygen, without an endotracheal tube. Others might have used a different approach. In any case, all should have been able to present a rationale for their choice.

How is the rationale for a given anesthetic management developed? We extract several *key words;* cholecystectomy, phenobarbital, and asthma, as shown in Table 2–1.

The reasoning for a somewhat unusual management, that is, no intubation for an upper abdominal incision and halothane for a juxtahepatic operation, becomes clear with this analysis.

There are other key words in this history, for instance, 40-year-old woman.

As in the case of phenobarbital, this key word itself can have several categories (see Table 2–2, which has two of the many possible subcategories for phenobarbital):

The *key-word* system leads to rational, teachable plans of action, development of alternatives, and assignment of priorities to therapeutic issues. For instance, a gynecologic history is needed regarding possible pregnancy and the use of contraceptive pills. The use of *beta*-2-adrenergic stimulating drugs reduces the likelihood of arrhythmias when halothane is employed because of its bronchodilating effects. Methoxyflurane is excluded because the history of phenobarbital intake suggests the activation of microsomal enzymes and consequently the excessive biotransformation of methoxyflurane into toxic breakdown products. As a result of these considerations of drug interaction, a third drug (for example, enflurane) may be chosen.

In the search for drug interactions and by the use of this approach, we can record a drug history using the familiar *review of systems*. There are many different ways to organize such an approach. It makes little difference which one adopts as long as one adheres to a method, which is the only way to minimize the chance of forgetting a system, a drug, or a problem.

3

MECHANISMS: GENERAL PRINCIPLES

WERNER E. FLACKE and JOAN W. FLACKE

Modern anesthesia is based on planned use of the effects and interactions of several, sometimes multiple, drugs. This is a significant departure from earlier times, when a single, "complete" anesthetic agent was employed to bring about the conditions required for the conduct of surgical and other diagnostic and therapeutic procedures. Of the several reasons for this change, the first is the recognition that clinical anesthesia combines several different conditions: analgesia, loss of consciousness and memory formation, skeletal muscle relaxation, and autonomic, especially cardiovascular, stability in the face of major stresses. Next is the increasing realization that general anesthetics are toxic. Finally, the introduction of so-called adjuvant drugs has made it possible to achieve several of the foregoing components of anesthesia by means other than the use of classic general anesthetic agents. Not only can muscle relaxation be produced by intravenous injection of neuromuscular blocking drugs, but almost any degree of analgesia can be achieved by large doses of potent analgesics. We can bring about clouding of consciousness and inhibition of memory formation by drugs other than general anesthetics.

Although each adjuvant drug needed to produce a part of the total syndrome of clinical anesthesia has its own drawbacks, the disadvantages of single-agent anesthesia are such that proponents of that practice have all but disappeared. Indeed, a return to it is unlikely unless new agents with properties that would increase their safety considerably become available.

These continuing developments in the simultaneous use of several drugs place a much greater burden on the anesthesiologist to understand drug interactions. It is not our purpose here to reexamine well-established practices. Although we shall discuss general principles of drug interaction that have a bearing on present-day anesthesia, we wish to focus mainly on unintentional and usually undesirable interactions whose mechanisms are often controversial and obscure.

The clinical significance of many drug interactions is often undetermined, and few of the questions posed have been answered definitively.[1,2] For example, the answer to the question whether to discontinue antihypertensive medication before anesthesia and operation was not presumable, but required observation and careful comparative evaluation.[3-5] This answer (not to discontinue) remains to be documented for the newer antihypertensive agents. The important issue of the optimal use of *beta*-adrenergic antagonists during anesthesia is still incompletely resolved and is the subject of debate.[6] Even such long-established practices as the use of anticholinergic agents in anesthesia are not unequivocally decided.[6a,b] Continuing careful work is needed to settle these and other questions. This is one reason for including in this chapter not only interactions of unquestioned significance but also those of unknown importance.

There are certain general difficulties and limitations in the discussion of drug interactions. First we have to *recognize* when the effects of a drug are altered by one or several other drugs, that is, whether or not an interaction has taken or is taking place. Frequently, finding the answer is not as easy as may appear at first.

Normal Variability

Drug responses, like other biological variables, can only be described statistically. Ideally, a drug response centers on a mean with a normal distribution. This is true for both "normal" and "abnormal" responses. A difference is statistically significant only when the mean responses of two comparable groups differ by more than twice the standard error. One must constantly be careful not to be misled by random variations within the norm.[7-9]

Strictly speaking, a drug interaction must be described in statistical terms before it can be accepted as scientifically proven. Often, however, a statistical description is not available in anesthesia, at least not initially. This is the rationale for case reports, which serve to alert the profession and perhaps to solicit confirmations or denials of such observations.

Other Factors Affecting Drug Responses

Apart from this "normal biologic variation," many factors that may affect a drug response are potentially recognizable. Perhaps the most important factor is the influence of *underlying disease*. (This is the first question one asks in the face of a possibly altered response. A definite answer is often impossible.) We also know that internal and external *environmental factors* may alter drug responses. For example, the effect of halothane on body temperature depends greatly on room temperature and humidity. Circadian rhythms, seasonal variations, climate, and diet may alter drug responses, but the clinical significance of these factors in anesthesia is often unknown. The importance of *genetic factors* has been appreciated by anesthesiologists for some time, particularly in connection with abnormal pseudocholinesterase and the response to succinylcholine, with porphyria, hemoglobinopathies, and malignant hyperpyrexia.[10-13] Although the incidence of each such abnormality is low, the list of recognized genetic factors and our understanding of them at the gene level is growing rapidly.

Special Aspects of Drug Interaction in Anesthesia

The anesthesiologist's role in medicine is unique because he or she:

(a) predominantly uses rapidly acting drugs;

(b) measures, often very precisely, the response to the drugs administered;

(c) frequently relies on drug antagonism; and

(d) is accustomed to titrating the dose or concentration of a drug.

Individual titration of dose according to the response obtained is important in administering potent drugs with steep dose-response relationships and a low therapeutic ratio. Unless the variability of the response to a given dose is minimal, titration is the only safe method for dealing with such drugs.

In anesthesia, interactions that result in a minor increase or decrease in responses are of little consequence and are dealt with routinely. The value of understanding and anticipating drug interactions for the anesthesiologist often lies in that this knowledge permits anticipation of the altered response.

Some examples of drug interactions can be found in the Case Reports at the end of this chapter.

TYPES OF DRUG INTERACTIONS

Drug interactions can be divided into three major categories: *in vitro* incompatibilities, physical or chemical, sometimes also called pharmaceutic interactions; interactions resulting from pharmacokinetic factors; and pharmacodynamic interactions.

This categorization is useful for organizing material but does not claim to reflect clinical reality. Actually, some interactions involve all three categories at once. The case of neuroleptic agents (phenothiazines and butyrophenones) may serve as an example. Their antipsychotic effects seem to be related to their ability to block dopamine and/or norepinephrine receptors, and perhaps muscarinic cholinoceptive, histamine, and 5-hydroxytryptamine receptors. They possess local anesthetic activity, and their clinical effects may include sedation or mild stimulation in addition to the desired antipsychotic effects. These agents also can induce extrapyramidal effects, cholestatic jaundice, dermatitis (both by a photosensitivity and an allergic mechanism), and blood dyscrasias. They may depress hepatic metabolism and act as inducers of hepatic microsomal enzymes. They inhibit the amine pump and thus reduce uptake of norepinephrine into adrenergic neurons as well as uptake of drugs that are substrates for the same transport mechanism. Neuroleptic drugs are bound to plasma proteins and may compete there for binding sites with other drugs. Thus these agents possess an enormous potential for interactions that involve every type of known pharmacokinetic and pharmacodynamic mechanism. Obviously, under these circumstances the analysis of a given interaction is difficult or sometimes impossible; nevertheless, an attempt to dissect the mechanisms is essential for prediction and prevention of other pharmacologic hazards. Fortunately, few other drugs are as prone to multiple interactions as are the antipsychotic agents.

Some authors divide adverse drug reactions into type A and type B.[13a] Type A reactions are the result of an exaggerated, but otherwise normal, pharmacologic action of a drug given in the usual therapeutic doses. Type B reactions are totally aberrant effects that are not to be expected from the known pharmacologic actions of a drug given in the usual doses to a patient whose body handles the drug in a normal way. Malignant hyperthermia, acute porphyria, and many allergic reactions fall into this category. A certain practical usefulness to this categorization cuts across the more rational, theoretically sounder classification we prefer. We also try to avoid classification by letters or numbers if instead we can classify by some informational dimension.

In Vitro Incompatibilities

This type of interaction occurs before a drug is absorbed systemically or administered parenterally.[14,15] It includes interactions between drugs in solution as well as in the gastrointestinal tract prior to absorption. The anesthesiologist is concerned with both problems. Premedication is often given by mouth. The most potent drugs used in anesthesia are administered intravenously, often into an infusion line along with drugs that are not a part of the anesthetic procedure, for example, antibiotics. One should never mix any drugs unless one is absolutely sure that no undesirable interaction can occur. In view of the long list of incompatibilities, it is sound policy to refer to the hospital pharmacist for this type of information. It must also be noted that the same generic drug may be formulated in different ways by different manufacturers, and that its formulation may affect compatibility with other agents. Table 3–1 is an example of

Table 3–1
Incompatibilities of Some Antibiotics in Infusion Solutions

Drug	Incompatible with:	Drug	Incompatible with:
Amphotericin B	Penicillin G Tetracyclines Diphenhydramine	Erythromycin gluceptate	Cephalothin Chloramphenicol Colistimethate Tetracyclines Aminophylline Barbiturates Phenytoin Heparin Vitamin B
Cephalothin (Keflin)	Chloramphenicol Erythromycin Kanamycin Polymyxin B Tetracyclines Vancomycin Aminophylline Barbiturates Calcium salts Phenytoin Heparin Norepinephrine Phenothiazines	Kanamycin sulfate	Cephalothin Methicillin Barbiturates Calcium gluconate Phenytoin Heparin
Chloramphenicol	Cephalothin Erythromycin Polymixin B Tetracyclines Vancomycin Aminophylline Barbiturates Diphenhydramine Phenytoin Hydrocortisone	Penicillin G	Amphotericin B Lincomycin Chlorpheniramine Chlorpromazine Dexamethasone Phenytoin Ephedrine Heparin Metaraminol Phenylephrine
Colistimethate	Cephalothin Erythromycin Hydrocortisone		

the incompatibilities of a number of antibiotic agents frequently given by infusion.

Drugs compounded in tablet and capsule form may interact after oral administration.[16,17] Chelation and inactivation of tetracyclines by antacids containing polyvalent cations, such as Ca^{++}, Mg^{++}, or Al^{+++}, are a typical case. Agents such as kaolin, pectins, charcoal, or hydrated aluminum silicate, which are used in the treatment of diarrhea because of their adsorbent properties, will also adsorb and inactivate many drugs and thus prevent their systemic uptake.[18] Cholestyramine interferes with absorption of warfarin, digitoxin, thyroid preparations, and thiazide diuretics.[19] The effect of changes in pH on the gastrointestinal absorption of aspirin is known even to television viewers. Drugs that affect gastrointestinal motility such as narcotic analgesic and anticholinergic or cholinomimetic drugs (metoclopramide) can modify or delay the absorption of orally administered preparations.[20-22] Metoclopramide is a new drug that is known to stimulate gastric motility and facilitate gastric emptying. Its exact mechanism of action is not clear although it is known to be a dopamine antagonist and to sensitize tissues to acetylcholine. Anticholinergic drugs block this effect. The influence of the drug upon drug absorption depends upon the site of absorption (stomach or small intestine) of the drug in question.[22a]

Pharmacokinetic Interactions

A good definition of pharmacokinetics is: "everything that happens to the drug in the organism." (Pharmacodynamics, on the other hand, is: "everything the drug does to the organism.") Thus pharmacokinetics includes processes of drug absorption (unless the drug is injected directly into the bloodstream), distribution, including the influence of plasma protein binding, and elimination, by excretion through the bile or kidney or by metabolic inactivation.

Hemodynamic Conditions. Since the intravenous route provides the fastest and most direct access to sites of drug action, it is essentially the only route used during anesthesia. The onset and duration of action of most drugs administered intravenously are more profoundly affected by distribution processes than by excretion and metabolism.[23] Intravenous induction agents, short-acting barbiturates, benzodiazepines, etomidate, and potent narcotics are typical examples. Some basic and simple principles are not always taken into account in practice. The concentration of the drug leaving the heart is a function of the rate of injection of a given dose and the volume into which the drug is injected, that is, the venous return over the period of injection. The rate of delivery to the tissues is determined by the concentration of unbound drug in the arterial blood and the tissue blood flow. Any drug that affects either cardiac output or flow distribution will affect the rate of drug delivery and the total amount delivered, especially to the brain and the myocardium, the two organs most closely involved both in the anesthesia desired and in the most serious potential adverse effect, myocardial depression. For a given rate of injection, the concentration of a drug in the arterial blood is a function of cardiac output. Although this is rarely determined before induction, one can make an educated guess as to the cardiovascular status of the patient and the likely changes that may be produced by the drug injected. For example, if thiopental is given to a patient with low cardiac output, a "normal" rate of injection will result in the delivery of a higher-than-normal drug concentration to the brain and the myocardium, where most of the output is being directed. There, the high concentration may further compromise cardiac function, if the low output is secondary to reduced cardiac competence. Another example is propranolol, or any other *beta*-adrenergic antagonist. In doses that are now used intravenously in anesthesia, propranolol acts entirely by attenuating or blocking adrenergic influences on the heart, influences either neurogenic or resulting from circulating catecholamines. Such deprivation does not affect the output of a heart with normal contractility, which is capable of accommodating venous return without adrenergic support. It may, however, decrease the output of a marginally competent heart dependent on neurogenic support to maintain output. It also reduces output elevated by abnormal sympathetic activity secondary to, for example, anxiety or pain. Of course, propranolol will blunt the normal sympathetic reflex response to any drug-induced decrease in cardiac output and blood pressure.

With inhalation anesthetic agents, the rate of rise of the anesthetic's concentration in the alveolar gas and the cardiac output (or pulmonary flow) are the important parameters for rate of uptake. The relative importance of these two processes with agents of low and high blood-gas solubility coefficients are too well known to be reviewed here.[24] It should be noted, however, that the processes can be influenced by prior drug therapy and preanesthetic medication, as discussed in the examples concerning cardiac output. Bronchodilator drugs decrease airway resistance and may improve the ventilation/perfusion ratio in patients with obstructive disease and hence accelerate the mean rate of rise of the anesthetic's concentration in the alveolar gas and the concentration in the arterial blood and in pulmonary venous blood. The opposite occurs with drugs that cause an increase in airway resistance. The most common example of the latter may again be propranolol, which permits unopposed bronchoconstriction by blocking the bronchodilator effect of sympathetic innervation mediated by *beta*-adrenergic receptors.

The retarding effect of epinephrine on the rate of absorption of local anesthetics exemplifies the general rule that perfusion determines the rate of absorption and mobilization of any drug from its tissue depot when other factors are equal.[25] The influence, however, of systemic changes in cardiovascular function on drug absorption after local administration is not as familiar. Such changes may be dramatic after intramuscular or subcutaneous administration of certain drugs to patients suffering decreased tissue blood flow, such as patients in shock or impending shock. In these cases, correction of cardiovascular failure leads to an improvement of tissue blood flow and mobilization of a previously stagnant tissue drug depot. Rebound respiratory depression from excessive morphine injected intramuscularly under combat conditions is well known; equally instructive are cases of subcutaneous epinephrine overdosage during acute circulatory failure. These problems are avoided by the IV route.

Protein Binding. Displacement from plasma protein binding of one drug by another is an important possible cause of drug interaction.[26] However, most examples of clinical significance have involved long-acting drugs. Perhaps the most debated example is the displacement of warfarin by phenylbutazone with an increase in free warfarin concentration and consequent slow increase in clotting time.[27] Although the importance of this example for anesthesiologists is limited, many drugs used in anesthesia have steep dose-response curves, are given in near-toxic doses, and are highly protein bound. Hence the potential for this type of interaction in anesthesia is strong. Displacement of quinidine and of phenytoin (diphenylhydantoin) has been reported and could represent an example of this type of interaction. The high protein binding of propranolol and its potential as a cause of myocardial depression makes this drug another candidate for displacement with harmful consequences.[19a] Unfortunately, no documentation for such consequences has been presented, probably because the situation in clinical anesthesia is so complex that the distinction of possible causes is difficult. Wardell has listed the requirements for demonstrating a displacement reaction:[28]

(a) *in vitro* demonstration of displacement,
(b) demonstration of displacement *in vivo*,
(c) demonstration that the time course of the toxic symptoms parallels the rise and subsequent fall in free drug concentrations, and
(d) elimination of other possible causes for the symptoms.

In anesthesiology one must also consider protein binding in connection with other circumstances. Plasma protein and drug concentrations may change massively and quickly during infusion of crystalloid solutions or infusion of whole blood and plasma preparations. Thus the concentration of free, that is, pharmacologically active, drug may change as the binding percentage rises and falls. This is likely to be of practical importance only with potent drugs that are highly protein bound.

Biotransformation. The majority of metabolic transformations of drugs occurs in the liver. Since these processes will be reviewed in Chapter 6, only a few general points will be made here.

Both inhibition and stimulation of metabolism of one drug by another can occur. The first is due to the acute interaction of two drugs competing for the same metabolic pathway; the second may be the consequence of previous prolonged administration of a drug producing enzyme induction. Although the usual result of metabolization of a drug is detoxification, that is, inactivation and increased renal excretion, there are also examples of the transformation of a drug to a more active form, for example, parathion, chloral hydrate, and cyclophosphamide. In anesthesia, metabolism is important in the formation of toxic metabolites. Hepatic metabolism may be influenced also by changes in liver blood flow produced by another drug.[23,36] The effect of propranolol-induced reduction in liver blood flow on drugs that depend heavily upon liver detoxification has been documented repeatedly.

Some drugs are not metabolized in the liver. The best-known example in anesthesia is, of course, the hydrolysis of succinyldicholine by plasma cholinesterase. Clinical doses of anticholinesterase drugs prolong the effect of the muscle relaxant.[29] Inadvertent inhibition of cholinesterases is probably most common today as the result of exposure to organophosphates used as pesticides. Fortunately, clinical signs of plasma cholinesterase inhibition are seen only when enzyme activity is severely depressed.[29]

Another important example of extrahepatic enzyme inhibition is the inhibitors of monoamine oxidases (known as MAO inhibitors or MAOI). These drugs were widely used in the treatment of depressive disorders then were largely displaced by tricyclic antidepressants and recently experienced another upsurge in therapeutic uses. MAO are widely distributed, especially in adrenergic nerve terminals, in liver and kidney, and metabolize monoamines like norepinephrine, dopamine, and 5-hydroxytryptamine. Because the main mechanism for termination of norepinephrine is reuptake into the nerve ending, MAOI do not prolong the effect of exogenously administered norepinephrine. However, the effect of indirectly acting sympathomimetics, of which tyramine is the prototype, is greatly potentiated, especially if the sympathomimetics themselves are substrates for MAO. This is the basis of the well-known "cheese reaction" elicited by foodstuffs containing tyramine.[30,31] For the anesthesiologist it is more important to know that sympathomimetics such as ephedrine, phenylephrine and dopamine are potentiated in patients on MAOI.[32,33]

Another significant effect of these drugs is the potentiation and alteration of the effect of meperidine.[34] The exact mechanism of the interaction is not clear, although inhibition of N-demethylation by MAOI has been demonstrated.[35] However, the effect of meperidine is not simply increased and prolonged; it is altered in character. This may be because MAOI are not specific for MAO alone, and their administration results in an increase in brain monoamines other than norepinephrine.[34] The interaction of different monoamines in the CNS (central nervous system) is far from fully understood.

Renal Excretion. Renal excretion is the route of elimination for drugs metabolized either slowly or not at all. The kidneys also excrete the products of drug metabolism after they have been metabolically altered to more polar or water soluble compounds which are more suitable for renal excretion. Because the role of the kidneys is discussed in more detail in Chapter 16, we outline here some general principles only.

Renal excretion proceeds by : (1) glomerular filtration (passive), with and without reabsorption, and (2) active tubular secretion. Substances filtered but not reabsorbed are those unable to cross cell-membrane barriers. Such polar substances, for example, quaternary ammonium compounds, are restricted to the extracellular space, and permeate the gastrointestinal-tract mucosa or the blood-brain barrier poorly, if at all. Therefore, the calculation of their excretion rate is a simple matter. The extracellular volume is cleared by glomerular filtration. In the normal case the glomerular filtration volume per minute is about one-one hundredth of the extracellular volume, so the extracellular fluid should be cleared in about 100 minutes.

Since the process is not linear but a first order (i.e., exponential) one, the half-time of excretion is not 50 but about 70 minutes.

Other approximations follow from this basic premise. Tubular secretion, clearing total renal plasma flow, is about five times the glomerular filtration rate; hence a drug restricted to the extracellular space but secreted by the kidney has a half-time of one-fifth of the above, that is, about 14 minutes.

Conversely, a highly lipid soluble drug (not metabolized) that crosses all membranes easily would be distributed in the total body water at least and be fully reabsorbed in the tubules. Thus its concentration in the final urine is only equal to that in the plasma, which is equal to that in the total body water. The half-time of excretion is about 20 days. If, as expected, the drug is also bound to tissue macromolecules or dissolved in body fats, its virtual volume of distribution can be many times the total body water volume and excretion would be accordingly prolonged. Such drugs cannot be excreted unless they are metabolized to a more polar derivative. This, rather than demonstrable toxicity, is the reason for the ban of DDT and caution with marihuana and its main active component tetrahydrocannabinol (THC).

These examples define the periods of time involved and give an approximation of the orders of magnitude of renal excretion for different drugs. Drugs secreted by the tubules and nonlipid-soluble (polar) drugs are subject to modification of excretion by other drugs within the perioperative period. In order to predict renal handling of a drug, it is necessary to know its physicochemical properties and its metabolic fate. Unfortunately, this information is still not easily available today. With it one can make useful predictions of the changes in renal excretion that will result from administration of other drugs that may produce changes in renal blood flow and filtration rate.[36] In drugs actively secreted, one must also consider interactions resulting from competition for the secretory process. However, the number of those interactions is small, and such information should be provided routinely by manufacturers.

The case of partially ionized weak acids and weak bases and the influence of the pH of urine on their excretion is often discussed, but its importance is limited because most of these drugs are metabolized in the liver.[37] (See Chap. 2.)

Pharmacodynamic Interactions

These are the most important from an anesthesiologic standpoint. Since drug selectivity is never absolute, and since every drug usually produces several effects, the variety of possible interactions almost defies organization. Any attempt to categorize must remain artificial and simplistic. The effect of a given combination should never be ascribed to a single type of interaction, unless there is solid evidence for excluding multiple mechanisms.

It is best to use different methods of organization that overlap and are not mutually exclusive. Even so, there are cases that cannot be definitively grouped because of our limited understanding of the exact mechanism of action of drugs. Categorization only helps to improve our thinking about general principles, which, in turn, may help to anticipate unknown and prospective interactions.

It is generally accepted that many drugs exert their effects by combining with specific "receptors." Hence we can distinguish among drug interactions at the same receptor, drug interactions involving different receptors, and drug interactions not mediated by receptors.

Drugs Acting on the Same Receptor. Pharmacologic receptors, i.e., molecular structures of high specificity, exist only for agents that occur physiologically, that is, neurotransmitters, hormones, and enzymes: acetylcholine (ACh), norepinephrine (NE), epinephrine (EPI), dopamine, 5-hydroxytryptamine, histamine, endorphins/enkephalins, angiotensin, pituitary hormones, corticosteroids, endoperoxides (prostaglandins, thromboxanes, prostacyclins), neuropeptides, and others. Only drugs that in chemical structure sufficiently resemble these physiologic agents can be expected to interact specifically with these receptors. Yet the number of these drugs is large, both agonists and antagonists: it includes analogs of acetylcholine such as carbachol or succinylcholine, sympathomimetics, morphine and related agents, and analogs of corticosteroids and of sex hormones. There is also the long list of drugs that do not mimic but block the effects of physiologically occurring agonists: atropine, curare-like agents, hexamethonium, *beta*-adrenergic antagonists, *alpha*-adrenergic antagonists, naloxone, aldosterone antagonists, and antiestrogens.

Drugs interacting with the same receptor can only elicit or block the same effects as the normal physiologic agonist, albeit of different magnitude and duration. However, one type of receptor may activate different effector systems: for example, ACh relaxes smooth muscle in the vascular bed but constricts airway and gastrointestinal smooth muscle. It depolarizes the endplate of skeletal muscle and of ganglionic and CNS postsynaptic membranes; it slows the rate of cardiac pacemakers and the rate of atrioventricular conduction. Nature can use the same neurotransmitter for different purposes because it has developed "delivery systems" (the nerve endings) that permit exquisite localization. Unfortunately, we have developed nothing like it, and in our crude hands receptor-specific agonists and antagonists given simply into the bloodstream produce a variety of effects. Thus atropine, given intravenously, will block all muscarinic cholinergic receptors wherever they are located. In addition to preventing bradycardia and conduction block, it may cause urinary retention and precipitate glaucoma. Furthermore, atropine is not alone in causing this type of effect. Many other drugs that are not used primarily for the purpose of blocking muscarinic receptors, such as antihistaminics, tricyclic antidepressants, some phenothiazines, benzodiazepines, pancuronium, gallamine, and meperidine have secondary properties similar to those of atropine. In a whole organism, or patient, many possibilities for drug interaction with agents of this type exist, even though we would like to think of such drugs as "receptor-specific."

As previously mentioned, interaction with a receptor may result in activation or block, i.e, *agonistic* or *antagonistic* activity. In principle, receptor-active compounds have two properties: *affinity* for the receptor and *intrinsic activity* (or *efficacy*) once the drug-receptor complex has been formed.[38,39] Affinity determines the potency of the drug; intrinsic activity can vary between maximal and zero. If a compound has sufficient affinity but no intrinsic activity it is an antagonist. With intermediate levels of intrinsic activity, compounds are partial agonists; in the presence of a full agonist, such compounds behave as partial antagonists.[40,41]

Paton has proposed a hypothesis that accounts for the differences in efficacy or intrinsic activity of drugs.[42,43] Though the hypothesis lacks proof, it deserves discussion, because it provides some intuitive framework for phenomena whose relatedness is not easily seen. Paton postulates that the magnitude of the drug response is related not to the concentration of the existing drug-receptor complexes (occupation theory) but to the rate of formation of complexes (rate theory). When the rate of drug-receptor interaction is sufficiently high, the drug elicits a response, that is, it is an agonist. When the rate is low, no response occurs, and the drug is an antagonist. Partial agonists show an intermediate behavior.

The hypothesis accounts for some well-known facts: the onset of action of agonists is faster than that of antagonists, for example, the response to ACh as opposed to the response to atropine, or the response to succinylcholine as opposed to that to curare-like agents. The difference between agonistic and antagonistic activity becomes a quantitative rather than a qualitative difference. Thus it should not be surprising that some compounds that are typical antagonists may behave like partial agonists under some conditions and in some tissues: this may account for the agonist activity of atropine, slowing heart rate and AV-conduction and producing vasodilation in certain skin areas (atropine blush).

In accordance with Paton's rate theory, antagonists dissociate from the receptor much more slowly than do agonists, as witnessed in every-day experience. The action of curare-like agents lasts longer than the action of depolarizing neuromuscular blocking agents; propranolol has a longer action than NE; the actions of atropine are prolonged (hours to days), whereas ACh is evanescent (even if its rapid enzymatic destruction is prevented).

Surmountable and Nonsurmountable Antagonists. The rate theory reduces the difference between agonist and antagonist drugs to the difference in their rate of association (and dissociation) with the receptor; hence the difference between surmountable and nonsurmountable drugs may also be viewed as an expression of the actions of time constants. An antagonist is considered surmountable if its rate of dissociation from the receptor during the presence of an agonist is sufficiently fast that equilibration between the two occurs during the presence of the agonist. However, several typical surmountable antagonists may behave as though nonsurmountable when they are tested in sufficiently high concentrations against agonists released by nerve activity.[44] For example, propranolol will cause a parallel shift to the right of the dose-response curve of an adrenergic agonist (for instance, NE) when the agonist is given by continuous infusion (or present in the bath fluid in an *in vitro* experiment). However, if the same agonistic response is produced by nerve stimulation, that is, by

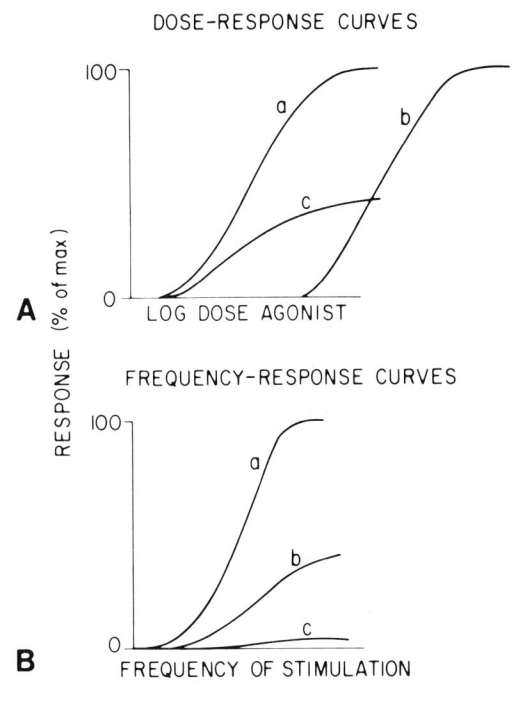

Fig. 3–1. *A*, Curve a is a typical dose-response curve to an agonist drug. Curve b shows the response to the same agonist in the presence of a surmountable, competitive antagonist. Curve c shows the response to the same agonist in the presence of a nonsurmountable antagonist. This example depicts the situation that occurs when there is complete equilibrium between the agonist and the antagonist molecules competing for the receptor. When the antagonist is surmountable and competitive, the maximum response (curve b) depends only on the ratio of agonist/antagonist and the agonist concentration can be increased at will by the experimenter. A nonsurmountable antagonist reduces the number of receptors available regardless of the concentration of agonist present, i.e., the maximum response is reduced (curve c).
B, Curve a describes the response to increasing frequency of nerve stimulation under control conditions. Even in the presence of a surmountable antagonist the maximal response is decreased (curves b and c). In this situation the concentration of agonist available cannot be increased at will, but depends on the ability of the nerve endings to release transmitter. Since this capacity is limited, the response will decrease above a certain concentration of antagonist, although the antagonist is surmountable in principle.

NE released from the nerve terminal, the antagonism appears nonsurmountable (Fig. 3–1). Presumably, the nerve is not capable of releasing the concentration of the transmitter needed to restore the equilibrium in favor of the agonist (transmitter) when the antagonist concentration exceeds a certain limit. Functionally, when the agonist is a nerve-derived transmitter, a "surmountable" antagonist may produce a "nonsurmountable" block. The frequency-response curve shift is skewed rather than parallel, and the ceiling of the response is decreased. The antagonist ultimately can produce a complete nerve-effector block, that is, a pharmacologic denervation. This occurs with propranolol and may occur with atropine, although the doses of atropine used clinically are not sufficient to cause this type of block.

True *nonsurmountable antagonists* are characterized by a very slow rate of dissociation or none at all. This is the case with phenoxybenzamine and Dibenamine (*alpha*-adrenergic antagonists) for which no significant reversal of the drug-receptor bond occurs during the lifetime of the receptor.[45] This means that a full response can be elicited again only after the regeneration of the receptor, that is, after 2 or 3 weeks. With this type of drug the rate of administration is unimportant, as long as successive doses are given while the effect of the previous dose is still present. The drugs are highly cumulative. Other examples of this irreversible type of antagonism are the organophosphate anticholinesterases and some monoamine oxidase inhibitors discussed previously. Echothiophate and isoflurophate are the only anticholinesterase organophosphates used clinically (as miotics), but exposure to insecticide organophosphates is common, especially among agricultural workers.

Drugs Acting on Different Receptors. Drugs may act on different receptors to produce the same or opposing effects. The receptors may be located on the same or on different cells in the same organ or in different organs or systems, but they must affect the same function.

Drugs acting on different receptors and exerting the same effect are said to be *additive*. (The terminology is often confusing, because the terms addition, summation, synergism, potentiation are not always used with the same meaning [See Chap. 1].) What is important about such a drug interaction is that different drugs that share the same type of desired activity may possess different toxic properties. In this case the desired effects will be additive, whereas the toxic effects, one hopes, would not.

If one drug exerts no effect by itself but increases the effect of another drug, the interaction is called *potentiation*. An example of this type is the effect of cocaine and cocaine-like drugs in potentiating the effects of NE. Cocaine inhibits uptake of NE into adrenergic nerve terminals, the major mechanism of dissipation of free NE, and thus increases and prolongs the NE concentration near the receptor sites. When cocaine is given to a patient, its effect depends upon the presence or absence of free NE.

In the case of drugs that exert opposite effects, the result of the interaction is *antagonism*. In contrast to the *pharmacologic antagonism* (on the same receptor) previously described, this type of antagonism is usually called *"functional"* or *"physiologic" antagonism*.[47] The latter is thus named because all physiologically occurring antagonisms are of this type. This applies to the well-known antagonism between sympathetic and parasympathetic innervation (or of sympathomimetic and parasympathomimetic drugs) in the heart, in the airways, and in the gastrointestinal tract, as well as to the antagonism between two nerve endings impinging on the same postsynaptic membrane (called in this case "postsynaptic inhibition"). Nature does not seem to have developed the idea of a pharmacologic interaction, although there is no *a priori* reason why this should be so.

Clinical examples of functional drug antagonism are few. One example is the case in which histamine and other vasodilator agents are released during an anaphylactic reaction or by a histamine-releasing agent and are "antagonized" by epinephrine or another vasoconstrictor. In this case, the antagonism is not between the drug causing the anaphylactic reaction (or the histamine release) and the vasoconstrictor directly, but between the released vasodilators and the constrictor.

More common and more important is the situation in which a drug or several drugs influence an existing physiologic antagonism, for example, when atropine or propranolol is used to influence heart rate or impulse conduction. In this case, the effect of the antagonist is not only a function of its dose (or rate of administration) but also of the magnitude of the existing tone of sympathetic or parasympathetic nerve activity, as well as of the magnitude of the physiologically opposing innervation. For example, the increase in heart rate after a given dose of atropine differs depending on the type of anesthesia, because sympathetic cardiac tone is variably affected by general anesthesia (and also by other conditions, such as surgical stimulation).

If both atropine and propranolol are used, the effect of the first will influence the effect of the second. Atropine tachycardia is not as marked in a patient treated with propranolol or other *beta*-blockers. Patients treated with a *beta*-blocker or a reserpine-type drug are more likely to develop reflex bronchospasm in response to mechanical stimulation or after anticholinesterase administration.[48] (The existence of a physiologic sympathetic bronchodilator tone was initially realized only after the introduction of *beta*-adrenergic antagonists.)

Recently, the function of sympathetic nerves has been found to be regulated by a peripheral negative feedback mechanism involving *alpha* receptors, and, perhaps, by muscarinic receptors and interaction with parasympathetic nerves.[49-51] Administration of an *alpha*-adrenergic antagonist increases the release of norepinephrine and the effect of sympathetic nerve activity.

Under normal conditions the transmitter, NE, may exert an inhibitory effect on its own release (negative feedback). Thus, the tachycardia seen after phentolamine-induced hypotension is due not only to the activation of baroreceptor reflexes and to an intrinsic positive chronotropic effect of the drug, but also to the increased release of NE resulting from the block of *alpha* receptors in the adrenergic terminal. Atropine also increases the release of NE, and some of the effects of atropine on the heart may be caused by increased sympathetic transmitter release.[52] Of course, this interaction occurs only where sympathetic and parasympathetic nerves are present simultaneously, such as in the heart.

Interactions at different receptors occur following inhibition of the amine pump that transports NE back into adrenergic nerve terminals. Cocaine produces its cardiovascular toxicity by this mechanism, as do the tricyclic antidepressants (see above).[53,54] This type of drug action results in potentiation of NE, and to a lesser extent EPI. (Isoproterenol is not taken up into adrenergic neurons and thus is not potentiated.) NE may be administered externally or released endogenously. Cocaine toxicity is the subject of the first case report in this chapter.

A consequence of the cocaine-like action of tricyclic antidepressants is their antagonism to antihypertensive agents of the adrenergic neuron-blocking type such as reserpine, guanethidine, and bethanidine. These drugs are substrates of the amine pump and exert their blocking effect on the adrenergic neuron after being concentrated in adrenergic nerve endings. The administration of tricyclic antidepressant results in loss of blood-pressure control by adrenergic neuron-blocking drugs.[55,56]

Recently, tricyclic antidepressants were found to jeopardize blood-pressure control in patients treated with clonidine.[57] The mechanism has not been elucidated, but it is possible that the increased level of free norepinephrine that results from the action of the antidepressants antagonizes the effect of clonidine on central *alpha* receptors, where clonidine is thought to exert its antihypertensive effect.

Drug Interactions not Mediated by Pharmacologic Receptors. The main drugs used in anesthesia, general and local anesthetic agents, do not act on specific receptors but produce their effects by physicochemical interactions and cause conformational changes of biologic macromolecules, proteins, and lipids, especially those in excitable membranes. This has now been demonstrated directly,[58-62] but the lack of receptor-specificity had been postulated long ago, because there are no specific structural requirements for anesthetic activity and no pharmacologic antagonists. In fact, physicochemical rather than chemical properties correlate best with anesthetic potency, for example, lipid solubility.[62]

Because of this, the effects of general anesthetics are roughly additive. Moreover, the effects of some drugs used for premedication are additive with general anesthetics. The addition of nitrous oxide reduces the anesthetic concentration of halothane and other inhalation agents required to achieve MAC (minimum alveolar concentration),[63,64] but the toxic dose is also lowered. Hence there is no significant increase in the therapeutic index (lethal dose 50/therapeutic dose 50).[65,66] The use of premedication, such as barbiturates and benzodiazepines, also reduces the required concentration of the general anesthetic, but in these cases the therapeutic index has not been determined.[67] Although the "sparing" effect of narcotic analgesics is clear, their effect on the therapeutic index depends on the parameter chosen.[63,64] They produce respiratory depression and a condition of complete analgesia by a receptor-specific effect.[68] Thus the combination of narcotic analgesics and general anesthetics represents an interaction between two types of drugs.

These two types of central nervous system (CNS) drugs must be distinguished. The first consists of general anesthetic agents, alcohol, sedative-hypnotics, and antiepileptic agents. For these agents there is no evidence for a specific receptor site.[26] This and the similar behavior of these drugs in certain *in vitro* test systems are evidence that they share a similar mechanism of action.[69] Shanes has coined for them the term "membrane stabilizers."[70] As expected, they have additive effects, both therapeutic and toxic. The second group of CNS drugs are known to affect receptor mechanisms. Morphine and other narcotic analgesics, the major tranquilizers, and the antidepressants belong to this group. Sufficient evidence has been accumulated to include the benzodiazepine group of drugs among the agents that exert their effect by interacting with specific receptors, in this case receptors involved in the action of gamma amino butyric acid (GABA) as CNS transmitter. Benzodiazepines do not simply act on pre- or postsynaptic receptors but affect the GABAergic system in some more complex fashion.[70a] Recently, a specific benzodiazepine antagonist has been found, a development that so far has not led to clinical applications.

Agents of the first group are capable of inducing tolerance, dependence, and withdrawal symptoms, and there is a high degree of cross-tolerance among them. Of the agents in the second group, only the narcotics cause physical addiction. Narcotic addiction and dependence on sedative-hypnotics are different entities, and there is no real cross-tolerance. In spite of the important differences between the CNS effects of the different drugs of the first group and various general anesthetics, their toxic actions are roughly additive.

General anesthetics act in principle on all cells and tissues of the body. As discussed previously, even receptor-specific drugs lack selectivity when given systemically, because appropriate receptors may occur in many tissues and organs. However, anesthetic agents can affect almost all tissues and organs because the macromolecules that are the target of their action are ubiquitous. Relative selectivity may result from differences both in the concentration of targets in different tissues and in the functional importance of affected macromolecules. This, and the functional complexity of the central nervous system, is what makes these agents suitable for clinical anesthesia.

A good example of the degree of parallelism between central and peripheral effects of general anesthetics is the strong correlation between direct myocardial depressant activity and anesthetic potency over a wide range of absolute potencies.[71,72] (The extent of autonomic compensation for the direct myocardial depressant effect determines the overall cardiac depression under clinical conditions.) Other examples of the peripheral effects of general anesthetics are: effects on neuromuscular and ganglionic transmission, on airway and vascular smooth muscle, on liver function, and on cardiac electrical events.[73,74]

Antiarrhythmic agents such as quinidine and procainamide are drugs used for their peripheral effects but known to possess CNS side effects. These agents are close to local anesthetics and overlap with them in clinical use. The peripheral effects of local anesthetics (from myocardial depression, to smooth muscle relaxation, to potentiation of neuromuscular block) are well known.

Depression of nerve function does not necessarily manifest itself in a general progressive and systematic decrease of all CNS activity. Inhibitory neurons and synaptic processes are important for overall function. Inhibition of such inhibitory processes by depressant drugs may lead to transient neuronal activation, which may even lead to convulsions, but ultimately overall depression supervenes.[75]

Time Sequence and Drug Interaction. The time course of action of a CNS drug is not related to the blood or tissue level in a simple fashion. With intravenous anesthetic agents, the blood level at the time of recovery from anesthesia is higher than the level at which anesthesia begins. This is known as "acute tolerance." On the other hand, the "calming" effect of a moderate, or sedative, dose of a sedative-hypnotic or the "antianxiety" effect of a tranquilizer often lasts longer than the plasma or tissue concentration. Preanesthetic medication should be given at the appropriate time, so that the blood level of the drug is past its peak at the time of induction. In this way the drug effect is greater than proportional to the blood level, and toxic or side effects of premedicant and anesthetic are less than arithmetically additive.

Recently cocaine was reported not to cause cardiac dysrhythmias during halothane anesthesia.[76] This is obviously at variance with our experience (see Case Report) and that of others.[87] The difference lies in the sequence of administration. In our case, the patient had absorbed cocaine and was undergoing a difficult operation, accompanied by considerable excitement and anxiety with sympathetic activation, when general anesthesia with halothane was induced. This sympathetic activity was potentiated by cocaine with disastrous consequences. In the study quoted,[76] cocaine was administered to patients already under halothane anesthesia. Sympathetic activity *during* halothane anesthesia is low. Hence there was little NE to be potentiated.

A special situation exists in patients with drug dependence resulting from chronic or subchronic administration of either the sedative-hypnotic or the narcotic-analgesic class.[77] It is common practice to maintain the state of dependence during anesthesia, since that is not the time to bring about withdrawal. This requires that the appropriate dose of the appropriate drug be given at the proper rate, which in the clinical situation is often not simple. The diagnosis of the type of drug required and the determination of the correct dose cannot always be made only on the basis of the patient's history but may require trial and titration. As mentioned, any sedative-hypnotic agent can be used to substitute for any drug of the "general CNS-depressant" class, including alcohol. Pentobarbital is the usual sedative-hypnotic used. Any narcotic can be used to substitute for any other narcotic, but the severity of withdrawal symptoms seems to be related to the rate of elimination of the narcotic. Methadone may offer an advantage because of its longer duration of action.

The administration of a narcotic antagonist, for example, naloxone, is dangerous in the case of a narcotic addict because the displacement of the narcotic from receptor sites is rapid, and an acute withdrawal syndrome is precipitated, the severity of which depends on the naloxone dose and on the intensity of the existing addiction. On the other hand, in the nonaddict, the *acute* effects of even a high dose of a narcotic may be terminated without risk. No recognizable withdrawal syndrome is thereby precipitated, except relatively rare exceptions that are characterized by massive sympathetic discharge.[78] These reactions have led to greater caution in the use of naloxone, but their basis or mechanism is not well understood.

Since the first edition of this book was written, a group of drugs acting by a novel mechanism of action has appeared.[78a,78b] These drugs act by inhibiting the flux of calcium ions through the so-called "slow channels." In this they resemble the local anesthetics which inhibit sodium flux through the "fast sodium channels." However, while there are few differences between different local anesthetic agents in their action on the sodium channels, there are distinct differences between different "calcium-channel blockers" (as they have come to be somewhat incorrectly called). Calcium channels play a role in electrophysiologic processes across excitable membranes, and ionized Ca^{++} is the mediator of contraction in all types of muscle. (Interestingly, the calcium-channel blockers do not affect contractility of skeletal muscle as does dantrolene, the drug of choice in malignant hyperthermia.) Calcium-channel blockers affect either predominantly electrophysiologic processes in the heart involving calcium currents making them useful as antidysrhythmic agents and accounting for their potential toxic effect by blocking AV-conduction, or they inhibit contractility of vascular smooth muscle. Some are more potent on the coronary vessels and others more on peripheral vascular beds. All have the potential to depress myocardial contractility. The group will be discussed in detail in Chapter 10.

Obviously, calcium-channel blockers are agents with properties that make them prime candidates for interaction with several other drugs used in anesthesia. Special care must be given to potential additive myocardial depressant action when these drugs are given in the presence of—or in addition to—*beta*-adrenergic antagonists as well as general anesthetic agents.

At least two calcium-channel blockers were used in Europe for some time—although their true mechanism of action was only slowly becoming clear. Perhaps, the delay to their introduction to the United States was due to a hesitancy to accept the idea that drugs having such a similar basic mechanism of action could indeed affect differentially closely related tissues, e.g., the smooth muscle of different vascular beds. Furthermore, ionized calcium is an essential part of a vast number of biologic processes from enzyme function to exocrine and endocrine secretion. It may be good to keep this in mind and to be alert for less frequent toxic effects or interactions with other drugs used during the perioperative period.

Other Drug Interactions. The classifications used cannot encompass all forms of drug interactions. Two of special importance to the anesthesiologists are discussed briefly.

It is well documented that several antibiotics, especially aminoglycosides and polymyxin B, may depress neuromuscular transmission and cause prolongation of the action of nondepolarizing neuromuscular blocking drugs.[79] The major site of action is on prejunctional nerve terminals. The antibiotics interfere with the synthesis and function of the bacterial cell wall. This action may extend as well to the motor nerve terminals and the end-plate, and may account for other toxic effects of the same antibiotics, especially their ototoxicity and nephrotoxic effect.

Another serious complication of anesthesia is malignant hyperpyrexia or hyperthermia.[81-84] There is evidence that different clinical and pathogenic forms of malignant hyperthermia occur, but the common denominator is the role of general anesthetic agents and the contribution of neuromuscular blocking drugs in triggering the syndrome. There is also good evidence for a genetic predisposition. The most dangerous form of the syndrome is due to dysfunction of the release and reuptake mechanisms of calcium in skeletal muscle. In view of the multiple roles of calcium in many enzymatic and membrane processes, it is possible that other functions involving calcium are also affected.

Biological effects produced by altered concentrations of the ionic milieu are also hard to categorize. These alterations may occur as a result of drugs such as diuretics, which mobilize tissue fluids and electrolytes and promote their renal excretion, or they could be due to the direct injection of parenteral fluids and ion solutions, for example, calcium and potassium.

Combination of Factors in Pharmacodynamic Drug Interactions. There are important clinical entities of drug interactions that cannot be readily discussed in the framework we have chosen, because they involve the intricate interaction of nondrug factors and of drugs belonging to different classes. We shall discuss the precipitation of cardiac arrhythmias as an example of this type of situation.

The following are presently considered to be causally related to the occurrence of cardiac dysrhythmias:[85,86] (1) the basic propensity of myocardial cells to discharge spontaneously; (2) the influence of autonomic transmitters or endogenous humoral agents, which may either directly affect the "automaticity" of aberrant foci or create the conditions for discharge by reducing the rate of the normal pacemaker and by slowing or blocking normal impulse conduction; (3) the influence of hypoxia and hypercarbia and of hypokalemia and hypercalcemia; (4) the role of ventricular wall tension, determined in turn by arterial pressure (afterload), diastolic filling (preload), and the contractility of the myocardium; and finally, (5) the direct effects of drugs, such as the sensitizing effects of some general anesthetics, the actions of digitalis, and the effects of antidysrhythmic drugs.

These factors and their combinations can be influenced in many ways by drugs, even those without a direct effect on the heart. For example, diuretics may cause hypokalemia and affect total circulating fluid volume. Apart from its possible sensitizing effect, a general anesthetic in interaction with surgical stimulation affects cardiac autonomic nerve activity, arterial and venous pressures, myocardial contractile force, and secondarily, ventricular volumes. Digitalis increases the susceptibility of the heart to dysrhythmias, especially in the presence of hypokalemia or hypercalcemia, though its positive inotropic actions may prevent ventricular dilatation or cardiac failure with secondary catastrophic decrease of myocardial perfusion. Many more examples could be given, but the point is clear: in preventing or treating cardiac dysrhythmias it is important to remember the variety of possible contributing factors and the ways in which they may be influenced by drug action. Dysrhythmias are more frequent during the induction period. This is partly due to the events such as afferent stimulation during laryngoscopy and intubation, injection of succinyl choline, and skin incision, but a contributing factor is the exposure of the heart to high concentrations of the anesthetic at a time when CNS depression is still insufficient to suppress autonomic reflex activity.

No one can be aware of every possible drug interaction. The volume of literature on drug interactions has greatly increased in recent years. Some reports are based on single case observations that do not fit into any logical framework. Other suggestions are simply extrapolations from *in vitro* experiments or animal observations that may or may not have relevance to clinical situations.

Acute Allergic Drug Reactions

Strictly speaking perhaps allergic drug reactions do not belong in a book entitled "Drug Interactions" although some allergic reactions may be viewed as interaction of a drug with itself. At any rate, regardless of semantics we have decided to include a short treatment of the subject for practical reasons. Allergic (anaphylactic) and anaphylactoid drug reactions occurring within a short interval after or during administration of anesthesia are not uncommon. Although we do not know of any statistics on their exact frequency in anesthesia, almost half of all drug reactions leading to hospital admissions are allergic in nature; thus, it stands to reason that their occurrence in the peri-anesthetic period is of a similar order of magnitude. Another reason to deal with allergic drug reactions is the fact that their happening is independent of the seriousness of a patient's underlying condition or disease. Hence, when an allergic reaction leads to death or permanent injury, it is especially tragic and traumatic in a healthy patient undergoing elective surgery. Finally, although allergic drug reactions may be relatively rare and thus unexpected, many such incidents are both serious and at the same time easily treated when promptly recognized and dealt with. The thought of a possible allergic drug reaction should be always present.

The term "allergic" means literally only that the reaction is "different," but in practice it is used to describe hyperreactions of the immediate, delayed, and even slowly developing type. (The latter are often the same as autoimmune disease.) The anesthesiologist is most frequently and most importantly involved only with acute or subacute reactions. Thus, we will only discuss reactions that are likely to present acutely in the peri-anesthetic period. This restriction seems to have been observed also by Stoelting who has recently written an excellent review article on the subject, to which the reader is directed for a more detailed treatment than will be possible here.[86a]

Following Stoelting we shall consider three types of acute reactions commonly described as "allergic," although only the first is clearly due to a change in sensitivity caused by previous exposure to the same or a closely related drug. This first mechanism is called anaphylactic or type I hypersensitivity and is mediated by immunoglobulin E antibodies. The second type does not require prior exposure and sensitization. It involves activation of the complement system either by the classic (by interaction of a drug with IgG or IgM antibodies) or by the alternate pathway. The third type of reaction is called anaphylactoid and is due solely to drug-induced release of mediators, most importantly histamine. For this reason this type is often referred to simply as a "histamine release" reaction. An allergic reaction may involve more than one of the above mechanisms.

This simultaneous involvement of more than one mechanism and the fact that all mechanisms ultimately result in release of common mediators may explain partly one important feature of allergic drug reactions: the pathophysiology and hence the symptomatology of reactions are similar and clinically indistinguishable regardless of the specific drug involved. It is not the pharmacodynamic effect of the drug itself that causes the manifestations but the mediators, which may either be present ready to be released or can be formed *de novo* as consequence of the administration of the drug. This fact has two important implications: the treatment of allergic drug reactions is the same regardless of the nature of the eliciting drug; and there is in most instances no obvious dose-response relationship.

The latter statement requires clarification. The reason for the apparent lack of a dose-response relationship is the fact that small amounts of drug (relative to the required pharmacologic dose) are sufficient to elicit a maximal response. If careful experiments are done in which the doses are scaled down to the appropriate range, a dose-response relationship can be demonstrated. The usually correct statement concerning the lack of dose-response relationship applies to most but not all situations. For example, a dose-response relationship has been described for some histamine release reactions, and inferred from the empirical observations that (1) allergic drug reactions are more frequent after IV than after IM injections (presumably because of the higher peak plasma levels that are likely after IV administration), and (2) patients sensitive to parenterally administered drug may tolerate oral administration. One should remember that drug administration by aerosol inhalation leads to rapid drug absorption.

While it is true that allergic drug reactions may be encountered in any patient, it is well established that patients with atopy and patients with a positive history of previous allergic reactions (e.g., to penicillin) are severalfold more likely to experience such reactions in the future. Thus, the drug allergy question during the preanesthesia visit must be taken seriously and may alert the anesthetist to be on guard. On the other hand, a negative history is no guarantee against a future allergic reaction. At the same time, the opposite also applies: a patient who has experienced an allergic reaction before may tolerate the same drug without reaction at another time. Also, the patient (and his/her physician or dentist) may have misdiagnosed an earlier episode; there are patients who claim allergic reactions to placebo, even to completely inert placebo preparations. Moreover, a positive (and true) history of hypersensitivity to a drug administration may have been due not to the drug itself but to an additive or solvent that may or may not be present in the formulation of the same drug coming from a different manufacturer.

The most serious and immediately life-threatening form of allergic drug reaction is that of anaphylactic shock with acute hypotension, erythema, and edema formation (which is, of course, most serious if it occurs in the mucosa of the larynx or bronchi and affects airway patency), loss of circulating intravascular fluid volume, bronchospasm, and possibly cardiac arrhythmias. The diagnosis of this reaction should be and usually is immediate, and therapy is usually equally obvious and especially easy in a patient who is as well monitored and controlled as patients under anesthesia are. Airway patency, adequate oxygenation, and volume replacement have the highest priority. If the patient is slow to respond, a bolus injection of intravenous epinephrine should be administered, followed by infusion if required.

Epinephrine is still the drug of choice, and any anesthesiologist who has other preferences must have good reasons to defend these. There are several rationales for the unique efficacy of epinephrine, but the main reason is clinical experience, not finely wrought pharmacologic explanations. One fact worth noting is the inhibition of further mediator release by epinephrine.

It may surprise some readers that we so strongly recommend a physiologic rather than pharmacologic antagonist. The reason is again mainly empirical, but it is also logical in view of the fact that several mediators in addition to histamine (slow reacting substance leucotrienes, prostaglandins, platelet activating factor) may contribute to producing the manifestations of acute allergic reactions. We do not have the space to discuss the nature and the effects of the different mediators that have been shown to be involved; at any rate the only pharmacological antagonists available at present are the antihistamines for both H_1 and H_2 receptors.

Pretreatment with both types of antihistamines combined has been shown to be effective in the prevention and treatment of histamine release reactions, but routine pretreatment cannot be justified. Although some forms of allergic reactions (urticaria, mild localized mucosal edemas) may respond to these pharmacologic antagonists alone, it should be remembered that even combined antihistamines are not effective in the treatment of bronchospasm. If there is an absolute contraindication to epinephrine, such as cardiac dysrhythmia during halothane anesthesia, aminophylline may be used to treat bronchospasm, and antihistamine agents may be effective in dealing with cardiac dysrhythmias secondary to an acute allergic drug reaction.

More subtle forms of allergic hypersensitivity reactions to a drug may explain some intra- and postoperative symptoms such as nausea and vomiting, fever, malaise, and even pulmonary complications. We can hope that future laboratory determinations of, e.g., immunoglobulins, will improve the diagnostic and eventually the therapeutic situation.

We feel that it is necessary to distinguish carefully between general observations of factors underlying drug interactions, which can be and must be verified and quantified, and the virtually limitless potential for juxtaposition and combination of factors that may be encountered in the individual clinical case. For example, the effect of cocaine and tricyclic antidepressants on the amine pump that transports endogenous catecholamines and antihypertensive drugs of the adrenergic neuron blocking type is a verifiable observation. However, whether this interaction will lead to a clinical manifestation in a specific case, that is, a hypertensive episode or loss of blood-pressure control, depends on the circumstances of that particular situation. The observation must be known, but for the evaluation of the individual case an understanding of the many potentially contributing factors is required.

We have tried to show on one hand the enormous complexity of drug interactions, and on the other the possibility of reducing the variety of potential interactions to a more manageable framework. The unavoidable corollary of this undertaking, the occasional oversimplification of complex entities, seems justified to us by the advantage of a more comprehensive perspective.

CASE REPORT

A 25-year-old, 70-kg man underwent an operation for correction of a deviated nasal septum. The operation was begun under local anesthesia. Four milliliters of 5% cocaine were used topically to anesthetize the nostrils, and the area of operation was infiltrated with 2% lidocaine, 5 ml, without epinephrine. After about 30 minutes, the patient became restless and complained of pain. Therefore, it was decided to administer general anesthesia. The anesthetist elected to use halothane with 50% nitrous oxide for both induction and maintenance of anesthesia. No atropine was given. During induction, about five minutes after the start of halothane 2 to 2.5%, the patient experienced severe cardiac dysrhythmias: first bradycardia, then multifocal ventricular extrasystoles, and finally ventricular fibrillation. In spite of strenuous efforts at resuscitation and defibrillation, the patient died in the operating room.

Comment. The cocaine used for local anesthesia was absorbed with time.[87] Even if only a part of the total dose of 200 mg was absorbed, it was sufficient to decrease reuptake of norepinephrine into the adrenergic nerve terminals. In the absence of high sympathetic activity there might not have been any manifestation of this pharmacologic condition. However, with the development of pain, causing an increase in sympathetic nervous activity, and the subsequent inhalation of halothane, there were additional factors: sensitization of the heart to catecholamines by halothane's reaching the heart in a high concentration, and pain, which further increased sympathetic cardiac-nerve activity. In the presence of previously administered cocaine, these conditions combined were sufficient to elicit severe and irreversible dysrhythmias. It is not clear whether acute hypertension leading to reflex bradycardia contributed to the result. The choice of halothane, administered after cocaine in the presence of pain, was tragic.

CASE REPORT

A 70-year-old, 70-kg man with angina pectoris and mild congestive heart failure was scheduled to undergo an open heart operation for replacement of the mitral valve and placement of bypass grafts to the left anterior descending and right coronary arteries. He was taking digoxin, 0.25 mg/day, and propranolol, 100 mg four times a day, with the last dose given three hours before the operation. Anesthesia was induced with morphine, 2 mg/kg, and diazepam, 10 mg. Nitrous oxide, 50%, was added to the oxygen after intubation, which was facilitated by intravenous curare, 24 mg. About two minutes after intubation, the patient's blood pressure fell to 80/50 mm Hg, his heart rate fell to 50/minute, and the central venous pressure remained low at about 4 to 5 mm Hg. (A Swan-Ganz catheter had not been placed and left heart filling pressures were not known.) He was given ephedrine intravenously in 5-mg increments until his pressure and pulse returned to acceptable levels without elevation of central venous pressure; the total dose of ephedrine was 50 mg. The operation proceeded satisfactorily and the patient was "put on the pump" without further difficulty.

Comment. Ephedrine acts directly as a pressor agent, and indirectly by the release of norepinephrine (NE) from the adrenergic nerve endings. Hence the improvement in blood pressure could have been caused by two kinds of drug interactions: (1) ephedrine constricted the peripheral, especially the venous, vascular bed, dilated as a result of histamine release by morphine. The action of ephedrine (and the NE it released) was on the adrenergic, not the histaminergic, receptors, that is, the antagonism was physiologic; (2) the improvement in heart rate and in myocardial contractility represented the action of the drug on the *beta*-adrenergic receptors in the heart, the same receptors in the vicinity of which an unknown concentration of propranolol was present. This was a pharmacologic drug antagonism. The presence of both physiologic and pharmacologic antagonists explains the need for such a large dose of the agonist (ephedrine) to surmount it. The dose required could only have been determined by titration. Epinephrine, had it been prepared in advance, might have been the better choice because it acts more rapidly and permits more rapid titration; however, ephedrine was at hand and proved sufficient.

Case Report Continued. The period of extracorporeal perfusion proceeded in a satisfactory manner. At the conclusion of the operation, the heart did not pump adequately and an isoproterenol infusion was necessary to allow the discontinuance of bypass. However, shortly after protamine was given (to reverse the residual heparin), cardiac performance improved and the isoproterenol was no longer needed.

Comment. At the time heparin was given prior to insertion of the cannulae there was a large increase in free (as opposed to bound) propranolol because of the interference by the heparin (probably mediated by free fatty acids[19a]) with the protein binding of propranolol. The concentration of free propranolol decreased again at the time protamine was given, and more protein became available again for binding. This represents a change in drug effect secondary to a change in protein binding and accounts for the apparent cardiotonic effects of the protamine.

Case Report Continued. The patient was taken to the intensive care unit in good hemodynamic condition with a blood pressure of 110/80, cardiac output of 6 liters per minute, a pulse of 80, a temperature of 36.5°C, and central venous pressure of 9 mm Hg. His chest was clear and blood gases were normal on controlled ventilation with oxygen, 40%. His peripheral circulation was good, as evidenced by pink, warm skin and strong pedal pulses. As he was still unconscious, he was given a dose of 0.2 mg naloxone IV (intravenously) with disastrous consequences: sudden awakening, apprehension, excitement, hypertension (but no tachycardia), and onset of severe pulmonary edema (rales, foam from endotracheal tube, deterioration of arterial blood gases). This was treated satisfactorily with morphine (required total dose 40 mg IV) and positive pressure ventilation with oxygen, 100%. The patient recovered uneventfully.

Comment. This course of events after the administration of naloxone represents once more two kinds of drug interactions: (1) the reversal of the morphine-induced central-nervous-system (CNS) depression by naloxone is an example of drug interaction on the same receptor; (2) however, the resultant awakening, accompanied by pain and excitement, in turn led to generalized sympathetic nervous system discharge, causing release of endogenous norepinephrine with its vasoconstrictor (*alpha*-adrenergic) as well as cardiac (*alpha*- and *beta*-adrenergic) effects. The result was the autotransfusion of large amounts of fluid from the dilated capacitance vessels of the peripheral vasculature into the central vascular compartment, which the recently traumatized left heart, still under the influence of the *beta*-adrenergic antagonist, was unable to handle. This combination of factors resulted in pulmonary edema. When analgesia, histaminergic peripheral vasodilation, and CNS sedation were again provided by means of more morphine, the situation reversed itself once more.

REFERENCES

1. Koch-Wester, J., and Greenblatt, D.J.: Drug interactions in clinical perspective. Eur. J. Clin. Pharmacol., 11:405, 1977.

2. Avery, G.S.: Drug interactions that really matter: A guide to major important drug interactions. Drugs, 14:132, 1977.
3. Alper, M.H., Flacke, W.E., and Krayer, O.: Pharmacology of reserpine and its implications for anesthesia. Anesthesiology, 24:524, 1963.
4. Ominsky, A.J., and Wollman, H.: Hazards of general anesthesia in the reserpinized patient. Anesthesiology, 30:443, 1969.
5. Prys-Roberts, C., Meloche, R., and Foex, P.: Studies of anesthesia in relation to hypertension I: Cardiovascular responses of treated and untreated patients. Br. J. Anaesth., 43:122, 1971.
6. Prys-Roberts, C.: Beta-receptor blockade and anesthesia. In Drug Interactions. Edited by D.G. Grahame-Smith. Baltimore. University Park Press, 1977.
6a. Eikard, B., and Andersen, J.R.: Arrhythmias during halothane anesthesia II: The influence of atropine. Acta Anaesthesiol. Scand., 21:245, 1977.
6b. Eikard, B., and Sørensen, B.: Arrhythmias during halothane anesthesia. I: The influence of atropine during induction with intubation. Acta Anaesthesiol. Scand., 20:296, 1976.
7. Smith, S.E., and Rawlins, M.: Variability in Human Drug Response. London, Butterworth, 1973.
8. Sjöqvist, F.: The role of drug interactions in interindividual variability of drug metabolism in man. Arch. Pharm., 297:S35, 1977.
9. Gilette, J.R.: Individually different responses to drugs according to age, sex, functional and pathological state. In Drug Responses in Man. Edited by G. Wolstenholme and R. Porter. London, Ciba Foundation, Churchill, 1967.
10. Vesell, E.S., and Page, J.G.: Genetic control of drug levels in man: Antipyrine. Science, 161:72, 1968.
11. Alexanderson, B., Price Evans, D.A., and Sjöqvist, F.: Steady state plasma levels of nortriptyline in twins: Influence of genetic factors and drug therapy. Br. Med. J., 4:764, 1969.
12. Bertler, A., and Smith, S.E.: Genetic influences in drug responses of the eye and the heart. Clin. Sci. Mol. Med., 40:403, 1971.
13. Kalow, W.: Genetic factors in relation to drugs. Annu. Rev. Pharmacol., 5:9, 1965.
13a. Davies, D.M. (Ed.): Textbook of Adverse Drug Reactions. Oxford, Oxford University Press, 1981.
14. Cadwallader, D.E.: Biopharmaceutics and Drug Interactions. Montclair, N.J., Rocom Press, 1974.
15. Griffin, J.P., and D'Arcy, P.F.: A Manual of Adverse Drug Interactions. Bristol, John Wright & Sons, 1975.
16. Prescott, L.F.: Drug interaction during absorption. Arch. Pharm., 297:S29, 1977.
17. Nimmo, W.S.: Drugs, diseases and altered gastric emptying. Clin. Pharmacokinet., 1:189, 1976.
18. Brown, D.D., and Juhl, R.P.: Decreased bioavailability of digoxin due to antacids and Kaolin-Pectin. N. Engl. J. Med., 295:1034, 1976.
19. Benjamin, D., Robinson, D.S., and McCormack, J.: Cholestyramine binding of warfarin in man and in vitro. Clin. Res., 18:336, 1970.
19a. Wood, M., Shand, D.G., and Wood, A.J.: Propranolol binding in plasma during cardiopulmonary bypass. Anesthesiology, 51:512, 1979.
20. Prescott, L.F.: Gastric emptying and drug absorption. Br. J. Clin. Pharmacol., 1:189, 1974.
21. Adjopon-Yamoah, K.K., Scott, D.B., and Prescott, L.F.: The effect of atropine on the oral absorption of lidocaine in man. Eur. J. Clin. Pharmacol., 7:397, 1974.
22. Nimmo, W.S., et al.: Inhibition of gastric emptying and drug absorption by narcotic analgesics. Br. J. Clin. Pharmacol., 2:509, 1975.
22a. Daniel, E.E.: Pharmacology of adrenergic, cholinergic, and drugs acting on other receptors in gastrointestinal muscle. In Handbook of Experimental Pharmacology. Mediators and Drugs in Gastrointestinal Motility II. Endogenous and Exogenous Agents. Edited by G. Bertaccini. Berlin, Springer-Verlag, 1982, pp. 249–322.
23. Nies, A.S.: The effects of hemodynamic alterations on drug disposition. Hemodynamic drug interactions. Neth. J. Med., 20:46, 1977.
24. Eger, E.I.: Anesthetic Uptake and Action. Baltimore, Williams & Wilkins, 1974.
25. Evans, E.F., et al.: Blood flow in muscle groups and drug absorption. Clin. Pharmacol. Ther., 17:44, 1975.
26. Goldstein, A., Aranow, L., and Kalman, S.M.: Principles of Drug Action. The Basis of Pharmacology. 2nd Edition. New York, John Wiley & Sons, 1974.
27. Aggeler, P.M., et al.: Potentiation of anticoagulant effect of warfarin by phenylbutazone. N. Engl. J. Med., 276:496, 1967.
28. Wardell, W.M.: Redistributional drug interactions: a critical examination of putative clinical examples. In Drug Interactions. Edited by P.L. Marselli, S. Garratini, and S.N. Cohen. New York, Raven Press, 1974.
29. Sunew K.Y., and Hicks, R.G.: Effects of neostigmine and pyridostigmine on duration of succinylcholine action and pseudocholinesterase activity. Anesthesiology, 49:188, 1978.
30. Blackwell, B., and Marley, E.: Interaction between cheese and monoamine oxidase inhibitors in rats and cats. Lancet, 1:530, 1964.
31. Blackwell, B., et al.: Hypertensive interactions between monoamine oxidase inhibitors and foodstuffs. Br. J. Psychiatry., 113:349, 1967.
32. Barar, F.S.K., et al.: Interactions between catecholamines and tricyclic monoamine oxidase inhibitor antidepressive agents in man. Br. J. Pharmacol., 43:472P, 1971.
33. Cocco, G., and Ague, C.: Interactions between cardioactive drugs and antidepressants. Eur. J. Clin. Pharmacol., 11:389, 1977.
34. Evans-Prosser, C.D.G.: The use of pethidine and morphine in the presence of monoamine oxidase inhibitors. Br. J. Anaesth., 40:279, 1968.
35. Clark, B., and Thompson, J.W.: Analysis of the inhibition of pethidine. N-demethylation by monoamine oxidase inhibitors and some other drugs with special reference to drug interactions in man. Br. J. Pharmacol., 44:89, 1972.
36. Freeman, J.: The renal and hepatic circulation in

anaesthesia. Ann. R. Coll. Surg. Engl., 46:141, 1970.
37. Prescott, L.F.: Clinically important drug interactions. In Drug Treatment. Edited by G.S. Avery. Sidney, Adis Press, 1976.
38. Stephenson, R.P.: A modification of receptor theory. Br. J. Pharmacol., 11:379, 1956.
39. Ariens, E.J., van Rossum, J.M., and Simons, A.M.: Affinity, intrinsic activity and drug interaction. Pharmacol. Rev., 9:218, 1957.
40. Furchgott, R.F.: Receptor mechanisms. Annu. Rev. Pharmacol., 4:21, 1964.
41. Waud, D.R.: Pharmacological receptors. Pharmacol. Rev., 20:49, 1968.
42. Paton, W.D.M.: A theory of drug action based upon the rate of drug receptor combination. Proc. R. Soc., Lond. [Biol.], 154:21, 1961.
43. Paton, W.D.M., and Rang, H.P.: A kinetic approach to the mechanism of drug action. In Advances in Drug Research. Edited by H.J. Harper and A.B. Simmonds. New York—London, Academic Press, 1966.
44. Flacke, W., and Flacke, J.W.: Effects of surmountable antagonists of cardiac responses to nerve stimulation. Proc. VII. Internat. Congress Pharmacol, Paris, July, 1978.
45. Nickerson, M.: Nonequilibrium drug antagonism. Pharmacol. Rev., 9:246, 1957.
46. Reference 46 has been deleted.
47. Ariens, E.J., Simonis, A.M., with van Rossum, J.M.: Drug receptor interaction: Interaction of one or more drugs with different receptor systems. In Molecular Pharmacology. Edited by E.J. Ariens. New York-London, Academic Press, 1964, Vol. I.
48. MacDonald, A.G., and McNeill, R.S.: A comparison of the effect on airway resistance of a new beta blocking drug ICI 50,172. Br. J. Anaesth., 40:508, 1968.
49. Langer, S.Z.: Presynaptic regulation of catecholamine release. Biochem. Pharmacol., 23:1793, 1974.
50. Stjärne, L.: Basic mechanisms and local feedback control of secretion of adrenergic and cholinergic neurotransmitters. In Handbook of Psychopharmacology. Edited by L.L. Iversen, S.D. Iversen, and S.H. Snyder. New York-London, Plenum Press, 1975, Vol. 6.
51. Starke, K.: Regulation of noradrenaline release by presynaptic receptor systems. Rev. Physiol. Biochem. Pharmacol., 77:2, 1977.
52. Löeffelholz, K., and Muscholl, E.: Inhibition by parasympathetic nerve stimulation of the release of the adrenergic transmitter. Naunyn Schmiedebergs Arch. Pharmacol., 267:181, 1970.
53. Trendelenburg, U.: Supersensitivity and subsensitivity to sympathomimetic amines. Pharmacol. Rev., 15:225, 1963.
54. Iversen, L.L.: Inhibition of noradrenaline uptake by drugs. J. Pharm. Pharmacol., 17:62, 1965.
55. Mitchell, J.R., et al.: Guanethidine and related agents. III. Antagonism by drugs which inhibit the norepinephrine pump in man. J. Clin. Invest., 49:1596, 1970.
56. Boakes, A.J., et al.: Interactions between sympathomimetic amines and antidepressant agents in man. Br. Med. J., 1:311, 1973.
57. Briant, R.H., Reid, J.L., and Dollery, C.T.: Interaction between clonidine and desipramine in man. Br. Med. J., 1:522, 1973.
58. Hubbell, W.L., et al.: The interaction of small molecules with spin labeled erythrocyte membranes. Biochim. Biophys. Acta, 219:415, 1970.
59. Koehler, L.S., Curley, W., and Koehler, K.A.: Solvent effects on halothane 19 Fe nuclear magnetic resonance in solvents and artificial membranes. Mol. Pharmacol., 13:113, 1977.
60. Eyring, H., Woodbury, J.W., and D'Arrigo, J.S.: A molecular mechanism of general anesthesia. Anesthesiology, 38:415, 1973.
61. Halsey, M.J.: Mechanisms of general anesthesia. In Anesthetic Uptake and Action. Edited by E.I. Eger, II. Baltimore, Williams & Wilkins, 1974.
62. Cuthbert, A.W.: Membrane lipids and drug action. Pharmacol. Rev., 19:59, 1967.
63. Saidman, L.J., and Eger, E.I., II: Effect of nitrous oxide and of narcotic premedication on the alveolar concentration of halothane required for anesthesia. Anesthesiology, 25:302, 1964.
64. Munson, E.S., Saidman, L.J., and Eger, E.I., II: Effect of nitrous oxide and morphine on the minimum anesthetic concentration of fluroxene. Anesthesiology, 26:134, 1965.
65. Wolfson, B., Keilar, C.M., and Lake, C.L.: Anesthetic index, a new approach. Anesthesiology, 38:583, 1973.
66. Wolfson, B., et al.: Anesthetic Indices—Further data. Anesthesiology, 48:187, 1978.
67. Perisho, J.A., Buechel, D.R., and Miller, R.D.: The effect of diazepam (Valium[R]) on minimum alveolar anesthetic requirement (MAC) in man. Can. Anaesth. Soc. J., 18:536, 1971.
68. Lowenstein, E., Hallowell, P., and Levine, F.: Cardiovascular response to large doses of intravenous morphine in man. N. Engl. J. Med., 281:1389, 1969.
69. Seeman, P.: The membrane actions of anesthetics and tranquilizers. Pharmacol. Rev., 24:583, 1972.
70. Shanes, A.M.: Electrochemical aspects of physiologic and pharmacologic action in excitable cells. Pharmacol. Rev., 10:59, 1958.
70a. Olson, R.W.: Drug interactions at the GABA receptor-ionophore complex. Ann. Rev. Pharmacol. Toxicol., 22:245, 1982.
71. Price, H.L., and Helrich, M.: The effect of cyclopropane, diethyl ether, nitrous oxide, thiopental, and hydrogen ion concentration on the myocardial function of the dog heart-lung preparation. J. Pharmacol. Exp. Ther., 115:206, 1955.
72. Brown, B.R., and Crout, J.R.: A comparative study of the effects of five general anesthetics on myocardial contractility. Anesthesiology, 34:236, 1971.
73. Richter, J., Landau, E.M., and Cohen, S.: The action of volatile anesthetics and convulsants on synaptic transmission: a unified concept. Mol. Pharmacol., 13:548, 1977.
74. Garfield, J.M., et al.: A pharmacological analysis of ganglionic actions of some general anesthetics. Anesthesiology, 29:79, 1968.

75. Mori, K., and Winters, W.: Neural background of sleep and anesthesia. Int. Anesthesiol. Clin., 12:76, 1975.
76. Chung, B., Naraghi, M., and Adriani, J.: Sympathomimetic effects of cocaine and their influence on halothane and enflurane anesthesia. Anesthesiology Rev., 5:16, 1978.
77. Dundee, J.W., and McCaughey, W.: Interaction of drugs associated with anesthesia. In Recent Advances in Anesthesia and Analgesia. Edited by C.L. Hewer. Boston, Little Brown, 1973.
78. Flacke, J.W., Flacke, W.E., and Williams, G.D.: Acute pulmonary edema following naloxone reversal of high-dose morphine anesthesia. Anesthesiology, 47:376, 1977.
78a. Fleckenstein, A.: Specific pharmacology of calcium in myocardium, cardiac pacemakers, and vascular smooth muscle. Ann. Rev. Pharmacol. Toxicol., 17:149, 1977.
78b. Calcium Antagonismus. Edited by A. Fleckenstein and H. Roskamm. Berlin, Springer, 1980, p. 270.
79. Pittinger, C., and Adamson, R.: Antibiotic blockade of neuromuscular function. Annu. Rev. Pharmacol., 12:169, 1972.
80. Fogdall, R., and Miller, R.D.: Prolongation of a pancuronium-induced neuromuscular blockade by polymyxin B. Anesthesiology, 40:84, 1974.
81. Denborough, M.A., and Lovell, R.R.H.: Anesthetic deaths in a family. Lancet, 2:45, 1960.
82. Britt, B.A., and Kalow, W.: Malignant hyperthermia: A statistical review. Can. Anaesth. Soc. J., 17:293, 1970.
83. Isaach, H., and Barlow, M.B.: Malignant hyperpyrexia. J. Neurol. Neurosurg. Psychiatry, 36:228, 1973.
84. Editorial: New causes for malignant hyperpyrexia. Br. Med. J., 4:488, 1974.
85. Katz, R.L., and Epstein, R.A.: The interaction of anesthetic agents and adrenergic drugs to produce cardiac arrhythmias. Anesthesiology, 29:763, 1968.
86. Hoffman, B.F.: The genesis of cardiac arrhythmias. In Mechanisms and Therapy of Cardiac Arrhythmias. Edited by L.S. Dreifus and W. Likoff. New York, Grune and Stratton, 1966.
86a. Stoelting, R.K.: Allergic reactions during anesthesia. Anesth. Analg., 62:41, 1983.
87. Adriani, J., and Campbell, D.: Fatalities following topical application of local anesthetics to mucous membranes. J.A.M.A., 162:1527, 1956.

4

PHARMACOKINETICS AND DRUG INTERACTIONS

ALDO N. CORBASCIO

The selection of the proper dose of a drug to achieve a specific pharmacologic effect is one of pharmacology's central concerns. Without a precise perception of how, when and how much of a drug should be administered, rational therapeutics would be a practical impossibility. Many of the therapeutic errors of the past were due to ignorance or neglect of quantitative factors in drug therapy. Hence a rational discourse concerning a drug requires a precise knowledge of certain intrinsic characteristics of the drug such as bioavailability, duration of action, peak effect, accumulation and rate of elimination from the body. Any concept of dose-effect relationship is based on a fundamental pharmacodynamic relationship between drug concentration at the site of action, or tissue phase, and the intensity of the effect.

The relationship between administered dose, tissue or receptor concentration and physiologic response is often quantitatively elusive and multifactorial, i.e., dependent upon the vagaries of the drug's absorption from the site of administration, its distribution in blood, its attachment to tissues and its metabolism and excretion.

The study of these factors is the province of pharmacokinetics, a relatively new discipline that deals with the behavior of drugs in the body, their distribution in tissues, their excretion and metabolism. The relationship between tissue or blood concentration of a drug and pharmacologic effect is the concern of pharmacodynamics. The distinction is often impossible to make, and a definite overlap exists frequently between these fields. A study of such factors is necessary not only for a safer use of a drug, but also for the possibility of developing better drugs or new therapeutic modalities.

Although the importance of pharmacokinetics cannot be overestimated, its development had to wait for the introduction of sensitive analytical methodologies and suitable mathematical models. The analytical techniques include gas chromatography, high-pressure liquid chromatography and mass spectroscopy. They possess a sensitivity in the picogram range (1×10^{-9} g). These models help us understand the kinetics of drugs in the body, and perhaps more importantly, they help clarify the impact of changes in kinetic parameters. The need for some kind of mathematical model that could serve as a general paradigm of drug action has encouraged the introduction of a number of mathematical concepts that have added some clarity—and occasional confusion—to the field.

This chapter can only touch on some of the principles of this important topic. For detailed information and understanding the reader is referred to two excellent books on the subject.[1,2]

Drug Dispositional Process

The route of administration is of primary importance to determine what portion of the drug will reach the plasma. Drugs administered by the oral route are subject to the uncertainties of gastric and enteral absorption. In general a considerable fraction of the drug absorbed through these routes will be delivered to the liver and subjected to sequestration and metabolism before the drug is able to reach the systemic circulation.

Drugs administered by the subcutaneous or intramuscular route can gain access to the general circulation and bypass the liver, provided they are injected in areas in which a sufficiently brisk blood flow exists. The example of subcutaneous morphine administered in combat conditions is well known, though worth recalling. When morphine sulfate is injected into a wounded soldier who has sustained a large blood loss from his wounds and is in borderline shock due to exposure, the drug is poorly absorbed, and no analgesia results. This induces the corpsman to administer another and possibly larger dose of morphine, which is also ineffective until the administration of fluids and plasma restores an adequate capillary flow, which promotes the absorption of the drug. The sudden mobilization, however, of the large morphine pool sequestered in peripheral tissue can lead to severe respiratory depression and often, death.

The main purpose of therapy is to deliver an accurate and effective concentration of a drug to a tissue receptor from which the drug will elicit the desired response without undesirable side effects. Since the response of tissues of individuals is highly variable, it is important to choose a dose that is likely to produce a therapeutic response in the largest possible number of patients. The ratio of the median lethal dose (LD_{50}) divided by the median effective dose (ED_{50}) is called the *therapeutic ratio*. This ratio, however, is generally too inclusive to provide an adequate guide to therapy.

BASIS OF PHARMACOKINETIC INTERACTIONS OF DRUGS

Some Pharmacokinetic Definitions

The *intensity of the effect* produced by a drug is approximately related to the fractions of the receptors occupied by the drug. A maximal effect occurs when all the receptors (R) are occupied by the agonist drug (D). Thus:

$$D + R \rightarrow DR \rightarrow Effect$$

Although a maximal saturation of receptors produces a maximal effect, a semimaximal occupation does not necessarily produce a semimaximal response. The greater the affinity of the drug for the receptor, the lower the drug concentration required to produce the maximal effect. This helps to define the *potency* of a drug.

The time required for the plasma concentration of a drug to diminish by 50% is defined as the *half-life* ($t_{1/2}$) of the drug. The measurement of this variable was inspired by the measurement of the decay of the radioactivity of isotopes. It provides the first definition as to the duration of action of a drug in the body and the time of its elimination and metabolism. In general, after 4 half-lives have been eliminated, most of the drug (94%) has left the circulation.

The *slope of the decline* in plasma concentration provides important information as to the rapidity of the process of elimination of the drug from plasma and the need of readministration of the drug in order to maintain a therapeutic level in plasma.

The *volume of distribution* of a drug in the body stems from the presumption (which is in fact a gross approximation) that the body behaves as a single compartment into which the drug is evenly distributed. The concentration of the drug in the body is expressed as the volume of water that could contain a dose of the drug if this were to distribute itself evenly into the whole volume. For example, antipyrine, which is dispersed evenly into body water without binding to plasma proteins, has a volume of distribution of 40 liters in a 70-kg man. This corresponds to the total body water for a normal man of this weight. The volume of distribution of chlorpromazine is 1,400 liters, a value which appears nonsensical unless one considers that the drug is irregularly distributed in the body water with selective concentration in certain compartments. Salicylate has a volume of distribution of 12L/70kg. This indicates that the drug is restricted to extracellular fluids (9L) and that it does not enter intracellular water.[3]

The volume of distribution does not relate to a specific anatomic space but instead relates plasma concentration to total amount of drug in the body. It provides some clue as to the ability of the drug to penetrate tissues. This may be important in the treatment of overdose.[3] Drugs with a small volume of distribution do not penetrate tissues and can be more readily removed by dialysis. Drugs with a high volume of distribution (e.g., digoxin 500L/70kg) cannot be readily mobilized by dialysis because they are sequestered in tissues. Drugs possess the ability to bind reversibly to nonspecific and nonfunctional sites located on plasma proteins, which function as a carrier and storage system. The type of binding can vary according to the type of chemical bond established between the drug and the carrier. It is usually labile (for example hydrogen bonds or van der Waals forces).

Binding to plasma albumin molecules is of great theoretical and practical interest. Drugs are carried in plasma in a free and a bound form. The free form is the active pharmacologically available fraction, while the bound form is pharmacologically inert. The two forms are in equilibrium. This means that as soon as the free form is metabolized or eliminated, a corresponding aliquot of the bound form will become available, owing to dissociation of the bound form from plasma proteins.

When one administers intravenously a drug that is extensively bound, the concentration of the pharmacologically active drug will depend upon the rate of injection. If the rate of injection is rapid, the binding capacity of plasma proteins will be exceeded, and a high concentration of free drug will be achieved. This tactic will magnify the intensity of the pharmacologic response in relation to the amount injected. Thiopental (80% protein bound) injected in this manner achieves a more rapid and pleasant induction.

When a drug is extensively bound to protein, any displacement by another drug can cause relevant pharmacologic effects. Interactions occur whenever the drugs administered concurrently compete for the same binding site on the protein. This is a source of clinically important drug interactions. The fact that two drugs are protein bound does not necessarily imply that one drug will displace the other, because each drug may bind to a different site of the protein molecule. For example, indomethacin can be displaced by aspirin but not by phenylbutazone. Anticoagulants such as warfarin are easily displaced by salicylates, phenylbutazone and other nonsteroidal anti-inflammatory agents with consequent danger of bleeding.

Disease (e.g., liver failure or nephrotic syndrome) can affect plasma albumin and thereby decrease drug binding. In addition, bilirubin can be extensively bound to plasma proteins and may influence binding of such agents as sulfonamides (other endogenous substances share this characteristic).

Drugs with a high degree of protein binding tend to prolong their sojourn in the body. Bound drugs are less available to the receptor and hence have a lower ther-

Table 4–1
Plasma Protein Binding of Some Drugs

Salicylates	59–80%
Phenylbutazone	95%
Meperidine	40%
Thiopental	80%
Phenobarbital	20%
Pentobarbital	37%

apeutic activity, but a prolonged effect. They are less liable to be distributed in tissues, less likely to cross the blood-brain barrier and less liable to be displaced by dialysis. See Table 4–1 for the relative binding of several typical drugs. The importance of protein binding is emphasized later in the chapter.

Some drugs show a definite propensity to distribute themselves selectively to certain tissues, e.g., tetracyclines in bone and teeth; digoxin in the heart, liver and kidney; chloroquine in the retina; and thiopental in CNS and fat. Clinically important displacements can occur only when the tissue depot constitutes a significant aliquot of body mass (e.g., body fat), because the drug that is displaced has a large sink to which to distribute (50L of body water). Hence the dilution effects are significant.

Measurements of plasma concentrations of a drug are useful in several areas. These include:

1. Determining appropriate dosage and frequency of administration.
2. Following the course of a drug whose therapeutic ratio is small (e.g., digitalis).
3. Verifying patient compliance.
4. Investigating causes of therapeutic failure at conventional doses (e.g., anticonvulsants).
5. Helping in cases of impairment of eliminatory processes (liver and kidney failure).
6. Detecting the onset of toxicity at doses in the therapeutic range.
7. Aiding in the diagnosis and management of drug overdose.

DISPOSITIONAL FACTORS AFFECTING DRUG CONCENTRATION AT RECEPTOR SITES

In some cases the occupancy of a limited number of receptors by an agonist induces a maximal response. This is true of "spare receptors," which can be quantified as that fraction of receptors that can be irreversibly blocked without affecting the height of the maximal response. This is important in some drug responses in which the receptor is coupled to an enzyme system. Occupation of a small portion of receptors can induce a maximal activation of the enzyme. This situation occurs typically at the neuromuscular junction, where there are a large number of cholinergic receptors, far in excess of the need to elicit a muscle action potential. It has been shown experimentally that a large fraction (80%) of the receptor sites can be blocked without any appreciable effect on neuromuscular transmission.[4]

The presence of a drug that can block the receptor without inducing any noticeable effect will displace the dose-response curve of the agonist to the right without affecting the shape or the ceiling of the pharmacological response. This type of drug is called an antagonist. The ratio of the dose of the agonist required to induce the same response in the presence of the antagonist is called the *dose ratio*, or D-R. The greater the degree of competitive blockade, the greater is the dose ratio.

Prolonged exposure of the receptor can decrease its responsiveness. Tachyphylaxis has been extensively studied with catecholamines and has been recently extended to the desensitization that occurs after prolonged exposure to *beta* blockers or insulin. For example, some forms of diabetes characterized by excessive production of insulin cause a deficiency of insulin receptors and a decreased tissue responsiveness to endogenous insulin.

The density of receptor population may be age dependent, as shown by Vestal et al.,[5] who have demonstrated that the cardiac chronotropic response to isoproterenol decreases progressively with age, such that elderly patients require doses of isoproterenol 4 to 5 times greater than younger subjects to increase their heart rate.

Pharmacokinetic factors may play a crucial role in diminishing or exaggerating the pharmacologic response to a drug. Reduction in the volume of distribution, rate of metabolism, or rate of excretion can induce an increase in the concentration of a drug at a receptor site. Small alterations in protein binding (2%) in drugs which are extensively bound to plasma proteins (90%) (warfarin, propranolol, diazepam) can induce a large increase of the free fraction of the drug with profound pharmacologic effects. In a drug less extensively bound to plasma proteins (70%) a 2% reduction of the bound fraction will cause only a small increase in pharmacologic response.

Orally administered drugs that are subject to removal or trapping by the liver are called *high-extraction drugs*. A typical example is propranolol, 78% of which is trapped and hydroxylated during its first pass through the liver. That this is a determining factor in the pharmacokinetics of propranolol is indicated by the fact that its intravenous dose is 1% or less than the oral dose. The extent of absorption of the unchanged drug into the systemic circulation is defined as the *systemic availability* of the drug.[6] The entity of the first-pass effect in the liver can be estimated by a formula as follows:

$$R = 1 - \frac{\text{i.v. dose}}{\text{Area}_{i.v.} F}$$

in which R is the ratio of areas under the plasma concentration curves after oral and intravenous dose and F is the flow rate through the liver (1.5 L/m) (Fig. 4–1).

The termination of the pharmacologic action of many drugs is due to their metabolism into inactive metabolites by the intervention of a large number of drug metabolizing enzymes, of which coenzyme P-450 is a major component. The liver is the major, though not the exclusive, site of drug metabolism. Several other important sites of metabolism have been identified in the lung, kidney and intestine. The prior administration of other drugs can increase or decrease the activity of drug-metabolizing enzymes. Stimulation of drug metabolism increases the clearance of the drug and tends to reduce both its plasma level and its duration of action.

The half-life of the drug and its duration of action will be similarly affected. Such interactions may be harmful if a drug whose blood concentration is critical to the survival of a patient is rapidly cleared from circulation (e.g., rapid elimination of an antiepileptic, an antidysrhythmic drug or anticoagulant).

The reduced effectiveness of anticoagulants that occurs during the simultaneous administration of barbiturates was probably the first such interaction detected clin-

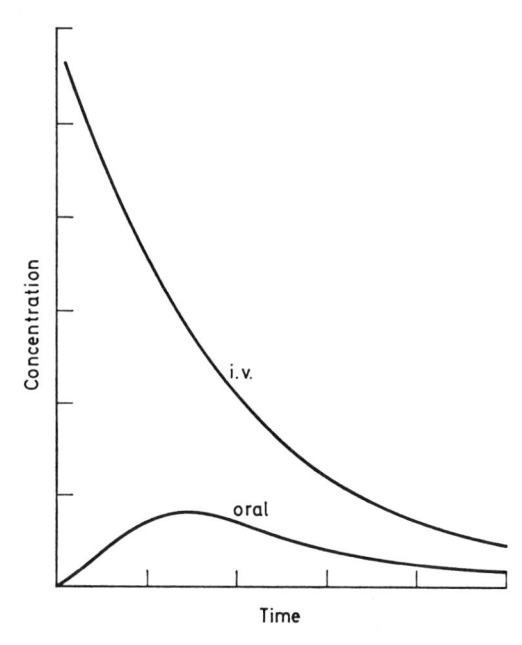

Fig. 4–1. First pass effect on systemic bioavailability. Drug concentration in the plasma after intravenous and oral administration of the same dose of a drug with a total clearance of 1.15 L/min after i.v. administration. It is assumed that the drug is eliminated only by biotransformation in the liver.

ically.[7] This observation has been amply confirmed and explained in terms of stimulation of liver drug-metabolizing enzymes by barbiturates (See Chapters 6 and 20). The administration of a barbiturate lowers the blood level and the therapeutic effects of dicoumarol and warfarin and shortens their respective half-lives.[8,9] Phenobarbital can reduce the serum levels of digoxin and shorten its half-life in some patients.[10] Barbiturates can also affect the elimination of chlorpromazine and tricyclic antidepressants and lower the plasma level of nortriptyline-treated patients.[11]

Ethanol is a well known inducer of hepatic drug-metabolizing enzymes (See Chapter 20). Its prolonged ingestion (3 months) in alcoholic subjects increases the clearance of warfarin, diphenylhydantoin and tolbutamide.[12]

Enzyme induction decreases the toxicity of meprobamate, pentobarbital, lidocaine, mepivacaine and prilocaine.[13] It has also been established experimentally that pretreatment of mice with phenobarbital or chlorcyclizine decreases the toxicity of alkylphosphates (malathion, parathion or EPN). This is probably due to liver induction of both true and plasma cholinesterases, which inactivate these compounds before they combine with tissue acetylcholinesterase.[14]

Hemodynamic Drug Interactions

The hemodynamic effects of one drug can affect substantially the absorption, steady-state level, and disposition of another. This is particularly true of drugs that are highly extractable by the liver, such as lidocaine, propranolol or propoxyphene. It has been found in monkeys that the clearance of lidocaine is reduced by the concomitant administration of propranolol.[15] In this case, *beta*-adrenergic blockade caused by propranolol decreased cardiac output and liver blood flow with a reduction of the rate of delivery of lidocaine to its site of hepatic metabolism.

Stenson and colleagues have shown that changes in hepatic blood flow secondary to a decrease in cardiac output influence blood levels of lidocaine in man.[16] The influence of circulatory events on lidocaine kinetics and disposition in monkeys was studied by Benowitz and associates.[16a] They showed that a 30% reduction in cardiac output secondary to acute hemorrhage impaired lidocaine extraction by the liver and decreased drug clearance by 40%, volume of distribution by 20%, and elimination half-life by 40%. The administration of isoproterenol induced an increase in cardiac output and hepatic blood flow with a 40% increase in the rate of drug clearance, a 30% increase in volume of distribution, and a slight increase in the half-life of lidocaine.

Hence the kinetics of a highly extracted drug will be profoundly influenced by hemodynamic factors. Any agent that interferes with or tends to reduce liver blood flow by a direct effect on its vasculature or by an indirect effect on its perfusion pressure is likely to influence to some degree its own duration of action and metabolic disposition, as well as the duration of action and metabolism of other drugs administered concomitantly.

The Importance of Protein Binding. The amount of free drug that finally reaches its tissue receptors is influenced by its binding to plasma and to tissues that are not part of the pharmacologic target. They constitute a large sink in which the drug is dispersed, as well as an important carrier system that dampens and modulates drug action.

Most acidic drugs tend to bind to serum albumin, which acts as a circulatory reservoir of bound drugs. Most studies on drug binding have been performed on such a system. Few studies deal with the binding of the drug to its pharmacologic target, i.e., a specific receptor. As discussed above, protein binding is vitally important, because drugs bound to a macromolecular transport system are generally inactive and become so only upon their release. Therefore only the unbound drug reaches the receptor, and drug response can be predicted more accurately in terms of the concentration of the free drug. The type of binding between the drug and the macromolecule carrier is usually labile (hydrogen bonds, hydrophobic bonds or dipole induced bonds). A tighter type of binding (covalent or ionic) would render it unavailable to the receptor and hence inactive. The degree of binding of the drug to the macromolecular complex is dictated by several factors such as 1. drug concentration, 2. protein concentration, 3. presence of competing drugs for the same binding sites, 4. affinity of the drug for the protein, and 5. the pH of the plasma.

In contrast to acidic drugs, basic drugs bind to lipoproteins, glycoproteins or *gamma*-globulins.[18] The total albumin content of the human body is approximately 0.4% of body weight (~ 300 g), while total body tissue comprises 40% of body weight (~30 kg).

The volume of distribution of a drug is dependent on plasma and tissue binding. If a drug is extensively bound to plasma protein and little to body tissues, its volume of distribution will be small (e.g., warfarin or phenylbutazone). Drugs that are extensively bound to body tissues have a large volume of distribution. A drug that is highly bound to plasma and tissue proteins will have a large volume of distribution with a small fraction of unbound circulating drug, while a drug that is not bound will produce high blood levels. The degree of binding will influence its steady-state levels and its elimination.

The degree of plasma protein binding exerts great influence on the hepatic metabolism of a drug. The rate of metabolism of a drug will depend on the amount of free, unbound drug that can reach liver metabolizing enzymes. Hepatic extraction will not be limited in this case by liver blood flow.

Renal clearance of drugs is subject to similar factors. Since drugs bound to albumin cannot filter through the intact kidney glomerular membrane, only the free fraction is available for filtration. If a drug is secreted by a tubular mechanism, only the free drug can be excreted in the urine. There is, however, an equilibrium between free and bound drug, and a decrease in the free-drug concentration is likely to induce dissociation of the protein-drug complex which may make more drug available for elimination.

The problems of tissue binding of drugs have not yet been approached with any degree of precision.[19] Gibaldi et al. have predicted that drugs with a large volume of distribution possess a biologic half-life that is inversely proportional to the free fraction of drug in tissues and is relatively unaffected by protein binding.

Highly bound drugs competing for the same carrier site on the protein can influence each other's binding and disposition by displacement. A small degree of displacement of a highly bound drug will cause a large increase in the free unbound fraction of the drug. The consequences of this may be important, particularly if the drug has a small volume of distribution. An increase in free drug will make more of it available for pharmacologic action, metabolism and excretion. This can significantly affect the half-life of the drug and the duration of its effects. Displacement of binding between highly bound drugs with a small volume of distribution can induce significant drug interactions especially if the therapeutic ratio is small.

Changes in the composition of plasma proteins (hypoalbuminemia), their physical state (glycosylation of hemoglobin in diabetes) or their body distribution (with burns, surgery, or pregnancy) can affect the kinetic parameters of many drugs in important ways, especially if several bound drugs are administered simultaneously, and if the capacity of the macromolecular carrier is exhausted. This phenomenon is particularly evident after repeated injections that achieve rapidly a high concentration of the drug in tissues with the highest perfusion (e.g., brain, is slow, with peak concentrations occurring within 15 to 30 minutes after intravenous injection. The elimination half-life from the CNS was correspondingly longer (3.0 hours) than from plasma (1.3 hours). They attributed the slow rate of uptake and elimination of morphine to its limited lipid solubility and its tendency to ionize at physiological pH.[29] In the brain, a normally lower tissue pH favors the ionization of morphine and its retention in neural tissue. This inevitably delays its exit from the CNS and its recirculation through the blood-brain barrier and its disposition in other tissues.

In renal failure a characteristic prolongation of the narcotic effect of morphine occurs. This is probably due to the accumulation of morphine glucuronides which normally are excreted exclusively via the kidney. Hug et al. have shown by intracerebral injection of such glucuronides that these metabolites are pharmacologically active and can produce narcosis and respiratory depression.

Morphine pKa is close to the range of blood pH. Hence any change in pH can induce significant changes in the degree of the drug's ionization, which in turn affects the ability of the drug to penetrate the blood-brain barrier, causing a corresponding enhancement of its CNS effects and prolonging its pharmacologic action.

Nishiateno et al.[29] have shown in the dog that an increase in plasma pH induced by hyperventilation favors the access and retention of morphine in the CNS. This effect may be adversely affected by the opposite vascular changes in blood flow (constriction) caused by hypocapnia. These observations are very important and deserve further study in man.

Morphine therefore behaves differently from highly soluble narcotics such as fentanyl. This is a typical case in which information obtained from peripheral kinetic data cannot be immediately translated into pharmacologic responses in the CNS.

Fentanyl. Fentanyl is a potent intravenous opiate analgesic that is 100 times more potent than morphine. It has a more rapid onset and shorter duration of action than morphine or meperidine. Owing to the low plasma levels in patients, it is difficult to quantitate accurately in biological fluids.

McCain and Hug[31] have shown that fentanyl has a rapid distribution half-life of 1.8 minutes and a slow distribution half-life of 13.3 minutes. The rapid distribution phase represents equilibration with highly perfused tissues (brain), while the slow distribution phase indicates equilibration of the highly perfused tissues with fat.

The drug is metabolized almost exclusively in the liver, as only 7% is excreted in the urine. It has a high intrinsic clearance (13.3 ml/kg/m), suggesting a high hepatic excretion rate and perfusion-dependent elimination. Oral fentanyl is largely ineffective, owing to its low bioavailability and a marked first-pass effect in the liver.

Its volume of distribution is similar to morphine and meperidine owing to high lipid solubility. Fentanyl concentrates in fat depots. This accounts for its large volume of distribution and is a rate limiting factor for its elimination from the body. It is moderately bound to plasma proteins, with a free fraction of 19% in plasma. Fentanyl protein binding is pH dependent, as the free, unbound fraction declines to 10% at a pH of 7.6. Because of its high lipid solubility, the drug gains access rapidly to the CNS and resembles heroin in the rapid onset of its pharmacologic action.

The rapid onset and termination of fentanyl anesthesia can be reconciled and explained in terms of pharmacodynamic findings in the dog.[32] A bolus intravenous injection achieves optimal CNS concentrations in the brain within 2 to 10 minutes. This coincides with the respiratory depression and narcotic effect, which correspond to the log of fentanyl concentration in plasma and CSF. As the plasma concentration declines, the drug leaves the CNS and redistributes to muscle and tissue. In this respect fentanyl behaves very much like thiopental. Multiple doses cause accumulation of the drug in the plasma and a decrease in the brain muscle and fat gradient with a marked increase and prolongation of narcotic effect.

Conclusion

The kinetic behavior of a drug in the body is subject to a multiplicity of variables, such as plasma and tissue protein binding, diffusion, sequestration in fat depots, and conversion to active and inactive metabolites. The level of a drug in plasma, however, correlates often in a linear fashion with the effect at the pharmacologically responsive target. Measurements of a steady state of a drug in plasma may be essential to develop an optimal dosage, prevent accumulation and monitor compliance.

These principles cannot be applied indiscriminately. A small number of important drugs that bind irreversibly or covalently with the receptor, such as alkylphosphates, LSD, reserpine, or MAO inhibitors, elude a clear kinetic correlation with their prolonged pharmacologic effect (hit and run drugs). Kinetic criteria do not apply to drugs whose effect depends on their diffusion to poorly perfused areas (e.g., antibiotics in necrotic tissues).

Drugs extensively bound to plasma proteins are subject to the vagaries of complex macromolecular carriers (e.g., hypoalbuminemia) and may require the measurement of the free fraction of the drug, a procedure that is often difficult and time consuming. The study of the effects on displacement of the binding of one drug versus another is still in its infancy, although it shows considerable promise in the explanation of many phenomena observed in the study of drug interactions.

REFERENCES

1. Prys-Roberts and Hug, C.C., Jr. (Eds.): Pharmacokinetics of Anaesthesia. London, Blackwell Scientific Publications, 1984, 358 pp.
2. Stanski, D.R., Watkins, W.: Drug Disposition in Anesthesia. New York, Grune and Stratton, 1982, 203 p.
3. Laurance, D.R., and Brenner, P.M.: Clinical Pharmacology. New York, Churchill Livingstone. 1980, p. 118.
4. Waud, B.E.: Neuromuscular blocking agents. Current problems in anesthesia and critical care medicine. Chicago, Year Book Medical Publishers, 1977.
5. Vestal, R.E., Wood, A.J.J., and Shand, D.G.: Reduced beta-receptor sensitivity in the elderly. Clin. Pharmacol. Therap., 26:181, 1979.
6. Levy, G., and Gibaldi, M.: Pharmacokinetics. Chap. 59 p. 23, Hand. Exp. Pharmacol. xxvii/3, New York, Springer Verlag, 1975.
7. Avellaneda, M.: Interferencia de los barbiturios en la accion del tromexan. Medicina, Buenos Aires, 15:109, 1955.
8. Conney, A.H., Sandur, M., and Burns, J.J.: Drug interactions in man. I. Lowering effect of phenobarbital on plasma levels of bishydroxy coumarin (dicumarol) and diphenylhydantoin (dilantin). Clin. Pharm. Ther., 6:420, 1965.
9. MacDonald, M.G., and Robinson, D.S.: Clinical observations of possible barbiturate interference with anticoagulation. J.A.M.A., 204:97, 1968.
10. Solomon, H.M., and Abrams, W.B.: Interactions between digitoxin and other drugs in man. Am. Heart J., 83:277, 1972.
11. Alexanderson, B.: Pharmacokinetics of nortriptyline in man after single and multiple oral doses: The predictability of steady-state plasma concentrations from single dose plasma-level data. Europ. J. Clin. Pharmacol., 4:82, 1972.
12. Carulli, N., et al.: Alcohol drug interactions in man: Alcohol and tolbutamide. Eur. J. Clin. Invest., 1:421, 1971.
13. Heinon, J.: The effect of drugs on the duration of toxic symptoms caused by sublethal doses of local anesthetics—an experimental study in mice. Acta Pharmacol. Toxicol., 21:155, 1964.
14. Welch, R.M., and Coon, J.M.: Studies on the effect of chlorcyclizine and other drugs on the toxicity of several organophosphate anticholinesterases. Pharmacol. Exp. Ther., 144:192, 1964.
15. Branch, R.A., Shand, D.G., Wilkinson, G.R., and Niel, S.A.: The reduction of lidocaine clearance by d-l propranolol. An example of hemodynamic drug interaction. J. Pharmacol. Exp. Ther., 184(2):515, 1973.
16. Stenson, R.E., Constantino, R.T., and Harrison, D.C.: Interrelationship of hepatic blood flow, cardiac output and blood levels of lidocaine in man. Circulation, 18:205, 1971.
16a. Benowitz, N., Rowland, M., Forsyth, R., and Melmon, K.L.: Circulatory influences on lidocaine disposition. Clin. Res., 21:467, 1973.
17. Branch, R.A., et al.: Increase in hepatic blood flow and d-propranolol clearance by glucagon in the monkey. J. Pharmacol. Exp. Ther., 187:581, 1983.
18. Piafsky, K.M.: Disease induced changes in plasma binding of basic drugs. Clin. Pharmacok., 5:246, 1980.
19. Gibaldi, M., Levy, G., and McNamara, P.J.: Effect of plasma protein and tissue binding on the bio-

logical half life of drugs. Clin. Pharmacol. Ther., 24:1, 1978.
20. Blaschke, T.F.: Protein binding and kinetics of drugs in liver diseases. Clin. Pharmacokin., 2:32, 1977.
21. Jusko, W.J., and Gretch, M.: Plasma and tissue protein binding of drugs in pharmacokinetics. Drug. Metab. Rev., 5:43, 1976.
22. Gibaldi, M.: Drug distribution in renal failure. Am. J. Med., 62:471, 1977.
23. Brodie, B.B., et al.: The phase of thiopental in man and a method for its estimation in biological material. J. Pharmacol. Exp. Ther., 98:85, 1950.
24. Shideman, F.E., et al.: The role of the liver in the detoxification of thiopental by man. Anesthesiology, 10:421, 1949.
25. White, P.F.: Effects of halothane anesthesia on the biodisposition of ketamine in rats. J. Pharmacol. Exp. Ther., 196:536, 1976.
26. Grant, I.S., et al.: Pharmacokinetic and analgesic effects of i.m. and oral ketamine. Br. J. Anaesth., 53:805, 1981.
27. Stanski, D.R., et al.: Kinetics of intravenous and intramuscular morphine. Clin. Pharmacol. Ther., 24:52, 1978.
28. Hug, C.C., et al.: Pharmacokinetics of morphine injected intravenously into the anesthetized dog. Anesthesiology, 54:38, 1981.
29. Nishiateno, K., Ngai, S.H., Finck, A.D., et al.: Pharmacokinetics of morphine post operatively, concentrations in serum and brain in the dog during hyperventilation. Anesthesiology, 47:407, 1977.
30. Finck, A.D., et al.: Pharmacokinetics of morphine. Effects of hypercarbia on serum and brain morphine concentrations in the dog. Anesthesiology, 47:407, 1977.
31. McCain, D.A., and Hug, C.C.: Intravenous fentanyl kinetics. Clin. Pharmacol. Ther., 28:106, 1980.
32. Hug, C.C., and Murphy, M.R.: Fentanyl disposition in cerebrospinal fluid and plasma and its relationship to respiratory depression in the dog. Anesthesiology, 50:342, 1979.

5

THE EFFECT OF pH

J.S. GRAVENSTEIN and A.H. ANTON

In the following pages we present an example of how a shift in pH can alter the pharmacologic effectiveness of drugs that are weak acids or weak bases. A pH shift can affect the (1) pharmacologic effectiveness, (2) absorption, (3) distribution, (4) renal excretion, and (5) metabolism of drugs. Although these categories are interrelated, it is helpful to discuss them separately.

CASE REPORT

A 20-year-old man was admitted to the hospital emergency ward in a coma. He had ingested an unknown quantity of tablets and capsules. It was known that the drugs included phenobarbital, meperidine, and amphetamine. After tracheal intubation, controlled ventilation and an intravenous infusion were established. An arterial blood-gas analysis showed a mixed metabolic-respiratory acidosis, with pH 7.00 and P_{CO_2} 60 mm Hg. The patient's arterial pressure was low (65/40 mm Hg) and his heart rate was high (115 beats/min).

The following questions are now raised: (a) Will gastric absorption of the drugs have progressed at an equal rate? (b) Is the acidemia equally beneficial (or detrimental) to a patient with barbiturate, opioid, and amphetamine intoxication? (c) Can renal excretion of these drugs be enhanced by therapeutic maneuvers?

PHARMACOLOGIC EFFECTIVENESS OF SHIFTS IN pH

In order to examine these questions and to consider the therapeutic consequences, it is necessary to review how pH changes are expressed and what such changes do to weak acids (such as barbiturates) and to weak bases (such as opioid and amphetamine).

The central issue is that these substances dissociate, the degree of dissociation being H-dependent. For phenobarbital, the products of this dissociation would be the ionized form of the drug,

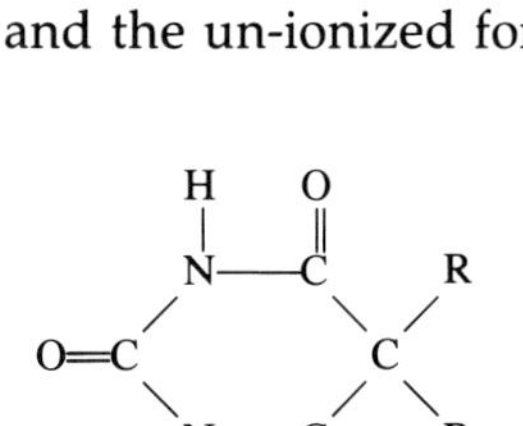

and H^+

and the un-ionized form:

51

Better known are the products of dissociation of carbonic acid:

$$\underset{H_2CO_3}{\text{un-ionized}} \rightleftharpoons \underset{HCO_3^-}{\text{ionized}} \text{ and } H^+$$

As a general rule, the un-ionized form is more lipid-soluble than the ionized form.[1-3] The un-ionized species, therefore, can cross cellular membranes and is more likely to reach across the blood-brain barrier to the brain, and in pregnancy to reach across the placenta to the fetus. While the un-ionized state favors the diffusion across cellular membranes, other factors are also important. There are, for example, differences in lipid-solubility among un-ionized drugs. For example, un-ionized phenobarbital is less lipid-soluble than un-ionized thiopental.

To express or calculate the degree of ionization, the anesthesiologist can use formulas that relate the concentration of hydronium ions to the proportion of the ionized and un-ionized species of any given weak acid or weak base. Instead of H_3O^+ (hydronium ion) we use, for the sake of convenience, the concentration of $[H^+]$ (hydrogen ion).

The $[H^+]$ in water—we are dealing with aqueous systems—is temperature-dependent. Water dissociates into $[H^+]$ and $[OH^-]$. At 25° C, pure water has an equal amount of both ions. The pKa is 7 and at the pH of 7 neutrality exists. As the temperature is raised in aqueous solutions, the equilibrium shifts and the pH falls.[4] In the ensuing discussion we ignore the temperature effect on pKa, since it is small and for the purpose of clinical decisions can be overlooked. Many pKa values reported in the literature refer to measurements at room temperature (usually 25° C). However, since we are not discussing precise physicochemical changes, it is enough to be aware of our imprecision. The following is our shorthand notation for the substances to be discussed:

ionized phenobarbital = PL⁻
un-ionized phenobarbital = PL
ionized meperidine = ME⁺
un-ionized meperidine = ME
hydrogen ion = H⁺
ionized lidocaine = LI⁺
un-ionized lidocaine = LI
ionized amphetamine = AM⁺
un-ionized amphetamine = AM

Since the degree of ionization is dependent on the $[H^+]$ in the aqueous system in which the drugs are dissolved, we utilize Henderson's equation, the simplest formulation that describes this relationship. For phenobarbital it reads:

$$[H^+] = K_a \cdot \frac{PL}{PL^-}$$

This formula states that a doubling of $[H^+]$ leads to a change of the ratio $\frac{PL}{PL^-}$ by a factor of 2. K_a is a constant. The value of K_a can be determined by assuming a 50% ionization at which point $\frac{PL}{PL^-}$ becomes 1. Thus K_a is the hydrogen ion concentration at which 50% of a weak acid is ionized. For phenobarbital, $K_a = 63$, that is, when a liter of aqueous solution has 63 nmol (nanomoles) $[H^+]$, there is as much PL as PL⁻. At that $[H^+]$, half of the present phenobarbital is available in the form that easily penetrates membranes. Reducing $[H^+]$ by half would also reduce $\frac{PL}{PL^-}$ by half.

It is easy to convert this simple relationship into familiar pH values as follows:

pH	4	5	6	7	8	9	10
[H⁺]nmol	100000	10000	1000	100	10	1	.1

In the upper scale we have shown pH units and in the lower scale the hydrogen-ion concentration in nanomoles per liter. As with any logarithmic scale, each full step on the scale (for example, from 6 to 7, or from 9 to 8) results in a tenfold change in the hydrogen ion concentration. A patient with a pH of 7.2 has ten times as many hydrogen ions in his blood as he would at a pH of 8.2.

The hydrogen ion concentration [H$^+$] shown in this example is expressed in nanomoles (1 nmol = 10^{-9} mol). At a physiologic pH of 7.4, we have 40 nanomoles, hence at pH 8.4 we have 4 nanomoles and at 6.4 we would count 400 nanomoles/liter of blood.

Since pH 7.4, is not shown on this scale, we have prepared an enlargement of the scale from pH 6.7 to 8.0.

pH	6.7 6.8 6.9 7.0 7.1 7.2 7.3 7.4 7.5 7.6 7.7 7.8 7.9 8.0
[H$^+$]nmol	200 160 128 100 80 64 50 40 32 25 20 16 12.5 10

This scale shows us that with each 0.3 unit shift in the pH scale (or any such logarithmic scale) we must multiply or divide by a factor of 2 on the scale for the hydrogen ion concentration. Thus if we move from pH 7.40 (40 nanomoles) to 7.1 (80 nanomoles), we shift by 0.3 pH units and increase the hydrogen concentration by a factor of 2.

Or, if we start with 55 nanomoles H$^+$ and increase to 110, the pH must shift by 0.3 units, that is, from pH 7.26 to 6.96. In order to enter data between 7.3 and 7.4 (or between any other units), we need to expand the scale further (see Table 5–1). For example, from a pH 7.3 in Row A, we can either increase pH by 0.3 units to 7.66 (See Row B, below pH 7.36) or decrease pH by 0.3 units to 7.06 (See Row C, below pH 7.36).

From these scales it is possible to approximate other values not shown. Since our ability to make precise pH measurements is limited and since in clinical practice a pH difference between, say, 7.29 and 7.31 rarely matters, we can conclude that without log table, slide rule, or calculator a conversion of H$^+$ into pH and vice versa is easy and sufficiently accurate to be clinically adequate. For intervals other than from 7.0 to 7.1, 7.3 to 7.4, and 7.7 to 7.8, we have to estimate to obtain fair approximations.

For interesting mathematical reasons, many researchers and clinicians in the field prefer to use logarithmic scales and expressions, and they use Hasselbalch's version of Henderson's equation, the so-called Henderson-Hasselbalch equation:

$$pH = pK + \log \frac{\text{ionized weak acid}}{\text{un-ionized weak acid}}$$

Where pH = $-\log[H^+]$
pK$_a$ = $-\log K_a$

We observe that in the Henderson-Hasselbalch equation used for weak acids the relation of ionized to un-ionized now shows as

$$\log \frac{\text{ionized weak acid}}{\text{un-ionized weak acid}}$$

Any increase in hydrogen ion concentration (= decrease in pH) results in an increase in the un-ionized fraction. What is true for the relation of [H$^+$] to pH is also true for the other side of the equation, where $\frac{PL}{PL^-}$ is converted into $\log \frac{PL^-}{PL}$. From this information we can prepare a table by following these steps: (1) by determining what the pK$_a$ of the weak acid is (here phenobarbital) (equal to K$_a$ of 63) = pK$_a$ = 7.2, and (2) by filling in the figures following the numbered steps on the left (Table 5–2).

RELATION OF SHIFT IN pH TO DRUG ABSORPTION

We can now return to our patient and make certain statements. Theoretically the absorption of PL from the acid medium of the stomach should be rapid (provided the drug is sufficiently lipid-soluble) if gastric pH is low.[5,6] At a gastric pH of 7.2, the PL$^-$/PL ratio is 1, at 6.2 it is .1/1, at 5.2 it is .01/1, at 4.2 it is .001/1, and at 3.2 it is .0001/1. At the assumed gastric pH 3.2 the drug is almost completely un-ionized,

Table 5-1

pH Values and the Calculated Values of Hydrogen Ion Concentration (Actual) as well as Suggested Approximations

pH	7.30	7.31	7.32	7.33	7.34	7.35	7.36	7.37	7.38	7.39	7.40	
[H+] nmol	50	49	48	47	46	45	44	43	42	41	40	(approximate)
	(50.12)	(48.98)	(47.86)	(46.77)	(45.71)	(44.67)	(43.65)	(42.66)	(41.68)	(40.7)	(39.8)	(actual)

From here it is easy to increase or decrease pH by 0.3 units:
Increase pH by 0.3 units from respective values in top row

pH	7.60		7.62		7.64		7.66		7.68		7.7	
[H+] nmol	25		24		23		22		21		20	

Decrease pH by 0.3 units from respective values in top row

pH	7.0	7.01	7.02	7.03	7.04	7.05	7.06	7.07	7.08	7.09	7.1	
[H+] nmol	100	98	96	94	92	90	88	86	84	82	80	

Table 5–2
*The Impact of a pH Change on the Ionization of a Drug**

$$pH = pk_a + \log \frac{\text{ionized weak acid}}{\text{un-ionized weak acid}}$$

Step	Instruction	Prepare in Advance	Result
4	up 0.3 pH units doubles PL⁻/PL ratio	8.1 = 7.2 + log	8 PL⁻ / 1 PL
8	up 0.3 pH units doubles PL⁻/PL ratio	8.0 = 7.2 + log	6.4 PL⁻ / 1 PL
12	up 0.3 pH units doubles PL⁻/PL ratio	7.9 = 7.2 + log	5 PL⁻ / 1 PL
3	up 0.3 pH units doubles PL⁻/PL ratio	7.8 = 7.2 + log	4 PL⁻ / 1 PL
7	up 0.3 pH units doubles PL⁻/PL ratio	7.7 = 7.2 + log	3.2 PL⁻ / 1 PL
11	up 0.3 pH units doubles PL⁻/PL ratio	7.6 = 7.2 + log	2.5 PL⁻ / 1 PL
2	up 0.3 pH units doubles PL⁻/PL ratio	7.5 = 7.2 + log	2 PL⁻ / 1 PL
6	up 0.3 pH units doubles PL⁻/PL ratio	7.4 = 7.2 + log	1.6 PL⁻ / 1 PL
10	up 0.3 pH units doubles PL⁻/PL ratio	7.3 = 7.2 + log	1.25 PL⁻ / 1 PL
1	Start with pK of substance. Ratio PL⁻/PL = 1	7.2 = 7.2 + log	1 PL⁻ / 1 PL
5	Down 1 pH unit 1/10 of PL⁻/PL ratio	7.1 = 7.2 + log	.8 PL⁻ / 1 PL
9	Down 1 pH unit 1/10 of PL⁻/PL ratio	7.0 = 7.2 + log	.64 PL⁻ / 1 PL

*To estimate the impact of a pH change on the ionization of a drug, follow the steps outlined. First prepare the list of pH and pK_a values. Then go to Step 1, i.e. the pK_a of the drug in question (phenobarbital) and write in the ratio of ionized to un-ionized, which at this point is $\frac{1}{1}$. Then follow the steps numbered on the left.

which facilitates absorption of weak acids, such as PL. If PL is absorbed, gastric lavage may not yield much PL.

The rules for dissociation of weak bases are essentially the same, except that in Henderson-Hasselbalch's equation the position of ionized to un-ionized is reversed.

$$pH = pK_a + \log \frac{\text{un-ionized weak base}}{\text{ionized weak base}}$$

Since ME has a pK_a of 8.5 and AM 9.8, we can estimate that in an acid pH of the stomach practically all ME and AM are in ionized form. Little may be absorbed and gastric lavage may yield more of these bases than of phenobarbital if both are taken in equal amounts at the same time. Of course, gastric activity may propel the drugs into a more alkaline small intestine where the pH is closer to the pK_a values of these drugs, and absorption may progress more rapidly.

There is evidence that the un-ionized part of the barbiturates is pharmacologically active, with respect to both its CNS and its cardiac effects.[7,8] Now we can say that an elevation of pH is beneficial because it reduces PL while it increases PL⁻. Theoretically, the patient's ratio at pH 7.0 should be about .64 PL⁻/1PL, that is, about 39% ionized. By raising pH to 7.4 the ratio should rise to 1.6 PL⁻/1PL or about 62% ionized. That rise should produce a noticeable lessening of the barbiturate-induced depression.

How is this pH shift accomplished? If we bring it about by hyperventilation alone, a rough estimate suggests that we have to double ventilation in order to reduce P_{CO_2} by a factor of 2, which in turn increases pH by about 0.3 units. This makes a few untrue suppositions, for example, it presupposes that HCO_3^- does not change when P_{CO_2} is altered. However, for a quick estimate our system works in this case as well (Table 5–3) and offers useful clinical approximations. H_2CO_3 is obtained by converting P_{CO_2} mm Hg into mEq/L by multiplying it by .03. Thus 60 mm Hg P_{CO_2} converts into 1.8 mEq/L H_2CO_3. At pH 7.0 the bicarbonate must be 14.4 mEq/L. Lowering P_{CO_2} to 30 mm Hg without changing the HCO_3^- (unlikely in real life) brings the pH to 7.3.

The advantage of correcting the acidosis with hyperventilation is that the intracellular pH experiences about the same shift in pH, since CO_2 readily diffuses across cell membranes.

The toxicity of some local anesthetics can also be reduced in this way[9,10] even though these drugs are weak bases. Their active form appears to be, perhaps exclusively, the ionized form.[11] Elevating intracellular pH therefore would cause these anesthetics to become less ionized and hence less toxic.

DRUG DISTRIBUTION IN RELATION TO SHIFT IN pH

There is a disadvantage in relying on P_{CO_2} alone for the pH shift. A simple three-compartment model of our patient's heart, blood, and urine illustrates the point (Fig. 5–1). The model assumes that the intracellular pH of the myocardium is 0.1 pH unit lower than that of the blood. That of the urine is even lower. Using the prepared format we can fill in the spaces. We need to assume a definite quantity of phenobarbital in the blood (ignoring protein binding).

The figure shows that the most alkaline compartment has the greatest amount of phenobarbital. The reason is that it has the greatest concentration of ionized weak acid. The un-ionized fraction can equilibrate across the membranes and is therefore the same in all compartments. For a weak base the situation is inverse. The most acidic compartment has the highest concentration of the ionized weak base and therefore has the greatest concentration of the drug (for example, meperidine and amphetamine here concentrate in the urine compartment). To look at it in another way, un-ionized material passively distributes itself, seeking an equilibrium. The pH in the

Table 5-3
The Effect of the Ratio of Bicarbonate (HCO_3^-) to P_{CO_2} ($P_{CO_2} \times 0.03$) on pH

$$pH = pK_a + \log \frac{\text{ionized weak acid}}{\text{un-ionized weak acid}}$$

3	up 0.3 pH units doubles HCO_3^-/H_2CO_3 ratio	$7.4 = 6.1 + \log$	$\frac{20\ HCO_3^-}{1\ H_2CO_3}$
		7.3 7.2	
2	up by 1 pH unit tenfold increase in HCO_3^-/H_2CO_3 ratio	$7.1 = 6.1 + \log$	$\frac{10\ HCO_3^-}{1\ H_2CO_3}$
6	up by 0.3 pH units doubles HCO_3^-/H_2CO_3	$7.0 = 6.1 + \log$	$\frac{8\ HCO_3^-}{1\ H_2CO_3}$
5	up by 0.3 pH units doubles HCO_3^-/H_2CO_3 ratio	$6.7 = 6.1 + \log$	$\frac{4\ HCO_3^-}{1\ H_2CO_3}$
4	down 1 pH unit 1/10 of HCO_3^-/H_2CO_3	$6.4 \times 6.1 + \log$	$\frac{2\ HCO_3^-}{1\ H_2CO_3}$
1	enter pH at pK of carbonic acid	$6.1 = 6.1 + \log$	$\frac{1\ HCO_3^-}{1\ H_2CO_3}$

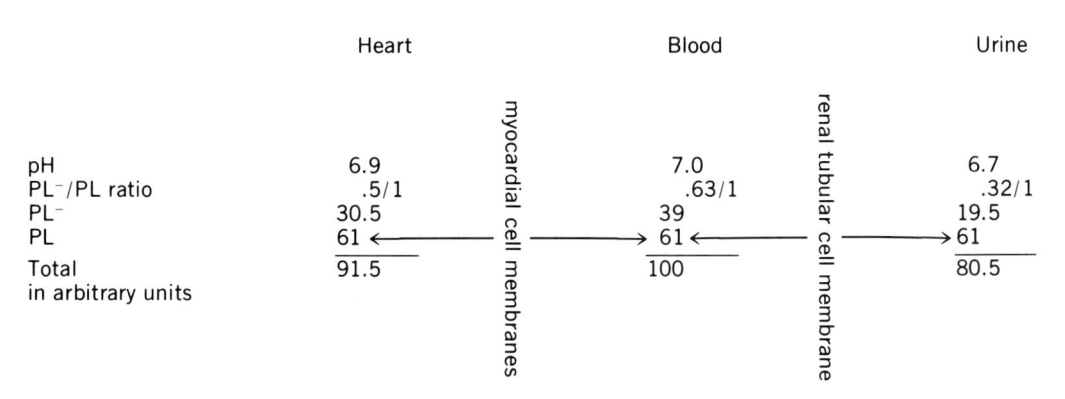

	Heart		Blood		Urine
pH	6.9		7.0		6.7
PL^-/PL ratio	.5/1	myocardial cell membranes	.63/1	renal tubular cell membrane	.32/1
PL^-	30.5		39		19.5
PL	61 ←	→	61 ←	→	61
Total in arbitrary units	91.5		100		80.5

Fig. 5–1. A simplified model showing a "heart," a "blood," and a "urine" compartment. The un-ionized species of phenobarbital (PL) equilibrates across the membranes separating the compartments. The ionized species does not cross.

different compartments then establishes how much total drug the compartment holds by forcing a certain amount (satisfying the Henderson-Hasselbalch equation) into the ionized form. Whatever is taken away from the un-ionized species in this process reestablishes a gradient, and more un-ionized drug flows into the compartment until equilibrium is established, as shown in Figure 5–1.

Now we decrease Pco_2 so that the pH in all compartments rises by 0.3 units (Fig. 5–2).

The total phenobarbital in these three compartments now is 88 + 100 + 72 = 260. At the lower pH it was 91.5 + 100 + 80.5 = 272. Therefore, we have reduced the cardiac PL total.

We repeat the treatment, but this time with $NaHCO_3$ (Fig. 5–3). It is ionized to a great degree and therefore does not penetrate rapidly intracellularly. Nonetheless, it is subject to glomerular filtration, and urine pH rises. The assumption is that we injected enough $NaHCO_3$ intravenously to obtain the result shown in Figure 5–3 without changing Pco_2.

THE EFFECT OF SHIFT IN pH ON RENAL EXCRETION

Total phenobarbital is again 272, but in this case urine concentration is high. If we alkalinize the urine further, more of the drug is trapped in the urine and carried away.[12,13] Alkalinization of urine and active diuresis are therefore important therapeutic goals.[14] The heart has less phenobarbital than in the example where Pco_2 was lowered, even though the PL, the most active form pharmacologically, is the same in both instances. We argue, then, that adequate ventilation with normalization of Pco_2 is desirable but that alkalinization should be accomplished with $NaHCO_3$.

We have omitted several features in order to simplify the presentation of the principles involved. For one, the pK_a of weak acids and bases needs to be close to physiologic pH values in order to realize clinically noticeable effects when pH is changed. For instance, a measurable effect of pH on the CNS (central nervous system) toxicity of local anesthetics was described by Englesson and Grevsten for a series of local anesthetics,[9,10] among them:

	pK_a
lidocaine	7.9
prilocaine	7.9
procaine	9.1
mepivacaine	7.7
bupivacaine	8.1

All of these have pK values not far removed from 7.4. For a drug such as benzocaine (pK_a = 2.8) a pH effect would

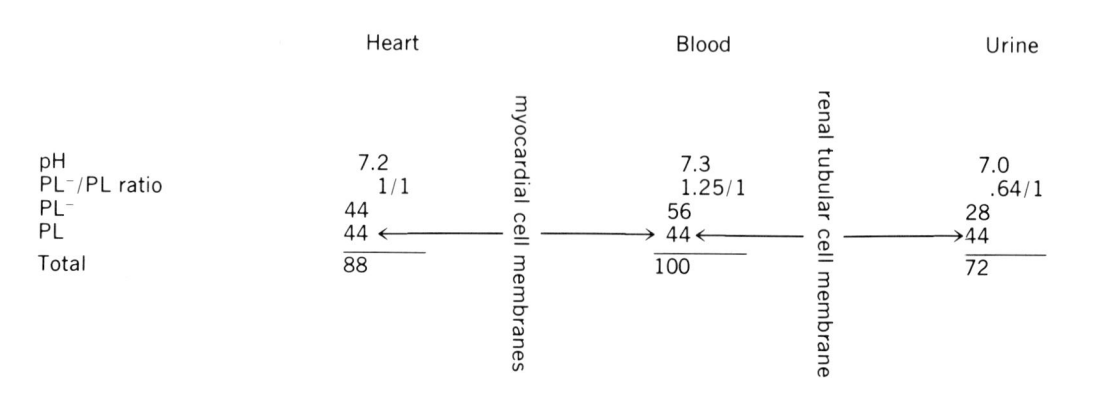

	Heart		Blood		Urine
pH	7.2		7.3		7.0
PL^-/PL ratio	1/1		1.25/1		.64/1
PL^-	44		56		28
PL	44 ←	myocardial cell membranes	→ 44 ←	renal tubular cell membrane	→44
Total	88		100		72

Fig. 5–2. As in Fig. 5–1, but after decreasing Pco_2.

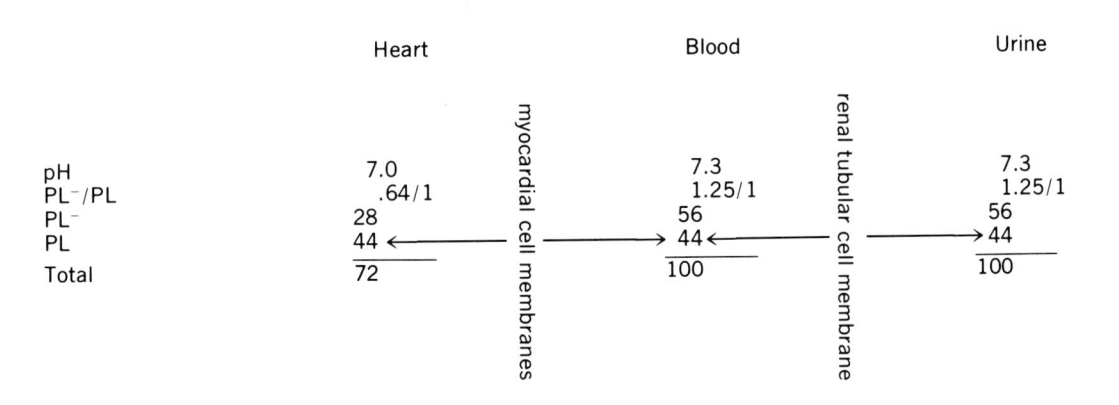

	Heart		Blood		Urine
pH	7.0		7.3		7.3
PL⁻/PL	.64/1		1.25/1		1.25/1
PL⁻	28		56		56
PL	44 ←	myocardial cell membranes	→ 44 ←	renal tubular cell membrane	→ 44
Total	72		100		100

Fig. 5–3. As in Fig. 5–1 after treatment with bicarbonate.

probably not become noticeable because benzocaine is almost completely un-ionized whether the pH is 6.8 (un-ionized to ionized $\frac{10000}{1}$) or 7.8 $\left(\frac{100000}{1}\right)$.

Benson and co-workers tested the pH effect *in vitro* in a series of opiates and their antagonists.[15] These drugs—all weak bases—have pK_a values between 7.59 (nalorphine) and 9.38 (cyclazocine). In all instances the drugs became more soluble as pH was increased (more un-ionized), and this has clinical implications. However, the progression of changes in the distribution coefficient was not as predictable as we have presented it, possibly because of differences in lipid-solubility (independent of ionization). For meperidine, pK_a 8.5, however, the distribution coefficient rose from 20.2 at pH 7.1 to 38.2 when the pH was raised to 7.4, that is, almost by the predicted factor of 2 with a 0.3 unit pH shift.

The importance of blood pH on the distribution of morphine, a weak base, was vividly demonstrated *in vivo* by Shulman, et al.[16] These investigators showed in rats that during alkalemia (pH 7.62), uptake of morphine sulfate by the brain was 2 to 3 fold greater than during acidemia (pH 7.16).

The protein binding of drugs may be affected by pH, but these effects are usually small in the physiologic pH range. For example, some barbiturates and muscle relaxants become more protein bound as pH rises within physiologic limits.[3,17,18] We are not aware, however, of any observation where this mild effect was shown to be clinically noticeable.

Amphetamine, as well as related ephedrines, are weak bases. Their excretion rate can be influenced by urine pH, as expected for drugs of that category.[18] Similar relationships have been demonstrated for local anesthetics and procainamide.[20,21]

Of therapeutic interest are the observations by Järnberg and his co-workers.[22] These investigators were able to show that fluoride could be cleared far more rapidly from the body if the urine was rendered alkaline. This effect was powerful. In patients with acid urine, peak plasma fluoride levels were 26.4 ± 7.9 μM, while in patients with alkaline urine these levels were 13.5 ± 2.4 μM. It is important to observe that the fluoride levels here determined in patients were the result of general anesthesia with enflurane.

Important to the physician in the emergency room is the study by Perez-Reyes and his co-workers who were able to increase the renal excretion of phencyclidine (angels' dust) by vigorous acidification of urine and diuresis.[23] We speculate that the elimination of ketamine may similarly be influenced by acidification of the urine.

RELATION OF SHIFT IN pH TO DRUG METABOLISM

If we alkalinize the blood and urine of our patients and thereby delay the excretion of the drugs that are weak bases, do we thereby increase the metabolism of these drugs?

Metabolism needs to be considered when it produces a pH-induced change in the relative ratio of the ionized and un-ionized fractions of a drug. Metabolism is a slow process, and we think more in terms of enzyme induction and inhibition. Depending on the drug, however, a shift in the pH can significantly influence not only a drug's urinary excretion rate but also its metabolic inactivation if its passage through the body is prolonged. This is due to a close relationship between the lipid-solubility of a drug and its metabolism by the hepatic microsomal enzyme system.[24] As described earlier, the un-ionized fraction is more lipid-soluble and therefore can reach the major drug-metabolizing machinery housed in the endoplasmic reticulum of the liver.

For example, we consider what happens to amphetamine as the pH of plasma and urine is changed. It is well known that the urinary excretion of amphetamine and other weak organic bases can be increased significantly in man under conditions that lead to the production of an acid urine.[25-28] Decreasing the pH of urine from 7 to 5 with only a minor change in plasma pH, for example, decreases the un-ionized fraction of amphetamine in urine one hundredfold and thereby favors a shift of drug from plasma into the flowing urine, even though it is already more than 99.9% ionized at pH 7.0. This is referred to as the ion-trapping mechanism and is effective in removing such drugs from the body. Thus, under conditions leading to an acid urine, Beckett et al. found that approximately 60% of ingested amphetamine is excreted within the first 16 to 48 hours, whereas in an alkaline urine only about 5% is excreted during the same interval.[25,26] The metabolic consequences of such pH-induced changes in the rate of excretion of amphetamine were recently studied by Davis et al. in four subjects either on an acid diet (urine pH 5.5 to 6.0) or after the administration of sodium bicarbonate (urine pH 7.5 to 8.0) (blood pH and gases were not measured).[28] The plasma half-life of amphetamine averaged seven hours in metabolic acidosis and increased almost threefold to 20 hours with the administration of sodium bicarbonate. Since more amphetamine remained in the body under alkaline conditions, one might have expected more opportunity for metabolism. That is what happened. During acid urine production, with an increase in the ionized fraction, less un-ionized amphetamine was available for metabolism, so that most of the administered drug was excreted unchanged, in about four times the amount of the deaminated product. Conversely, during metabolic alkalosis, more un-ionized amphetamine was metabolized and the excretion of the deaminated metabolite approximated that of the unchanged parent compound. Thus the longer amphetamine remains in the body, that is, the higher the urinary pH, the more it is metabolized. In addition, the greater are its pharmacologic effects, since metabolism is slow.[25]

We can speculate on the clinical implications of this relationship. If the effects of weak acidic or basic drugs are mainly terminated by metabolism, a shift in the acid-base status or a depression of renal or liver function by pathologic condition or by anesthesia could make more drug available than could be metabolized. This could result in an increased amount of active drug in the body and possible toxicity. Since enzymes function optimally at a certain pH, to what extent would an altered (pathologic or iatrogenic) acid-base status modify the efficiency with which an enzyme inactivates a drug? How many incidents of drug toxicity attributed to "biologic variation" may be due to an increase in bioavailability because of a change in acid-base status?

Although the number of such incidents is small, the results described above with amphetamine suggest that the relationship of toxicity, drug metabolism, and acid-base status deserves closer attention. A candidate for such pH-mediated differences in metabolism is meperidine with its pK_a of 8.5, close to physiologic values. Since some meperidine is demethylated into a toxic normeperidine in man, a patient with active enzyme systems and delayed meperidine excretion may show unexpected signs of toxicity.[29]

Our patient raises many issues related to the pH effect on drugs, their action, and their disposition. In our example, treatment with bicarbonate and artificial ventilation is in order. It hastens the renal elimination of phenobarbital and helps to reduce its effects on the brain and the heart. At the same time we inhibit, through alkalinization, the elimination of meperidine and amphetamine. Both drugs may become subject to more metabolic biotransformation, a slow process at best. Nevertheless, the undesirable effects of meperidine and amphetamine are more acceptable and are more readily treated than those of the barbiturates.

REFERENCES

1. Goldstein, A., Aronow, L., and Kalman, S.M.: Principles of Drug Action. 2nd Ed. New York, John Wiley & Sons, 1974.
2. Gilman, A.S., Goodman, L.S., and Gilman, A.: Goodman and Gilman's The Pharmacological Basis of Therapeutics. 6th Ed. New York, Macmillan, 1980.
3. Eger, E.I., II: Anesthetic Uptake and Action. Baltimore, Williams & Wilkins, 1974.
4. Hills, A.G.: Acid Base Balance, Chemistry, Physiology, Pathophysiology. Baltimore, Williams & Wilkins, 1973.
5. Schanker, L.S.: On the mechanism of absorption of drugs from the gastrointestinal tract (a review). J. Med. Pharm. Chem., 2:343, 1960.
6. Hogben, C.A.M., et al.: Absorption of drugs from the stomach. II. The human. J. Pharmacol. Exp. Ther., 120:540, 1957.
7. Waddell, W.J., and Butler, T.C.: The distribution and excretion of phenobarbital. J. Clin. Invest., 36:1217, 1957.
8. Hardman, H.F., Moore, J.I., and Lum, B.K.B.: A method for analyzing the effect of pH and the ionization of drugs upon cardiac tissue with special reference to pentobarbital. J. Pharmacol. Exp. Ther., 126:136, 1959.
9. Englesson, S.: The influence of acid-base changes on central nervous system toxicity of local anaesthetic agents. I. Acta Anaesthesiol. Scand., 18:79, 1974.
10. Engelsson, S., and Grevsten, S.: The influence of acid-base changes on central nervous system toxicity of local anesthetic agents. II. Acta Anaesthesiol. Scand., 18:88, 1974.
11. Ritchie, J.M., and Greengard, P.: On the active structure of local anesthetics. J. Pharmacol. Exp. Ther., 133:241, 1961.
12. Milne, M.D., Scribner, B.H., and Crawford, M.A.: Non-ionic diffusion and the excretion of weak acids and bases. Am. J. Med., 24:709, 1958.
13. Weiner, I.M., and Mudge, G.H.: Renal tubular mechanisms for excretion of organic acids and bases. Am. J. Med., 36:743, 1964.
14. Lassen, N.A.: Treatment of severe acute barbiturate poisoning by forced diuresis and alkalinisation of the urine. Lancet, 2:338, 1960.
15. Benson, D.W., Kaufman, J.J., and Koski, W.S.: Theoretic significance of pH dependence of narcotics and narcotic antagonists in clincial anesthesia. Anesth. Analg. (Cleve.), 55:253, 1976.
16. Shulman, D.S., and Kaufman, J.J.: Eisenstein MM and Rapoport SI: Blood pH and brain uptake of ^{14}C-morphine. Anesthesiology, 61:540, 1984.
17. Cohen, E.N., Corbascio, A., and Fleischli, G.: The distribution and fate of d-tubocurarine. J. Pharmacol. Exp. Ther., 147:120, 1965.
18. Hughes, R.: The influence of changes in acid-base balance on neuromuscular blockade in cats. Br. J. Anaesth., 42:658, 1970.
19. Wilkinson, G.R., and Beckett, A.H.: Absorption, metabolism and excretion of the ephedrines in man. I. The influence of urinary pH and urine volume output. J. Pharmacol. Exp. Ther., 162:139, 1968.
20. Eriksson, E., and Granberg, P.O.: Studies on the renal excretion of Citanest[R] and Xylocaine.[R] Acta Anaesthesiol. Scand. [Suppl.], XVI:79, 1965.
21. Weily, H.S., and Genton, E.: Pharmacokinetics of procainamide. Arch. Intern. Med., 130:366, 1972.
22. Järnberg, P.O., Ekstrand J., and Irestedt, L.: Renal fluoride levels during and after enflurane anesthesia are dependent on urinary pH. Anesthesiology, 54:48, 1981.
23. Perez-Reyes, M., Di Guiseppe, S., Brine, D.R., et al.: Urine pH and phencyclidine excretion. Clin. Pharmacol. Ther., 32:5, 635, 1982.
24. Conney, A.H.: Pharmacological implications of microsomal enzyme induction. Pharmacol. Rev., 19:317, 1967.
25. Beckett, A.H., Rowland, M., and Turner, P.: In-

fluence of urinary pH on excretion of amphetamine. Lancet, 1:303, 1965.
26. Beckett, A.H., and Rowland, M.: Urinary excretion kinetics of amphetamine in man. J. Pharm. Pharmacol., 17:628, 1965.
27. Astatoor, A.M., et al.: The excretion of dextroamphetamine and its derivatives. Br. J. Pharmacol., 24:293, 1965.
28. Davis, J.M., et al.: Effects of urinary pH on amphetamine metabolism. Ann. N.Y. Acad. Sci., 179:493, 1971.
29. Stambaugh, J.E., et al.: A potentially toxic drug interaction between pethidine (meperidine) and phenobarbitone. Lancet, 1:398, 1977.

| 6 |

THE ROLE OF THE LIVER

BURNELL R. BROWN, JR. and GEORGE E. McLAIN, JR.

Within the last two decades, clinical pharmacology has been complicated by the realization that the pharmacodynamics of one drug can rarely be considered independent from that of other drugs. In practice, the surgical patient frequently receives several drugs, each given for a particular therapeutic purpose. When these drugs are combined, the possibilities of interaction become astronomic. The science of drug interactions is new, and our meager knowledge is outstripped by the pragmatics of vogues of current therapy. It is the purpose of this chapter to review briefly some of the typical drug interactions mediated specifically by the liver.

DRUG BIOTRANSFORMATION IN THE LIVER

The liver is the largest organ of the body and has manifold functions. It is unique because the hepatocyte, its major cell type, is histologically consistent but is functionally inconsistent, i.e., capable of undergoing a variety of biochemical reactions. From a strictly pharmacologic point of view, one of the major tasks of the liver is the biotransformation of drugs. Within the framework of this goal, numerous drug interactions may occur.

Although the lung and the kidney actively participate in the biotransformation of xenobiotics, the bulk and degree of activity of the liver dictate that it be considered the primary organ involved in this function. The reason for biotransformation is simple. Many drugs, particularly CNS (central nervous system)-active ones administered during the course of anesthesia, are lipophilic, because of their intrinsic physicochemical structure. Penetration of the blood-brain barrier by a drug is controlled by its affinity for lipids. Thus inhalation anesthetics, barbiturates, tranquilizers, sedatives, and analgesics must be able to penetrate into the brain to produce the desired pharmacologic result. Except for inhalation anesthetics, which are eliminated primarily through the lungs, excretion of drugs is entirely by the renal route. The tubular epithelium of the nephron is essentially a complex lipid layer. Thus centrally active drugs are secreted by the glomeruli of the nephron unit but rapidly reenter the systemic circulation because they are taken up by the tubular epithelium. It has been estimated that the half-life of an extremely lipophilic "fixed" (nonvolatile) drug, such as thiopental, would be approximately 20 years if no biotransformation occurred. The essence of drug biotransformation is the conversion of a lipid-soluble compound into one of increased polarity, or water solubility, so that it may be easily eliminated by the kidneys.

Electron microscopy of the hepatocyte reveals loose sheets of contiguous membranes and channels within the cytoplasm, termed the endoplasmic reticulum.[3] The endoplasmic reticulum is rich in lipids, particularly unsaturated ones such as arachidonic acid, coupled as esters to phosphatidylcholine and phosphatidylethanolamine. Such a biochemical structure mandates that lipid-soluble drugs will be found in high concentrations in the endoplasmic reticulum once entry into the hepatocyte occurs. Most of the enzymes of biotransformation are located within this organelle.[1] If the endoplasmic reticulum is extracted from the hepatocyte by cell disruption and ultracentrifugation, the endoplasmic reticulum can be isolated for *in vivo* studies. This process, however, converts the endoplasmic reticulum from contiguous sheets into membrane fragments that coalesce into spheres, the so-called microsomes. Thus the enzymes of biotransformation may appropriately be termed microsomal enzymes, although microsomes are artifacts, which do not exist *in vivo*.

There are four chemical reactions by which lipophilic drugs are converted into water-soluble, or polar ones: (1) *Oxidation*, (2) *Conjugation*, (3) *Hydrolysis*, and (4) *Reduction*. The most commonly employed processes are oxidation and conjugation. Hydrolysis is uncommon and is dependent on the drug substrate's possession of an ester group. Reduction is a rare form of biotransformation. In an attempt to increase polarity, a drug may undergo several sequential reactions, such as oxidation followed by conjugation. A classic example of this is found in the biotransformation of pentobarbital. Initially, aliphatic hydroxylation occurs. This is followed by conjugation with glucuronic acid, a highly polar congener of glucose. In addition to facilitating excretion, biotransformation usually results in the termination of pharmacologic activity of the drug. This is not universally the case, however. Drug metabolites may be as active as, and sometimes more active than, the parent compound.

Strictly speaking, oxidation is defined not only as the addition of molecular oxygen, but also as the removal of an electron, or relative diminution of electronegativity. A variety of reactions occurs under the general heading of oxidation, such as (1) *Hydroxylation (OH group addition)*, (2) *Dealkylation (CH_3 and C_2H_5 group removal)*, (3) *N-oxidation (N to N–O) O-dealkylation (C_2H_5O to OH)*, and (5) *Dehalogenation*. Oxidative biotransformation is accomplished in the endoplasmic reticulum of the hepatocyte by a series of enzymes termed *mixed-function oxygenases*. This enzymatic system is particularly adapted to metabolism of foreign drugs, pollutants, and carcinogens (collectively, xenobiotics). A few naturally occurring endogenous compounds are metabolized by the system (for example, steroids) but in general it acts only on xenobiotics.[2]

The prominent features of the drug-metabolizing enzymes are: (1) *Lack of substrate specificity*, (2) *Low turnover number* and (3) *Ability to be induced*. A unique property, which differentiates this system from other enzymatic reactions of the body, is the low order of substrate specificity. This means that the same series of enzymes can biotransform many structurally unrelated compounds. Drugs of different structures, such as general inhalation anesthetics, acetaminophen, meperidine, barbiturates, benzodiazepines, and phenothiazines, are biotransformed by a single group of enzymes. The disadvantage of this apparently simple arrangement is that the reactions proceed slowly, defined biochemically as a low-turnover number. Thus the metabolic half-time of drugs is measured in terms of hours rather than milliseconds as is common in many enzymatic reactions such as the acetylcholine-acetylcholinesterase system.

In order to compensate for the low-turnover number, the microsomal enzymes have the capacity to increase drug metabolic rates by the process of induction.[4-6] This sometimes misunderstood concept is really straightforward and teleologically appealing: when the enzymes are chronically stimulated by certain drugs or environmental pollutants, the content and hence the activity of the enzymes increase. There are at least 300 drugs and chemicals known to produce microsomal enzyme induction. Chronology is important in assessing induction status. The inducing agents work both by increasing the synthesis of new enzymatic protein and by decreasing catabolic rates; thus, the content of enzyme increases. This phenomenon takes time. A good example of a clinically employed drug that induces biotransformation enzymes is phenobarbital. A single dose of the barbiturate produces clinically insignificant induction and maximal induction does not occur until the drug has been administered for four to five days. When the drug is discontinued, microsomal enzyme levels fall to normal in approximately 48 to 72 hours. Since the microsomal enzyme systems are not substrate-specific, induction of them by one drug usually results in an increased rate of biotransformation of many other drugs. Induction would seem to be nature's defense mechanism to prevent pharmacologic overdosage when the body is assailed chronically by foreign substances.

At least two changes are seen following drug induction: (1) decreased pharmacologic activity and half-life of other drugs; and (2) increased enzyme and protein content of the endoplasmic reticulum of the hepatocytes, as seen by electron microscopy.[7]

Figure 6-1 illustrates the enzymes of oxidative biotransformation.[8] Cytochrome P-450 is the terminal enzyme of the system. The overall reaction involves a combination of drug and molecular oxygen with cytochrome P-450. Reducing equivalents (electrons) derived from reduced nicotinamide-adenine dinucleotide (NADPH) are transferred to this enzyme-O_2-substrate complex by means of the enzyme NADPH cytochrome C reductase. After activation of diatomic, molecular oxygen to the monatomic species, one oxygen atom is reduced to water, the other incorporated into the drug.

A concept that must be discussed is the description of induction and its effects on the enzymes of biotransformation as an entirely quantitative phenomenon. This is not true—qualitative changes also occur. Cytochrome P-450 is not a single entity but a mixture of enzymes, many of which have not yet been identified. Thus an inducing drug may stimulate one subset of cytochrome P-450 enzymes and not another. For example, phenobarbital treatment of animals not only increases the rate and amount of biotransformation of methoxyflurane, but also qualitatively stimulates metabolism toward the pathway of free fluoride production. Qualitative differences explain why some inducing drugs are more selective than others, and why some inducers such as 3-methylcholanthrene stimulate such a narrow spectrum of biotransformation of other drugs. A corollary of this fact has to do with the genetics of drug biotransformation, since there are variations in the rates and quality of biotransformation in different individuals.[9] Perhaps this is explained by genetic differences in the quality and quantity of the isoenzymes contained in cytochrome P-450.

HEPATIC DRUG INTERACTIONS

Several mechanisms of drug interactions occurring in the liver can be explained by alterations in the drug-metabolizing enzyme sequence.

Inhalation Anesthetics

Any inhibition of one drug biotransformation by another may result in prolon-

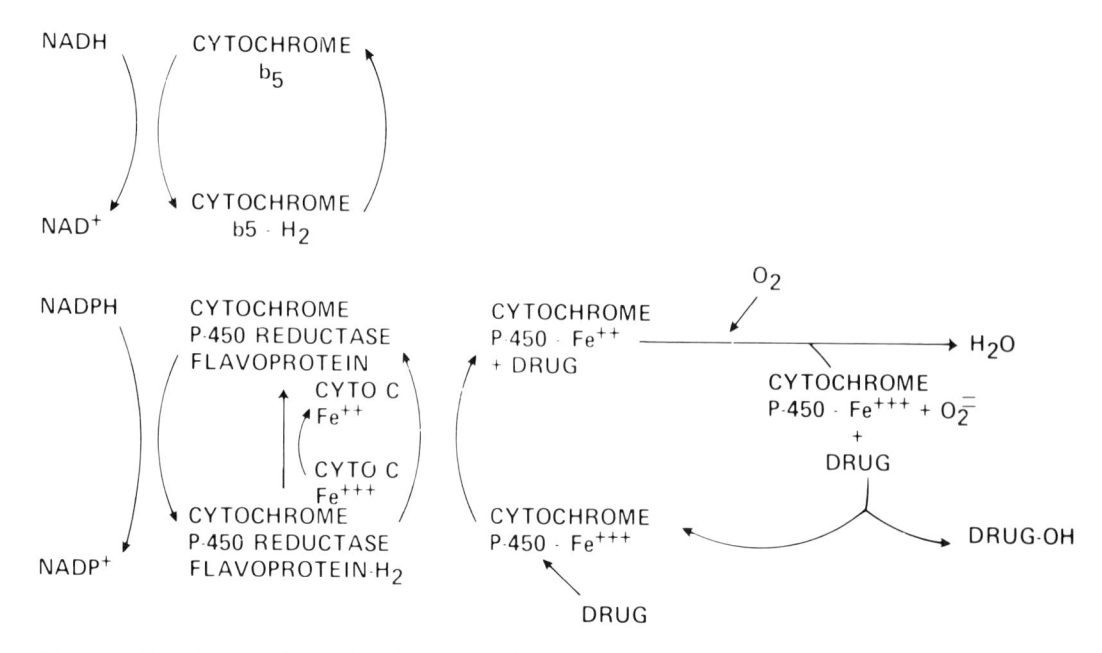

Fig. 6–1. The microsomal oxidation electron transfer system.

gation of the half-life and the potentiation of one or both of the drugs. The inhalation anesthetics in common use (for example, halothane) are lipophilic substances. The cytochrome P-450 system is imbedded in the matrix of the endoplasmic reticulum, which is a lipid-rich area. Following an accumulation of inhalation anesthetics, there is inhibition of biotransformation of the barbiturate.[10,11] This inhibition is noncompetitive, leading to the speculation that the effect is allosteric. Glucuronide conjugation reactions are also inhibited by anesthetics, but not to the same degree as oxidative drug metabolism.[12] If drugs with a short metabolic half-life, such as pentazocine, lidocaine, and hexobarbital, are injected into animals equilibrated with anesthetic concentrations of halothane, the half-life is prolonged. However, this is not entirely due to enzymatic inhibition. Most inhalation anesthetics decrease splanchnic blood flow, so that the distribution of fixed drugs to the liver is impaired. The prolonged half-life is thus a resultant both of reduced enzymatic biotransformation and of decreased hepatic bioavailability. This is seen in man with the combination of halothane and pentobarbital. The net clinical effect is a prolongation and intensification of the pharmacologic action of fixed drugs given during the course of inhalation anesthesia. The general implications have not been studied in great detail in man.

Combinations of Fixed Agents

Because of the nature of cytochrome P-450, with its intrinsic low substrate specificity, any particular drug is liable to inhibit the biotransformation of another, and thus increase its potency. This has been repeatedly demonstrated *in vitro* with many fixed drugs, including barbiturates, narcotics, and tranquilizers.[13] There are reasons to believe that fixed drugs act competitively to inhibit metabolism, but the exact enzyme kinetics in a complex system such as this are unknown. Also unknown is the precise clinical relevance of this type of interaction. The terms used by clinicians to describe this mechanism are "potentiation," "synergism," and "addition" (see Chap. 1).

Induction

A partial list of drugs capable of inducing liver microsomal enzymes is *(1) Barbiturates, (2) Glutethimide, (3) Phenylbutazone, (4) Chloral hydrate, (5) Meprobamate, (6) Chlordiazepoxide, (7) Phenytoin (Diphenylhydantoin), (8) Cortisone, (9) Ethanol, (10) Diphenylhydramine, (11) Polychlorobiphenyls, (12) DDT, Lindane, (13) Cigarette smoke, and (14) Cannabis.* It must be remembered that all inducing substances do not produce identical increases in cytochrome P-450, because of the variability and multiplicity of the isoenzymes of that system. For example, ethanol is not only quantitatively a weaker inducing drug than phenobarbital, but qualitatively it induces a narrower spectrum of enhanced biotransformation of other drugs. In clinical practice, a careful history is perhaps the best way to determine whether drug induction is present, but this is not absolute since genetic factors may either inhibit or enhance induction.

The classic drug interaction in the induced patient results in decreased effectiveness of a drug given simultaneously with the inducer. In the clinical situation, this would be defined as tolerance. A typical example is the barbiturate user, who requires increasing amounts of the drug to achieve a euphoric state. Repeated ingestion of the barbiturate leads within days to enzyme induction, consequent increased biotransformation rate, and shortened half-life with anesthetics; tolerance to preoperative medications may be noted, as well as an increased requirement for intravenous barbiturates and sedatives. Narcotics are not considered inducing drugs, and tolerance to these addictive drugs is not predicated on this mechanism, although on the other hand, the inducing drugs can enhance biotransformation of certain narcotics.

Occasionally abrupt reduction of the induced state can lead to problems, as illustrated by the following example.[14] Patients suffering from myocardial infarction may simultaneously receive sodium warfarin as an anticoagulant and a sedative, such as phenobarbital. The phenobarbital acts as a potent enzyme-inducer, stimulating the rapid biotransformation of sodium warfarin. Thus while on this regimen, the patient requires a larger dose of sodium warfarin than normal to maintain desired prothrombin levels. When the inducing drug, phenobarbital, is discontinued, microsomal enzyme levels fall abruptly. Now the same dose of sodium warfarin becomes an overdose since biotransformation has returned to a normal rate. Prothrombin time is prolonged and bleeding occurs with a possible fatal outcome (see Chap. 20).

Abnormal Shunting of Biotransformation

This category of hepatic drug interaction is rare. A clinical example is observed when a monoamine oxidase (MAO) inhibitor and meperidine are combined. There have been numerous case reports to the effect that when patients on chronic MAO-inhibitor therapy receive conventional amounts of parenteral meperidine (50 to 100 mg), a sudden reaction consisting of hypertension, convulsions, and hyperthermia is frequenty produced. Although the mechanism is not established, it has been hypothesized that MAO inhibitors block the normal route of meperidine biotransformation to meperidinic acid, and that this causes meperidine to form normeperidine, a convulsant.[15]

VISCEROTOXICITY AND ANESTHETIC DRUG INTERACTIONS

An unusual drug reaction encountered in clinical anesthesia is postanesthetic hepatic necrosis. Whether this represents a true drug interaction in humans is speculative, although there are abundant animal data to support the hypothesis. Halothane is used as an example in the following discussion, since more work has been done with it in this regard than with any other anesthetic.

It is now recognized that enzyme-inducing drugs cause increased rates and amounts of biotransformation of volatile inhaled anesthetics.[16] Obviously, volatile anesthetics differ from fixed drugs in that the former are primarily eliminated by the lungs, whereas the latter require biotransformation to decrease activity and to facilitate renal elimination. In general, biotransformation, whether induced or not, is helpful, since it shortens a prolonged pharmacologic action and provides a defensive compensatory mechanism against chronic drug accumulation. In halogenated volatile anesthetics, this may not always be so, as in the case of methoxyflurane. It is established that the biotransformation of methoxyflurane leads to the formation of a free fluoride ion, which can damage the renal tubule, and produce renal impairment of the high-output failure type.[17] Less well known is that inducing drugs enhance biotransformation both qualitatively and quantitatively. Thus extrapolating from animal data, the use of this anesthetic in a patient with a drug history conducive to the induced state may be hazardous regardless of dose.

It is not certain whether hepatotoxicity is a consequence of drug interaction. Animals pretreated with phenobarbital are more susceptible to carbon tetrachloride and chloroform hepatotoxicity than untreated ones.[18] Free radicals and reactive intermediates produced in quantity from these halogenated alkanes by the induced enzymes attack liver macromolecules, resulting in centrolobular necrosis. Ordinarily, the oxidative biotransformation of halothane is benign. The products formed are trifluoroacetic acid and bromide and chloride ions, all innocuous.[19] However, metabolites of great potential reactivity have been observed in the urine and exhaled air of both persons and animals following a conventional exposure to halothane.[20,21] There is strong experimental evidence to indict an abnormal, reductive pathway of halothane that may produce reactive intermediates leading to hepatic necrosis. Two animal models of "halothane hepatotoxicity" have been produced.[22-24] In the first, a single dose of a mixture of polychlorobiphenyls is given to the animals. These compounds greatly induce both oxygen- and nonoxygen-dependent subunits of cytochrome P-450. When these animals are subsequently anesthetized with 1% halothane in 99% oxygen, typical centrolobular necrosis occurs. The second model involves pretreatment with phenobarbital followed by anesthesia with 1% halothane in a hypoxic environment ($F_IO_2 = 0.14$). Again, centrolobular necrosis results. Another factor contributing to the nonoxygen-dependent or "reductive" biotransformation of halothane is the known propensity of the anesthetic to decrease liver blood flow by direct action on splanchnic vessels, primarily by the constriction of the hepatic artery.

Although unproven, "halothane hepatitis" could be envisioned as a possible drug interaction. In the following hypothetical example, an obese 40-year-old woman is scheduled for an elective hysterectomy. Halothane is used satisfactorily as the primary anesthetic. However, within a few days, the patient develops symptoms of a vaginal cuff abscess. The gynecologist gives antibiotics as therapy. Because of apprehension on the patient's part, he also prescribes sedatives and hypnotics—enzyme inducing drugs—for several days. We shall assume that this patient initially possessed a genetically determined small quantity of a cytochrome P-450 isoenzyme variant that biotransforms halothane through reductive pathways to reactive products.[25] However, the amount of this particular enzyme and hence the amount of reactive metabolites produced are small during the first exposure to halothane. Therefore, no overt liver damage is noted. Owing to the failure of antibiotic therapy for the abscess, the patient requires a second operation. At this time, however, the inducing drugs have changed her pharmacologic environment. The enzyme responsible for biotransformation of halothane to reactive metabolites was of low concentration and a low order of activity initially. Now it has been activated and increased by the inducing drugs. A short reexposure to halothane for drainage of the abscess may lead to the production of reactive metabolites in sufficient quantity to initiate an autocatalytic destruction of liver macromolecules, leading to centrolobular necrosis and jaundice. We repeat, the existence of this drug interaction has not been proven in man, but animal data support this possibility. Such speculation does not imply that a patient with a history of ingestion of a known inducing drug should not receive halothane. Induction of the metabolism of halothane through normal metabolic pathways is apparently harmless. The difference is that this theoretic patient initially had a genetically abnormal cytochrome P-450 variant that could be induced. It must be reiterated that induction of normal cytochrome P-450 does not ordinarily lead to such a catastrophic event.

Another area of current research is the role of immune mechanisms in supporting what may be an initial biotransformation reaction. Antibodies to halothane metabolites—haptenes—coupled with hepatic proteins can be found in plasma of individuals who have suffered from putative halothane hepatitis.[26,27] From data such as these, one might speculate that there may be initiation of hepatic injury from the aforementioned metabolic considerations. In certain persons, however, perpetuation and increasing severity of the lesion are via the mechanism of an immune complex. Although it has been stated that liver damage from a drug such as halothane may be solely ascribed to hypoxia,[28] the human experience seems to preclude hypoxia as the major cause of post-halothane liver necrosis. Obviously, the issue is not settled as yet.

In summary, the liver is the primary site of a multiplicity of drug interactions. In our drug-oriented society, most of these interactions go unnoticed during clinical anesthesia. We lack sufficiently sophisticated monitoring to detect these events at the molecular level. The anesthesiologist thus perceives them grossly in the form of patient tolerance to drugs or prolonged effects of drugs, but the intelligent practitioner should be aware of latent dangers. Viscerotoxicity following halogenated anesthetics, particularly hepatic necrosis, may be a rare, unpredictable form of subtle drug interaction. If this is true, an intensive study for its detection and prevention may be required.

REFERENCES

1. Gillette, J.R., Brodie, B.B., and LaDu, B.N.: The oxidation of drugs by liver microsomes: on the role of TPNH and oxygen. J. Pharmacol. Exp. Ther., *119*:532, 1957.
2. Cooper, D.Y., et al.: Photochemical action spectrum of the terminal oxidase of mixed function oxidase systems. Science, 147:400, 1965.
3. Claude, A.: Microsomes, endoplasmic reticulum and interaction of cytoplasmic membranes. *In* Microsomes and Drug Oxidation. Edited by J.R. Gillette, et al. New York, Academic Press, 1969.
4. Conney, A.H.: Pharmacological implications of microsomal enzyme induction. Pharmacol. Rev., *19*:317, 1967.
5. Remmer, H., and Merker, H.J.: Effects of drugs on the formation of smooth endoplasmic reticulum and drug metabolizing enzymes. Ann. N.Y. Acad. Sci., *123*:79, 1965.
6. Brown, B.R., Jr.: Hepatic microsomal enzyme induction. Anesthesiology, *39*:178, 1973.
7. Fouts, J.R., and Rogers, L.A.: Morphologic changes in stimulation of microsomal drug metabolizing enzyme activity of phenobarbital, chlordane, benzpyrene, or methylcholanthrene in rats. J. Pharmacol. Exp. Ther., *147*:112, 1965.
8. Gillette, J.R., Davis, D.C., and Sasame, H.C.: Cytochrome P-450 and its role in drug metabolism. Annu. Rev. Pharmacol., *12*:51, 1972.
9. Vesell, E.S., et al.: Genetic control of drug levels and of the induction of drug-metabolizing enzymes in man. Individual variability in the extent of allopurinol and nortryptiline drug metabolism. Ann. N.Y. Acad. Sci., *179*:152, 1971.
10. Baekeland, F., and Greene, N.M.: Effect of diethyl ether on tissue distribution and metabolism

of pentobarbital in rats. Anesthesiology, *19*:724, 1958.
11. Brown, B.R., Jr.: The diphasic action of halothane on the oxidation metabolism of drugs by the liver: An in vitro study in the rat. Anesthesiology, *35*:241, 1971.
12. Brown, B.R., Jr.: Effects of inhalation anesthetics on hepatic glucuronide conjugation: A study of the rat in vitro. Anesthesiology, *37*:483, 1972.
13. Rubin, A., Tephly, T.R., and Mannering, G.J.: Kinetics of drug metabolism by hepatic microsomes. Biochem. Pharmacol., *13*:1007, 1964.
14. Goss, J.E., and Dickhaus, D.W.: Increased bishydroxy coumarin requirements in patients receiving phenobarbital. N. Engl. J. Med., *273*:1094, 1965.
15. Rogers, K.J., and Thornton, J.A.: The interaction between monoamine oxidase inhibitors and narcotic analgesics in mice. Br. J. Pharmacol., *36*:470, 1969.
16. Van Dyke, R.A.: Metabolism of volatile anesthetics, II. Induction of microsomal dechlorinating and ether-clearing enzymes. J. Pharmacol. Exp. Ther., *154*:364, 1966.
17. Mazze, R.I., Trudell, J.R., and Cousins, M.J.: Methoxyflurane metabolism and renal dysfunction: Clinical correlation in Man. Anesthesiology, *35*:247, 1971.
18. Brown, B.R., Jr., Sipes, I.G., and Sagalyn, A.M.: Mechanisms of acute hepatotoxicity: chloroform, halothane, and glutathione. Anesthesiology, *41*:554, 1974.
19. Rehder, K., et al.: Halothane biotransformation in man: A quantitative study. Anesthesiology, *28*:711, 1967.
20. Cohen, E.N., et al.: Urinary metabolites of halothane in man. Anesthesiology, *43*:392, 1975.
21. Makai, S., et al.: Volatile metabolites of halothane in the rabbit. Anesthesiology, *47*:248, 1977.
22. Sipes, I.G., and Brown, B.R., Jr.: An animal model of hepatotoxicity associated with halothane anes thesia. Anesthesiology, *45*:622, 1976.
23. Sipes, I.G., Brown, B.R., Jr., and McLain, G.E.: Unpublished observations.
24. Widger, L.A., Gandolfi, A.J., and Van Dyke, R.A.: Hypoxia and halothane metabolism in vivo. Anesthesiology, *44*:197, 1976.
25. Brown, B.R., Jr., Sipes, I.G., and Baker, R.K.: Halothane hepatotoxicity and the reduced derivative 1,1,1-trifluoro-2-chloroethane. Environ. Health Perspect., *21*:185, 1977.
26. Vergani, D., et al.: Antibodies to the surface of halothane altered rabbit hepatocytes in patients with severe halothane-associated hepatitis. N. Engl. J. Med., *303*:66, 1980.
27. Gandolfiaj: Unpublished observation.
28. Shingu, K., Eger, E.I., II, and Johnson, B.H.: Hypoxia may be more important than reductive metabolism in halothane induced hepatic injury. Anesth. Analg., *61*:824, 1982.

7

SYMPATHOMIMETIC DRUGS

K.C. WONG and JOEL D. EVERETT

The integrity of the sympathetic nervous system is essential for the optimal homeostatic control of the cardiovascular system. Anesthesiologists rely on routine monitoring of the arterial blood pressure as an expression of adequate perfusion of vital organs. This fundamental concept is clinically useful. However, adequate pressure does not always reflect adequate blood flow, since the arterial blood pressure is the product of cardiac output and peripheral vascular resistance, and since cardiac output is the product of stroke volume and heart rate. Stimulation of the sympathetic nervous system can be induced by (1) reflex or direct stimulation of sympathetic nerves to cause a release of norepinephrine from adrenergic nerve terminals, (2) endogenous release of catecholamines (epinephrine and norepinephrine) from the adrenal medulla, or (3) exogenous administration of sympathomimetic drugs. Regardless of the mode of sympathetic stimulation, the caliber of blood vessels, the strength of cardiac contraction, and the heart rate or rhythm are usually affected. Thus arterial blood pressure is regulated by sympathetic activities.

Anesthesiologists not infrequently must anesthetize a patient who has been exposed to drugs that alter the normal physiology of the sympathetic nervous system. Furthermore, all anesthetics and other drugs used by the anesthesiologist affect the sympathetic system to varying degrees. Interactions between these drugs and anesthetics constitute a complex problem for optimal patient care. Rational use of sympathomimetic agents is made only after proper appreciation of the normal physiology of the adrenergic nervous system and of the drugs and anesthetics that alter normal adrenergic responses.

This chapter deals with adrenergic mechanisms, agents that influence normal adrenergic mechanisms, the influence of anesthetics on sympathomimetic drugs, and sympathomimetic drugs in hypotension or shock.

ADRENERGIC MECHANISMS

CASE REPORT

A healthy 22-year-old man was anesthetized with halothane–N_2O–O_2 for an operation on maxillofacial injuries consequent to a motorcycle accident. The only relevant history was a habitual use of cocaine by inhalation. An uneventful induction and oral tracheal intubation were performed following the intravenous injection of thiopental and succinylcholine. Anesthesia was maintained with halothane and N_2O–O_2. During the operation cocaine (10%) was applied topically on the nasal mucosa to minimize bleeding. Prior to the application of cocaine the patient had stable vital signs except for transient episodes of junctional rhythm (formerly nodal) observed on the electrocardiogram (ECG). However, after cocaine was applied, he developed tachycardia, hypertension, and ventricular extrasystoles. Frequent measurements of arterial blood pressure by an arm cuff showed a systolic blood pressure of between 150 and 200 mm Hg. The 3-liter flow of N₂O, 60% of the inspired gas mixture, was replaced by an equal-volume flow of O₂. Three divided doses of propranolol totaling 3 mg were administered over a period of 15 minutes. The blood pressure and cardiac rhythm gradually returned to normal within five minutes.

First we must ask why the patient developed episodes of junctional rhythm following the administration of halothane-N₂O and prior to the topical application of cocaine on the nasal mucosa. Halothane anesthesia induces cardiac junctional rhythm both in man and in experimental animals.[1-6] Halothane depresses the sinoatrial node and the atrial conduction *in vitro* and enhances nodal activity *in vivo*;[1,2,4-6] both mechanisms can promote the development of junctional rhythms.[7-9] Moreover, the heart is more susceptible to circulating or exogenously administered catecholamines during halothane anesthesia.[10-12]

Tachycardia and hypertension frequently occur immediately following the induction of anesthesia and endotracheal intubation. This response represents a reflex increase in sympathetic tone due to endotracheal intubation. With the further deepening of anesthesia, the sympathetic response usually subsides. Thus junctional rhythm is frequently seen following induction and endotracheal intubation of a patient anesthetized with halothane and during periods in which anesthetic depth may be inadequate to suppress sympathetic responses. Normally, junctional rhythms do not require treatment unless they induce hypotension and ventricular dysrhythmias. Repeated cocaine intake may exaggerate the pharmacological actions of catecholamines. This change may account for the development of junctional rhythms.

It is unclear whether N₂O augments the dysrhythmic effects of halothane in man. Nitrous oxide alone possesses an inherent adrenergic stimulatory effect.[13] The addition of N₂O to halothane, ether, and morphine in man produces a predominant *alpha*-adrenergic stimulatory response.[14-16] However, the interaction of N₂O with fluroxene produced a mixed *alpha* and *beta* response.[17] In dogs, the addition of 50% N₂O to halothane, enflurane, or methoxyflurane significantly reduced the dose of epinephrine required to induce ventricular dysrhythmias in comparison with similar studies, in which N₂O was not added. Furthermore, in dogs anesthetized with 1.1 MAC halothane, only the combination of 50% N₂O:50% O₂:halothane significantly reduced the amount of epinephrine needed to produce ventricular dysrhythmias.[17b] The addition of either 50% N₂ or 50% helium had no effect.

The second question is why the topical application of cocaine caused hypertension, tachycardia, and ventricular dysrhythmias in this patient. A discussion of the normal disposition of catecholamines in the body is necessary for a better understanding of the interaction of cocaine and halothane.

Disposition of Catecholamines (Fig. 7–1)

Uptake by Adrenergic Nerve Endings. Norepinephrine and epinephrine are released from the adrenergic nerve endings and the adrenal medulla, respectively. The released catecholamines interact with receptor sites to elicit adrenergic responses. Catecholamines are removed in part by reuptake into the nerve terminal. This active transport (reuptake) of the catecholamines from the extracellular fluid into the intraneuronal (cytoplasmic) sites is the most important pathway of termination of adrenergic responses.[18,19] Other sympathomimetics to be discussed may also depend on this mechanism for terminating their adrenergic actions.

Catechol-O-Methyl Transferase (COMT). Catechol-O-methyl transferase is an enzyme that is widely distributed in the soluble cytoplasmic fraction of cells and plasma. It has no selective localization within adrenergic nerves. This enzyme

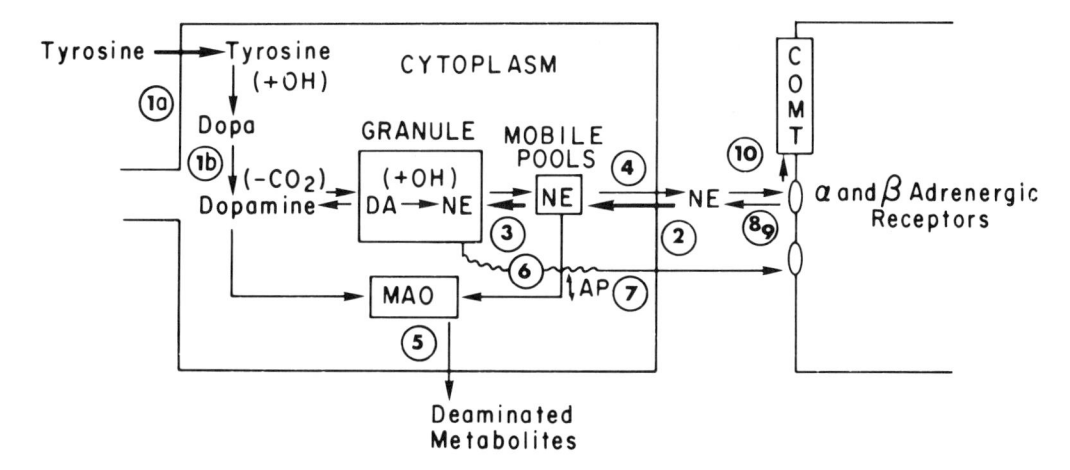

Fig. 7-1. Synthesis, uptake, release and actions of norepinephrine (NE) at adrenergic nerve terminals. Dopamine (DA) nerve action potential (AP).

1. a. Synthesis blocked *(alpha-*methyl-p-tyrosine) b. Synthesis of false transmitters *(alpha-*methyldopa → methylnorepinephrine).
2. Active transport (extracellular fluid → cytoplasm) blocked by cocaine, imipramine, chlorpromazine, ouabain, ketamine.
3. Blockade of transport system of storage granule membrane (reserpine). Destruction of NE by mitochondrial MAO.
4. Displacement of transmitter from axonal terminal (amphetamine, tyramine, ephedrine).
5. Inhibition of enzymatic breakdown of transmitter (pargyline, nialamide, tranylcypromine).
6. Depletion of norepinephrine from granule (guanethidine).
7. Prevention of release of transmitter (bretylium).
8. Transmitter interaction with postsynaptic receptor (phenylephrine, isoproterenol).
9. Blockade of endogenous transmitter at postsynaptic receptor [phenoxybenzamine *(alpha);* propranolol *(beta);* practolol *(beta* 1); butoxamine *(beta* 2)].
10. Inhibition of COMT (pyrogallol). (Adapted from Gilman, A.G., Goodman, L.S., and Gilman, A.: *Goodman & Gilman's The Pharmacological Basis of Therapeutics.* 6th Ed. New York, Macmillan, 1980.)

transfers a methyl group to the 3-hydroxy position of the catechol nucleus (Fig. 7-2). The methoxy derivative of the catecholamine has only a fraction of the pharmacologic activity of its parent structure.[19,20] COMT is a slow mechanism for terminating catecholamine response.

Monoamine Oxidase (MAO). Monoamine oxidase is mainly an intramitochondrial enzyme present in all sympathetic nerve endings. MAO cleaves the amino group of catecholamines and oxidizes the terminal carbon to pharmacologically inactive acid (mandelic acid) (Figs. 7-1, 7-2). MAO is believed to be important in maintaining proper levels of catecholamine in sympathetic nerve terminals. Inhibition of MAO leads to some accumulation of norepinephrine in adrenergic nerve endings that has clinical implications in the anesthetic management of patients taking MAO inhibitors (sometimes known as MAOI).[18,19,21,22]

Catecholamine-Induced Cardiac Dysrhythmias

There are three important components to catecholamine-induced dysrhythmias: (1) *alpha-*adrenergic stimulation, which produces peripheral vascular constriction, (2) vagal stimulation which suppresses the rate of spontaneous depolarization of the sinoatrial node and of atrioventricular (AV) conduction, and (3) myocardial *beta-*adrenergic stimulation, which produces tachycardia and increases automaticity of excit-

Fig. 7–2. Disposition of monoamines.

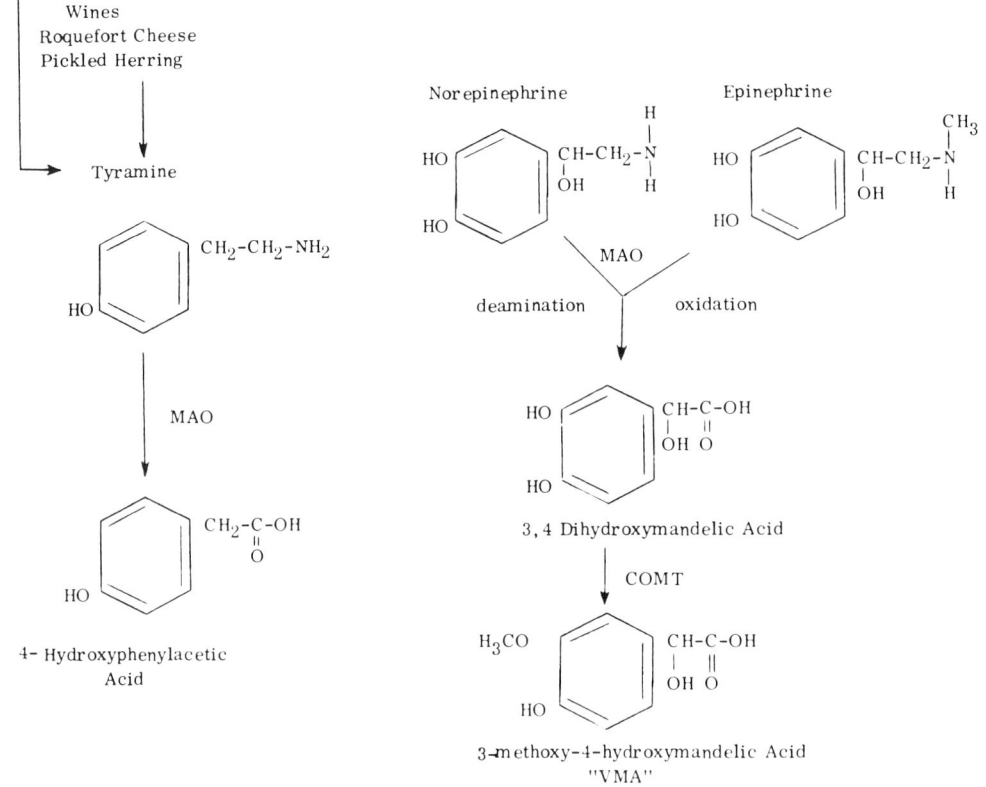

MAO Inhibitors (Pargyline, Nialamide, Tranylcypromine)
1. Increase available catecholamine in the nerve terminal.
2. Increase available tyramine for displacement of catecholamine from the nerve terminal

able cardiac cells. Cardiac dysrhythmias can develop without the simultaneous presence of all three components, especially in patients with preexisting myocardial ischemia (occurring, for example, with myocardial infarction, congestive heart failure, hypotension or hypertension, congenital or acquired heart disease, or cardiac trauma). Rational treatment of cardiac dysrhythmias during anesthesia requires the correct diagnosis of its cause. Before making the diagnosis, the physician should focus immediate attention on oxygen delivery to the patient and adequate maintenance of blood pressure. Most supraventricular dysrhythmias with acceptable blood pressures are self-limiting, provided the anesthetic depth, oxygen delivery, and tissue perfusion are satisfactory. Junctional rhythm with bradycardia frequently responds to intravenous atropine, 0.2 to 0.4 mg, whereas junctional rhythm without bradycardia may respond to intravenous succinylcholine, 20 mg/70 kg.[5] Intravenous lidocaine (4 mg/ml; 4 mg/min) or 1 to 2 mg/kg bolus is an effective treatment for ventricular extrasystoles.[23,24] Catecholamine-induced ventricular extrasystoles may be more specifically antagonized by propranolol administered in 1-mg doses.[25,26]

Factors (Non-Pharmacological) that Increase Sympathetic Activity

1. *Carbon dioxide.* Hypercapnia induces a direct adrenal medullary release of epinephrine.[27–29]

2. *Pheochromocytoma.* Large amounts of catecholamines are released by this adrenal medullary tumor.[30,31]
3. *Hyperthyroidism.* Thyroid hormone potentiates the cardiovascular responses to catecholamines.[32-34]
4. *Congestive heart failure.* Patients with uncompensated myocardial failure have elevated blood levels of circulating catecholamines with a simultaneous reduction in myocardial catecholamine content.[35-38]
5. *Sympathectomy.* Denervated sympathetic organs are hypersensitive to exogenously administered catecholamines.[39]
6. *Spinal cord transection.* The sympathetic nervous system is hypersensitive to certain stimuli (for example, cold and bladder distension).[40]

Since discussion of these factors is beyond the scope of this chapter, the indicated references should be consulted for detailed information.

AGENTS THAT INFLUENCE NORMAL ADRENERGIC MECHANISMS

The biosynthesis of catecholamines and some enzyme inhibitors is summarized in Table 7–1. *Alpha*-methyldopa, MAO inhibitors, and disulfiram are enzyme inhibitors with important clinical anesthetic implications.

Agents that Decrease Sympathetic Activity

Disulfiram (Antabuse). Disulfiram is used to treat chronic alcoholism.[41] Chronic therapy with disulfiram causes an accumulation of acetaldehyde in the body following ingestion of alcohol. Acetaldehyde is produced by the initial oxidation of ethanol by alcohol dehydrogenase in the liver and is oxidized further to acetic acid. Disulfiram not only inhibits the rate of oxidation of acetaldehyde, but also inhibits dopamine *beta*-hydroxylase, which is needed for the synthesis of norepinephrine from dopamine.[42,43] Severe hypotension has been reported during general anesthesia with halogenated agents in patients on chronic disulfiram therapy.[43a] Immediate therapy may consist of: (1) discontinuation of the halogenated agent, (2) intravascular volume expansion and (3) administration of direct-acting alpha-sympathomimetics, for example, phenylephrine or methoxamine.[43a]

Alpha-methyldopa (Aldomet). *Alpha*-methyldopa is a decarboxylase inhibitor that interferes with the formation of dopamine (Fig. 7–1). It is structurally similar

Table 7–1
Biosynthesis and Metabolism of Catecholamines

		Enzyme	Enzyme Inhibitors
Phenylalanine ↓ Tyrosine	←	hydroxylase	
↓ DOPA	← rate limiting	hydroxlyase	← *alpha*-methyl-p-tyrosine
↓ Dopamine	←	decarboxylase	← *alpha*-methyldopa (Aldomet)
↓ Norepinephrine	← rate limiting	*beta*-hydroxylase	← disulfiram (Antabuse)
↓ Epinephrine	←	N-methyltransferase	
↓ Metanephrine	←	COMT	← Pyrogallol, Tropolone
↓ Vanillylmandelic acid	←	MAO	← MAO Inhibitor (Pargyline)

to DOPA and allows *alpha*-methyldopa to act as a false transmitter. The decarboxylated *alpha*-methyldopa *(alpha*-methylnorepinephrine) is stored in the adrenergic nerve terminal and is released by neural stimulation. However, *alpha*-methylnorepinephrine has only a fraction of the potency of normally synthesized catecholamines. More importantly, alpha-methyldopa also inhibits central outflow of adrenergic impulses to the periphery.[44] *Alpha*-methyldopa does not significantly inhibit the synthesis of norepinephrine, as demonstrated by normal urinary vanillylmandelic acid excretion during *alpha*-methyldopa therapy.[45] Moderate hypotension caused by *alpha*-methyldopa is characterized by a decline in cardiac output, whereas peripheral vascular resistance is significantly reduced.[45–48] *Alpha*-methyldopa is commonly used to treat patients with moderate hypertension (diastolic pressure 100 to 120 mm Hg) and can theoretically exert a hypotensive effect during general or regional anesthesia.[44] However, there are no published data to indicate the incidence or even the existence of alarming hypotension in the anesthetized patient who has been taking *alpha*-methyldopa. Adequate volume replacement with balanced electrolyte solution and/or blood or blood products prevents hypotension. Preoperative interruption of *alpha*-methyldopa therapy is unnecessary, although careful intraoperative monitoring is essential.

Reserpine (Serpasil). Reserpine is an alkaloid of rauwolfia serpentina that exerts its antihypertensive effect by depletion of catecholamine storage granules in the adrenergic nerve terminals of the brain, the heart, and the blood vessels (Fig. 7–1).[50–53] Depletion is slower and less complete in the adrenal medulla. It is commonly used to treat patients with mild hypertension (diastolic pressure of 90 to 100 mm Hg), for which reserpine's sedative and bradycardiac effects are desirable.[44] The latency of onset of orally administered reserpine is about one week; a full effect is achieved in three to four weeks. Likewise, reserpine's cardiovascular and other effects may persist for two to four weeks following its withdrawal. The parenteral injection of reserpine exerts a hypotensive effect in 15 to 30 minutes, with a maximal response in two to four hours.

Earlier reports indicated the need for the discontinuance of reserpine therapy two weeks prior to the administration of anesthesia. The reasons given for the withdrawal of rauwolfia therapy were (1) the depletion of catecholamine stores can produce profound hypotension during general anesthesia,[54–55] (2) the cardiovascular response to exogenous administration of sympathomimetic drugs may be unpredictable,[54–58] and (3) reserpine may exert a neurodepressant action on reflex baroreceptor mechanisms.[54–58]

Munson and Jenicek observed no significant increase in the incidence or severity of hypotension during anesthesia of reserpined treated patients was continued up to the day of anesthesia in comparison with patients whose therapy was discontinued 10 to 14 days before elective surgical procedures.[59] They concluded, therefore, that rauwolfia therapy need not be discontinued before anesthesia and surgical procedures, although it is important for the anesthesiologist to be aware of the patient's drug intake and to consider this in anesthetic management.[59] Katz et al. drew similar conclusions from observations conducted in 100 patients undergoing rauwolfia therapy.[60]

Hypertensive patients are frequently hypovolemic.[60,61,62] All general anesthetics produce a direct depressant effect on the cardiovascular system. Therefore, an anesthetic that causes the least cardiovascular depression when compared with others of equal potency is the best choice. "Balanced anesthesia" (narcotic-N_2O-O_2-relaxant) generally produces less hypotension than inhalational anesthesia.[62a] In our experience, patients who are adequately controlled by the oral administration of reserpine alone require no interruption of therapy. Hypotension may be minimized by intravascular replacement prior to and during anesthetic induction.[58–60,63,64] Suggested guidelines for the hypovolemic patient include the infusion of 15 ml/kg of balanced crystalloid solution during the night before an operation and 7 to 10 ml/kg of crystalloid solution during induction of anesthesia. Patients with total serum protein of less than 5 g/L (normal = 6 to 9 g/L) are also benefited by the infusion of 5% Purified Protein Fraction (that is, 12.5 g albumin/250 ml) to reduce intravascular fluid shift to the interstitial space. Vasopressors should be used only for temporary support of arterial blood pressure, and the vasopressor chosen should not entirely depend on the endogenous release of stored catecholamines.[65–68]

Continuous arterial pressure and ECG recordings are useful for the optimal care of any patient with a labile cardiovascular system.

Guanethidine (Ismelin). Guanethidine is one of the most potent antihypertensive drugs used today. Thus its use has been generally limited to patients with a diastolic pressure in excess of 120 mm Hg.[44] Its potent hypotensive effect is the result of at least two pharmacologic actions on the sympathetic nervous system: (1) blockade of postganglionic adrenergic nerve transmission and (2) displacement of norepinephrine from granular storage (Fig. 7–1).[69–71] Guanethidine has little effect on the catecholamine content of the adrenal medulla and penetrates the central nervous system (CNS) poorly following systemic administration. The hypotensive effects of guanethidine reach a maximum in 10 to 14 days. Similarly, its hypotensive effects persist for several days after its withdrawal. The therapeutic benefit of guanethidine can be antagonized by tricyclic antidepressants.[72]

Important anesthetic considerations for the management of patients undergoing prolonged guanethidine therapy are related to the drug's pharmacologic actions. Hypotension is accentuated by CNS depressants. Guanethidine induced sympathectomy may result in increased fluid accumulation and decreased myocardial performance, leading to overt heart failure. However, withdrawal of guanethidine in a severely hypertensive patient may result in undesirable rebound hypertension.

Clonidine (Catapres). Clonidine is a potent antihypertensive drug that is frequently used in the treatment of moderate to severe hypertension. Clonidine is structurally similar to tolazoline (Priscoline) and likewise has been shown to have some *alpha*-adrenergic blocking activity.[73] Clonidine's antihypertensive effect is attributed to the inhibition of the bulbar sympathetic cardiovascular and vasoconstrictor centers.[74–75] Severe rebound hypertension has been reported when clonidine therapy is terminated abruptly.[76] This rebound hypertension may also occur following the patient's emergence from general anesthesia.[77] Gradual replacement of clonidine with another antihypertensive agent several days before an operation may be helpful.[77] However, continued clonidine therapy without interruption, including the day of an operation, is also recommended.

Since clonidine is only absorbed from the GI tract, postoperative management of the patient receiving this agent preoperatively requires the use of another antihypertensive agent. The use of propranolol for replacement of clonidine is not recommended because it may increase peripheral vascular resistance while decreasing positive inotropy.[77a]

Beta-*Adrenergic Blocking Drugs.* The *beta*-adrenergic receptors were first described by Ahlquist in 1948 and have been further differentiated pharmacologically into *beta* 1 and *beta* 2 receptors.[78,79,80] Stimulation of *beta* 1 receptors produces positive inotropic and chronotropic effects on the heart, whereas stimulation of *beta* 2 receptors results in vasodilation of pulmonary and peripheral vasculature. Propranolol blocks both *beta* 1- and *beta* 2-adrenergic receptors. Blockade of these receptors results in reduced inotropy and chronotropy, decreased velocity of mechanical systole, prolonged AV conduction, and hypotension.[25,26,81] In the presence of preexisting partial heart block the administration of propranolol may cause complete AV dissociation and cardiac arrest. Propranolol causes *beta*-adrenergic blockade and leaves vagal and *alpha*-adrenergic mechanisms intact, thus allowing peripheral vascular resistance to increase by reflex compensatory mechanisms.[82] Propranolol is used in the treatment of cardiac dysrhythmias, angina pectoris, and the cardiovascular manifestations of thyrotoxicosis.[83] Propranolol is a useful adjunct to other antihypertensive agents, since it inhibits release of renin from the juxta-glomerular apparatus.[81]

Anesthetic management of a patient who has cardiac disease and who requires propranolol for the control of angina pectoris now requires that plasma levels of *beta*-blockers be maintained at optimal therapeutic levels before and throughout surgery. Its plasma half-life in man is approximately three hours.[84] No plasma level or atrial depressant effect from propranolol can be found 48 hours after discontinuation.[85] Propranolol and its active metabolite, 4-hydroxypropranolol, are primarily excreted in the urine.

Sudden withdrawal of propranolol is associated with recurrence of angina, dysrhythmias, and even myocardial infarction.[86-88] Although previous work suggested that propranolol should be discontinued prior to surgery, recent experience indicates that such practices are unnecessary or even dangerous in patients who have severe myocardial insufficiency.[86-89]

Drug Interactions with Propranolol. The positive inotropic effect of digitalis is not antagonized by propranolol, although both drugs can depress AV conduction. Propranolol is considered effective in treating digitalis-induced dysrhythmias.[25] However, caution should be observed when these two drugs are used concurrently, because their additive effect on AV conduction may lead to complete heart block.

Large doses of morphine are known to release histamine and increase airway resistance in man.[16,90] *Beta*-adrenergic blockade also increases airway resistance. There is potential danger of an additive effect when morphine and propranolol are used concurrently. Propranolol should not be administered to patients with bronchospastic or obstructive airway disease.

Calcium-channel antagonists (verapamil and nifedipine) have become increasingly important in the management of supraventricular dysrhythmias and coronary insufficiency, respectively. An increasing number of patients come to surgery while receiving propranolol and a calcium-channel antagonist concurrently. Since calcium ions are required for cardiac as well as smooth muscle contraction, the interaction of propranolol with calcium-channel antagonists has an additive depressant effect on AV conduction as well as on myocardial contractility. Furthermore, the general clinical impression is that patients receiving this drug combination tend to have a decreased peripheral vascular resistance following cardiopulmonary bypass.

Anesthetic agents such as diethyl ether and cyclopropane release endogenous catecholamines. Elevation of peripheral resistance in the presence of myocardial depression can be detrimental to the left ventricle. On the other hand, the judicious administration of halothane, the narcotics, or methoxyflurane has been used successfully for cardiac operations in patients taking propranolol.[91] Although enflurane is also used advantageously in cardiac operations, it can induce hypotension during induction. This response, however, may not be consequent to a direct myocardial depressant effect. Hypotension during induction is common, which probably is not from myocardial depression per se.[92-94] All inhalational agents which reduce peripheral vascular resistance are expected to have an additive effect with calcium-channel antagonists. For example, recent data suggest that the combination of nifedipine, propranolol, and halothane clinically reduces peripheral vascular resistance and mean arterial pressure in anesthetized patients.[94a]

Chlorpromazine and Lithium Carbonate. Twenty percent of all prescriptions written in the United States are for medications intended to treat psychiatric disorders.[95] Chlorpromazine, the prototype of the phenothiazine derivatives, is still widely used. Chlorpromazine produces many pharmacologic actions including antihyperthermia, antihistamine, CNS sedation, antiemesis, and *alpha*-adrenergic inhibition.[96] The last is the result of the blockade of postsynaptic *alpha*-adrenergic receptors and reuptake of norepinephrine into adrenergic nerve terminals (Fig. 7–1). Orthostatic hypotension and reflex tachycardia are common in patients taking chlorpromazine. Discontinuance is probably unnecessary if the drug is required for maintaining psychiatric equilibrium in the patient. Since it also possesses a CNS-depressant action, the effect of preoperative sedatives may be potentiated. Intraoperative management is not a major problem, but the anesthesiologist should be aware of the potential hypotensive additive effects of general anesthetics and of narcotic analgesics in combination with chlorpromazine and other phenothiazines. Direct-acting *alpha*-adrenergic stimulants (methoxamine or phenylephrine) would be more effective than indirect-acting *alpha*-adrenergic stimulants in overcoming the phenothiazine-induced hypotension.

Lithium carbonate is becoming popular in the treatment of various psychiatric disorders.[97] Lithium inhibits acetylcholine synthesis and release from the cholinergic nerve terminal. It also replaces sodium during cellular depolarization and antagonizes the pressor response to norepinephrine in man.[98] Lithium carbonate has been shown to potentiate the neuromuscular blocking actions of pancuronium, succinylcholine, and decamethonium.[99,100] (See Chap. 19.)

General Guidelines. Reasons for uninterrupted antihypertensive therapy:
1. Temporary withdrawal of antihypertensive drugs may be helpful, but it does not insure a more stable anesthetic course.
2. Withdrawal of drugs in patients with severe hypertension may precipitate:
   a. Renal damage by diastolic pressures above 140 mm Hg.
   b. Cardiac failure from left ventricular strain.
   c. Cerebral vascular accident.
   d. Decreased blood volume.
   e. Inconveniences of delay to the patient and the hospital.

When antihypertensive therapy is not interrupted, the following considerations are helpful:
1. Prophylactic intravascular replacement with crystalloids and plasma expanders.
2. Importance of assuring a smooth induction of anesthesia.
3. Avoidance of abrupt postural changes and excessive intra-abdominal manipulation.
4. Avoidance of abrupt increases in anesthetic concentration.
5. Avoidance of playing "catch-up" in blood loss.

Agents that Increase Sympathetic Activity

Monoamine Oxidase (MAO) Inhibitors (Pargyline, Phenelzine, Tranylcypromine). The MAO inhibitors block oxidative deamination (Figs. 7–1 and 7–2) of naturally occurring monoamines. These inhibitors do not inhibit synthesis of biogenic amines, which accumulate in the adrenergic nerve terminal.[22] After the administration of a large dose of MAO inhibitor, norepinephrine, epinephrine, dopamine, and 5-hydroxytryptamine levels increase in the brain, heart, intestine, and blood.[101] Successful treatment of psychotic depressions may be related to their ability to elevate endogenous amines. Although MAO inhibitors may be present in the body for a short time only, they produce long-lasting, irreversible inhibition of the enzyme. Regeneration of MAO after the discontinuance of drug therapy may require weeks.

Acute overdosage may produce agitation, hallucinations, hyperpyrexia, convulsions, hypertension, or hypotension. Orthostatic hypotension is common in patients taking MAO inhibitors. The action of sympathomimetic amines is potentiated by MAO inhibitors; adrenergic drugs with partial or complete indirect actions (for example, ephedrine, amphetamine, tyramine) may produce exaggerated release of neuronal catecholamines.[101] The ingestion of cheese, wine, and pickled herring, which have a high tyramine content, can precipitate a hypertensive crisis.[21] Reflex sympathetic stimulation is similarly intensified. MAO inhibitors can also prolong and intensify the effects of CNS depressants including alcohol, barbiturates, anesthetics, and potent analgesics, although the mechanism of this potentiating effect of MAO inhibitors is unclear.[101] Adverse CNS interactions, such as convulsions, coma, and hyperthermia, have been reported wtih tricyclic antidepressants, especially imipramine and amitriptyline.[102] A 2-week wash-out period is advisable when introducing a tricyclic antidepressant into a MAO-treated patient. Hyperpyrexia, hypertension, convulsions and coma have been reported in patients who are given MAO inhibitors and meperidine.[102a,b,c]

The current recommendation that MAO inhibitors should be discontinued for at least 2 weeks prior to elective surgery is based upon clinical impressions and limited case reports suggesting the complications resulting from the interactions of MAO inhibitors and intraoperative drugs.[102d] There has been a paucity of hard data to substantiate this recommendation. Evan-Prosser demonstrated no significant adverse effects on 15 patients who were given analgesic doses of meperidine or morphine while taking MAO inhibitors.[102e] A recent study in dogs showed that tranylcypromine (Parnate) pre-treatment did not elevate plasma catecholamine levels. The reflex hypertensive response to enflurane anesthesia, however, was significantly greater than the response to fentanyl anesthesia.[102f] We have also demonstrated that pargyline pre-treatment does not reduce the dysrhythmogenic threshold of epinephrine in halothane anesthetized dogs.[102g] Thus the appropriate anesthetic management of patients treated with MAO inhibitors is undefined. With the advent of continuous and more detailed monitoring systems and of agents that spare the cardiovascular system, such patients have been successfully managed with fentanyl-nitrous-relaxant or regional anesthesia. In general narcotics which release significant amounts of endogenous catecholamines and histamine (morphine and meperidine) should be avoided because these patients are hemodynamically labile and do not possess the benefits of full homeostasis. If hypertensive episodes occur, agents that produce *alpha*-adrenergic blockade (chlorpromazine, phentolamine), ganglionic blockade (trimethaphan, pentolinium), or direct vasodilation (nitroprusside) may be used.

Other Antidepressants

Tricyclic Antidepressants. Imipramine, desipramine, amitriptyline, and other closely related drugs have almost replaced MAO inhibitors in the treatment of psychotic depression because there are fewer side effects associated with the continued use of the tricyclic antidepressants.[103] The mechanism by which imipramine exerts its antidepressant action in psychotic depression is not clear. All tricyclic antidepressants block the reuptake of norepinephrine by adrenergic nerve terminals (Fig. 7–1).

Synthesis and release of other catecholamines are not affected. About two to five weeks must elapse before the CNS-therapeutic effects of the drug are evident. With a reduction in catecholamine storage and a demonstrable anticholinergic effect of these drugs, orthostatic hypotension, tachycardia, and cardiac dysrhythmias are commonly observed.[103] The most frequent ECG change following imipramine therapy is inversion or flattening of the T wave. The combined use of imipramine and guanethidine may result in cardiac standstill.[104] The concurrent administration of MAO inhibitors and tricyclics can produce convulsions, coma, and hyperpyrexia.[102] Other drug interactions include the potentiation of CNS depressants, the antagonism of the antihypertensive effects of guanethidine, and the potentiation of the pressor effects of sympathomimetic amines.[105] Similarly, imipramine is expected to augment intraoperatively induced sympathetic activity.[106] Imipramine has been shown to produce tachycardia and hypertension during the anesthetic management of patients concurrently receiving halothane and pancuronium.[106a] Dogs pretreated with imipramine exhibited a decreased threshold to epinephrine-induced dysrhythmias.[102g] In spite of these unusual problems, the discontinuance of tricyclic antidepressants prior to an operation is probably unnecessary.

Amphetamine. Amphetamine is structurally similar to sympathomimetic amines except that it has a powerful CNS-stimulating action in addition to its peripheral *alpha*- and *beta*-adrenergic stimulatory effects. The acute toxic effects of amphetamine are an extension of its therapeutic effects and are usually the result of overdosage. The CNS effects commonly include restlessness, hyperreflexia, fever, and irritability. The cardiovascular effects may include hypertension, tachycardia, cardiac dysrhythmias, and circulatory collapse.

There is a lack of published data on the interaction of amphetamine and anesthetics on the CNS and cardiovascular systems. With normal anorectic and cerebral-stimulating doses, no serious anesthetic problems are likely. Chlorpromazine is helpful in controlling CNS symptoms and hypertension resulting from an acute amphetamine overdose. Amphetamine has been shown to increase anesthetic requirement in dogs by virtue of its CNS-stimulatory effects.[106b] The depletion of CNS catecholamines with repeated amphetamine intake may reduce the required anesthetic dose.[106b]

Cocaine. Cocaine is an alkaloid of *Erythroxylon coca*. It was introduced as a local anesthetic in clinical practice in 1884 by Koller.[107]

The structural similarities of cocaine, procaine, and atropine may account for some of the important pharmacologic actions of cocaine (Fig. 7–3), such as (a) local anesthesia, (b) CNS stimulation, (c) peripheral vascular constriction and tachycardia, (d) reduced uptake of catecholamines at adrenergic nerve endings (Fig. 7–1) and subsequent potentiation of the responses of sympathetic innervated organs to epinephrine and norepinephrine.

The significant vasoconstrictor property of cocaine is desirable for hemostasis in

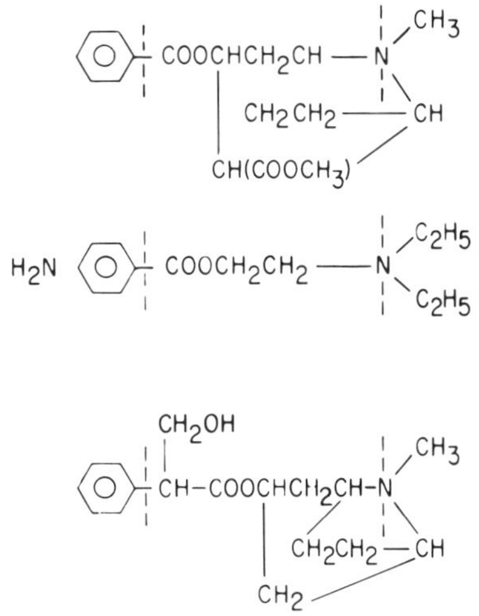

Fig. 7–3. Structural comparison of cocaine, procaine, and atropine.

otolaryngologic surgery. The addition of epinephrine to cocaine for additional vasoconstriction is of questionable value, especially when one considers the hazards of hypertension and cardiac dysrhythmias produced by the cocaine-epinephrine interaction.[108] Anderton and Nassar showed that, in patients undergoing nasal operations and anesthetized with halothane-N$_2$O-O$_2$, the topical administration of cocaine, 20 mg, dissolved in 2 ml of saline solution without epinephrine produces adequate nasal decongestion without serious cardiovascular problems.[109]

The fatal dose of cocaine in man is estimated at 1.2 g, but the usual maximal dose in clinical practice is about 200 mg.[110] Toxic effects have been reported from doses as low as 20 mg.[110] Habitual use of cocaine could enhance intrinsic sympathetic activity in man as well as potentiate the effects of sympathomimetic agents.

ANESTHETIC INFLUENCE ON SYMPATHOMIMETIC AGENTS

In 1895, Oliver and Schaefer first showed that adrenal extract produced ventricular fibrillation in a dog anesthetized with chloroform.[111] The pioneering work of Meek et al. used a dysrhythmogenic dose of 10 µg/kg epinephrine diluted in 5 ml of normal saline solution, which was injected into dogs at the rate of 1 ml/10 sec.[112] Electrocardiographic changes were carefully monitored. More recently, other researchers have used the onset of ventricular extrasystoles as the endpoint following incremental doses of epinephrine.[113–117] Epinephrine-induced cardiac dysrhythmias are a useful method of evaluating the dysrhythmogenicity of anesthetics. Although there are other chemical or mechanical means of inducing cardiac dysrhythmias, the use of epinephrine has particular clincial relevance during anesthesia. Intraoperative cardiac dysrhythmias are frequently associated with imbalance of the autonomic nervous system, usually a preponderance of sympathetic activity.

Epinephrine is commonly used to reduce surgical bleeding. The well-known publications of the Columbia group recommend that the hemostatic dose of epinephrine in adults during halothane-N$_2$O-O$_2$ anesthesia should not exceed 10 ml of 1:100,000 in any given 10-minute period nor 30 ml per hour.[10] Ten milliliters of 1:100,000 epinephrine is equal to 100 µg or to about 1.5 µg/kg/10 min (for a 70-kg person). This dosage guide may be safely used for other halogenated inhalation anesthetics, since the combination of halothane and epinephrine is more dysrhythmogenic than these others. It is convenient to use a commercially prepared, diluted lidocaine-epinephrine solution, for example, lidocaine 0.5% with epinephrine 1:100,000. Evidence suggests that the addition of lidocaine may reduce the severity of potential dysrhythmias induced by epinephrine.[115] However, under conditions of increased endogenous sympathetic activity, hyperthyroidism or hypercapnia, for example, the dysrhythmogenicity of epinephrine is enhanced.

Because of different experimental designs, it is difficult to compare the results from different studies. In spite of this, some conclusions are evident. Diethyl ether is still the least sensitizing drug, whereas cyclopropane is the most sensitizing to epinephrine-induced or intraoperative dysrhythmias (Table 7–2). The halogenated ethers are less sensitizing than halothane. The mechanism for this "sensitizing" effect on the myocardium is not understood; the elevation of arterial blood pressure, the slowing of the sinoatrial rate, and the increase of myocardial automaticity are components that contribute to catecholamine-induced dysrhythmias, as discussed. A relative ranking of drug sensitivity to epinephrine-induced dysrhythmias is listed, as follows (1 = least sensitive, 5 = most sensitive):

Diethyl ether	1
Fluroxene (Fluoromar)	2

Table 7-2
Dosage of Epinephrine Required to Produce Ventricular Dysrhythmias in Man and Dog

Anesthetic	Species	Dosage (µg/kg)	Investigator
Diethyl ether	Dog	10*	Meek et al. (1937)[112]
	Man	10–20†	Wong et al. (1974 and unpublished data)[120]
Fluroxene	Dog	43–48	Joas & Stevens (1971)[116]
	Dog	10*	Wong et al. (1977)[185]
Isoflurane	Dog	22–37	Joas & Stevens (1971)[116]
	Man	6.72 ± 0.66	Johnston et al. (1976)[115]
Methoxyflurane	Dog	14.0 ± 4.7	Munson & Tucker (1975)[113]
	Dog	10–50	Bamforth (1961)[117]
	Man	1–2‡	Hudon (1961)[123]
Enflurane	Dog	17.1 ± 7.2	Munson & Tucker (1975)[113]
	Man	10.9 ± 8.9	Johnston et al. (1960)[115]
Halothane	Dog	4.6 ± 3.3	Munson & Tucker (1975)[113]
	Dog	5–8	Joas & Stevens (1971)[116]
	Man	2.11 ± 0.15	Johnston et al. (1976)[115]
	Man	1.7§	Katz et al. (1962)[10]
Cyclopropane	Dog	1–2	Dresel et al. (1960)[119]
	Man	up to 7 in 30 min**	Matteo et al. (1963)[122]
	Dog	10	Meek et al. (1937)[112]

* Occasional nodal rhythm.
† Occasional ventricular dysrhythmias. Stable cardiac rhythm during induced hypothermia of infants requiring cardiac surgery.
‡ Occasional wandering pacemaker.
§ Recommended safe dose.
** Ventricular dysrhythmias in 30% patients.

Isoflurane (Forane)	2
Methoxyflurane (Penthrane)	3
Enflurane (Ethrane)	3
Halothane (Fluothane)	4
Cyclopropane	5

The dog is more resistant than man to the dysrhythmogenic effect of epinephrine (Table 7–2). However, there is a qualitative similarity between the two species in their response to the effects of anesthetic-epinephrine interaction. It is the general clinical impression that balanced anesthesia (that is, narcotic-N$_2$O-muscle relaxant) produces minimal disturbance of the cardiovascular system. Similarly, dogs anesthetized with a narcotic (morphine, fentanyl or meperidine), N$_2$O, and pancuronium demonstrated virtually no ventricular tachycardia from intravenous epinephrine; in contrast, dogs anesthetized with halothane or enflurane-N$_2$O-pancuronium were prone to develop ventricular tachycardia during the epinephrine challenge.[17a] Minimal anesthesia consisting of 70% N$_2$O and d-tubocurarine or gallamine also protected dogs from epinephrine-induced ventricular tachycardia or fibrillation.[118]

SYMPATHOMIMETIC ANESTHETICS

Phencyclidine (Ketamine)

Ketamine produces anesthesia by the stimulation of the medulla and limbic systems of the brain and by the simultaneous depression of the cortex.[124–126] The cardiovascular system is stimulated by anesthetic doses of ketamine, which causes a significant elevation in cerebrospinal fluid (CSF) pressure, heart rate, and mean arterial blood pressure. The work of Traber et al.

suggests that this stimulation of the cardiovascular system may be of central origin and thereby require an intact sympathetic system. Whether ketamine causes depression of baroreceptors is uncertain.[127–131]

Ketamine blocks the neuronal reuptake of catecholamines (Fig. 7–1) in a manner similar to that of cocaine.[132,133] Ketamine probably enhances the dysrhythmogenicity of epinephrine in dogs anesthetized with halothane-N_2O-O_2.[134] In larger doses, direct myocardial depression occurs.[130] We found that ketamine potentiates the inotropic effects of norepinephrine, epinephrine, and tyramine, whereas it antagonizes isoproterenol and dopamine intropy.[135] A possible explanation for this difference is that there are two neuronal uptake processes for vasoactive amines. Uptake 1 (intraneuronal) has greater affinity for norepinephrine; Uptake 2 (extraneuronal) has greater affinity for isoproterenol. Cocaine and ketamine preferentially block the Uptake 1 process.

Ketamine should be used with caution in patients who have hypertension or myocardial disease or who are taking drugs that increase sympathetic tone (e.g., thyroxine).

Dioxolanes (Dexoxadrol and Etoxadrol)

The dioxolanes possess pharmacologic properties similar to those of ketamine but are structurally quite dissimilar from ketamine. Etoxadrol (CL-1848C, Cutter Laboratories), 0.75 mg/kg, was administered intravenously to 11 adult male volunteers. The duration of unconsciousness induced by this single dose was from 50 to 85 minutes. Analgesia and amnesia usually exceeded the duration of unconsciousness. Cardiac output, heart rate, and arterial blood pressure were significantly elevated for 120 minutes following drug injection with minimal undesirable psychologic side effects.[136] No subject experienced hallucination in the postarousal period. The clinical use of this longer-acting ketamine-like drug awaits further studies in man.

SYMPATHOMIMETIC AGENTS IN SHOCK

CASE REPORT

A 55-year-old man involved in an automobile accident arrived at the emergency room in shock. The only significant historical data were digoxin and furosemide intake for over five years for "heart trouble." He was complaining of severe pain in the left upper quadrant of the abdomen and rebound tenderness. Cuff arterial blood pressure, taken from the brachial artery, was 60/40 mm Hg with a thready pulse of 160/min. His skin was pale, cold, and clammy to the touch. Laboratory tests showed a hematocrit of 24% and serum potassium concentration of 2.8 mEq/L. No urine was obtainable for analysis. The ECG showed a depressed ST segment with first-degree AV block and occasional ventricular extrasystoles. Roentgenograms revealed fracture of ribs 7, 8, and 9 on the right side; the flat and upright films of the abdomen suggested increased opacity with demonstrable air under the diaphragm. Bloody fluid was aspirated by paracentesis. A presumptive diagnosis of ruptured spleen and bowel with hemorrhagic shock was made. Preoperative preparation of the patient was carried out in the surgical intensive care unit for a scheduled exploratory laparotomy and splenectomy.

However, before the patient was brought to the operating room, he developed episodes of ventricular fibrillation in the intensive care unit. Electrical countershock was effective in defibrillating the heart, but each time ventricular fibrillation recurred after a few minutes of regular cardiac rhythm. Assuming that there was continued intra-abdominal bleeding perpetuating the labile cardiovascular state, the physicians rushed the patient to the operating room. Upon arrival, the following were noted: (1) the patient's trachea had been intubated (during the cardiopulmonary resuscitation) and the lungs mechanically ventilated; (2) one liter of 5% dextrose in water and a unit of albumin were running into a peripheral venous catheter; (3) one liter of dilute epinephrine (1 µg/ml) in 5% dextrose in water was being administered through a central venous pressure (CVP) catheter; (4) the bladder was catheterized, but there was no urine in the receptacle; (5) no auscultatory pressures were obtainable from a pressure cuff around the upper arm, but there was a palpable carotid pulse; (6) his temperature was 34.5°C, and (7) the patient was still conscious.

Diazepam 10 mg and pancuronium 7 mg were administered intravenously while another intravenous catheter was established. The patient was mechanically ventilated with 100% O_2 and the operation began. Intravenous replacement now consisted of albumin and 5% dextrose in lactated Ringer's solution with KCl 40 mEq/L added. The patient continued to exhibit ventricular extrasystoles. When the radial pulse became palpable, a percutaneous catheter was placed in the radial artery for continuous pressure monitoring. An immediate arterial blood gas yielded Po₂—120 mm Hg, Pco₂—24 mm Hg, pH—7.2 and negative base excess—8.4 mEq/L; serum [Na]—142 mEq/L and serum [K]—2.7 mEq/L. The metabolic acidosis was corrected following two injections of NaHCO₃ 50 mEq, and the respiratory alkalosis was corrected by reduction of mechanical ventilation.

The epinephrine solution was replaced by dopamine (5 to 10 μg/kg/min). Following infusion of four units of warmed whole blood, two liters of crystalloid solution, and two units of albumin, there was evidence of urine formation and of increased need for anesthesia. Serum [K] had increased from 2.7 to 3.4 mEq/L without additional intravenous KCl. The number of ventricular extrasystoles appearing on the ECG reduced to one to two per minute. Hemorrhage was controlled after the removal of the ruptured spleen and the operation was successful. The patient was discharged after 22 days of hospitalization.

What may be some of the contributing factors to the patient's repeated occurrences of ventricular fibrillation prior to the operation? The main factors to be considered are hypotension, hypoxia, acidosis, hypothermia, hypocapnia, and hypokalemia. Adverse responses to epinephrine and other catecholamines are common under such circumstances. These factors will be discussed further.

The pathophysiology of low perfusion states will be reviewed before the discussion of the sympathomimetic drugs. Comments will then be directed toward the anesthetic management of the hypotensive patient.

Pathogenesis of Shock

Shock is a state of inadequate tissue perfusion. The low-flow state in vital organs is the final common denominator in all forms of shock, which results from failure of one or more of the following separate but interrelated factors:[137] (1) the pump (heart), (2) the content and volume of the intravascular space (blood), (3) the arteriolar tone, and (4) the venous tone. Thus it is clinically useful to classify shock in terms of (1) primary pump failure—cardiogenic shock, (2) reduction of intravascular volume—hypovolemic shock, and (3) changes in arteriolar or venous tone—neurogenic and/or septic shock.

Microcirculation. The result of inadequate tissue perfusion is the lack of tissue-blood exchange of gases and metabolic substrates that occurs primarily at the terminal vascular bed, that is, in the arterioles, capillaries, and venules (Fig. 7-4). The arterioles are especially sensitive to sympathetic stimulation. Changes in the caliber of the arterioles provide for the maintenance of blood pressure and volume flow through the capillary beds. However, without adequate intra-arterial volume, arteriolar constriction would reduce capillary perfusion. The venous system normally contains about two-thirds of the total intravascular volume. Sympathetic stimulation also increases venous tone, thus delivering more blood to the arterial system. Humoral agents, pH, and acidic metabolites are important factors in the regulation of capillary blood flow through actions exerted on terminal arterioles, pre- and postcapillary sphincters, venules, and capillaries, where transcapillary exchange occurs.[138-142] Cardiac filling and regulation of active (arterial) blood volume are governed by the muscular venules and veins.

Vasomotion is a unique feature of the microcirculation that provides a cyclic opening and closing of the pre- and postcapillary sphincters to change the perfusion pattern of capillary beds. Vasomotion is probably the most important vasomotor determinant of capillary blood flow and transcapillary exchange. It can be influenced by local tissue and humoral agents as well as by physical factors.[138-142]

The terminal-phase shock represents, therefore, a decompensation of the physiologic controls of microcirculation. Since this is a simplistic approach to a complex problem, the reader is referred to several excellent sources for more complete treatment of the subject.[137-144]

Classification of Sympathomimetic Agents

Alpha- *and* **Beta-***Adrenergic Receptors.* In 1948, Ahlquist postulated the existence

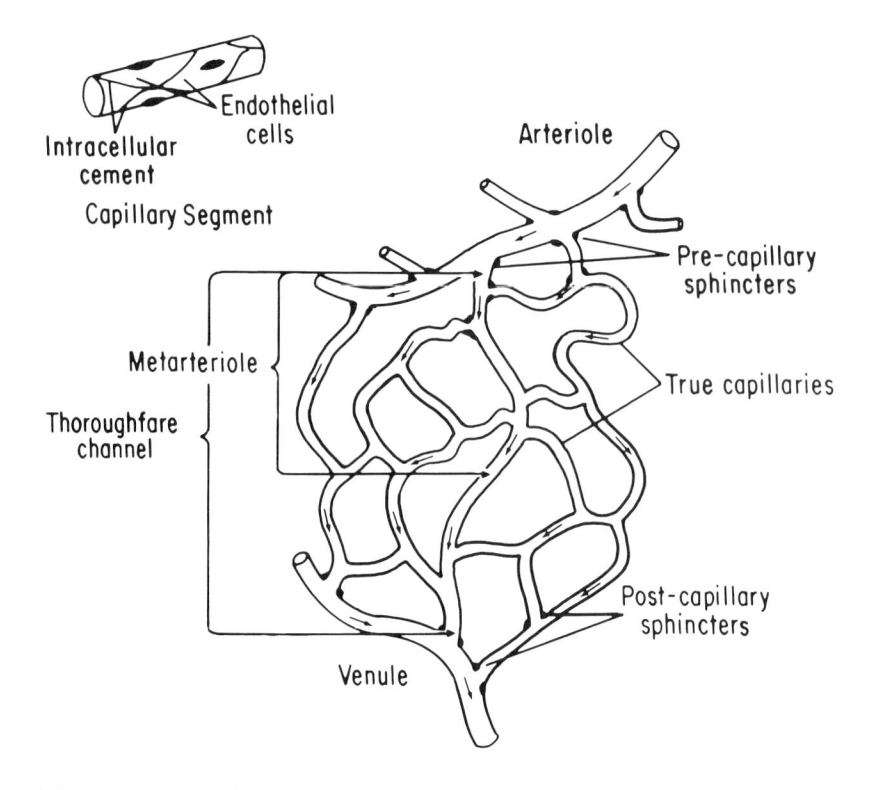

Fig. 7-4. Schematic drawing of the microcirculation. See details in text. (Adapted from Zauder, H.L.: *Pharmacology of Adjuvant Drugs.* (Clincial Anesthesia Series.) Philadelphia, F.A. Davis, 1973.)

of *alpha-* and *beta-*adrenergic receptors in the sympathetic section of the nervous system.[78] The stimulation of *alpha-*adrenergic receptors leads to vasoconstriction of the vasculature. The *alpha-*receptors are further divided into *alpha* 1, the postsynaptic vasoconstrictor receptor, and *alpha* 2, the presynaptic inhibitory adrenoreceptor. The stimulation of the *alpha* 2-receptor is believed to inhibit the release of norepinephrine from the adrenergic nerve terminal. This concept is supported by the observation that phenoxybenzamine blocks *alpha* 1, in preference to *alpha* 2-receptors; therefore, the prevention of vasoconstriction at the postsynaptic receptor is accompanied by pre-synaptic release of norepinephrine.[144a] Circulating norepinephrine inhibits while epinephrine stimulates *alpha* 2-receptors.[144a]

The stimulation of *beta-*adrenergic receptors leads to positive inotropic and chronotropic effects on the heart, vasodilation, and bronchodilation. *Beta-*adrenergic receptors have been further differentiated more recently into 2 subsets, *beta* 1 (cardiac stimulation) and *beta* 2 (subserving bronchial and peripheral vasodilation).[79,80]

The action of dopamine on adrenergic receptors is different from that of the other catecholamines. The renal vasodilatory effect of dopamine is not antagonized by *beta-*adrenergic blockers, atropine, or antihistamines. Thus the term "dopaminergic receptor" is used to describe its actions.

Direct Versus Indirect Action. Direct action implies a drug-receptor interaction without the release of endogenous catecholamines from the adrenergic nerve terminals for its pharmacologic action. Direct-acting sympathomimetic amines are catecholamines—epinephrine, norepinephrine, isoproterenol, and dopamine; and adrenergic amines—methoxamine and phenylephrine. Indirect action implies that the drug acts primarily at a catecholamine storage site and requires the presence of endogenous catecholamines. Indirect-acting sympathomimetics include tyramine (an endogenous amine), amphetamine, and the more clinically useful agents ephedrine, metaraminol, and mephentermine.

Sympathomimetic Drug Actions

The use of sympathomimetic amines as an adjunct during anesthesia is intended to improve tissue perfusion. The rational choice of a drug can be made only following the diagnosis of the cause of the hypotension or shock. Is it pump failure, hypovolemia, increased vascular capacitance, or a combination of these? The choice should be further weighed against its efficacy in patients with a history of any drug therapy that influences the normal adrenergic mechanism. The vasoactive drugs should also be compatible with the anesthetic regimen. The rationale for the use of sympathomimetic agents should focus on the temporary support of the circulatory system until the cause can be corrected.

Common causes of hypotension during anesthesia are excessive depth of anesthesia, hypoxia, intravascular volume deficit, and surgical manipulation. Less common causes include myocardial infarction, pulmonary embolism, and cerebral vascular accident. The pharmacologic actions and dysrhythmogenicity of several sympathomimetic agents used to treat hypotensive states are summarized in Table 7–3. Those agents with similar actions are expected to have similar interactions with drugs as well as pathophysiologic conditions discussed in this chapter. Table 7–3 is intended to assist the reader with the appropriate selection of a vasoactive agent. The pharmacologic actions of vasoactive agents are discussed briefly.

Catecholamines. All catecholamines are direct-acting agents. All except isoproterenol are synthesized in the body (Fig. 7–1). They are called "catechol" because they all possess a dihydroxybenzene (catechol) moiety.

Epinephrine (Adrenalin). Epinephrine, predominantly *beta* at low concentrations, stimulates both *alpha* and *beta* receptors. In higher doses through *alpha*-adrenergic stimulation it constricts arterioles, precapillary sphincters, veins, and large arteries. Epinephrine is useful for cardiopulmonary resuscitation because it takes advantage of its positive inotropic and chronotropic effects (*beta*-receptor stimulation) and of the increase in coronary blood flow.[145] However, it is generally believed that acidosis antagonizes the cardiovascular-stimulant actions of epinephrine and must be corrected in order to maximize the effect of epinephrine and other sympathomimetic amines. Unpublished data from our laboratory suggest that the infusion of lactic acid to anesthetized dogs may be far more detrimental to cardiovascular dynamics than the infusion of HCl. The infusion of HCl to reduce serum pH to 7.0 did not reduce the mean arterial pressure to the same extent as that observed at a pH of 7.2 during lactic acid infusion. The reduced response to catecholamine stimulation may be related to lactic acidosis rather than to a low pH in the anesthetized animal. Hypothermia, hypercapnia, hypoxia, and hypokalemia potentiate epinephrine-induced cardiac dysrhythmias. Ventricular fibrillation should be corrected by countershock before the administration of intravenous bolus epinephrine for resuscitation. The simultaneous administration of lidocaine, 1 to 3 mg/kg, helps to reduce cardiac excitability and automaticity.

Epinephrine should be reserved for the most difficult cases during anesthesia and is generally contraindicated in patients with severe coronary disease. Epinephrine is the most dysrhythmogenic of the catecholamines and is frequently used for hemostasis during an operation. Its interaction with halothane is of great concern to the anesthesiologist, as discussed.

Table 7-3
Adrenergic Drugs Used in Hypotension or Shock

Drugs	Action Receptor	Action Type	VC	VD	CS	Cardiac Output	Intravenous Dose	Arrhythmogenicity
Catecholamines								
Epinephrine	α & β	Direct	++++	+++	++++	Increased	0.1–0.25 mg	+++++
Norepinephrine	α & β	Direct	+++++	0	+++	Unchanged or decreased	2–8 μg/min	+++++
Isoproterenol	β₁ & β₂	Direct	0	+++++	++++	Increased	2–4 μg/min	++++
Dopamine	α & β	Direct & some indirect	++	++*	++	Increased	50–200 μg/min	+++
Sympathomimetics								
Methoxamine	α	Direct	++++	0	0	Decreased	5–10 mg	+
Phenylephrine	α	Direct	++++	0	0	Decreased	0.1–0.5 mg	++
Ephedrine	α & β	Indirect & some direct	++	+	+++	Increased	10–25 mg	++
Metaraminol	α & β	Indirect & some direct	+++	++	+	Decreased	0.5–5.0 mg	++
Mephentermine	α & β	Indirect	+	+++	++	Increased	5–15 mg	+

VC = vasoconstriction; VD = vasodilation; CS = cardiac stimulation
* Renal and mesenteric vasodilation caused by stimulation of "dopaminergic receptors."

Norepinephrine (Levophed). This agent causes marked and sustained vasoconstriction by means of its action on *alpha*-adrenergic receptors.[145,146] By means of *beta*-adrenergic stimulation, it also causes a positive inotropic and chronotropic effect. Its *alpha*-stimulating effect is dominant, and causes hypertension by an increase in peripheral vascular resistance with compensatory vagal reflex bradycardia. Cardiac output may decrease or remain unchanged. Coronary blood flow is elevated, as with epinephrine. The circulating volume may be reduced following the prolonged use of norepinephrine, probably owing to an increase in postcapillary vasoconstriction and a loss of protein-free fluid caused by the increased capillary pressure.

Norepinephrine should only be administered intravenously in dilute concentrations (4 μg/ml). The infusion site should be checked frequently for possible extravasation into the tissues, since local necrosis and sloughing of the skin is a dreaded complication. Sometimes without obvious extravasation, blanching along the course of the infused vein is seen. Infusion of an *alpha*-adrenergic blocker (for example, phentolamine, 5 to 10 mg) in the norepinephrine-extravasated tissue may reduce the severity of tissue ischemia. Stellate ganglion block of the same side of the infiltrated arm may also improve circulation to the ischemic area.

Norepinephrine also has significant arrhythmogenic effects. Like epinephrine, intraoperative use of norepinephrine should be reserved for the most severe cases only. Norepinephrine has been used in patients who devleop hypotension from loss of vasomotor tone as a consequence of spinal anesthesia or surgical sympathectomy, but other less hazardous vasopressor agents such as ephedrine and methoxamine are effective and should be used in preference to norepinephrine.[147]

Isoproterenol (Isuprel). Isoproterenol is almost a pure *beta*-adrenergic stimulant possessing both *beta* 1 and *beta* 2 stimulatory effects. Its bronchodilating effect makes it important as an aerosol mist in the treatment of asthma and other bronchoconstricting diseases.

The potent cardiac stimulatory action of isoproterenol is accompanied by peripheral vasodilation. Cardiac output is raised by an increase in the venous return to the heart, combined with the positive inotropic and chronotropic actions of the drug. The increase in cardiac output usually maintains systolic pressure, but mean arterial pressure may be reduced. Renal blood flow is elevated in patients in cardiogenic or septicemic shock, where intravascular volume is not reduced.[145,148] *Beta*-adrenergic stimulation increases AV conduction. Since isoproterenol is devoid of *alpha*-adrenergic stimulating activity, reflex bradycardia (more frequently observed with epinephrine and norepinephrine) does not occur. Thus isoproterenol is effective in treating atrioventricular heart block and for cardiac resuscitation, as well as in supporting the cardiovascular system during open heart operations.[145,149]

Isoproterenol is also helpful in treating cor pulmonale and pulmonary embolism.[150-152] The dysrhythmogenicity of isoproterenol is less than that of epinephrine or norepinephrine.[145,153]

Dobutamine (Dobutrex). Dobutamine acts directly on *beta*-receptors in the heart to produce a positive inotropic effect and to a lesser extent a positive chronotropic effect. Dobutamine has proved useful for direct cardiac stimulation during cardiogenic shock.[153a] In contrast to dopamine, dobutamine does not have an effect on the dopaminergic receptors in the renal vascular system and, therefore, does not produce renal vasodilation.[153b]

Terbutaline. Terbutaline is a moderately selective *beta* 2-agonist that possesses less pronounced cardiac stimulatory effects. It is a sympathomimetic agent administered orally or subcutaneously for the treatment of obstructive airway disease.

Dopamine (Intropin). Dopamine is the immediate precursor in the endogenous synthesis of norepinephrine in the body (see earlier discussion). Like other catecholamines, it exerts a positive inotropic action. Cardiac output is increased but there is little change in arterial blood pressure or heart rate. Peripheral vascular resistance is usually decreased. Dopamine produces mesenteric and renal vasodilation. Renal blood flow, glomerular filtration rate, urine flow, and sodium excretion are enhanced.[145,148,154–156]

The drug is less likely than other catecholamines to cause cardiac dysrhythmia or tachycardia, but these are dose-related phenomena, as tachycardia is not uncommon during open heart operations when dopamine is used to support the circulation.[153] Tachycardia is less likely to develop if dopamine is infused at a rate of less than 5 μg/kg/min.[155]

The advantage of dopamine over other catecholamines is its ability to maintain renal blood flow while providing a stimulatory effect on the myocardium. It is well known that renal perfusion is sacrificed during low-perfusion states in an attempt by the body to shunt more blood to the brain and the heart. Urinary output is thus an important monitor for assessing the adequacy of organ perfusion. Dopamine is commonly used for circulatory support and the treatment of shock.[140–145,157–159]

Noncatecholamines

Methoxamine (Vasoxyl) and Phenylephrine (Neo-Synephrine). Both sympathomimetic amines act directly on *alpha* receptors and are almost pure peripheral vasoconstrictor agents. They are devoid of cardiac stimulatory actions at the usual concentrations used to treat hypotension.[145,160,161] Reflex vagal bradycardia is common with both agents; therefore, these drugs are used clinically to relieve attacks of paroxysmal atrial tachycardia. Most vascular beds are constricted; renal, splanchnic, and cutaneous blood flows are reduced, but coronary blood flow may increase as the result of increased mean arterial pressure and increased coronary filling time (that is, reflex bradycardia). Cardiac dysrhythmias are infrequently observed during anesthesia. Large doses of phenylephrine given during halothane anesthesia produce ventricular dysrhythmias in dogs.[162] These drugs are useful for the temporary treatment of acute hypotension resulting from the discrepancy between intravascular volume and peripheral vascular capacitance.

Methoxamine and phenylephrine are useful for common clinical situations such as hypotension associated with spinal anesthesia;[147] controlled hypotension, which does not correct itself when the hypotensive agent (for example, nitroprusside or trimethaphan) has been removed; and low-perfusion pressure during cardiopulmonary bypass when there appears to be adequate intravascular volume.

Ephedrine. Ephedrine is an alkaloid occurring in various plants of the genus *Ephedra* and has been used in China for over 5,000 years. The Chinese herb containing ephedrine and called *Ma huang* (yellow astringent) was introduced into Western medicine by Chen and Schmidt in 1924.[163] These researchers reported the cardiovascular effects of the alkaloid and noted its similarities to epinephrine.

Ephedrine is a partially indirect-acting sympathomimetic amine that exerts its effects by the release of endogenous catecholamines from the adrenergic nerve terminals and the adrenal medulla. Some direct effect also exists.[145,164] Thus both *alpha-* and *beta-*adrenergic receptors are stimulated by ephedrine.

The cardiovascular stimulatory effects of ephedrine diminish with rapidly repeated doses. The mechanism of this tachyphylactic response is not clear, but the depletion of catecholamine stores is a factor. The drug usually elevates both systolic and diastolic pressures in man. Cardiac output is increased, provided there is adequate venous return to the heart.

Effects on renal circulation appear to be a dose-dependent phenomenon: at lower concentrations, *beta*-adrenergic effects are more prominent, wtih the result that renal blood flow is increased; whereas at high concentrations, *alpha*-adrenergic stimulation predominates and produces constriction of renal blood vessels.[145,165] Splanchnic circulation is reduced.

Placental blood flow is maintained by ephedrine in concentrations effective for supporting the maternal circulation, thus making this sympathomimetic drug the drug of choice in treating hypotension in the parturient patient.[166,167] One intravenous dose of ephedrine (10 to 25 mg) maintains an adequate pressure for seven to ten minutes, with little tendency to overshoot.

The effects of ephedrine on cardiac electrophysiology are complex. Local effects of the drug include an increase in the excitability of ventricular muscle that is manifested by ventricular tachycardia and fibrillation, and an increase in idioventricular rhythm.[168,169] However, in the anesthetized dog ephedrine prevents the atrial fibrillation induced by epinephrine and the ventricular fibrillation induced by an electrical current applied to the ventricle. Cardiac dysrhythmias have been demonstrated in the dog with halothane and ephedrine,[11] but no apparent problem is associated with the administration of ephedrine during methoxyflurane anesthesia.[170]

Metaraminol (Aramine). Metaraminol has both direct and indirect actions and overall effects similar to those of norepinephrine.[145] Its pressor action is of longer duration than its cardiac stimulant action; therefore, in man its *alpha*-adrenergic or pressor effects predominate.[171] Both systolic and diastolic pressures are elevated. Metaraminol increases venous tone and reduces cerebral blood flow. The effect of metaraminol on renal blood flow depends on the preexisting condition of the patient; for instance, it reduces renal blood flow in hypotensive individuals.[172] Pulmonary vasoconstriction results in elevated pulmonary blood pressure even when cardiac output is reduced.

Metaraminol depletes effectively nonepinephrine stores in adrenergic nerve terminals.[173] Consequently, its continuous infusion leads to reduced cardiovascular response. Furthermore, metaraminol is taken up by the adrenergic nerve terminal and acts as a false transmitter, although it is much less potent than endogenous catecholamines. Hypotension may result from the prolonged use of metaraminol.[173,174] It may be useful to think of metaraminol as a "potent ephedrine."

Mephentermine (Wyamine). Mephentermine is pharmacologically similar to ephedrine and metaraminol because it acts in part by releasing catecholamines. Hence it induces cardiac excitation, vasodilation, and vasoconstriction. The cardiac effects of mephentermine are more consistent than its vascular effects. Cardiac output is increased in normal subjects as well as in patients suffering from shock.[175,176] Systemic vascular resistance may increase, decrease, or remain unchanged. Coronary blood flow is usually increased as the result of increased blood pressure and local vasodilation.[177,178]

The responses of the renal and splanchnic circulations to intravenous mephentermine are variable. Cardiac dysrhythmias induced by halothane in man may be prevented by mephentermine,[162] which is less likely to produce renal vasoconstriction and cardiac dysrhythmias than other sympathomimetic amines that stimulate *alpha* and *beta* receptors. It also abolishes cardiac dysrhythmias induced by digitalis and myocardial infarction.[159,179] Thus the use of mephentermine has advantages over metaraminol in the treatment of hemorrhagic or cardiogenic shock.[177]

Anesthetic Management of Hypotension or Shock

Sympathomimetic agents should support the cardiovascular system until the cause of hypotension has been adequately treated. An accurate diagnosis of the cause of hypotension allows a more rational choice of drug therapy. It should be reemphasized that common causes of hypotension during anesthesia are excessive depth of anesthesia, hypoxia, intravascular loss, and surgical manipulation. The previous administration of drugs that interfere with endogenous catecholamine stores or metabolism of catecholamines can also affect the patient's tolerance to anesthetics and sympathomimetic amines. Careful monitoring and preparation are important to successful anesthetic management.

When a patient has hemorrhaged sufficiently to cause severe hypotension or shock, his defensive mechanisms shunt most of his remaining blood volume to the brain and heart; there is a concomitant increase in sympathetic tone with the release of norepinephrine, angiotensin, and vasopressin. To institute proper treatment, the anesthesiologist should monitor several physiologic parameters: direct arterial pressure, central venous pressure, urinary output, temperature, and ECG. The anesthesiologist should also make a repeated determination of hematocrit, blood gases, and osmolality of plasma and urine. Direct measurements of cardiac output with oxygen-transport calculations are becoming more common in this context. The use of a Swan-Ganz catheter in the pulmonary artery allows the sampling of mixed venous blood from which venous PO_2 or oxygen saturation can be determined.[180] A venous PO_2 of less than 30 mm Hg (normal—40) or a venous oxygen saturation of less than 60% (normal—75%) indicate a severe decrease in cardiac output and/or an increase in tissue extraction of oxygen.[181,182]

Mixed venous oxygen saturation is especially useful when acid-base disturbance is severe or when large quantities of stored bank blood with reduced 2,3-DPG (diphosphoglycerate) are transfused, because both alkalosis and a reduction of 2,3-DPG of red blood cells can decrease P-50 (that is, the PO_2 at which 50% of the hemoglobin is saturated).[181–183] Pulmonary shunt of 20 to 30% is not uncommon in the shocked patient. Frequent arterial blood-gas determinations, with an appropriate inspired concentration of oxygen to maintain the arterial PO_2 above 100 mm Hg, are desirable. Positive end-expiratory pressure is often necessary to improve the ventilation-perfusion ratio of the lungs in order to reduce pulmonary shunting.

The central venous pressure is used as an estimate of adequate intravascular volume replacement and right atrial filling pressure; 15 cm H_2O may be used as the upper limit of venous pressure. Pulmonary wedge pressure measured with a Swan-Ganz catheter is helpful when a filling pressure of 15 cm H_2O does not improve cardiac output or arterial pressure. Pulmonary wedge pressure can help to differentiate circulatory overload from the left ventricular failure.[180] The normal mean pulmonary capillary wedge pressure is 8 to 12 mm Hg.

Continuous urinary output monitoring from a catheter placed in the bladder is the most useful method of assessing organ perfusion.

The first and most important aspect of treating a patient in shock is intravascular volume replacement. Crystalloid solutions are helpful but should not be used singly, since redistribution of crystalloid solutions can produce excessive fluid in the interstitial space. Intravascular colloidal osmotic pressure should be maintained by the administration of albumin or plasma substitutes to minimize pulmonary edema. Whole blood should be administered without exceeding a hematocrit of 40%. Body temperature may decrease, necessitating the use of warm intravascular replacements. Hypothermia can reduce peripheral perfusion, potentiate cardiac dysrhythmias, produce acidosis, and depress the nervous system.[184] Hyperventilation leads to respiratory alkalosis (hypocapnia) and hypokalemia, which produce vasoconstriction (reduced perfusion) and irritable myocardium, respectively. Cardiac output can be increased with inotropic drugs. Dopamine, isoproterenol, and norepinephrine, chosen judiciously, may improve the efficiency and the distribution of perfusion. Large doses of glucocorticoids may be helpful.[185]

The ultimate choice of general anesthetic agents may not be important, since a patient in shock requires far less anesthetic than a normotensive one. The compatibility of the anesthetic chosen with the sympathomimetic agent used to support circulation is important. Unfortunately, there are little relevant published data. In general, sympathomimetic agents with greater *beta*-adrenergic activity are more dysrhythmogenic than agents with primarily *alpha*-adrenergic activity (Table 7–2), and the interaction of inhalation anesthetics that are ether derivatives is less dysrhythmogenic than that of inhalation anesthetics that are not ether derivatives. The use of narcotics as the primary anesthetic agent with O_2 supplemented by non-depolarizing muscle relaxants appears to have clinically minimal cardiovascular depressant effects. Potent sympathomimetic drugs should be administered in a dilute solution, with microdrip control to minimize overdosing as manifested by cardiac dysrhythmias or excessive hypertension.

Finally, special care should be exerted in the anesthetic management of the hypokalemic patient. Recent data suggest a causal relationship exists between hypokalemia from *beta* 2-receptor stimulation and exogenous epinephrine. Infusion of physiologic concentrations of epinephrine in human volunteers reduced plasma potassium by 0.82 mEq/L, but the hypokalemic response was antagonized by *beta* 2-receptor blockade.[186] In the dog, depletion of body potassium induced by lowering its serum concentration facilitate the ventricular tachycardia or fibrillation upon the intravenous infusion of epinephrine.[187] Furthermore, hypokalemic dogs have been shown to be more difficult to resuscitate than normokalemic dogs following asphyxia.[188]

Although it is generally believed that an elective surgical patient should go to surgery with plasma potassium concentration of at least 3.0 mEq/L,[189] there are no published data to substantiate this requirement. Patients who are digitalized and hypokalemic are prone to develop cardiac arrhythmias, especially in the presence of respiratory alkalosis.[189-192] A preliminary prospective study in surgical patients suggests that the incidence of dangerous cardiac arrhythmias in chronically hypokalemic patients is no different from that observed in normokalemic ones.[193] Thus, the question of what is a safe plasma potassium level before the patient may be anesthetized is still unsettled. Other factors should be considered. The rate and magnitude of potassium loss, the contemplated surgery and the physical status of the patient will help to decide when potassium therapy is appropriate.[189] Potassium therapy is not innocuous, since one in 200 patients receiving potassium may suffer a morbid or fatal episode of hyperkalemia.[193]

Hyperkalemia can also potentiate the arrhythmogenic effects of catecholamines. A disproportionate increase in serum potassium concentration with respect to intracellular potassium can inhibit repolarization of the cardiac cell. This cardiac effect is reflected on the ECG as an elevation of the T wave, a depression of the ST segment, and a prolongation of the PR interval. Further increases in serum potassium can lead to complete heart block and cardiac arrest. Important in enhancing catecholamine-induced dysrhythmias is vagal (cholinergic) stimulation, which suppresses the spontaneous depolarization of the sinoatrial node and of AV conduction (see earlier discussion). Hyperkalemia, then, mimics excessive cholinergic stimulation to the heart, allowing ventricular dysrhythmias to develop more readily. Direct-acting *alpha*-adrenergic stimulants are more desirable for managing the hyperkalemic, hypotensive patient (Table 7–2). Common causes of hyperkalemia in the operating room are (1) inappropriate exogenous intravenous replacement, (2) the administration of old blood that contains increased potassium concentration,[194,195] and (3) the use of succinylcholine in patients with severe burns, trauma, or spinal cord injury.[196-198]

The rational use of sympathomimetic agents for circulatory support is based on a proper appreciation of the pharmacology and pathophysiology of the sympathetic nervous system. Drugs that influence the normal adrenergic mechanisms must be considered in relation to possible interactions with certain general anesthetics. We took a simplified approach to the complex subject of low-flow state or shock and pointed out common problems that lead to circulatory failure. Optimal anesthetic management of the patient in shock requires recognition and treatment of the cause; temporary circulatory support can be provided by a properly chosen sympathomimetic agent in conjunction with a compatible anesthetic regimen.

REFERENCES

1. Hauswirth, O., and Schaer, H.: Effects of halothane on the sinoatrial node. J. Pharmacol. Exp. Ther., 158:36, 1967.
2. Atlee, J.L. III, and Rusy, B.F.: Halothane depression of A–V conduction studied by electrograms of the bundle of His in dogs. Anesthesiology, 36:112, 1972.
3. Biscoe, T.J., and Millar, R.A.: The effect of halothane on carotid sinus baroreceptor activity. J. Physiol. (Lond.), 173:24, 1964.
4. Price, H.L., Linde, H.W., and Morse, H.T.: Central nervous actions of halothane affecting the systemic circulation. Anesthesiology, 24:770, 1963.
5. Galindo, A., Wyte, S.R., and Wetherhold, J.W.: Junctional rhythm induced by halothane anesthesia—Treatment with succinylcholine. Anesthesiology, 37:261, 1972.
6. Reynolds, A.K., Chia, J.F., and Pasquet, A.F.: Halothane and methoxyflurane—A comparison of their effects on cardiac pacemaker fibers. Anesthesiology, 33:602, 1970.
7. Pick, A., and Langendorf, R.: Recent advances in the differential diagnosis of V–A junctional arrhythmias. Am. Heart J., 76:553, 1968.
8. Hamlin, R.L., and Smith, R.: Effects of vagal stimulation on S–A and A–V nodes. Am. J. Physiol., 215:560, 1968.
9. Russell, R., and Warner, H.R.: Effect of combined sympathetic and vagal stimulation on heart rate. Physiologist, 10:295, 1967.
10. Katz, R.L., Matteo, R.S., and Papper, E.M.: The injection of epinephrine during general anesthesia with halogenated hydrocarbons and cyclopropane in man. 2. Halothane. Anesthesiology, 23:597, 1962.
11. Takaori, M., and Loehning, R.W.: Ventricular arrhythmias during halothane anesthesia: Effect of isoproterenol, aminophylline and ephedrine. Can. Anaesth. Soc. J., 12:275, 1965.
12. Katz, J.H., and Bigger, T.: Cardiac arrhythmias during anesthesia and operation. Anesthesiology, 33:193, 1973.
13. Eisele, J.H., and Smith, N.T.: Cardiovascular effects of 40 percent nitrous oxide in man. Anesth. Analg. (Cleve.), 51:956, 1972.
14. Smith, N.T., et al.: The cardiovascular and sympathomimetic response to the addition of nitrous oxide to halothane in man. Anesthesiology, 32:410, 1970.
15. Smith, N.T., et al.: The cardiovascular responses to the addition of nitrous oxide to diethyl ether in man. Can. Anaesth. Soc. J., 19:42, 1972.
16. Wong, K.C., et al.: The cardiovascular effects of morphine sulfate with oxygen and with nitrous oxide in man. Anesthesiology, 38:542, 1973.
17. Smith, N.T., et al.: The cardiovascular responses to the addition of nitrous oxide to fluroxene in man. Br. J. Anaesth., 44:142, 1972.
17a. Puerto, B.A., Wong, K.C., et al.: Epinephrine-induced dysrhythmias: comparison during anaesthesia with narcotics and with halogenated inhalation agents in dogs. Can. Anaesth. Soc. J., 26:263, 1979.
17b. Liu, W.S., et al.: Epinephrine-induced arrhythmias during halothane anesthesia with the addition of nitrous oxide, nitrogen, or helium in dogs. Anesth. Analg., 61:414, 1982.
18. Axelrod, J.: The formation, metabolism, uptake and release of noradrenaline and adrenaline. In The Clinical Chemistry of Monoamines. Edited by H. Varley and A.H. Gawenlock. Amsterdam, Elsevier Publishing Co., 1963.
19. Blaschko, H., and Muscholl, E. (Eds.): Catecholamines. Vol. 33, Handbook of Experimental Pharmacology. Berlin, Springer-Verlag, 1972.
20. Axelrod, J.: Methylation reactions in the formation and metabolism of catecholamines and other biogenic amines: The enzyme conversion of norepinephrine (NE) to epinephrine (E). Pharmacol. Rev., 18:95, 1966.
21. Marley, E., and Blackwell, B.: Interactions of monoamine oxidase inhibitors, amines and foodstuff. Adv. Pharmacol. Chemother., 8:185, 1970.
22. Perks, E.R.: Monoamine oxidase inhibitors. Anesthesia, 19:376, 1964.
23. Rosen, M.R., Hoffman, B.F., and Andrew, L.W.: Electrophysiology and pharmacology of cardiac

arrhythmias. V. Cardiac antiarrhythmic effects of lidocaine. Am. Heart J., *89*:526, 1975.
24. Collinsworth, K.A., Kalman, S.M., and Harrison, D.C.: The clinical pharmacology of lidocaine as an antiarrhythmic drug. Circulation, *50*:1217, 1974.
25. Shand, D.G.: Propranolol. N. Engl. J. Med., *293*:280, 1975.
26. Nies, A.S., and Shand, D.G.: Clinical pharmacology of propranolol. Circulation, *52*:6, 1975.
27. Price, H.L.: Effect of carbon dioxide on the cardiovascular system. Anesthesiology, *21*:652, 1960.
28. Tenney, S.M., and Lamb, T.W.: Physiologic consequences of hypoventilation and hyperventilation. In Handbook of Physiology. Section 3, Respiration. Washington, D.C., American Physiology Society, 1965, Vol. II.
29. Gross, B.A., and Silver, I.A.: Central activation of the sympathetico-adrenal system by hypoxia and hypercapnia. J . Endocrinol., *24*:91, 1962.
30. Brunjes, S., Johns, V.J., and Crane, M.G.: Pheochromocytoma. N. Engl. J. Med., *262*:393, 1960.
31. Goldfien, A.: Pheochromocytoma: Diagnosis and anesthetic and surgical management. Anesthesiology, *24*:462, 1963.
32. Brewster, W.R., et al.: The hemodynamics and metabolic inter-relationships in the activity of epinephrine, norepinephrine and the thyroid hormones. Circulation, *13*:1, 1956.
33. Parsons, V., and Ramsey, I.: Thyroid and adrenal relationships. Postgrad. Med. J., *44*:377, 1969.
34. Murray, J.F., and Kelly, J.J.: The relation of thyroidal hormone level to epinephrine response: A diagnostic test for hyperthyroidism. Ann. Intern. Med., *51*:309, 1959.
35. Chidsey, C.A., Braunwald, E., and Morrow, A.G.: Catecholamine excretion and cardiac stores of norepinephrine in congestive heart failure. Am. J. Med., *39*:442, 1965.
36. Chidsey, C.A., et al.: Myocardial norepinephrine concentration in man. Effects of reserpine and of congestive heart failure. N. Engl. J. Med., *269*:653, 1963.
37. Braunwald, E.: The sympathetic nervous system in heart failure. Hosp. Pract., *5*:31, 1970.
38. Chidsey, C.A., and Braunwald, E.: Sympathetic activity and neurotransmitter depletion in congestive heart failure. Pharmacol. Rev., *18*:685, 1966.
39. Trendelenburg, U.: Supersensitivity and subsensitivity to sympathomimetic amines. Pharmacol. Rev., *15*:225, 1963.
40. Johnson, B., et al.: Autonomic hyperreflexia: A review. Milit. Med., *140*:345, 1975.
41. Morgan, R., and Cagan, E.J.: Acute alcoholic intoxication reaction and methyl alcohol intoxication. In The Biology of Alcoholism. Vol. 3, Clinical Pathology. Edited by B. Kissin and H. Begleiter. New York, Plenum Press, 1974.
42. Goldstein, M., et al.: Inhibition of dopamine *beta*-hydroxylase by disulfiram. Life Sci., *3*:763, 1964.
43. Goldstein, M., and Nakajima, K.: The effects of disulfiram on the repletion of brain catecholamine stores. Life Sci., *5*:1133, 1966.
43a.Diaz, J.H., and Hill, G.E.: Hypotension with anesthesia in disulfiram-treated patients. Anesthesiology, *51*:366, 1979.
44. Sellers, A.M., Itskovitz, H.D., and Lindauer, M.A.: Systemic arterial hypertension. In Cardiac and Vascular Diseases. Edited by H.L. Conn, Jr., and O. Horwitz. Philadelphia, Lea & Febiger, 1971. Vol. II.
45. Tyce, G.M., Sheps, S.G., and Frock, E.V.: Determination of urinary metabolites of catecholamines after the administration of methyldopa. Mayo Clin. Proc., *38*:571, 1963.
46. Onesti, G., et al.: Pharmacodynamics and clinical use of *alpha*-methyldopa in the treatment of essential hypertension. Am. J. Cardiol., *9*:863, 1962.
47. Onesti, G., et al.: Pharmacodynamic effects of *alpha*-methyldopa in hypertensive patients. Am. Heart J., *67*:32, 1964.
48. Dollery, C.T.: Methyldopa in the treatment of hypertension. Prog. Cardiovasc. Dis., *8*:278, 1965.
49. Weil, M.H., Barbour, B.H., and Chesne, R.B.: *Alpha*-methyldopa for the treatment of hypertension: Clinical and pharmacodynamic studies. Circulation, *28*:165, 1963.
50. Kalsner, S., and Nickerson, M.: Effects of reserpine on the disposition of sympathomimetic amines in vascular tissue. Br. J. Pharmacol., *35*:394, 1969.
51. Alper, M.H., Flacke, W., and Krayer, O.: Pharmacology of reserpine and its implications for anesthesia. Anesthesiology, *24*:524, 1963.
52. Sannerstedt, R., and Conway, J.: Hemodynamic and vascular responses to antihypertensive treatment with adrenergic blocking agents. A review. Am. Heart J., *79*:122, 1970.
53. Gaffney, T.E., Chidsey, C.A., and Braunwald, E.: Study of the relationship between the neurotransmitter store and adrenergic nerve block induced by reserpine and guanethidine. Circ. Res., *12*:264, 1963.
54. Ziegler, C.H., and Lovette, J.B.: Operative complications after therapy with reserpine and reserpine compounds. J.A.M.A., *176*:916, 1961.
55. Coakley, C.S., Alpert, S., and Boling, J.S.: Circulatory responses during anesthesia of patients on rauwolfia therapy. J.A.M.A., *161*:1143, 1956.
56. Naylor, W.G.: A direct effect of reserpine on ventricular contractility. J. Pharmacol. Exp. Ther., *139*:222, 1962.
57. Freedman, D.X., and Benton, A.J.: Persisting effects of reserpine in man. N. Engl. J. Med., *264*:529, 1961.
58. Dingle, H.R.: Antihypertensive drugs and anesthesia. Anaesthesia, *21*:151, 1966.
59. Munson, W.M., and Jenicek, J.A.: Effect of anesthetic agents on patients receiving reserpine therapy. Anesthesiology, *23*:741, 1962.
60. Katz, R.L., Weintraub, H.D., and Papper, E.M.: Anesthesia, surgery and rauwolfia. Anesthesiology, *25*:142, 1964.
61. Rocklin, D.B., Shohl, T., and Blakemore, W.S.:

Blood volume changes associated with essential hypertension. Surg. Gynecol. Obstet., *111*:569, 1960.
62. Finnerty, F.A., Bucholz, J.H., and Guillauden, R.L.: Blood volumes and plasma protein during levarterenol-induced hypertension. J. Clin. Invest., 37a:425, 1958.
63. Papper, E.M.: Selection and management of anaesthesia in those suffering from diseases and disorders of the heart. Can. Anaesth. Soc. J., *12*:245, 1965.
64. Ominsky, A.J., and Wollman, H.: Hazards of general anesthesia in the reserpinized patient. Anesthesiology, *30*:443, 1969.
65. Aviado, D.M.: Sympathomimetic drugs. Springfield, Ill., Charles C Thomas, 1970.
66. Zaimis, E.: Vasopressor drugs and catecholamines. Anesthesiology, *29*:732, 1968.
67. Rosenblum, R.: Physiologic basis for the therapeutic use of catecholamines. Am. Heart J., *87*:527, 1974.
68. Eger, E.I., and Hamilton, W.K.: The effect of reserpine on the action of various vasopressors. Anesthesiology, *20*:641, 1959.
69. Fries, E.D.: Guanethidine. Prog. Cardiovasc. Dis., *8*:183, 1965.
70. Page, I.H., Hurley, R.E., and Dustan, H.P.: The prolonged treatment of hypertension with guanethidine. J.A.M.A., *175*:543, 1961.
71. Fielden, R., and Green, A.L.: A comparative study of the noradrenaline-depleting and sympathetic-blocking action of guanethidine and (−)-β-hydroxy-phenethylquanidine. Br. J. Pharmacol. Chemother., *30*:155, 1967.
72. Mitchell, J.R., et al.: Guanethidine and related agents. III. Antagonism by drugs which inhibit the norepinephrine pump in man. J. Clin. Invest., *49*:1596, 1970.
73. Goodman, L.S., and Gilman, A.: The Pharmacological Basis of Therapeutics. 5th Edition. New York, Macmillan, 1975, p. 710.
74. Van Zwieten, P.A.: The central action of antihypertensive drugs medicated via central *alpha*-receptors. J. Pharm. Pharmacol., *25*:89, 1973.
75. Werner, U., Starke, K., and Schumann, H.J.: Actions of clonidine and 2-(2-methyl-6-ethyl-cyclohexylamino)-2-oxazoline on postganglionic autonomic nerves. Arch. Int. Pharmacodyn. Ther., *195*:282, 1972.
76. Hansson, L., et al.: Blood pressure crisis following withdrawal of clonidine (Catapres, Catapresan) with special reference to arterial and urinary catecholamine levels and suggestions for acute management. Am. Heart J., *85*:605, 1973.
77. Brodsky, J.D., and Bravo, J.J.: Acute postoperactive clonidine withdrawal syndrome. Anesthesiology, *44*:519, 1976.
77a.Bruce, D.L., et al.: Preoperative clonidine withdrawal syndrome. Anesthesiology, *51*:90, 1979.
78. Ahlquist, R.P.: A study of adrenotropic receptors. Am. J. Physiol., *153*:586, 1948.
79. Lands, A.M., Luduena, F.P., and Buzzo, H.J.: Differentiation of receptors responsive to isoproterenol. Life Sci., *6*:2241, 1967.
80. Levy, B., and Wilkenfield, B.E.: Selective interactions with *beta*-adrenergic receptors. Fed. Proc., *29*:1362, 1970.
81. Epstein, S.E., and Braunwald, E.: *Beta*-adrenergic receptors blocking drugs. Mechanism of action and clinical application. N. Engl. J. Med., *275*:1106, 1175, 1975.
82. Nies, A.S., Evans, G.H., and Shand, D.G.: Regional hemodynamic effects of *beta*-adrenergic blockade with propranolol in the unanesthetized primate. Am. Heart J., *85*:97, 1973.
83. Malcolm, J.: Adrenergic *beta*-receptor inhibition and hyperthyroidism. Acta Cardiol. (Brux.), *15*:320, 1972.
84. Shand, D.G., Nuckolls, E.M., and Oates, J.A.: Plasma propranolol levels in adults with observations in four children. Clin. Pharmacol. Ther., *11*:112, 1970.
85. Faulkner, S.L., et al.: Time required for complete recovery from chronic propranolol therapy. N. Engl. J. Med., *293*:280, 1975.
86. Nellen, M.: Withdrawal of propranolol and myocardial infarction. Lancet, *1*:558, 1973.
87. Diaz, R.G., et al.: Myocardial infarction after propranolol withdrawal. Am. Heart J., *88*:257, 1974.
88. Alderman, E.L., et al.: Coronary artery syndrome after sudden propranolol withdrawal. Ann. Intern. Med., *81*:625, 1974.
89. Kaplan, J.A., et al.: Propranolol and cardiac surgery: A problem for the anesthesiologist? Anesth. Analg. (Cleve.), *54*:571, 1975.
90. Eckenhoff, J.E., and Oech, S.R.: The effects of narcotics and antagonists upon respiration and circulation in man. Clin. Pharmacol. Ther., *1*:483, 1960.
91. Viljoen, J.F., Estafanous, F.G., and Kellner, G.A.: Propranolol and cardiac surgery. J. Thorac. Cardiovasc. Surg., *64*:826, 1972.
92. Graves, C.L., and Downs, N.H.: Cardiovascular and renal effects of enflurane in surgical patients. Anesth. Analg. (Cleve.), *53*:898, 1974.
93. Dobkin, A.B., et al.: Ethrane (compound 347) anesthesia: A clinical and laboratory review of 700 cases. Anesth. Analg. (Cleve.), *48*:477, 1969.
94. Shimosato, S., and Etsten, B.E.: Effect of anesthetic drugs on the heart: A critical review of myocardial contractility and its relationship to hemodynamics. Clin. Anesth., *3*:17, 1969.
94a.Fahmy, N.R., and Lappas, D.G.: Interaction of nifedipine, propranolol and halothane in humans. Anesthesiology, *59*:A39, 1983.
95. Goodman, L.S., and Gilman, A.: The Pharmacological Basis of Therapeutics. 5th edition. New York, Macmillan, 1975, p. 152.
96. Webster, R.A.: The antiadrenaline activity of some phenothiazine derivatives. Br. J. Pharmacol. Chemother., *25*:566, 1965.
97. Schou, M.: Lithium in psychiatric therapy and prophylaxis. J. Psychiatr. Res., *6*:67, 1968.
98. Goodman, L.S., and Gilman, A.: The Pharmacological Basis of Therapeutics. 5th Edition, New York, Macmillan, 1975, p. 791.
99. Borden, H., Clarke, M., and Katz, H.: The use of pancuronium bromides in patients receiving

lithium carbonate. Can. Anaesth. Soc. J., 21:79, 1974.
100. Hill, G.E., Wong, K.C., and Hodges, M.R.: Lithium carbonate and neuromuscular blocking agents. Anesthesiology, 46:122, 1977.
101. Goodman, L.S., and Gilman, A.: The Pharmacological Basis of Therapeutics. 5th Edition. New York, Macmillan, 1975, p. 180.
102. Goodman, L.S., and Gilman, A.: The Pharmacological basis of Therapeutics. 5th Edition. New York, Macmillan, 1975, p. 174.
102a. Palmer, H.: Potentiation of pethidine (correspondence). Br. Med. J., 2:944, 1960.
102b. Papp, C., and Benaim, S.: Toxic effects of iproniazid in a patient with angina. Br. Med. J., 2:1070, 1958.
102c. Shee, J.C.: Dangerous potentiation of pethidine by iproniazid and its treatment. Br. Med. J., 2:507, 1960.
102d. Jenkins, L.C., and Graves, H.B.: Potential hazards of psychoactive drugs in association with anaesthesia. Can. Anaesth. Soc. J., 12:121, 1965.
102e. Evans-Prosser, C.D.G.: The use of pethidine and morphine in the presence of monoamine oxidase inhibitors. Br. J. Anaesth., 40:279, 1968.
102f. Braverman, B., Ivankovich, M.D., and McCarthy, R.: The effects of fentanyl and vasopressors on anesthetized dogs receiving MAO inhibitors. Anesth. Analg. (In Press).
102g. Wong, K.C., et al.: Influence of imipramine and pargyline on the arrhythmogenicity of epinephrine during halothane, enflurane or methoxyflurane anesthesia in dogs. Life Sciences, 27:2675, 1980.
103. Klerman, G.L., and Cole, J.O.: Clinical pharmacology of imipramine and related antidepressant compounds. Pharmacol. Rev., 17:101, 1965.
104. Williams, R.B., and Sherter, C.: Cardiac complications of tricyclic antidepressant therapy. Ann. Intern. Med., 74:395, 1971.
105. Jenkins, L.C., and Graves, H.B.: Potential hazards of psychoactive drugs in association with anaesthesia. Can. Anaesth. Soc. J., 12:121, 1965.
106. Boaker, A.J., et al.: Interactions between sympathomimetic amines and antidepressant agents in man. Br. Med. J., 10:311, 1973.
106a. Edwards, R.P., et al.: Cardiac responses to imipramine and pancuronium during anesthesia with halothane or enflurane. Anesthesiology, 50:421, 1979.
106b. Johnston, R.R., Way, W.L., and Miller, R.D.: The effect of CNS catecholamine-depleting drugs on dextroamphetamine-induced elevation of halothane MAC. Anesthesiology, 41:57, 1974.
107. Koller, K.: Ueber die Vervendung des Conceins zur Anasthesirung. Auge. Wien. Med. Bul., 7:1352, 1884.
108. Adriani, J.: Appraisal of Current Concepts in Anesthesiology. St. Louis, C.V. Mosby Co., 1968, Vol. 4.
109. Anderton, J.M., and Nassar, W.Y.: Topical cocaine and general anaesthesia: An investigation of the efficacy and side effects of cocaine on the nasal mucosae. Anaesthesia, 30:809, 1975.
110. Goodman, L.S., and Gilman, A.: The Pharmacological Basis of Therapeutics, 5th Edition. New York, Macmillan, 1975, p. 386.
111. Oliver, G., and Schaefer, E.A.: The physiological effects of extracts of the suprarenal capsules. J. Physiol. (Lond.), 18:230, 1895.
112. Meek, W.J., Hathaway, H.R., and Orth, O.S.: The effects of ether, chloroform and cyclopropane on cardiac automaticity. J. Pharmacol. Exp. Ther., 61:240, 1937.
113. Munson, E.S., and Tucker, W.K.: Doses of epinephrine causing arrhythmia during enflurane, methoxyflurane and halothane anesthesia in dogs. Can. Anaesth. Soc. J., 22:495, 1975.
114. Tucker, W.K., Rackstein, A.D., and Munson, E.S.: Comparison of arrhythmic doses of adrenaline, metaraminol, epinephrine and phenylephrine during isoflurane and halothane anaesthesia in dogs. Br. J. Anaesth., 46:392, 1974.
115. Johnston, R.R., Eger, E.I. II, and Wilson, C.: A comparative interaction of epinephrine with enflurane, isoflurane and halothane in man. Anesth. Analg. (Cleve.), 55:709, 1976.
116. Joas, T.A., and Stevens, W.: Comparison of the arrhythmic doses of epinephrine during Forane, halothane and fluroxene anesthesia in dogs. Anesthesiology, 35:48, 1971.
117. Bamforth, B.J., et al.: Effect of epinephrine on the dog heart during methoxyflurane anesthesia. Anesthesiology, 22:169, 1961.
118. Wong, K.C., et al.: Antiarrhythmic effects of skeletal muscle relaxants. Anesthesiology, 34:458, 1971.
119. Dresel, P.E., MacCannell, K.L., and Nickerson, M.: Cardiac arrhythmias induced by minimal doses of epinephrine in cyclopropane-anesthetized dogs. Circ. Res., 8:948, 1960.
120. Wong, K.C., et al.: Deep hypothermia and ether anesthesia for open-heart surgery in infants—A clinical report of eight years' experience. Anesth. Analg. (Cleve.), 53:765, 1974.
121. This reference has been deleted.
122. Matteo, R.S., Katz, R.L., and Papper, E.M.: The injection of epinephrine during general anesthesia with halogenated hydrocarbons and cyclopropane in man. 3. Cyclopropane. Anesthesiology, 24:327, 1963.
123. Hudon, F.: Methoxyflurane. Can. Anaesth. Soc. J., 8:544, 1961.
124. Domino, E.F., Chodoff, P., and Corssen, G.: Pharmacologic effects of CI-581: A new dissociative anesthetic in man. J. Clin. Pharmacol. Ther., 6:279, 1965.
125. Corssen, G., and Domino, E.F.: Dissociative anesthesia. Anesth. Analg. (Cleve.), 45:29, 1966.
126. Wilson, R.D., et al.: Evaluation of CL-1848C: A new dissociative anesthetic in normal human volunteers. Anesth. Analg. (Cleve.), 49:236, 1970.
127. Traber, D.L., Wilson, R.D., and Priano, L.L.: Differentiation of the cardiovascular effects of CI-581. Anesth. Analg. (Cleve.), 47:769, 1968.
128. Traber, D.L., and Wilson, R.D.: Involvement of the sympathetic nervous system in the pressor response to ketamine. Anesth. Analg. (Cleve.), 48:248, 1969.

129. Traber, D.L., Wilson, R.D., and Priano, L.L.: Blockade of the hypertensive response to ketamine. Anesth. Analg. (Cleve.), 49:420, 1970.
130. Dowdy, E.G., and Kaya, K.: Studies of mechanism of cardiovascular response to CI-581. Anesthesiology, 29:931, 1968.
131. Slogoff, S., and Allen, G.W.: The role of baroreceptors in the cardiovascular response to ketamine. Anesth. Analg. (Cleve.), 53:704, 1974.
132. Nedegaard, O.: Cocaine-like effect of ketamine on vascular adrenergic neurons. Eur J Pharmacol., 23:152, 1973.
133. Miletick, D.J., et al.: The effect of ketamine on catecholamine metabolism in the isolated perfused rat heart. Anesthesiology, 39:271, 1973.
134. Kolhntop, D.E., Liao, J-C, and Van Bergen, F.H.: Effects on pharmacologic alterations of adrenergic mechanisms by cocaine, tropolone, aminophylline and ketamine on epinephrine-induced arrhythmias during halothane-nitrous oxide anesthesia. Anesthesiology, 46:83, 1977.
135. Hill, G.E., et al.: Interaction of ketamine with vasoactive amines at normothermia and hypothermia in the isolated rabbit heart. Anesthesiology, 48:315, 1978.
136. Chen, G.: Sympathomimetic anaesthetics. Can. Anaesth. Soc. J., 20:180, 1973.
137. Shires, G.T.: Principles in the management of shock. In Care of the Trauma Patient. New York, McGraw-Hill, 1966.
138. Altura, B.M.: Chemical and humoral regulation of blood flow through the precapillary sphincter. Microvasc. Res., 3:361, 1971.
139. Zweifach, B.W.: Functional Behavior of the Microcirculation. Springfield, Ill., Charles C Thomas, 1961.
140. Shepro, D., and Fulton, G.P. (Eds.): Microcirculation As Related to Shock (Symposium). New York, Academic Press, 1966.
141. Shoemaker, W.C.: Shock: Chemistry, Physiology and Therapy. Springfield, Ill., Charles C Thomas, 1967.
142. Hershey, S.G., and Altura, B.M.: Vasopressors and low-flow states. In Clinical Anesthesia. Edited by J.F. Artusio, Jr. Vol 10, Pharmacology of Adjuvant Drugs. Philadelphia, F.A. Davis, 1973.
143. Hardaway, R.M., III: Clinical Management of Shock: Surgical and Medical. Springfield, Ill., Charles C Thomas, 1968.
144. Nickerson, M.: Drug therapy of shock. In Shock: Pathogenesis and Therapy (Ciba Foundation Symposium). Edited by K.D. Bock. Berlin, Springer-Verlag, 1962.
144a. Langer, S.Z.: Pre-synaptic regulation of the release of catecholamines. Pharmacol. Rev., 32:337, 1980.
145. Aviado, D.M.: Sympathomimetic Drugs. Springfield, Ill., Charles C Thomas, 1970.
146. Dundee, J.W.: L-noradrenaline as vasoconstrictor. Br. Med. J., 1:547, 1952.
147. Bromage, P.R.: Vasopressors. Can. Anaesth. Soc. J., 7:310, 1960.
148. McNay, J.L., and Goldberg, L.I.: Comparison of the effects of dopamine, isoproterenol, norepinephrine and bradykinin on canine renal and femoral blood flow. J. Pharmacol. Exp. Ther., 151:23, 1966.
149. Redding, J.S., and Pearson, J.W.: Resuscitation from asphyxia. J.A.M.A., 182:283, 1962.
150. Halmagyi, D.F.J., et al.: Effect of isoproterenol in "severe" experimental lung embolism with and without post-embolic collapse. Am. Heart J., 65:208, 1963.
151. Halmagyi, D.F.J., Horner, F.J., and Starzecki, B.: Acute cor pulmonale and shock. Med. J. Aust., 2:143, 1965.
152. McDonald, I.G., et al.: Isoproterenol in massive pulmonary embolism: Haemodynamic and clinical effects. Med. J. Aust., 2:201, 1968.
153. Gilbert, J.L., et al.: Effects of vasoconstrictor agents on cardiac irritability. J. Pharmacol. Exp. Ther., 123:9, 1958.
153a. Tuttle, R.R., and Mills, J.: Dobutamine: Development of a new catecholamine to selectively increase cardiac contractility. Circulation Research, 36:185, 1975.
153b. Goldberg, L.I.: Newer catecholamines for treatment of heart failure and shock: an update on dopamine and a first look at dobutamine. Prog. Cardiovasc. Dis., 19:327, 1977.
154. Goldberg, L.I.: Dopamine—Clinical uses of an endogenous catecholamine. N. Engl. J. Med., 291:707, 1974.
155. Goldberg, L.I.: Cardiovascular and renal actions of dopamine: Potential clinical applications. Pharmacol. Rev., 24:1, 1974.
156. Allwood, M.J., Cobbold, A.F., and Gensburg, J.: Peripheral vascular effects of noradrenaline, isoproprylnoradrenaline and dopamine. Br. Med. Bull., 19:132, 1963.
157. Kuhn, L.A.: Shock in myocardial infarction—Medical treatment. Am. J. Cardiol., 26:578, 1970.
158. Bernstein, A., et al.: The treatment of shock accompanying myocardial infarction. Angiology, 14:559, 1963.
159. Bernstein, A., et al.: Treatment of shock in myocardial infarction. Am. J. Cardiol., 9:74, 1962.
160. Eckstein, J.W., and Abboud, F.M.: Circulatory effects of sympathomimetic amines. Am. Heart J., 63:119, 1962.
161. Schmid, P.G., Eckstein, J.W., and Abboud, F.M.: Comparison of the effects of several sympathomimetic amines on resistance and capacitance vessels in the forearm of man. Circulation (Suppl. 3), 34:3, 1966.
162. Catehacci, A.J., et al.: Serious arrhythmias with vasopressors during halothane anesthesia in man. J.A.M.A., 183:662, 1963.
163. Chen, K.K., and Schmidt, C.F.: The action of ephedrine, the active principle of the Chinese drug, Ma huang. J. Pharmacol. Exp. Ther., 24:339, 1924.
164. Zaimis, E.: Vasopressor drugs and catecholamines. Anesthesiology, 29:732, 1968.
165. Moyer, J.H., Morris, G., and Beazley, L.: Renal hemodynamic response to vasopressor agents in treatment of shock. Circulation, 12:96, 1955.
166. James, F.M., III, et al.: An evaluation of vasopressor therapy for maternal hypotension dur-

166. ing spinal anesthesia. Anesthesiology, 33:25, 1970.
167. Eng, M., et al.: The effects of methoxamine and ephedrine in normotensive pregnant primates. Anesthesiology, 35:354, 1971.
168. Seevers, M.H., and Meek, W.J.: The cardiac irregularities produced by ephedrine after digitalis. J. Pharmacol. Exp. Ther., 53:295, 1935.
169. Meek, W.J., and Seevers, M.H.: The cardiac irregularities produced by ephedrine and a protective action of sodium barbital. J. Pharmacol. Exp. Ther., 51:287, 1934.
170. Sphire, R.D.: Hypotension and other problems associated with methoxyflurane administration. Anesth. Analg. (Cleve.), 45:737, 1966.
171. Livesay, W.R., Moyer, J.H., and Chapman, D.W.: The cardiovascular and renal hemodynamic effects of aramine. Am. Heart J., 47:745, 1954.
172. Moyer, J.H., Morris, G., and Snyder, H.: A comparison of cerebral hemodynamics response to aramine and norepinephrine in the normotensive and hypotensive subjects. Circulation, 10:265, 1954.
173. Shore, P.A.: The mechanism of norepinephrine depletion by reserpine, metaraminol and related agents. The role of monoamine oxidase. Pharmacol. Rev., 18:561, 1966.
174. Crout, J.R., et al.: The antihypertensive action of metaraminol in man. Clin. Res., 13:204, 1965.
175. Udhoji, V.M., and Weil, M.H.: Vasodilator action of a pressor amine mephentermine in circulatory shock. Am. J. Cardiol., 16:841, 1965.
176. Andersen, T.W., and Gravenstein, J.S.: Mephentermine and ephedrine in man. A comparison study on cardiovascular effects. Clin. Pharmacol. Ther., 5:281, 1964.
177. Brofman, B.L., Hellerstein, H.K., and Caskey, W.H.: Mephentermine—An effective pressor amine. Am. Heart J., 44:396, 1952.
178. Welch, G.H., et al.: The effect of mephentermine sulfate on myocardial oxygen consumption, myocardial efficiency and peripheral vascular resistance. Am. J. Med., 24:871, 1958.
179. Regan, T.J., et al.: Sympathomimetics as antagonists of strophanthidin's ionic and arrhythmic effects. Circ. Res., 11:17, 1962.
180. Swan, H.J.C., and Ganz, W.: Use of balloon flotation catheters in critically ill patients. Surg. Clin. North Am., 55:501, 1975.
181. Martin, W.E., et al.: Continuous monitoring of mixed venous oxygen saturation in man. Anesth. Analg. (Cleve.), 52:784, 1973.
182. Stanley, T.H., and Isern-Amaral, J.: Periodic analysis of mixed venous oxygen tension to monitor the adequacy of perfusion during and after cardiopulmonary bypass. Can. Anaesth. Soc. J., 21:454, 1974.
183. Scheinman, M.M., Brown, M.A., and Rappaport, E.: Critical assessment of use of central venous oxygen saturation as a mirror of mixed venous oxygen in severely ill cardiac patients. Circulation, 40:165, 1969.
184. Wong, K.C.: Physiology and pharmacology of hypothermia. West. J. Med., 138(2):227, 1983.
185. Antonaccio, M.J.: Cardiovascular pharmcology. New York, Raven Press, 1977.
186. Brown, M.J., Brown, D.C., and Murphy, M.B.: Hypokalemia from beta$_2$-receptor stimulation by circulating epinephrine. New Engl. J. Med., 309:1414, 1983.
187. Wong, K.C., et al.: Chronic hypokalemia on epinephrine-induced dysrhythmias during halothane, enflurane, or methoxyflurane with nitrous oxide anesthesia in dogs. Anaesth. Sinica, 21:139, 1983.
188. Wong, K.C., Port, J.D., and Steffins, J.: Cardiovascular responses to asphyxial challenge in chronically hypokalemic dogs. Anesth. Analg., 62:991, 1983.
189. Wong, K.C., and Vitez, T.S.: Electrolyte imbalance. Seminars in Anesthesia 2(3):161, 1983.
190. Wright, B.D., and DiGiovanni, A.J.: Respiratory alkalosis, hypokalemia and repeated ventricular fibrillation associated with mechanical ventilation. Anesth. Analg. (Cleve.), 48:467, 1969.
191. Lawson, N.W., Butler, G.H., and Rat, C.T.: Alkalosis and cardiac arrhythmias. Anesth. Analg., 52:951, 1973.
192. Surawicz, B., and Gettes, L.S.: Effect of electrolyte abnormalities on the heart and circulation. In Cardiac and Vascular Diseases. Edited by H.L. Conn, Jr., and O. Horwitz. Philadelphia, Lea & Febiger, 1971.
193. Vitez, T.S., Soper, L.E., and Soper, P.B.: Chronic hypokalemia does not increase anesthetic dysrhythmias. Anesth. Analg., 61:221, 1982.
194. Burke, G.R., and Gulyassy, P.F.: Surgery in the patient with renal disease and related electrolyte disorders. Med. Clin. North Am., 63:1191, 1979.
195. Miller, R.D.: Complications of massive blood transfusions. Anesthesiology, 39:82, 1973.
196. Bunker, J.P.: Metabolic effects of blood transfusion. Anesthesiology, 27:446, 1966.
197. Tolmic, J.D., Joyce, T.H., and Mitchell, G.D.: Succinylcholine danger in the burned patient. Anesthesiology, 28:467, 1967.
198. Mazze, R.I., Escue, H.M., and Houston, J.B.: Hyperkalemia and cardiovascular collapse following administration of succinylcholine to traumatized patient. Anesthesiology, 31:540, 1969.
199. Tobey, R.E.: Paraplegia, succinylcholine and cardiac arrest. Anesthesiology, 32:359, 1970.

We express deep appreciation for the technical aid of Ms. Vicky Larsen in preparing this manuscript.

| 8 |

ANTIBRONCHOSPASTIC DRUGS

HARRY G.G. KINGSTON, HALL DOWNES, and CAROL A. HIRSHMAN

Asthma is the name given to a group of diseases characterized by reversible airway obstruction, which subsides either spontaneously or in response to drug therapy. This airway obstruction results from a combination of mucosal edema, secretions in the airway and bronchial smooth muscle constriction. Three major groups of drugs are used to treat asthma: Theophylline and similar agents, *beta* 2-sympathomimetics and steroids. The therapeutic range for both theophyllines and sympathomimetics is narrow. Toxic effects on the cardiovascular and nervous systems may be enhanced by drugs in common use in anesthetic practice. The following two case reports from the anesthetic literature are examples of interactions important to the anesthesiologist in the operating room.

CASE REPORT[*1]

A 65-kg, 57-year-old housewife was admitted for bronchoscopy and open lung biopsy of one of three right middle lobe pulmonary nodules, 10 years after radical mastectomy for adenocarcinoma involving her right breast and at least one axillary lymph node. Past medical history revealed episodic shortness of breath about every 6 months over the last 20 years. The episodes were characterized by wheezing, were often related to exposure to cats, dust, furnace cleaning or horseriding, and were usually improved on leaving the farm or by subcutaneous epinephrine administration in a local emergency room. She had never been hospitalized for asthma, nor did she have symptoms or signs suggestive of angina, myocardial ischemia, or congestive cardiac failure. She was anesthetized three times previously, each time her anesthesiologist told her she 'went too deep' with thiopental and advised her not to receive it again. She knew of no history of asthma during or following anesthesia.

Pulmonary function tests on admission demonstrated a decreased vital capacity (2.8L predicted, 2.5L actual), increased residual volume (1.7L predicted, 2.8 L actual), and decreased FEV_1 (70% of actual vital capacity). These values did not improve after inhalation of 0.5% isoproterenol. Nevertheless, an infusion of 40 mg/hr of aminophylline was begun. Five hours later, with the infusion still at 40 mg/hr, the preoperative evaluation was made by the anesthesiologist. Physical examination was unremarkable except for a right radical mastectomy scar. Her chest was clear. Blood pressure lying and standing was 130/80 mm Hg, with a pulse rate of approximately 88. Jugular venous pressure (estimated by neck vein examination) was 4 cm H_2O. Laboratory data included a normal ECG, a hematocrit of 35.2%, normal electrolytes and blood urea nitrogen, an arterial PO_2 of 71 mm Hg while the patient was breathing room air, with a PCO_2 of 36 mm Hg and pH of 7.44.

The potential of an interaction between aminophylline and anesthetic agents was discussed with the pulmonary consultant and it was agreed to stop the aminophylline infusion 2 hours prior to the patient's scheduled arrival in the operating room. In addition, the pulmonary consultant ordered a blood sample drawn for serum aminophylline concentration. After the blood was drawn (but before the result was available), he increased the aminophylline infusion to 55 mg/hr. Three hours before induction of anesthesia the patient ingested 15 mg of diazepam. Anesthesia was induced using a mask and 3L/min of N_2O 2L/min of O_2 with gradually increasing concentrations of halothane, while

---

*By permission from Roizen, M.F., and Stevens, W.: Multiform ventricular tachycardia due to the interaction of aminophylline and halothane. Anesth. Analg., 57:738, 1978.

ECG and arterial pressure were monitored continuously. When the inspired halothane concentration reached 2%, ventilation was controlled. Her blood pressure remained 160/90 mm Hg as it was on her arrival in the operating room. Five minutes after induction at the time when the inspired halothane concentration had been 2.5% for approximately 1½ minutes, multiform ventricular tachycardia developed with a rate of 160 to 170 beats per minute. Blood pressure fell to 110/60 mm Hg. Ventilation was controlled with 1.5% halothane and 98.5% oxygen. We gave 100 mg of lidocaine IV and drew a sample of arterial blood. One and one-half minutes later, cardiac rhythm returned to normal sinus rate and her blood pressure to 130/80. Operation and subsequent hospital course were otherwise uneventful. Arterial gases at the start of the multiform ventricular tachycardia were PO_2 102 mm Hg, PCO_2 27 mm Hg and pH 7.41. A 12-lead ECG obtained in the recovery room showed no change from the control record obtained before anesthesia. Subsequently, the laboratory reported the preoperative plasma aminophylline level drawn while the patient was receiving 40 mg/hr of aminophylline to be 21 μg/ml (therapeutic level 10 to 20 μg/ml).

This case serves to illustrate the potential cardiovascular toxicity of a halothane-theophylline interaction. The serum theophylline level during anesthesia is unknown since the theophylline infusion rate had been increased from 40 to 55 mg/h (after the blood sample for theophylline level had been drawn) and subsequently discontinued 2 to 2.5 hours before induction. Although it is possible that the serum theophylline level could have slightly exceeded the therapeutic range, ventricular tachycardia did not begin until 5 minutes after the administration of halothane.

CASE REPORT[*,2]

A 50-year-old, 50-kg woman was scheduled for a vocal cord stripping because of the development of hoarseness over a 3-month period. She had a history of alcohol abuse and chronic obstructive pulmonary disease with a marked bronchospastic component, for which she was being treated with 300 mg qid of a long-acting theophylline preparation. The patient denied a history of seizures. Four previous general anesthetic procedures had been uncomplicated. Physical examination was unremarkable. Preoperative laboratory tests were normal.

---
[*]Adapted with permission from Hirshman, C., et al.: Ketamine-aminophylline-induced decrease in seizure threshold. Anesthesiology, 56:464, 1982.

Ninety minutes before surgery, an IV infusion of aminophylline (1 mg·kg⁻¹·h⁻¹) was started to which a premedicant dose of diazepam 5 mg IM was added. Ketamine, 100 mg, was given IV over a 2-minute period for induction of anesthesia. With the patient breathing spontaneously, 1.5% halothane in oxygen was started. The patient developed random eye and limb movements. Approximately 2 to 3 minutes later, the patient became impossible to ventilate and developed a heart rate of 200 beats/min. Extensor spasm and opisthotonic posturing of the extremities, neck, and jaw ensued. Succinylcholine, 80 mg, was administered. Halothane was discontinued because of multifocal premature ventricular contractions (PVCs) and runs of ventricular tachycardia. The extensor seizures ceased. Ventilation via a mask became possible and intubation of the trachea was accomplished without difficulty. No wheezing was audible. Within minutes, ventilation again became impossible and the extensor spasm returned. Pancuronium 3 mg, IV, was given to facilitate controlled ventilation. Cardiac abnormalities continued despite 7.5 mg diazepam and 100 mg lidocaine. With continuous chest auscultation, 0.75 mg propranolol was given over a 5-minute period, at which time heart rate decreased from 180 to 120 beats per minute and PVCs resolved. Blood gases at this time were normal. The serum theophylline level was 19 μg/ml (therapeutic level 10 to 20 μg/ml). Surgery was cancelled. The patient was transferred to the recovery room and mechanically ventilated. The patient was alert and the trachea was extubated without problems 2 hours later.

This case demonstrates the occurrence of both ventricular tachydysrhythmias and generalized sezures at normally therapeutic levels of theophylline during ketamine-halothane anesthesia.

THEOPHYLLINE

Preparations

Theophylline is a methylxanthine derivative closely related to caffeine and theobromine. Since the water solubility of theophylline is low, concentrated aqueous solutions for IV use are usually prepared by compounding theophylline with a pharmacologically inactive base such as ethylenediamine, salicylate, choline or glycinate (Table 8–1). Similar compounds are also available as tablets for oral use, although theophylline itself is rapidly and completely absorbed from the gastrointestinal tract. Aminophylline contains 2 molecules of theophylline to one of ethylenediamine,

Table 8-1
Common Theophylline Preparations

Base	Generic Name
Ethylenediamine	aminophylline
Calcium salicylate	theophylline calcium salicylate
Choline	oxytryphylline
Sodium glycinate	theophylline sodium glycinate

The content of theophylline in these compounds differs widely and should be checked prior to anesthesia when a patient is receiving one of these compounds.

75 to 85% of the total dose being anhydrous theophylline.[3] Although other bases are employed to prepare water soluble theophylline compounds, theophylline alone is available in the anhydrous form or as the mono- and dihydrates. Since therapeutic plasma levels refer to *anhydrous* theophylline, it is important to recognize that the content of anhydrous theophylline in commercially available preparations varies from 48 to 100%,[4] and that appropriate adjustments in dose need be made.

Substitution of polar functional groups on the N-7 position in theophylline results in a number of theophylline congeners that are usually more water soluble and also less potent. An example of this is dyphylline, or 7-(2,3-dihydroxypropyl) theophylline. These congeners, which are chemically distinct from theophylline, do not share the same dose-response characteristics as theophylline. Their therapeutic and toxic levels are unknown. Furthermore, laboratory methods currently used to monitor serum theophylline levels do not detect the presence of these chemically distinct analogs.

Mechanism of Action

The mechanism of action of theophylline has been traditionally attributed to inhibition of phosphodiesterase with a resulting increase in intracellular levels of cAMP. This action, however, is pronounced only at high drug concentrations, and may not be the major component of its pharmacologic effect.[5,6] Other mechanisms that may contribute to the clinical effects of theophylline include altered intracellular calcium fluxes,[7] increased binding of cAMP to its specific binding protein,[8] release of endogenous catecholamines,[9,10] and antagonism of adenosine[11] or prostaglandins.[12]

Therapeutic and Toxic Effects

The principal therapeutic effects of theophylline are bronchodilation for the treatment of asthma and respiratory stimulation for the treatment of apnea in preterm infants. In addition, theophylline is useful in the treatment of pulmonary edema, although the physiologic mechanisms involved are poorly understood. Respiratory stimulation in preterm infants is produced at lower plasma levels (3 to 5 mg/L)[13] than bronchodilation in adult asthmatics (5 mg/L), and as the serum level is increased above 20 mg/L, toxic effects become more frequent.[14-16] In the range of 5 to 20 mg/L, the degree of bronchodilation increases progressively in proportion to the log of the serum level,[17] hence the efficacy of theophylline as a bronchodilator in asthmatics may be limited by toxicity rather than by a ceiling effect. The usual therapeutic range is between 10 and 20 mg/L, but the intensity of bronchodilation is significantly greater at the upper border of this range than at the lower.[18] On the other hand, while toxicity is uncommon at theophylline levels between 15 and 20 mg/L and is virtually absent at levels below 15 mg/L,[15] at levels above 25 mg/L, 75% of patients show evidence of toxicity.[15]

Theophylline, like caffeine, produces central nervous system stimulation, and is classified appropriately as an analeptic agent. This action, which has been attributed to an antagonism of the inhibitory effects of adenosine,[11] is therapeutically useful for respiratory stimulation, but may also induce seizures, which are associated with a significant mortality.[14] In the absence of other drugs, theophylline-induced seizures usually indicate high blood levels, with an average value around 50 mg/L.[14] However, it is important to recognize that minor symptoms of toxicity do not necessarily precede frank seizures,[14] and that monitoring of serum theophylline levels is the only reliable method of assessing the risk of theophylline toxicity.

Nausea and vomiting are common complications of therapy with theophylline, whether administered orally or intravenously.[19] When administered orally, part of its emetic effect reflects gastric irritation; but theophylline also directly stimulates central emetic mechanisms. When the drug is given IV, nausea and vomiting represent early signs of toxicity, and occur at blood levels slightly above the therapeutic range. The absence of a significant emetic effect cannot be taken as evidence of nontoxic blood levels.

Theophylline has positive inotropic and chronotropic effects on the myocardium,[20,21] and in addition releases catecholamines from endogenous stores[9,10] and increases circulating levels of catecholamines.[22] Since theophylline is also a vasodilator, these cardiac stimulant effects may not be accompanied by an increase in blood pressure. Tachycardia and ventricular dysrhythmias are common adverse effects signifying toxic blood levels.[15,16] In addition, rapid IV injection of theophylline can cause hypotension; direct injection into central venous catheters is particularly likely to produce such effects.

Allergy to theophylline preparations containing ethylenediamine has been reported to induce urticaria and dermatitis.[23]

Pharmacokinetics. Although theophylline is well absorbed from the gastrointestinal tract, oral preparations show substantial variation in bioavailability. The use of enteric-coated preparations in particular results in unpredictable and incomplete absorption. This is also true of rectal suppositories, which are often employed when vomiting interferes with oral medication. In the latter circumstance, the physician should maintain a high index of suspicion since vomiting may be an early sign of theophylline toxicity.

The apparent volume of distribution of theophylline is equivalent to about half of body weight,[23] so that for each mg/kg of dose, serum theophylline levels increase by 2 mg/L. Since the apparent volume of distribution varies among individuals, the initial loading dose is calculated to enter the low-end of the therapeutic range. The loading dose recommended by Mitenko and Ogilvie,[17] 4.5 mg/kg of theophylline (5.6 mg/kg of aminophylline) given over 20 minutes, would produce a serum theophylline concentration of 9 mg/L if the apparent volume of distribution was exactly 50% of body weight, and 15 mg/L if the volume of distribution was only 30% of body weight. Theophylline is 60% protein-bound. Reduced protein binding increases the volume of distribution in patients with hepatic disease, in the elderly and in premature infants. To check the adequacy of this initial dose, a blood sample can be drawn 30 minutes after injection, when the distribution phase is largely completed.[23]

Theophylline is metabolized by the liver to 1,3-dimethyl uric acid and 1-methyl uric acid, both relatively inactive compounds, and to 3-methylxanthine, which is half as potent a bronchodilator as theophylline. Elimination of theophylline depends principally upon hepatic microsomal metabolism rather than renal excretion, and most pharmacokinetic interactions involving theophylline, whether drug-drug interactions or drug-disease interactions, are based on an altered hepatic metabolism.[23-25] The metabolism of theophylline is highly variable among individuals and is readily influenced by medications and environmental or dietary factors (Table 8–2). The mean half-life of theophylline is about 8 hours in healthy, nonsmoking adults, but is reduced by half in smokers and is more than doubled in patients with severe liver disease or pulmonary edema. In children, from 6 months to teenage, the mean half-life is about half that seen in the healthy,

Table 8-2
Theophylline Elimination[23]

Increased Clearance	Decreased Clearance
Cigarette smokers	Elderly
Marijuana abusers	Newborn infants
High protein, low carbo- hydrate diet	Cirrhosis and cholestasis Cardiac failure
Charcoal broiled beef	Viral respiratory disease
Drug interactions	Drug interactions

non-smoking adult; however, neonates and especially premature neonates metabolize theophylline slowly.[26] In addition, 50% of the drug in neonates is excreted unchanged in the urine and a significant proportion is converted to caffeine. This has diagnostic significance when the toxic effects of theophylline appear to be present even though serum levels are within the accepted therapeutic range.[23]

To appreciate the clinical significance of these differences, it is important to recognize that the steady-state serum level is directly proportional to the elimination half-life. Therefore, if the half-life is doubled, the eventual steady-state serum level will also double. Since the therapeutic range for serum theophylline levels is narrow, failure to consider differences in theophylline elimination will lead to a considerable incidence of drug toxicity.

Early studies by Mitenko and Ogilvie[17] indicated that a constant IV infusion of theophylline of 0.72 mg/kg/h (0.9 mg/kg/h of aminophylline) following the loading dose would maintain the serum theophylline concentration in the therapeutic range. This infusion rate, however, produces excessively high serum levels in patients who metabolize theophylline more slowly than "normal," and more recent studies[27,28] have proposed slower infusion rates for many groups of patients. The uncertainty surrounding theophylline half-life in a particular patient emphasizes the importance of serum theophylline determinations in adjusting theophylline dose.

From the standpoint of preoperative evaluation, a serum theophylline level should reflect a reasonably steady-state situation, and may be misleading if the theophylline dose has been recently changed. When a new maintenance infusion rate is begun, it takes one half-life for the serum level to change half way from the old to the new steady state. Therefore, a preoperative sample obtained an hour after an increase in the theophylline infusion rate will provide a poor guide to the probable level during anesthesia on the following day.

Drug Interactions. Drug interactions involving theophylline are common and can involve both pharmacokinetic and pharmacodynamic factors. Significant pharmacokinetic interactions usually are based on induction or inhibition of drug metabolism. For the anesthesiologist it is appropriate to consider drug interactions under two headings: (1) Interactions with drugs commonly used in the preoperative and postoperative management of surgical patients and (2) interactions with drugs used during the course of anesthesia. Since there are excellent up-to-date reviews[23,25] of drug interactions involving theophylline, the following section will only consider a few drugs that are commonly employed in the perioperative period and that can have a marked effect on theophylline metabolism.

A. *Drugs used in the pre- and postoperative period*

 1. *Cimetidine* slows elimination of a variety of drugs by directly inhibiting microsomal drug metabolizing enzymes, and by reducing hepatic blood flow. Cimetidine markedly slows the elimination of theophylline[29,30] and produces about a two-fold increase in steady-state serum theophylline levels.[31,32] Furthermore, a significant decrease in the elimination of theophylline is apparent within 1 day from the institution of therapy with cimetidine.[30] Since cimetidine is one of the

most common prescription drugs, and may be ordered as part of the preanesthetic medication, cimetidine-theophylline interactions are particularly important to the anesthesiologist. The new H_2 antagonist, ranitidine, does not appear to affect the metabolism of theophylline.[33]

2. *Macrolide antibiotics:* Troleandomycin, and to a lesser extent erythromycin, retard the elimination of theophylline. However, since erythromycin must be administered for several days to significantly impair theophylline clearance,[34] there is no evidence to suggest that initiation of therapy in the immediate preoperative period will affect theophylline levels during the course of anesthesia.

3. *Propranolol:* Although propranolol is usually avoided in known asthmatics, it can, like cimetidine, markedly decrease theophylline clearance within the first day of therapy.[35]

4. *Phenytoin:* In contrast to the preceding drugs, phenytoin administered for 10 to 15 days markedly shortens the half-life of theophylline[36] and requires an increase in theophylline dose. Sustained administration of anticonvulsant doses of phenobarbital can also decrease theophylline half-life, although the effect is less pronounced.[37]

B. *Drugs Used Intraoperatively*

The effect of anesthetic drugs on theophylline disposition has rarely been studied in humans, and our limited knowledge is derived from experimental animals only.[38,39] In the only study comparing theophylline disposition in awake and anesthetized dogs,[39] induction of anesthesia with halothane or enflurane immediately following a brief infusion of theophylline produced a slight prolongation of the distribution phase without any significant difference in the elimination phase—as sampled for 32 minutes. Conversely, the aminophylline infusion did not affect the uptake of halothane or enflurane. However, an investigation interval longer than 32 minutes, as well as human studies, are needed before any firm conclusions can be reached as to the effect of anesthetics on the clinical pharmacokinetics of theophylline.

In contrast to the nearly complete absence of information on pharmacokinetic interactions between theophylline and drugs used during anesthesia, pharmacodynamic interactions have been reported frequently in the clinical literature or studies in animal experiments. Such interactions involve ketamine, inhalational anesthetics and the neuromuscular blocking agents.

1. *Ketamine*

Ketamine has been recommended for induction of anesthesia in asthmatics[40] on the basis of early clinical studies. More recently, in a dog model of asthma, ketamine was shown to be superior to thiopental in preventing antigen-induced increases in airway resistance.[41] This effect was chiefly attributable to sympathomimetic action, since it was prevented by pretreatment with propranolol. The sympathomimetic actions of ketamine probably reflect both central nervous system stimulation[42] and decreased re-uptake by peripheral adrenergic terminals.[43,44] Although induction of anesthesia with ketamine may be associated with increased levels of catecholamines,[45,46] the effects of ketamine on cardiac rhythm are controversial,[47] and experimental studies have suggested both sensitization to catecholamines and antidysrhythmic effects. In dogs receiving IV theophylline, subsequent injection of ketamine did not produce dysrhythmias even when the serum level of theophylline was in the toxic range.[48]

However, as discussed in the second case report, in patients receiving theophylline, induction of anesthesia with ketamine can result in seizures. While high doses of theophylline in human subjects can elicit seizures, studies in mice have demonstrated that ketamine and aminophylline, which individually did not lower the electroshock seizure threshold, caused a significant reduction in seizure threshold when administered together.[2] Thus, in asthmatic patients receiving aminophylline, either ketamine should be avoided or antiseizure medication should be included in the premedication to avoid precipitation of seizures.

2. *Inhaled Anesthetics*

Even prior to anesthesia, theophylline can elicit potentially fatal tachydysrhythmias.[16,49] In addition, methylxanthines cause release of endogenous catecholamines,[9,10] which may subsequently interact with commonly used inhaled agents. Since halothane is often recommended as an agent of choice for the anesthetic management of asthmatic patients[50,51] and is known to sensitize the heart to catecholamine-induced dysrhythmias,[52] potentially dangerous dysrhythmias may occur in the asthmatic patient because of an interaction between theophylline and halothane.[1,53]

In dogs, administration of aminophylline *after* induction of halothane anesthesia did not produce dysrhythmias, provided that the serum theophylline levels did not exceed the therapeutic range of 10 to 20 μg/ml;[54] higher levels of aminophylline, however, caused ventricular dysrhythmias. Our first case report demonstrates that ventricular dysrhythmias can occur during halothane anesthesia in man at serum theophylline levels only slightly above the therapeutic range, and should emphasize the importance of monitoring and stabilizing theophylline levels in the preoperative period.

Studies of halothane-theophylline interaction in dogs suggest that the following circumstances are especially likely to be associated with serious dysrhythmias:

a. High doses and serum levels of theophylline[54]

b. Light rather than deep anesthesia with halothane[55]

c. A fast heart rate[56]

d. Administration of ephedrine[53,57]

e. Induction of anesthesia *immediately following* IV injection of a loading dose of theophylline, even though plasma serum levels are within the therapeutic range.[56]

The last two circumstances, in particular, suggest that many halothane-theophylline interactions are actually halothane-theophylline-epinephrine interactions, since both ephedrine and an IV loading dose of theophylline are known to release endogenous catecholamines.

When enflurane[58] and isoflurane[59] were tested in dogs under the same conditions employed to study halothane-theophylline interactions, induction of anesthesia immediately following large doses of intravenous theophylline did not produce dysrhythmias, even though the highest theophylline dose produced a mean peak serum level of 93 mg/L. This is in agreement with previous studies of epinephrine-induced dysrhythmias which showed that substantially higher doses of epinephrine were required to produce dysrhythmias during enflurane or isoflurane anesthesia than during halothane anesthesia.[60,62]

In summary, to reduce the likelihood of dysrhythmias during anesthesia in patients receiving theophylline, a serum theophylline level should be measured in the preoperative period. This level should reflect a steady-state blood level resulting from a previously established dosage regimen, rather than the rapidly changing serum levels that follow an initial IV loading dose or a constant infusion that has been recently started or changed in rate. If the serum levels are within the therapeutic range, halothane represents an acceptable inhalational agent, although continuous EKG monitoring is recommended. If the serum level is greater than the therapeutic range, theophylline should be discontinued, sufficient time allowed for the serum drug level to decline, and a new serum level within the therapeutic range should be verified before induction of anesthesia.

We wish to again emphasize that the serum half-life of theophylline shows marked variation among individuals, and those with high serum levels are likely to be those whose theophylline has the longest half-lives. Therefore, any rigid recommendations as to the time necessary for decline of toxic levels into the therapeutic range will inevitably be in error in some patients. In an "average" patient with a theophylline half-life of about 8 hours and a serum level only slightly above the therapeutic range (21 to 25 mg/L), the serum theophylline level should have decreased into the therapeutic range within 8 hours after theophylline is discontinued. However, for a patient with severe liver disease, a theophylline half-life of 16 hours, and a serum level of 40 µg/L, an 8-hour interval would not be sufficient to allow the drug level to decline into the therapeutic range.

When serum levels are not available or the patient has a condition requiring urgent surgery, enflurane or isoflurane are safer alternatives for maintenance of anesthesia. If intraoperative wheezing necessitates IV administration of aminophylline, it should be diluted in 50 ml of saline solution and infused over a 20-minute period. Administration into a central line should be discouraged, since this has been a frequent cause of cardiac arrest.[63]

Finally, it should be remembered that halothane and theophylline have been used in animals as "a model" of malignant hyperpyrexia.[64]

3. *Muscle Relaxants*

Studies in animals[65] and man[66] have demonstrated that theophylline may antagonize nondepolarizing muscle block. The cause for this is not apparent but may be a direct presynaptic effect at the neuromuscular junction.

Pancuronium may be associated with tachycardia either because of its vagolytic[67] properties or because of an indirect sympathomimetic effect.[68] Supraventricular tachycardia has been reported following administration of pancuronium in patients receiving aminophylline, although serum theophylline levels were in the therapeutic range.[69] While this does not represent a contraindication to the use of pancuronium, it is prudent to remember that tachydysrhythmias are possible when this combination of drugs is used, and that animal studies suggest that theophylline-induced ventricular dysrhythmias are more likely to occur in subjects with marked tachycardia.[56]

Reversal of neuromuscular blockade with anticholinesterases such as neostigmine may precipitate bronchospasm by cholinergic mechanisms, but this can be prevented or reversed by intravenous atropine administration.[70]

SYMPATHOMIMETIC BRONCHODILATORS

The important sympathomimetic bronchodilators are either catecholamines or structurally related analogs. The pharmacology and interactions of catecholamines are discussed in Chapter 7, and we shall focus on the selective *beta* 2-agonists (Table 8–3) whose principal use is in the treatment of asthma. The therapeutic effect of these bronchodilators reflects a relatively selective action on *beta* 2-adrenoceptors, but all such drugs that are currently available also act to some extent as *beta* 1-receptors and can elicit tachycardia and cardiac dysrhythmias if given in a high enough dose. The apparent separation between the desired *beta* 2-effect (bronchodilation) and the unwanted *beta* 1-effect (cardiac stimulation) is influenced by the route of administration, and is more pronounced when the drugs are administered by the aerosol than by the intravenous route.

The selective *beta* 2-agonists differ chemically from isoproterenol and the endogenous catecholamines in the functional groups substituted on the phenyl ring and the terminal amine of the phenylethylamine skeleton common to most sympathomimetic drugs. Because of these differences, most selective *beta* 2-agonists are poor substrates for the enzymatic systems that rapidly metabolize catecholamines.[71] Furthermore, they do not appear to be subject to the rapid uptake into neuronal and extraneuronal stores that is chiefly responsible for terminating the action of endogenous catecholamines. As a result, most of the selective *beta* 2-agonists have a much longer duration of action than epinephrine or isoproterenol and can also be administered by the oral route (Table 8–3). While these pharmacokinetic differences are usually an advantage from the standpoint of ease of administration, they also mean that any adverse effect is likely to be much more persistent than with isoproterenol or a catecholamine. Potential adverse effects

Table 8–3
*Comparison of Some Sympathomimetic Bronchodilators**

	Isoproterenol	Metaproterenol	Terbutaline	Albuterol
Chemical structure	catechol amine	resorcinol	resorcinol	saligenin
Onset of action	rapid	rapid	slow	slow
Significant effect (hrs)	1–2	3–5	3–7	4–6
Comparative oral dose (mg)	—	20	5	4
Comparative aerosol dose (mg)	0.1	0.65	0.25	0.10

*According to data contained in reference 71

are those common to all *beta*-adrenoceptor agonists and include tachydysrhythmias, central nervous system stimulation, urinary retention, hypokalemia and inhibition of premature labor.

The selective *beta* 2-agonists also are frequently used for uterine relaxation in pregnancy. Pulmonary edema has occurred as a rare complication in unanesthetized[72,73] as well as anesthetized[74] patients in this group. The pathophysiologic mechanisms are not known but may be partly attributable to overhydration.

Prolonged use of *beta*-receptor agonists can result in desensitization, or tolerance. This can occur over a period of 1 to 2 weeks and requires a roughly equivalent time for restoration of normal responsiveness following termination of drug therapy.[75] Since desensitization apparently results from a decrease in the number[76,77] or affinity[78,79] of *beta*-receptors, tolerance to *beta*-adrenergic stimulants does not necessarily involve a loss of responsiveness to methylxanthines.[80]

Despite the common use of selective *beta* 2-agonists in the treatment of asthma, relatively little is known about their interaction with other drugs, and, to our knowledge, their interactions with anesthetic agents have not been studied. There are well-documented interactions, however, between catecholamines and anesthetics, which are discussed in Chapter 7. It would be reasonable to assume that the same interactions may occur with selective *beta* 2-agonists, especially if administered intravenously.

Even the interactions between *beta*-agonists and methylxanthines are relatively poorly understood, despite the prevalence of such combined therapy. While the therapeutic effect may be augmented, their toxicity is also likely to be enhanced, and a recent warning in the FDA drug bulletin has called attention to the increased incidence of adverse cardiac effects in laboratory animals receiving both *beta*-agonists and methylxanthines.[81] The extent of the clinical risk of toxic interactions between these two classes of bronchodilators has remained highly controversial.[82–84]

While most of the selective *beta* 2-agonists can be administered orally, parenterally, or as inhaled aerosols, the aerosol route has two great advantages: First, high concentrations can be achieved at the site of action in the airway, thereby maximizing the therapeutic effect and minimizing the undesirable *beta* 1 side effects. Second, the onset of action by this route is almost as rapid as with intravenous administration.

There are two ways in which aerosols can be used effectively in the operating room. The easiest method involves using a metered aerosol preparation which can be administered via a T-connector placed between the anesthesia circuit and the endotracheal tube. Pressure on the canister releases a fixed amount of drug which is then deposited into the airway during inspiration. When metered aerosol preparations are not available, aerosols can be administered by a hand-held nebulizer placed in the inspiratory limb of an anesthesia circuit via a T-piece connector.

Each manufactured product provides a different dose, and the manufacturer's dosage recommendations should be used as a guide. It is important to realize that when a patient has an endotracheal tube in place, a higher percentage of the drug will be deposited in the lung and, therefore, the dose must be adjusted to avoid overdosage.

CORTICOSTEROIDS

Although the anti-asthmatic actions of glucocorticoids are poorly understood, their effects can be dramatic and their margin of safety very great—at least from the standpoint of acute administration. However, one must recognize that the beneficial effects of these drugs in asthma do not appear for some hours. There is relatively little risk in the short-term use of steroids, and there are no known direct interactions between corticosteroids and anesthetic drugs, at least not in clinical practice. The major acute adverse effect of steroid administration appears to be precipitation of hyperosmolar nonketotic coma in patients with severe diabetes mellitus.[71]

Hydrocortisone has been the standard product for parenteral treatment of bronchospasms, and there is little evidence to suggest that other glucocorticoids offer any advantage for acute use. For chronic administration, however, aerosol preparations of steroids such as beclomethasone can sometimes control the asthmatic symptoms with much less risk of adrenal cortical suppression.

Interaction between corticosteroids and other classes of drugs used to treat asthma are the subject of considerable current interest. Corticosteroids "facilitate" the bronchodilator action of *beta*-agonists[85,86] and have restored responsiveness in subjects who had become tolerant to their effects.[86] On the other hand, there are suggestions that acute administration of large doses of corticosteroids can alter the disposition of theophylline. Thus in 5 out of 6 patients in status asthmaticus who were receiving theophylline infusions with stable serum drug levels, the IV administration of a large dose of hydrocortisone (500 mg followed 6 hours later by 3 further 200-mg increments at 2-hour intervals) was associated with a roughly two-fold increase in serum levels of theophylline.[87] In contrast, studies in healthy individuals suggest that corticosteroids may actually slightly enhance theophylline elimination.[88] Although further studies are needed, the clinician should be alert for possible changes in theophylline kinetics associated with corticosteroid administration.

CONCLUSION

Asthma is a common class of diseases affecting 2 to 5% of the population. A large proportion of these patients are on a regular intake of theophylline, sympathomimetics and steroids, either ordered by a physician or obtained as proprietary preparations available over the counter. Since there is a potential for life-threatening drug interactions with these drugs, the anesthesiologist should critically scrutinize the preoperative medications of patients with asthma and carefully plan the anesthetic regimen to minimize drug-associated complications.

REFERENCES

1. Roizen, M.F., and Stevens, W.C.: Multiform ventricular tachycardia due to the interaction of aminophylline and halothane. Anesth. Analg., 57:738, 1978.
2. Hirshman, C.A., Krieger, W., Littlejohn, G., Lee, R., and Julien, R.: Ketamine-aminophylline-induced decrease in seizure threshold. Anesthesiology, 56:464, 1982.
3. Ogilvie, R.I.: Clinical pharmacokinetics of theophylline. Clin. Pharmacokinet., 3:267, 1978.
4. Ellis, E.F., and Eddy, E.D.: Anhydrous theophylline equivalence of commercial theophylline formulations. J. Allergy Clin. Immunol., 53:116, 1974.
5. Fredholm, B.B., Brodin, K., and Strandberg, K.: On the mechanism of relaxation of tracheal muscle by theophylline and other cyclic nucleotide phosphodiesterase inhibitors. Acta Pharmacol. Toxicol., 45:336, 1979.
6. Bergstrand, H.: Phosphodiesterase inhibition and theophylline. Eur. J. Respir. Dis., 61(Suppl 109):37, 1980.
7. Kolbeck, R.C., Speir, W.A., Carrier, G.O., and Bransome, E.D.: Apparent irrelevance of cyclic nucleotides to the relaxation of tracheal smooth muscle induced by theophylline. Lung, 156:173, 1979.
8. Miech, R.P., Niedzwicki, J.G., and Smith, T.R.: Effect of theophylline on the binding of cAMP to soluble protein from tracheal smooth muscle. Biochem. Pharmacol., 28:3687, 1979.
9. Peach, M.J.: Stimulation of release of adrenal catecholamine by adenosine 3':5'-cyclic monophosphate and theophylline in the absence of extracellular Ca^{++}. Proc. Natl. Acad. Sci. (USA), 69:834, 1972.
10. Poisner, A.M.: Direct stimulant effect of aminophylline on catecholamine release from the adrenal medulla. Biochem. Pharmacol., 22:469, 1973.
11. Snyder, S.H., Katims, J.J., Annau, Z., et al.: Adenosine receptors and behavorial actions of methylxanthines. Proc. Natl. Acad. Sci., 78:3260, 1981.
12. Horrobin, D.F., Manku, M.S., Franks, D.J., et al.: Methyl xanthine phosphodiesterase inhibitors behave as prostaglandin antagonists in a perfused

rat mesenteric artery preparation. Prostaglandins, 13:33, 1977.
13. Milsap, R.L., Krauss, A.N., and Auld, P.A.M.: Efficacy of low-dose theophylline. Seminars in Perinatology, 5:321, 1981.
14. Zwillich, C.W., Sutton, F.D., Neff, T.A., et al.: Theophylline-induced seizures in adults: correlation with serum concentrations. Ann. Intern. Med., 82:784, 1975.
15. Jacobs, M.H., Senior, R.M., and Kessler, G.: Clinical experience with theophylline: relationships between dosage, serum concentration and toxicity. J.A.M.A., 235:1983, 1976.
16. Hendeles, L., Bighley, L., Richardson, R.H., et al.: Frequent toxicity from i.v. aminophylline infusions in critically ill patients. Drug Intel. Clin. Pharm., 11:12, 1977.
17. Mitenko, P.A., and Ogilvie, R.I.: Rational intravenous doses of theophylline. N. Engl. J. Med., 289:600, 1973.
18. Vozeh, S., Kewitz, G., Perruchoud, A., et al.: Theophylline serum concentration and therapeutic effect in severe acute bronchial obstruction: The optimal use of intravenously administered aminophylline. Am. Rev. Respir. Dis., 125:181, 1982.
19. Rall, T.W.: Central nervous system stimulants: the xanthines. In The Pharmacological Basis of Therapeutics, 6th Ed. Edited by Alfred G. Gilman, Louis S. Goodman and Alfred Gilman. New York, Macmillan, 1980.
20. Marcus, M.L., Skelton, C.L., Grauer, L.E., et al.: Effects of theophylline on myocardial mechanics. Am. J. Physiol., 222:1361, 1972.
21. Persson, C.G.A., Erjefält, I., Edholm, L-E, et al.: Tracheal relaxant and cardiostimulant actions of xanthines can be differentiated from diuretic and CNS-stimulant effects: role of adenosine antagonism? Life Sci., 31:2673, 1982.
22. Higbee, M.D., Kumar, M., and Galant, S.P.: Stimulation of endogenous catecholamine release by theophylline: a proposed additional mechanism of action for theophylline effects. J. Allergy Clin. Immunol., 70:377, 1982.
23. Hendeles, L., and Weinberger, M.: Theophylline: a "state of the art" review. Pharmacotherapy, 3:2, 1983.
24. Jusko, W.J., Gardner, M.H., Mangione, A., et al.: Factors affecting theophylline clearances: age, tobacco, marijuana, cirrhosis, congestive heart failure, obesity, oral contraceptives, benzodiazepines, barbiturates, and ethanol. J. Pharm. Sci., 68:1358, 1979.
25. McElnay, J.C., Smith, G.D., and Helling, D.K.: A practical guide to interactions involving theophylline kinetics. Drug Intel. Clin. Pharm., 16:533, 1982.
26. Simons, F.E.R., Rigatto, H., and Simons, K.J.: Pharmacokinetics of theophylline in neonates. Seminars in Perintology, 5:337, 1981.
27. Jusko, W.J., Koup, J.R., Vance, J.W., et al.: Intravenous theophylline therapy: Nomogram guidelines. Ann. Intern. Med., 86:400, 1977.
28. Hendeles, L., and Weinberger, M.: Guidelines for avoiding theophylline overdose. N. Engl. J. Med., 300:1217, 1979.
29. Jackson, J.E., Powell, J.R., Wandell, M., et al.: Cimetidine decreases theophylline clearance. Am. Rev. Respir. Dis., 123:615, 1981.
30. Reitberg, D.P., Bernhard, H., and Schentag, J.J.: Alteration of theophylline clearance and half-life by cimetidine in normal volunteers. Ann. Intern. Med., 95:582, 1981.
31. Campbell, M.A., Plachetka, J.R., Jackson, J.E., et al.: Cimetidine decreases theophylline clearance. Ann. Intern. Med., 95:68, 1981.
32. Weinberger, M.M., Smith, G., Milavetz, G., et al.: Decreased theophylline clearance due to cimetidine. N. Engl. J. Med., 304:672, 1981.
33. Powell, J.R., Rogers, J.F., Wargin, W.A., et al.: The influence of cimetidine vs ranitidine on theophylline pharmacokinetics. Clin. Pharmacol. Ther., 31:261 (abstract), 1982.
34. Prince, R.A., Wing, D.S., Weinberger, M.M., et al.: Effect of erythromycin on theophylline kinetics. J. Allergy Clin. Immunol., 68:427, 1981.
35. Conrad, K.A., and Nyman, D.W.: Effects of metoprolol and propranolol on theophylline elimination. Clin. Pharmacol. Ther., 28:463, 1980.
36. Marquis, J-F., Carruthers, S.G., Spence, J.D., et al.: Phenytoin-theophylline interaction. N. Engl. J. Med., 307:1189, 1982.
37. Landay, R.A., Gonzalez, M.A., and Taylor, J.C.: Effect of phenobarbital on theophylline disposition. J. Allergy Clin. Immunol., 62:27, 1978.
38. Stirt, J.A., Berger, J.M., Ricker, S.M., et al.: Aminophylline pharmacokinetics and cardiorespiratory effects during halothane anesthesia in experimental animals. Anesth. Analg., 59:186, 1980.
39. Berger, J.M., Stirt, J.A., and Sullivan, S.F.: Enflurane, halothane and aminophylline-uptake and pharmacokinetics. Anesth. Analg., 62:733, 1983.
40. Corssen, G., Gutierrez, J., Reves, J.G., et al.: Ketamine in the anesthetic management of asthmatic patients. Anesth. Analg., 51:588, 1972.
41. Hirshman, C.A., Downes, H., Farbood, A., et al.: Ketamine block of bronchospasm in experimental canine asthma. Br. J. Anaesth., 51:713, 1979.
42. Wong, D.H.W., and Jenkins, L.C.: An experimental study of the mechanism of action of ketamine on the central nervous system. Canad. Anaesth. Soc. J., 21:57, 1974.
43. Montel, H., Starke, K., Gorlitz, B-D, et al.: Tierexperimentelle Untersuchungen zur Wirkung des Ketamins auf periphere sympathische Nerven. Anaesthetist, 22:111, 1973.
44. Nedergaard, O.A.: Cocaine-like effect of ketamine on vascular adrenergic neurones. Eur. J. Pharmacol., 23:153, 1973.
45. Baraka, A., Harrison, T., and Kachachi, T.: Catecholamine levels after ketamine anesthesia in man. Anesth. Analg., 52:198, 1973.
46. Zsigmond, E.K., Kothary, S.P., Matsuki, A., et al.: Diazepam for prevention of the rise in plasma catecholamines caused by ketamine. Clin. Pharm. Ther., 15:223, 1974.
47. White, P.F., Way, W.L., and Trevor, A.J.: Keta-

mine—its pharmacology and therapeutic uses. Anesthesiology, 56:119, 1982.
48. Stirt, J.A., Berger, J.M., Roe, S.D., et al.: Cardiovascular effects of ketamine following administration of aminophylline in dogs. Anesth. Analg., 61:685, 1982.
49. Helliwell, M., and Berry, D.: Theophylline poisoning in adults. Br. Med. J., 2:1114, 1979.
50. Shnider, S.M., and Papper, E.M.: Anesthesia for the asthmatic patient. Anesthesiology, 22:886, 1961.
51. Gold, M.I.: Anesthesia for the asthmatic patient. Anesth. Analg., 49:881, 1970.
52. Hall, K.D., and Norris, F.H.: Fluothane sensitization of dog heart to action of epinephrine. Anesthesiology, 19:631, 1958.
53. Barton, M.D.: Anesthetic problems with aspirin-intolerant patients. Anesth. Analg., 54:376, 1975.
54. Stirt, J.A., Berger, J.M., Ricker, S.M., et al.: Arrhythmogenic effects of aminophylline during halothane anesthesia in experimental animals. Anesth. Analg., 59:410, 1980.
55. Takaori, M., and Loehning, R.W.: Ventricular arrhythmias induced by aminophylline during halothane anaesthesia in dogs. Can. Anaesth. Soc. J., 14:79, 1967.
56. Stirt, J.A., Berger, J.M., Roe, S.D., et al.: Halothane-induced cardiac arrhythmias following administration of aminophylline in experimental animals. Anesth. Analg., 60:517, 1981.
57. Takaori, M., and Loehning, R.W.: Ventricular arrhythmias during halothane anaesthesia: effect of isoproterenol, aminophylline and ephedrine. Can. Anaesth. Soc. J., 12:275, 1965.
58. Stirt, J.A., Berger, J.M., Roe, S.D., et al.: Safety of enflurane following administration of aminophylline in experimental animals. Anesth. Analg., 60:871, 1981.
59. Stirt, J.A., Berger, J.M., and Sullivan, S.F.: Lack of arrhythmogenicity of isoflurane following administration of aminophylline in dogs. Anesth. Analg., 62:568, 1983.
60. Joas, T.A., and Stevens, W.C.: Comparison of the arrhythmic doses of epinephrine during forane, halothane and fluroxene anesthesia in dogs. Anesthesiology, 35:48, 1971.
61. Tucker, W.K., Rackstein, A.D., and Munson, E.S.: Comparison of arrhythmic doses of adrenaline, metaraminol, ephedrine and phenylephrine during isoflurane and halothane anaesthesia in dogs. Br. J. Anaesth., 46:392, 1974.
62. Johnston, R.R., Eger, E.I., and Wilson, C.: A comparative interaction of epinephrine with enflurane, isoflurane, and halothane in man. Anesth. Analg., 55:709, 1976.
63. Camarata, S.J., Weil, M.H., Hanashiro, P.K., et al.: Cardiac arrest in the critically ill: I. A study of predisposing causes in 132 patients. Circulation, 44:688, 1971.
64. Varagic, V.M., Prostran, M., and Kentera, D.: Interaction of halothane and aminophylline on the isolated hemidiaphragm of the rat. Eur. J. Pharmaco., 61:35, 1980.
65. Dretchen, K.L., Morgenroth, V.H., Standaert, F.G., et al.: Azathioprine: effects on neuromuscular transmission. Anesthesiology, 45:604, 1976.
66. Doll, D.C., and Rosenberg, H.: Antagonism of neuromuscular blockade by theophylline. Anesth. Analg., 58:139, 1979.
67. Saxena, P.R., and Bonta, I.L.: Mechanism of selective cardiac vagolytic action of pancuronium bromide. Specific blockade of cardiac muscarinic receptors. Eur. J. Pharmacol., 11:332, 1970.
68. Docherty, J.R., and McGrath, J.C.: Sympathomimetic effects of pancuronium bromide on the cardiovascular system of the pithed rat: a comparison with the effects of drugs blocking the neuronal uptake of noradrenaline. Br. J. Pharmacol., 64:589, 1978.
69. Belani, K.G., Anderson, W.W., and Buckley, J.J.: Adverse drug interaction involving pancuronium and aminophylline. Anesth. Analg., 61:473, 1982.
70. Miller, M.M., Fish, J.E., and Patterson, R.: Methacholine and physostigmine airway reactivity in asthmatic and nonasthmatic subjects. J. Allergy. Clin. Immunol., 60:116, 1977.
71. Ziment, I.: Respiratory Pharmacology and Therapeutics. Philadelphia, W.B. Saunders Co., 1978, pp. 119–122.
72. Guernsey, B.G., Villarreal, Y., Snyder, M.D., et al.: Pulmonary edema associated with the use of betamimetic agents in preterm labor. Am. J. Hosp. Pharm., 38:1942, 1981.
73. Martin, A.J.: Severe unwanted effects associated with betasympathomimetics when used in the treatment of premature labour: causes, incidence and preventive measures. Br. J. Clin. Prac., 35:325, 1981.
74. Ravindran, R., Viegas, O.J., Padilla, L.M., et al.: Anesthetic considerations in pregnant patients receiving terbutaline therapy. Anesth. Analg., 59:391, 1980.
75. Nelson, H.S.: *Beta* adrenergic agonists. Chest 82 suppl:33S, 1982.
76. Mukherjee, C., Caron, M.G., and Lefkowitz, R.J.: Catecholamine-induced subsensitivity of adenylate cyclase associated with loss of *beta*-adrenergic receptor binding sites. Proc. Natl. Acad. Sci. USA, 72:1945, 1975.
77. Mickey, J.V., Tate, R., Mullikin, D., et al.: Regulation of adenylate cyclase-coupled *beta* adrenergic receptor binding sites by *beta* adrenergic catecholamines *in vitro*. Mol. Pharmacol., 12:409, 1976.
78. Lin, C-S., Hurwitz, L., Jenne, J., et al.: Mechanism of isoproterenol-induced desensitization of tracheal smooth muscle. J. Pharmacol. Exp. Ther., 203:12, 1977.
79. Avner, B.P., and Noland, B.: *In vivo* desensitization to *beta* receptor mediated bronchodilator drugs in the rat: decreased *beta* receptor affinity. J. Pharmacol. Exp. Ther., 207:23, 1978.
80. Avner, B.P., and Jenne, J.W.: Desensitization of isolated human bronchial smooth muscle to *beta*-receptor agonists. J. Allergy Clin. Immunol., 68:51, 1981.
81. Interactions between methylxanthines and *beta* adrenergic agonists. FDA Drug Bull., 11:19, 1981.
82. Nicklas, R.A., Whitehurst, V.E., and Donohoe,

R.F.: Combined use of *beta*-adrenergic agonists and methyl xanthines. N. Engl. J. Med., *307*:557, 1982.
83. Wilson, J.D., and Sutherland, D.C.: Combined *beta* agonists and methylxanthines in asthma. N. Engl. J. Med., *307*:1707, 1982.
84. Isles, A.F., and Newth, C.J.L.: Combined *beta* agonists and methylxanthines in asthma. N. Engl. J. Med., *309*:432, 1983.
85. Shenfield, G.M., Hodson, M.E., Clarke, S.W., et al.: Interaction of corticosteroids and catecholamines in the treatment of asthma. Thorax, *30*:430, 1975.
86. Ellul-Micallef, R., and Fenech, F.F.: Effect of intravenous prednisolone in asthmatics with diminished adrenergic responsiveness. Lancet, *2*:1269, 1975.
87. Buchanan, N., Hurwitz, S., and Butler, P.: Asthma—a possible interaction between hydrocortisone and theophylline. S. African Med. J., *56*:1147, 1979.
88. Hansten, P.D.: Theophylline and corticosteroids. Drug Interactions Newsletter, *4*:17, 1984.

BETA-ADRENERGIC BLOCKERS

EDWARD LOWENSTEIN and PIERRE FOËX

Drugs that antagonize the *beta* functions of the sympathetic nervous system (*beta*-adrenergic blockers) are widely used in medicine. Their introduction caused major concern to the anesthesiologist, who approached the *beta*-blocked patient with trepidation. Indeed, the initial experience seems to confirm the anesthesiologist's worst fears.[1,2] These fears, however, have now been dispelled and the opposite view now prevails, namely, that the discontinuance of *beta*-adrenergic blocking agents is inadvisable, and that their prophylactic administration may be beneficial.[3,5] In this chapter we examine the reasons for this dramatic reversal of opinion.

THE SYMPATHETIC NEUROEFFECTOR JUNCTION

The adrenergic neuroeffector junction consists of a postganglionic nerve terminal, a synaptic gap, and an effector cell. The effector cell contains the adrenergic receptors, which are specific cellular structures capable of the selective binding of agonists and antagonists (Fig. 9–1). The mediator, bound to the neuron, is released into the synaptic gap when a nerve action potential traverses the nerve terminal. As more of the mediator is released, more becomes bound to the receptor by the law of mass action. When a sufficient number of receptors is occupied by the mediator, the effect caused by that receptor occurs by the "all or none" principle. The effect is often mediated by the adenyl cyclase system acting as the "second-messenger." The binding is reversible, since the mediator may be metabolized in the junction, diffused into capillaries, or become rebound to the nerve terminals. When a mimetic drug is administered, it may act either directly or indirectly (Fig. 9–1).

Recent research has identified the *beta*-adrenergic receptor.[6] In man, the mediators of the *beta*-adrenergic nervous system are norepinephrine (neurotransmitter) and epinephrine (hormonal transmitter).

Antagonists of this system act by competitive inhibition. This term implies that agonists and antagonists compete for the same binding sites, and that their success in securing these depends on the specific affinity of the drug for the sites and the number of molecules available for binding. Furthermore, it implies that the binding is reversible, that the antagonist may be overcome by sufficient quantities of agonist (and is therefore never "complete"), and that the slope of the dose-response curve is unchanged by the antagonist.

The binding process is further complicated because the prolonged occupation of the receptor by a *beta* agonist (isoproterenol) leads in a few hours to "inactivation," or a functional reduction in the number of *beta*-adrenergic receptors (similar to

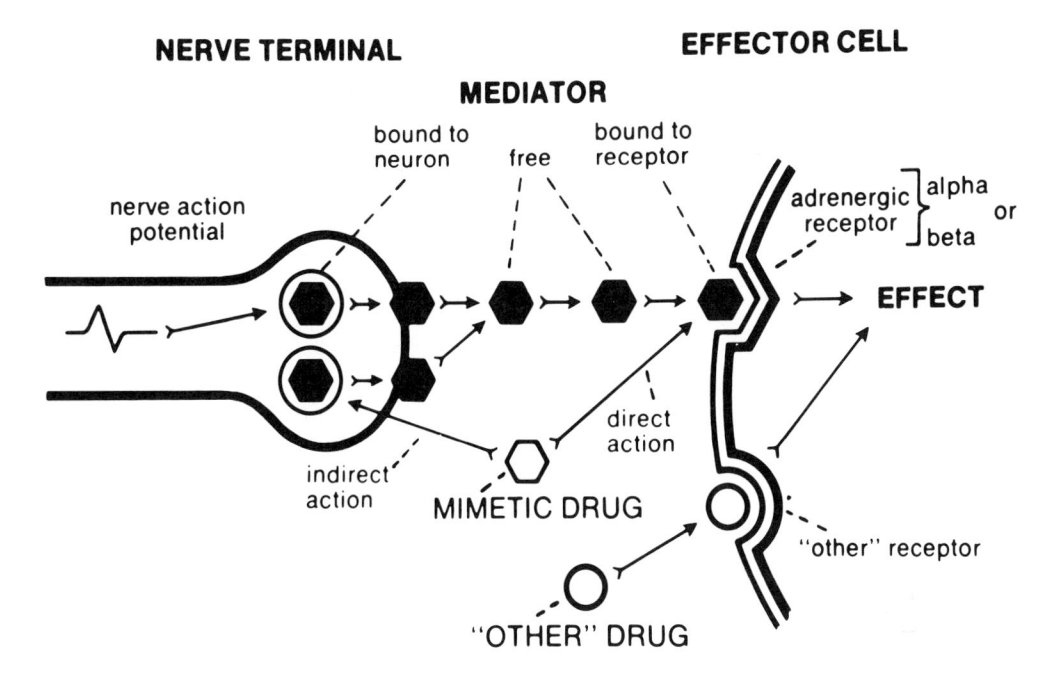

Fig. 9–1. A schematic representation of the sympathetic neuroeffector junction. See text for details. (From Moran, N.C.: The role of *alpha*- and *beta*-adrenergic receptors in the control of the circulation and in the actions of drugs on the cardiovascular system. *In* Cardiovascular Therapy. Edited by H.I. Russek and B.L. Zohman. Baltimore, Williams & Wilkins, 1971.)

epinephrine resistance in asthma). Furthermore, there is evidence that the chronic occupation of *beta* receptors by *beta* antagonists can *increase* the number of *beta* receptors (Fig. 9–2).[7] This means that the prolonged administration of a *beta*-blocker could induce catecholamine hypersensitivity, which might cause problems on withdrawal of the *beta*-blocker. Hypersensitivity has been convincingly demonstrated, and may indeed be due to this mechanism.[7]

CLASSIFICATION OF ADRENERGIC RECEPTORS

The adrenergic receptors were initially divided into *alpha* and *beta* categories by Ahlquist.[8] In 1967 Lands further subdivided the *beta*-adrenergic system into *beta* 1 and *beta* 2 receptors.[9] The primary actions of *beta* 1 receptor stimulation are exerted on the heart, whereas the primary actions of *beta* 2 receptor stimulation are arteriolar vasodilation, bronchodilation, and metabolic effects. Recent ligand binding studies indicate there is less homogeneity of receptor subtypes within organs than was thought previously.

Further subdivision of the *beta* 1 receptors may be warranted. This is suggested by the synthesis of relatively chronotropic-selective stimulating drugs,[10] as well as by the longer persistence of chronotropic over inotropic blockade after the discontinuance of propranolol.[11]

The specific effects of *beta* stimulation on the heart involve myocardial and electrophysiologic functions (Fig. 9–3). The former include increased ventricular ejection rate, decreased ejection time, and decreased ventricular volume, whereas the latter include increased automaticity, increased conduction velocity, and decreased atrioventricular node refractoriness. The myocardial effects are therefore associated with increased inotropy, and

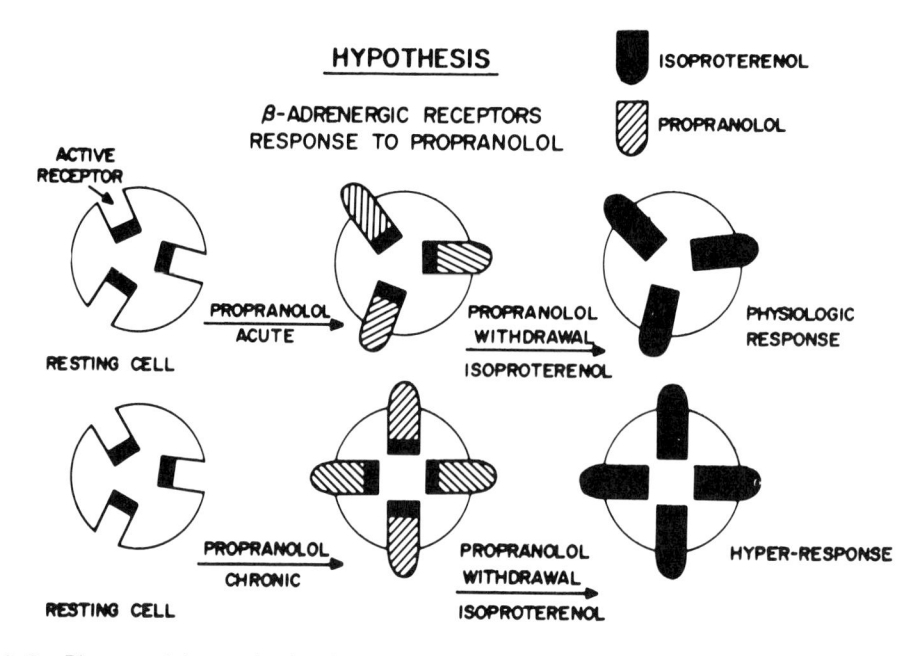

Fig. 9–2. Diagram of the mechanism for hypersensitivity of the *beta*-adrenergic nervous system following cessation of chronic propranolol therapy, as hypothesized by Boudoulas, H., et al.: Hypersensitivity to adrenergic stimulation after propranolol withdrawal in normal subjects. Ann. Intern. Med., 87:433, 1977. Top: When propranolol is administered on a short-term basis, active receptors are occupied by the antagonist. Following cessation, receptors are no longer occupied, and isoproterenol is associated with a response of normal magnitude. Repeated propranolol therapy (bottom) is associated with an increase in the number of receptors. Cessation of administration leaves an increased number of active, unbound receptors, so that isoproterenol administration causes an exaggerated response.

the electrophysiologic effects with increased heart rate and ventricular irritability.

Whether there is a direct effect of *beta*-adrenergic stimulation on the coronary arteries is a question that is undecided, and under intense, current investigation. Coronary dilation does occur, but it is considered by many to be due to autoregulation caused by local metabolic factors that are secondary to the increased contractile state and heart rate associated with *beta*-adrenergic stimulation.

Most sympathetically active compounds, whether endogenous or exogenous, have both *alpha*- and *beta*-stimulating capabilities. For example, although norepinephrine is frequently considered to have only vasoconstrictor (*alpha*-adrenergic) properties, its potent *beta*-adrenergic activity is apparent when the *alpha*-adrenergic system is blocked. Isoproterenol is a pure *beta*-adrenergic stimulating compound and methoxamine appears to be a pure *alpha*-adrenergic compound. These drugs represent the exception rather than the rule.

PROPERTIES OF *BETA*-ADRENERGIC BLOCKING DRUGS

As a group, *beta*-adrenergic blockers have three principal actions on the cardiovascular system. These include actions mediated by the *beta*-adrenergic nervous system, plus other actions:
1. Receptor subtype selectivity.
2. Intrinsic sympathomimetic activity (ISA).
3. Membrane-stabilizing or "quinidine-like" activity.

One must consider the relative actions

CARDIAC EFFECTS BETA STIMULATION

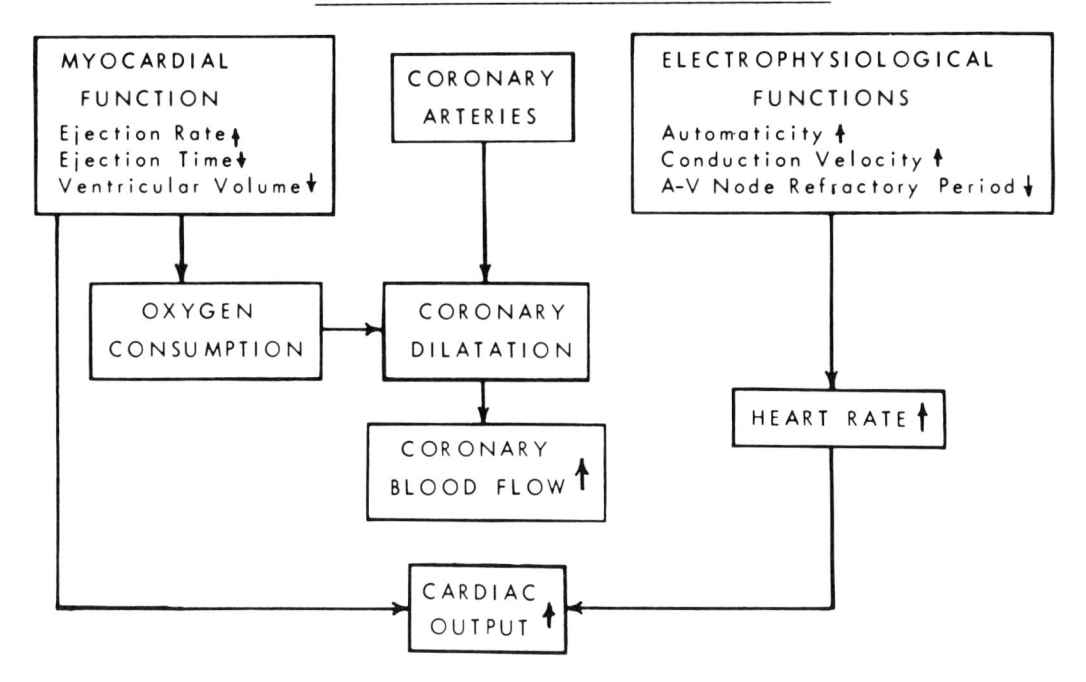

Fig. 9–3. Cardiac effects of *beta*-adrenergic stimulation. See text for details.

of each specific drug in order to predict its effect. For example, it is theoretically possible to synthesize either cardioselective (*beta* 1) or cardiac-sparing (*beta* 2) *beta*-adrenergic blocking drugs. Practolol is an example of the former, whereas butoxamine is an example of the latter. However, the terms "cardiac-sparing" and "cardioselective" are relative because when sufficiently high doses are administered, both *beta* 1 and *beta* 2 systems are affected. The clinical impact of the reported 10 to 40-fold *beta*-1 and *beta*-2 receptor selectivity is less than would be anticipated, since the serum levels achieved often negate this selectivity.

Despite these considerations, several *beta*-adrenergic blocking drugs are classified as "cardioselective," e.g., atenolol, metoprolol, practolol. Others block *beta*-1 and *beta*-2 receptors, e.g., propranolol, nadolol, pindolol, timolol. Labetalol blocks not only the *beta* receptors, but also the *alpha* receptors.

Some *beta*-adrenergic blocking drugs are pure antagonists, i.e., atenolol, metoprolol, propranolol, nadolol, timolol, while others are also partial agonists, e.g., practolol and pindolol. Partial agonists fit the receptor but elicit only part of the effect a pure agonist would elicit. However, because of receptor occupation, they prevent the effect of a pure agonist. Partial agonists can be considered as exhibiting intrinsic sympathomimetic activity (ISA). They produce less reduction in heart rate and inotropy than do pure antagonists.

Some *beta*-adrenergic blocking drugs have relatively important membrane stabilizing effects, particularly when given in large doses. Membrane stabilization, when it occurs, causes myocardial depression. However, with the usual clinical doses, depression of the myocardium is *not* caused by membrane stabilization but by removal of the inotropic effect of *beta*-adrenoceptor stimulation.

At present, six *beta*-adrenergic blocking drugs are available for clinical use in the United States: propranolol, metoprolol, atenolol, nadolol, pindolol and timolol.

They can be classified according to receptor subtype selectivity and presence or absence of agonist characteristics (ISA) (Table 9–1). Practolol, long a mainstay in Great Britain, is no longer available for chronic administration.

ABSORPTION AND ELIMINATION

Besides being absorbed rapidly, most lipophilic *beta*-blockers are almost completely absorbed from the gastrointestinal tract. The more hydrophilic drugs, atenolol and nadolol, are absorbed to a much lesser extent (Table 9–2). Because of degradation in the liver, the dose available to the systemic circulation after oral administration may be substantially reduced. This is termed the first-pass effect. The most lipophilic drugs have the lowest bioavailability.

Protein binding of *beta*-adrenoceptor blockers is variable. If protein binding is great, relatively high plasma concentrations are necessary to achieve adequate blockade since only the unbound fraction is active. Elimination may be via hepatic metabolism and/or renal excretion. The most lipophilic *beta*-adrenergic blockers have a total body clearance that approaches liver blood flow (Table 9–2).

Data on bioavailability are important in predicting the intravenous dose when patients are switched from oral to intravenous administration, as often occurs during the perioperative period. If bioavailability is high, as with atenolol, whose bioavailability is 50%, the intravenous dose *should* be about one-half the oral dose. Conversely, if bioavailability is low, as with nadolol, whose bioavailability is 25%, the intravenous dose should be about 25% of the oral dose. In practice it is necessary to titrate the drugs until the desired effect has been achieved. Because of the important role of the liver for the clearance of some *beta*-adrenergic blockers, accumulation may occur in liver diseases. The elimination half-life is shortest for metoprolol, pindolol, timolol and propranolol (3 to 4h), intermediate for atenolol (6 to 9h) and longest for nadolol (14 to 24h). An authoritative, concise review of the pharmacokinetics of *beta*-blockers has recently been written by Frishman.[12]

Propranolol, the only *beta*-adrenergic blocker available in the United States for nearly a decade, will probably become far less popular despite a fine record of efficacy. In large measure, this is because first-pass extraction by the liver results in 20-fold variation in plasma level at any given oral dose. In addition, it requires four doses a day, whereas other blockers such as timolol and atenolol can induce a reliable *beta* blockade with a twice-a-day regimen, while nadolol is effective with a once-a-day regimen.

CLINICAL APPLICATIONS

Nonsurgical Indications for Use of *Beta*-Adrenergic Blockers

As is often the case with newly popular drugs, *beta*-blockers were tried for many conditions, with or without justification. For example, on the basis of a double-blind crossover trial in which *beta* blockade appeared to improve the musical performance of solo string musicians, it was recommended that such drugs be considered when "career prospects or livelihood"

Table 9–1

	Cardioselective	Non Selective
Pure antagonists (no ISA)	atenolol metoprolol	propranolol nadolol timolol
Partial agonists (with ISA)	practolol	pindolol

Table 9-2

	Gastrointestinal absorption (%)	Bioavailability (%)	Metabolism, excretion
atenolol	40–50	40–50	renal
metoprolol	>95	50	hepatic
nadolol	25	25	renal
pindolol	>90	50–100	hepatic & renal
propranolol	>90	±30	hepatic
timolol	>90	50	hepatic & renal

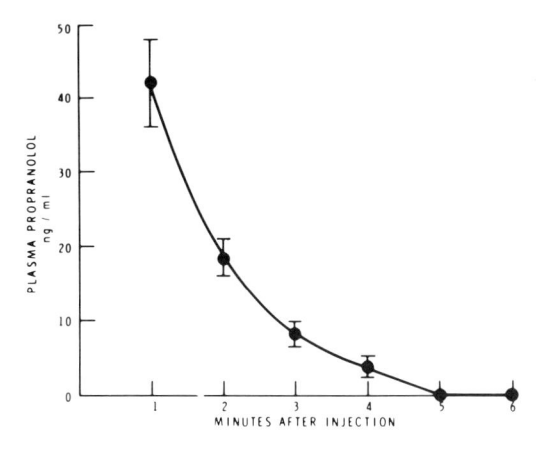

Fig. 9–4. Plasma propranolol concentration following administration of 1 mg intravenously in man. Although the drug is no longer detectable after five minutes, the duration of action appears to be between 15 and 30 minutes. (From Romagnoli, A., and Keats, A.S.: Plasma and atrial propranolol after preoperative withdrawal. Circulation, 52:1123, 1975.)

were at stake.[19] More conventional indications include hypertrophic ventricular outflow tract obstruction of both the left ventricle (idiopathic hypertrophic subaortic stenosis, asymmetrical septal hypertrophy, disproportionate upper septal thickening,) and the right ventricle,[20] digitalis toxicity, essential hypertension (in combination with other drugs or by itself),[13,14,21] thyrotoxicosis, myocardial infarction, angina pectoris, hyperdynamic septic shock,[22] migraine headache, and opiate addiction.

The sensitivity of essential hypertension to propranolol depends on the nature of the disease.[13] High- and normal-renin-associated hypertension responds to modest (160 mg/day) doses of propranolol. Low-renin hypertension responds only to higher doses (320 mg/day and greater). Patients with low-renin hypertension may receive up to 3 g/day of propranolol to the time of an operation.[13]

Ischemic heart disease (angina pectoris, postmyocardial infarction dysrhythmias, acute myocardial infarction) constitutes the best documented and most common indication for the administration of *beta*-adrenergic blockers. *Beta*-blockers clearly prolong the lifespan, enhance exercise tolerance in angina pectoris, help salvage ischemic myocardium in the presence of acute myocardial infarction, and effectively treat life-threatening dysrhythmias, particularly atrial tachydysrhythmias.[24] The consequence of these many indications is the large number of surgical patients with a history of recent *beta*-blocker intake.

ANESTHETICS AND *BETA*-BLOCKERS: A RATIONALE FOR CAUTION

Figure 9–5 schematically illustrates the function of the normal heart and the *beta*-adrenergically blocked heart. The normal heart easily handles its ordinary work load and has a large reserve besides. *Beta*-adrenergic blockade, by inhibiting the response of the heart to endogenous or exogenous neurohumoral influences, limits the ability of the heart to respond to an increased load. In addition, *beta* 2-mediated vasodilation is prevented unless selective blockade of cardiac receptors has been achieved. As noted above, this is possible even when a relatively cardioselective drug has been administered. On the other hand, *alpha*-mediated vasoconstriction is not affected. Thus, although the heart may

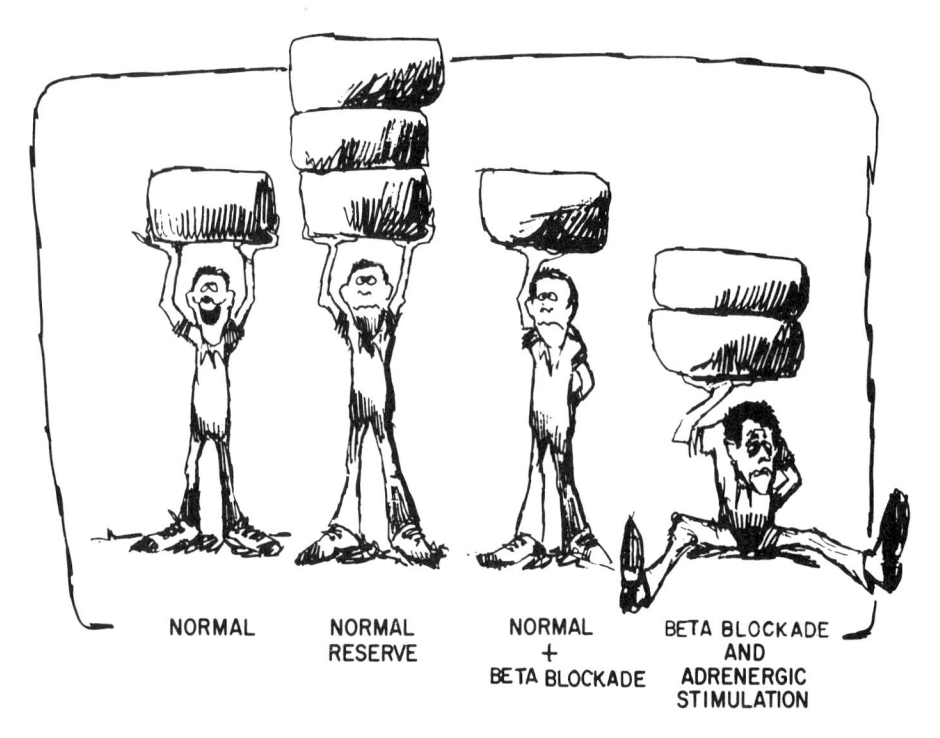

Fig. 9-5. Schematic illustration of the action of propranolol upon the normal heart. The heart is represented by the man, and the load (work) performed by the boulders he is lifting. Beta-adrenergic blockade "ties one hand behind the heart's back." This allows the heart to accomplish a normal amount of work but causes it to collapse when required to perform more, as in the presence of a catecholamine with *alpha*-agonist properties. See text for details.

be able to tolerate a normal work load, it may not be able to fulfill the demands of the additional flow or pressure associated with stress. The combination of an insufficient inotropic and chronotropic response to catecholamines and unopposed vasoconstriction may lead to heart failure and cardiovascular collapse. This is unusual in a heart with normal contractility. The heart with a history of failure, with cardiomyopathy, or with segmental wall motion abnormalities is most susceptible to these events.

There are many perioperative interventions and situations that may provoke sympathoadrenal discharge. Although some anesthetic agents may induce the liberation of catecholamines, surgical or nonsurgical stimulation (for example, preoperative apprehension, surgical incision, retraction, blood loss, tracheal intubation, postoperative pain) may challenge the heart with *alpha* and *beta* stimulation. Since the *beta* receptors are already occupied by the blocking agent, the heart's ability to increase its contractile state or heart rate is impaired. Since the *alpha* receptors are not occupied, the peripheral arteriolar circulation may constrict, increasing the work demand of the heart. Thus the "handicapped" heart, with one hand symbolically tied behind its back (Fig. 9-5), may collapse.

Initial clinical experiences confirmed the fear of anesthetizing patients who were *beta* blocked. For example, 5 mg propranolol was associated with bradycardia and hypotension when administered intravenously in the presence of diethyl ether, an anestheteic known to rely on the liberation of endogenous catecholamines to maintain circulatory stability.[1] Cardiogenic shock refractory to optimal therapy was reported at the conclusion of cardiopulmonary bypass in patients who had received large doses of propranolol until shortly before their operations.[2]

The fears of anesthetists regarding *beta*-blocked patients involve (1) the latent imbalance of the sympathetic system during *beta* blockade, (2) the clinical inability to reverse *beta* blockade, and (3) the misconception that *beta*-blockers in normal clinical doses cause direct myocardial depression by membrane stabilization.

Mechanisms of *Beta*-Adrenergic Blocking Agents in the Presence of Ischemic Heart Disease

Beta-adrenergic blockers appear to benefit ischemic or potentially ischemic myocardium by correcting, minimizing, or preventing an imbalance between myocardial oxygen demand and myocardial oxygen supply. The principal determinants of myocardial oxygen demand include myocardial wall tension, which is proportional to the ventricular systolic pressure and the ventricular volume, the contractile state of the heart, and the heart rate.[25] (Under most circumstances, the left ventricle, which performs "pressure work," is responsible for the major portion of myocardial oxygen demand. When severe right ventricular hypertension or hypertrophy is present, the right ventricle may have similar requirements.) Thus propranolol may decrease or prevent increases in left ventricular systolic pressure and heart rate, and may reduce the contractile state, all of which decrease myocardial oxygen demand (Table 9–3). On the other hand, the drug may dilate the ventricles and increase systolic ejection time, both of which increase myocardial oxygen demand. The balance between the beneficial and detrimental effects on the net myocardial oxygen balance is the primary determinant of whether the response is beneficial or detrimental.[26]

Table 9–3
Effects of Beta-Blockers in Relation to Myocardial Oxygen Consumption ($M\dot{V}O_2$)

		$M\dot{V}O_2$
1.	Decrease (prevent increase) left ventricular systolic pressure	↓
2.	Decrease (prevent increase) heart rate	↓
3.	Decrease (prevent increase) contractile state	↓
4.	Increase systolic ejection period	↑
5.	Cause left ventricular dilation	↑

Propranolol may also affect myocardial oxygen supply by two mechanisms. See text for details.

In addition, *beta*-adrenergic blockers may promote intramyocardial redistribution of blood flow to those areas most ischemic, a type of "Robin Hood" effect (Fig. 9–6). This concept was originally postulated by McGregor.[27] Although decreased coronary artery blood flow and increased coronary vascular resistance are documented after propranolol, this is thought to occur only in normal, nonischemic situations. Local metabolic regulation supervenes in the presence of ischemia.

Thus *beta* blockade relieves myocardial ischemia and angina pectoris by reestablishing a balance between myocardial oxygen demand and myocardial oxygen supply, which is limited in the patient with ischemic heart disease (Fig. 9–7).

Intraoperative Administration of *Beta*-Adrenergic Blocking Agents

Intraoperative situations occur in which it is theoretically desirable to administer a *beta*-adrenergic blocker. Experience proves that in this instance theory and practice coincide. These situations include sinus tachycardia, consequent to the administration of atropine, gallamine, and pancuronium; the prevention of tachycardia, hypertension, ventricular dysrhythmias, and myocardial ischemia during laryngoscopy

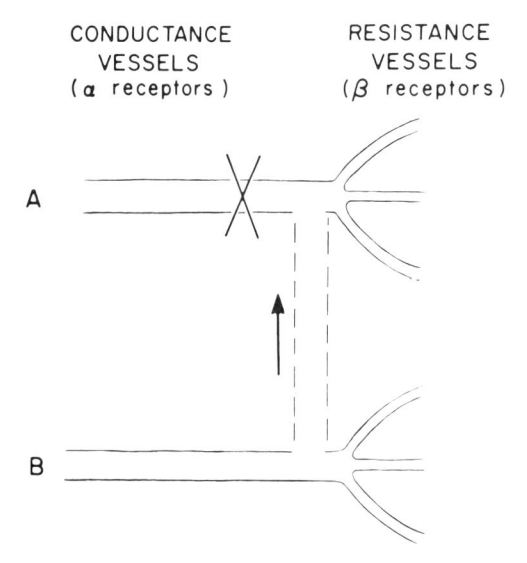

Fig. 9-6. Schematic diagram of the mechanism by which *beta*-adrenergic blockers may redistribute blood flow from normal to ischemic areas of myocardium. Occlusion in vascular bed A renders tissues ischemic, and thus reduces local resistance by producing maximal vasodilation. Collaterals (dashed lines) are the only source of blood for the ischemic area. *Beta* blockade enhances vascular resistance in nonischemic bed B, which results in favoring blood flow through the collaterals from B to A. Experimental confirmation of this hypothesis has been presented by Pitt. (From *Cardiovascular Beta Adrenergic Responses*. Edited by A.A. Kattus, G. Ross, and V. Hall. (UCLA Forum in Medical Sciences, No. 13). Los Angeles, University of California Press, 1970.)

and tracheal intubation of patients with hypertensive heart disease[5] (Fig. 9-8); a tachycardia in patients with evidence of acute myocardial ischemia (Fig. 9-9); an increase in heart rate and ventricular irritability consequent to catecholamine release secondary to the manipulation of a pheochromocytoma (only in the presence of *alpha*-adrenergic receptor blockade); and hyperthyroid crisis.

The administration of a *beta*-blocker prior to cardiopulmonary bypass in patients with ventricular hypertrophy, particularly in patients with severe aortic valve disease, is associated with a decrease in the incidence of ischemic contracture of the ventricle ("stone heart").[28] The dose of propranolol recommended in adults is 1 to 2 mg. The acute hemodynamic effects of such a dose are minor under these circumstances. In some centers the success of this regimen has led to its routine use prior to aortic cross-clamping and cardiopulmonary bypass in patients without ventricular hypertrophy. No objective evidence that this practice is beneficial exists, and the proven efficacy of cold cardioplegia has decreased the incidence of this maneuver.

The administration of *beta*-blockers is indicated also for the relief of life-threatening ventricular or atrial tachydysrhythmias (Fig. 9-10). In some centers propranolol is used initially for the relief of ventricular irritability, although lidocaine is still generally preferred. Atrial tachydysrhythmias are particularly devastating in patients with cardiac diseases (coronary artery disease, aortic stenosis). Propranolol is effective in these situations. Verapamil, a calcium-channel blocker, is now often used as a second line of defense.

The suggested dose-rates at which propranolol is administered intravenously vary greatly. Prys-Roberts recommends a 5 mg bolus in adults, and the earlier Swedish studies with ether and halothane anesthesia also used this regimen.[1,30] In most hospitals, increments of 0.25 to 1 mg to a total dose of .075 to 0.15 mg/kg maximum in adults are used. In children, the increments are smaller but the maximum total dose range is similar. Experience in the United States with intraoperative *beta*-adrenergic blocker administration other than propranolol is minimal. Other drugs may have advantages in certain situations. For instance, halothane induced systolic shortening (ischemic ventricular dysfunction) in an area of ventricle supplied by a critically narrowed coronary artery is improved by oxprenolol (a *beta*-blocker with ISA).[28a] Nonselective *beta*-adrenergic blockers have not yet been tested. Esmolol, an ultrashort-acting *beta*-blocker (elimination half-life 9 min) potentially provides the ability to rapidly alter the intensity of blockade.[28b]

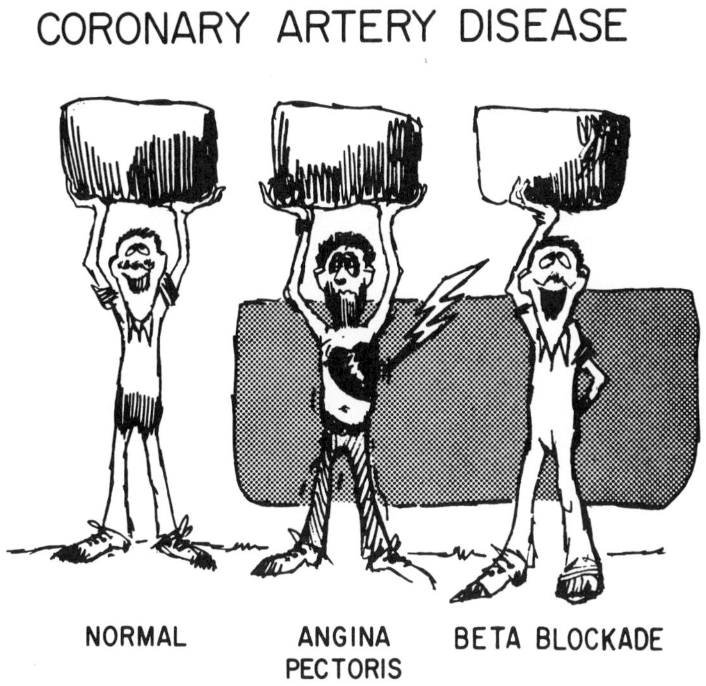

CORONARY ARTERY DISEASE

Fig. 9–7. Schematic representation of the situation pertaining in the presence of coronary artery disease. Angina pectoris occurs when the heart is performing a normal amount of work; *beta* blockade allows the same amount of work to be accomplished without evidence of myocardial ischemia.

Contraindications to *Beta*-Adrenergic Blockade

The primary contraindications to *beta*-adrenergic blockade are congestive heart failure, second- or third-degree heart block, and asthma. It is important to differentiate congestive heart failure, in which the heart is dependent on a catecholamine drive to maintain an adequate cardiac output, from acute elevations in left ventricular filling pressure associated with tachydysrhythmias. In the former, a *beta*-blocker may be disastrous; in the latter it may be lifesaving (Fig. 9–11). Some have argued that a *beta*-blocker with ISA is less likely to cause heart failure, but this hypothesis has not yet been proved. A *beta*-blocker should not be administered in the presence of second- or third-degree heart block unless pacing capabilities are immediately available. Low-dose atenolol (25 mg/day initial dose in adults), a drug with a maximum 40-fold selectivity for the *beta* 1 receptor, is a reasonable choice in asthmatic patients in whom *beta*-blockade is mandatory. At present, no cardioselective *beta*-blocker for use in patients with asthma is available in the United States for therapy in patients with asthma. Bronchoconstriction has been described in asthmatic patients even when a cardioselective drug has been employed,[29] emphasizing that cardioselectivity is a relative term.

Reversal of Propranolol-Associated Circulatory Depression (Table 9–4)

In most instances, circulatory depression associated with *beta*-adrenergic blockade consists of the combination of bradycardia and hypotension, which is usually relieved by atropine.[1,30] If readily available, as in cardiac surgical situations, cardiac pacing (preferably atrial) is equally effective. If bradycardia is not present, calcium chloride, up to 7 mg/kg by intravenous bolus, usually reverses hypotension. Whether

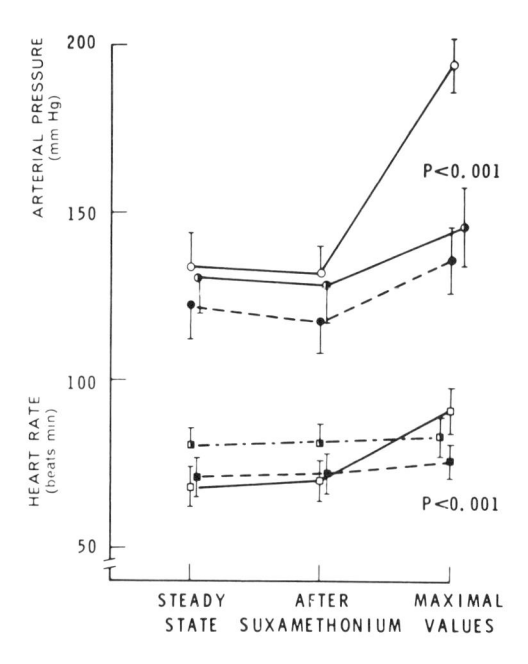

Fig. 9–8. Response of arterial blood pressure and heart rate to suxamethonium (succinylcholine) administration followed by laryngoscopy and tracheal intubation ("maximal values") during a standard anesthetic in three groups of patients with essential hypertension. Patients designated by the solid and half-filled squares and circles had received a beta-blocking drug, whereas those designated by the open circles and squares had not. The heart rate and blood pressure increases normally associated with laryngoscopy were attenuated by beta blockade. Incidence of ischemic ECG changes was reduced from 38 to 4%. (From Prys-Roberts, C., et al.: Studies of anesthesia in relation to hypertension. V. Adrenergic beta-receptor blockade. Br. J. Anaesth., 45:671, 1973.)

this response is due to enhanced myocardial contractility or to increased systemic vascular resistance is not known. This is more effective than isoproterenol, a nonselective beta agonist which is effective only in large doses. For example, in the presence of normal doses of propranolol (80 to 240 mg/day), the standard dose of isoproterenol must be increased 25 to 50 times[17] (see Table 9–5). The inotropic response may be less affected, but still required eight and 13 times the preblockade dose of isoproterenol in two patients receiving 160 and 240 mg/day.[17] If selective blockade of the cardiac beta receptors has been achieved, isoproterenol will cause marked vasodilation accompanied by hypotension before inotropy is augmented. In this situation, a relatively selective beta-1 agonist, such as dobutamine or prenalterol, should be used. Dopamine is a poor choice since the large doses needed to reverse beta-1 blockade may cause substantial vasoconstriction. On a long-term basis, digitalis is sometimes used to prevent the circulatory depression caused by large doses of propranolol, although this has little relevance to anesthesia. In spite of its theoretical contraindication, low doses of epinephrine (<2 μg/min) are sometimes used to reverse hypotension. The effect on cardiac output and systemic vascular resistance under these circumstances is not adequately defined.

Interactions Between Anesthesia and Beta-Adrenergic Blockade

The study of the interaction between anesthesia and beta-adrenergic blockade raises two questions: First, is there an additive and/or synergistic interaction between the circulatory-depressant action of the beta-adrenergic blocking agents and that of the anesthetic agents? Second, should beta-blockers be withheld or withdrawn prior to cardiac or noncardiac operations? These questions have been investigated in animals, and much information has been accumulated by experience in man.

Anesthetic agents can be divided into those that depend on the release of endogenous catecholamines to counteract their depressant effects (and therefore to maintain circulatory stability), and those that do not. There is certainly some overlap between these categories. Ether and cyclopropane typify anesthetic agents that depend on endogenous catecholamine liberation to support the circulation. Although narcotic anesthesia is often associated with catecholamine liberation during operations, circulatory competence is not dependent on this release. The modern com-

	NORMAL (Post-Induction)	BEFORE PROPRANOLOL	AFTER 0.1 mg PROPRANOLOL	AFTER 0.2 mg PROPRANOLOL
HR	81	107	102	84

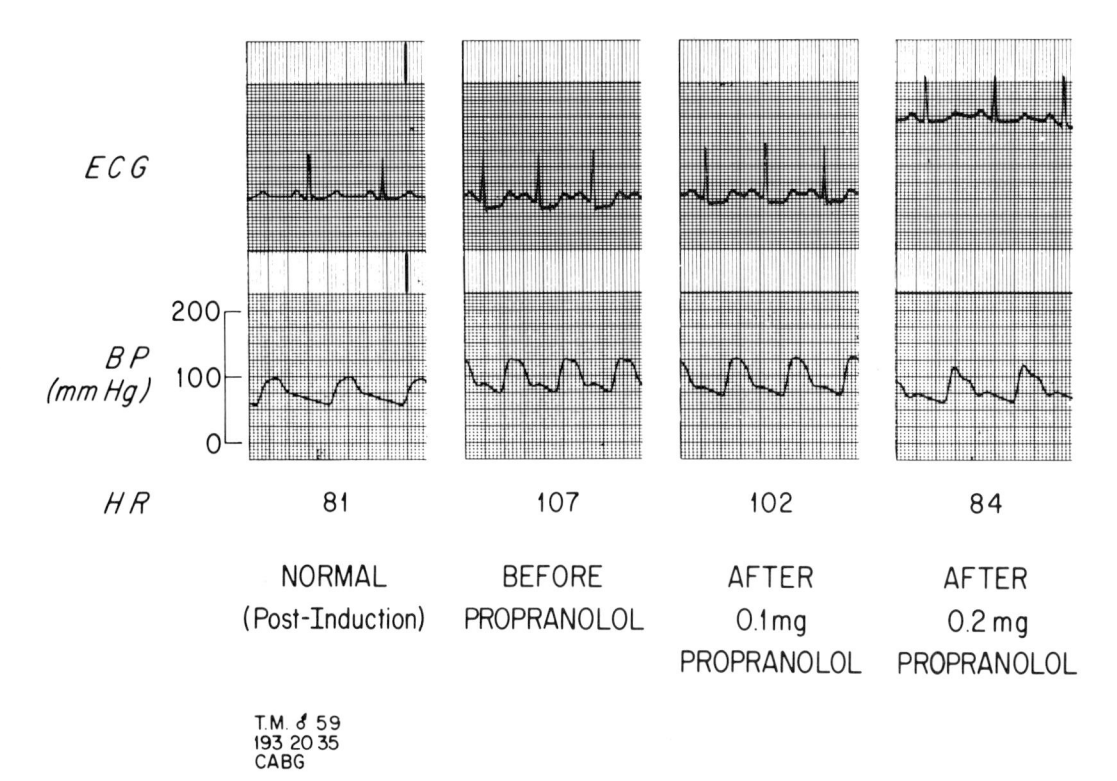

T.M. ♂ 59
193 20 35
CABG

Fig. 9–9. Relief of electrocardiographic evidence of myocardial ischemia by propranolol administration. A modest rise in heart rate (81 to 107) and blood pressure (110/55 to 125/75), consequent to surgical stimulation was associated with a 2 mm depression of ST segment. Two 0.1 mg increments of propranolol were associated with return of blood pressure and heart rate to pre-ischemic levels, and restoration of ST segment to normal.

monly used inhalation anesthetics do not depend on catecholamine liberation for circulatory stability.

For the reasons cited previously, it appears prudent to avoid *beta*-adrenergic blockade during ether and cyclopropane, since they depend on catecholamine release for the maintenance of circulatory integrity. In healthy volunteers, a 5 mg bolus of propranolol injected intravenously during ether anesthesia induced decreased heart rate, stroke volume, cardiac output, and increased systemic vascular resistance. The single episode of severe circulatory depression (hypotension, bradycardia) observed was reversed by atropine. Although data on intravenous induction agents are presently insufficient, ketamine appears to be similar to ether anesthesia in its dependence on endogenous catecholamines for circulatory integrity. Thus it may be wise to avoid the combination of *beta*-adrenergic blockers and this drug.

Those anesthetic agents that do not depend on catecholamine release for circulatory stability include halothane,[33] opioids, methoxyflurane, trichloroethylene, enflurane, and isoflurane. Clinical and experimental data indicate that the combination of *beta*-blockers with either narcotics or halothane is safe. For instance, the circulatory response to halothane in the normovolemic or hypovolemic animal is similar at several levels of halothane anesthesia, whether or not the animal has received a *beta*-adrenergic blocker.[34] Kopriva et al. reported the response of two groups of patients with ischemic heart disease to an anesthetic regimen consisting of thiopental, succinylcholine, nitrous oxide, hal-

RESOLUTION OF CHAOTIC RHYTHM POST-BYPASS BY PROPRANOLOL

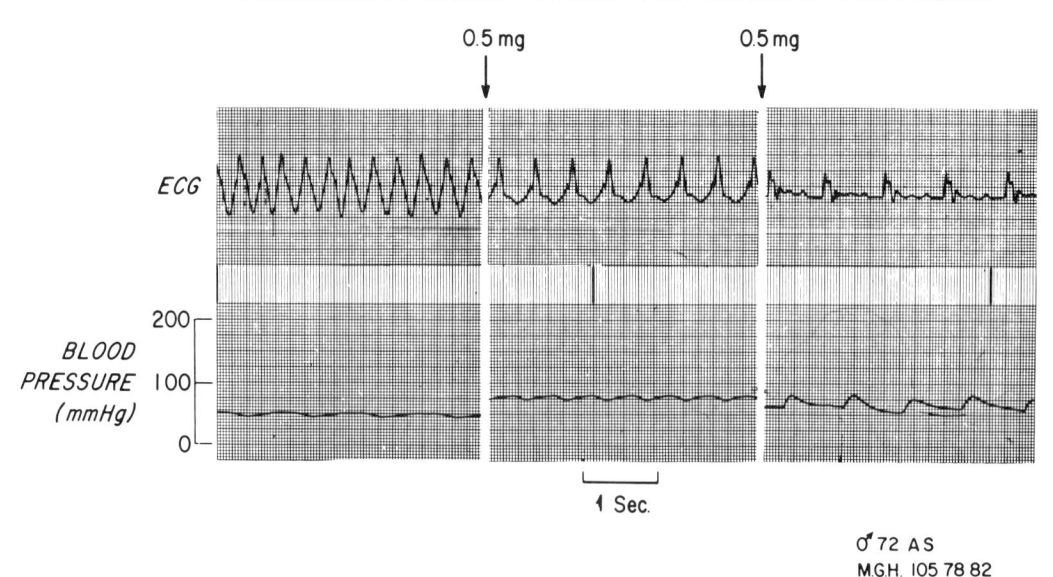

Fig. 9–10. Resolution by propranolol of chaotic ventricular rhythm prior to termination of cardiopulmonary bypass. Left panel: Chaotic rhythm persisted despite multiple attempts at electrical defibrillation and drug therapy including lidocaine, procaine amide, phenytoin, and bretylium tosylate at termination of cardiopulmonary bypass. Center panel: Propranolol (0.5 mg) produced an organized ventricular rhythm. Right panel: A further 0.5 mg propranolol was associated with sinus rhythm with AV and intraventricular block, increased ventricular ejection as indicated on the blood pressure tracing, and effective heart action. The patient's further course was uneventful.

Table 9–4

1. Bradycardia
    atropine
    pacing
2. Pharmacologic reversal
    cardioselective blocker: dobutamine, prenalterol
    nonselective blocker: isoproterenol
3. Action beyond the block
    digitalis
    calcium chloride
4. Empiric
    epinephrine in low doses

othane, and pancuronium.[35] One group received an average of 140 mg propranolol per day until a few hours before general anesthesia, whereas the other group did not receive the drug. The only difference between the groups was the lower heart rate in the group treated with propranolol. No differences in mean arterial pressure, cardiac output, stroke volume, or systemic vascular resistance were present in response to anesthesia or endotracheal intubation. Ventricular filling pressures were not measured in this study. Slogoff et al.[36] compared the response to isoproterenol beta-adrenergic stimulation of propranolol-blocked dogs receiving either halothane or morphine anesthesia. The researchers demonstrated that propranolol is associated with dose-related decreases in heart rate, cardiac index, stroke volume index, and left ventricular contractility, as well as increases in mean aortic pressure, systemic vascular resistance, and pulmonary capillary wedge pressure. However, no increased sensitivity to any measured effect of propranolol, expressed as the slope of the log dose-response curve, was observed. The researchers concluded that there was no potentiation by morphine or halothane of the effects of propranolol.

Studies with enflurane, trilene, and methoxyflurane, however, cause concern. For

Table 9-5
Effect of Beta Blockade on Subsequent Response to Isoproterenol in Man

Dose Propranolol (mg/day)	Chronotropic Multiple	Chronotropic Absolute	Inotropic Multiple	Inotropic Absolute
80	× 50	(40 μg)	—	—
160	× 23	(42 μg)	× 13	(17 μg)
240	× 38	(34 μg)	× 8	(6 μg)

Effect of *beta* blockade with oral propranolol (80 to 240 mg/day) on the subsequent response to intravenous isoproterenol in three subjects with coronary artery disease. Note the enormous increase in the dose of isoproterenol (23 to 50 times the original dose) required to increase heart rate by the same increment as before blockade. The dose required to increase contractility is also greatly elevated, but the increase is less than that required to elevate heart rate. (Data from Faulkner, S.L., et al.: Time required for complete recovery from chronic propranolol therapy. N. Engl. J. Med., 289:607, 1973.)

instance, enflurane is associated with marginally greater impairment of left ventricular function than halothane anesthesia in the normovolemic propranolol *beta*-adrenergically blocked dog. However, withdrawal of 20% of estimated blood volume is tolerated poorly by the circulation during enflurane anesthesia.[37] The degree of circulatory depression produced under these circumstances would be clinically unacceptable. Enflurane is widely used to anesthetize patients receiving propranolol for cardiac operations, and there is little evidence that unacceptable circulatory depression is induced. The disparity between these animal studies and the clinical experience may be dose related. The adverse response to enflurane was observed

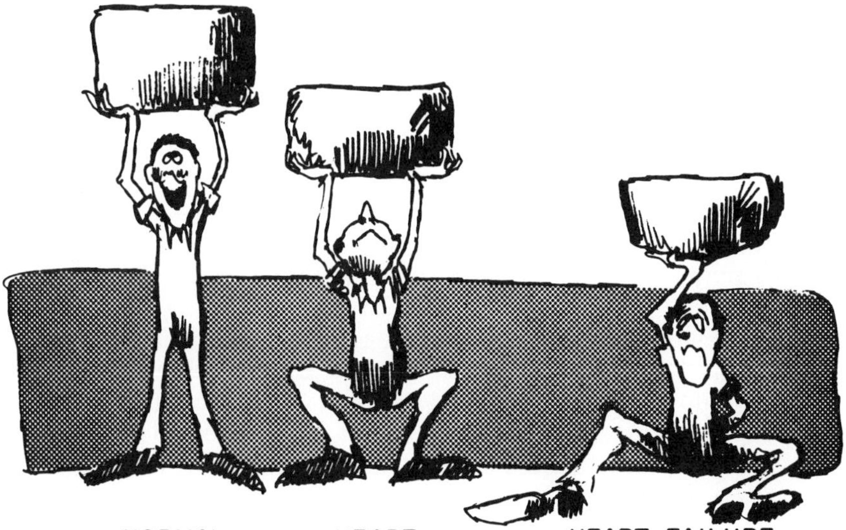

Fig. 9-11. Schematic diagram of the effect of *beta*-blocker administration in heart failure. Chronic heart failure is associated with progressive dependence on catecholamines for maintenance of circulatory integrity. Blockade induces acute interruption of this support, and collapse may occur without increasing the burden of the heart. Compare situation here to that depicted in the normal heart (Fig. 9-5) and the heart with coronary artery disease (Fig. 9-7).

at 3% end expired concentration, whereas 2% was well tolerated.[37a] Interestingly, response to enflurane in dogs in which *beta* blockade was achieved by oxprenolol, which possesses ISA was not different from dogs not *beta* blocked.[37b]

Trichloroethylene anesthesia in the normovolemic *beta*-blocked dog, pretreated for three weeks with 20 mg/kg/day of propranolol orally, did not inhibit adequate cardiovascular function.[38] However, the response to graded hemorrhage was associated with a decrease in cardiac output that precluded recovery in some animals. The cause of the circulatory collapse appeared to be direct myocardial depression, since normal left ventricular filling pressures were associated with inadequate stroke volumes.

The adverse interactions between trichloroethylene and methoxyflurane are only of historical interest. The most alarming observations were made with the combination of methoxyflurane 0.4% and practolol.[39] Three of ten dogs receiving practolol under these circumstances died within 15 minutes. These were the only deaths encountered by the investigators at Oxford when using this model. In the seven survivors, cardiac output and left ventricular dP/dt decreased, and left ventricular end-diastolic pressure increased in the presence of normal heart rate, blood pressure, and systemic vascular resistance. The clinical applicability of these studies is indicated by the report of a series of cardiac surgical patients who demonstrated irreversible circulatory depression at the termination of cardiopulmonary bypass after having received methoxyflurane.[2]

In contrast, experimental evidence suggests that isoflurane might be the ideal anesthetic agent to employ in the presence of *beta*-adrenergic blockade. Philbin and Lowenstein found no difference in cardiac output, arterial blood pressure, systemic vascular resistance, heart rate, or left ventricular filling pressure in dogs anesthetized with one and two MAC (minimum alveolar concentrations) isoflurane before and after administration of 0.5 mg/kg propranolol[31,40] (Fig. 9–12).

Sensitive indices of ventricular performance are only minimally depressed when 0.3 mg/kg propranolol is administered to dogs receiving isoflurane.[32] Thus, although isoflurane may be associated with a minor *beta*-adrenergic receptor-stimulating effect, its clinical importance remains unclear.

The studies performed to date in both man and animals thus indicate that myocardial depression from anesthetic agents and *beta*-adrenergic blockers is additive, and that a spectrum of tolerance to the combination of different anesthetic agents and a *beta*-blocker exists (see Fig. 9–13). The clinical implications of the data are that an absolute indication for the use of methoxyflurane, diethyl ether, trichloroethylene, or cyclopropane must exist before these drugs should be used in combination with *beta*-adrenergic blockers. Caution should be exercised when using high doses of enflurane in the presence of *beta* blockade. Halothane, narcotics, and isoflurane appear to be appropriate choices.

DISCONTINUANCE PRIOR TO ANESTHESIA AND OPERATION

By and large, whether to discontinue *beta*-adrenergic blockade prior to the administration of general anesthesia no longer is a controversial issue. The proponents of discontinuance believe that circulatory depression from the anesthetic-*beta*-blocker combination is possibly fatal. Those opposed to discontinuance feel strongly about the hazards of the former course of action. They base their arguments on the following factors: (1) if a patient needs *beta* blockade for relief of angina pectoris and myocardial insufficiency, withdrawal of a drug essential to the patient is irrational and hazardous, particularly in view of the formidable stress of the perioperative period;[4,41,42] and (2) the discontinuance of a *beta*-adrenergic blockade

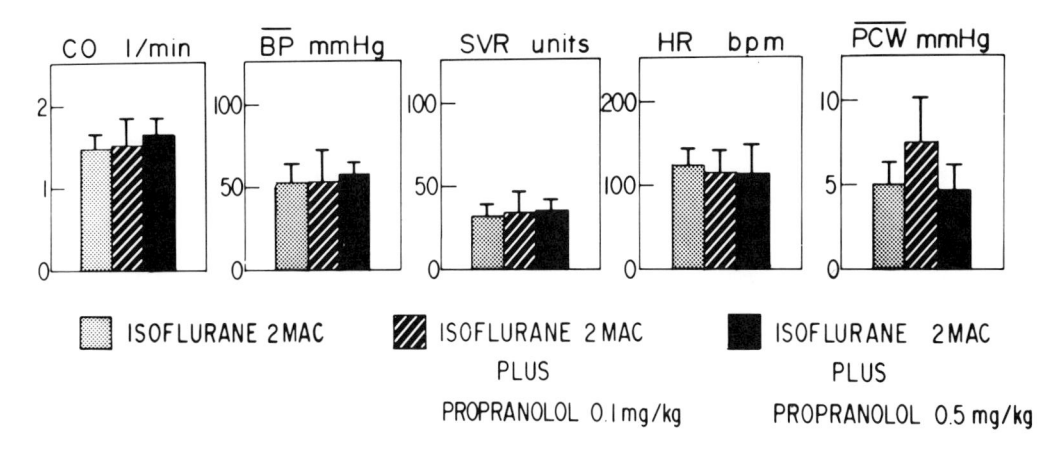

Fig. 9–12. Hemodynamic effect of propranolol during 2MAC isoflurane anesthesia in the dog. There was no detectable difference in cardiac output, arterial blood pressure, systemic vascular resistance, heart rate, and pulmonary capillary wedge pressure among three groups of dogs receiving isoflurane anesthesia, despite the absence of propranolol in one group, a modest dose (0.1 mg/kg) in a second group, and a large dose (0.5 mg/kg) in the third. The data suggest that isoflurane administration is associated with little if any *beta*-adrenergic agonism. (From Philbin, D.M., and Lowenstein, E.: Lack of *beta*-adrenergic activity of isoflurane in the dog: A comparison of circulatory effects of halothane and isoflurane after propranolol administration. Br. J. Anaesth., 48:1165, 1976.)

may lead to a situation analogous to denervation supersensitivity.[7]

Obviously, *beta* blockade can be safely discontinued in patients who did not initially present a valid indication for it. Mainly anecdotal clinical data exist to support the contention that *beta*-adrenergic blockers should be withheld or decreased in dose. Since some of these recommendations come from respected anesthesiologists in highly regarded clinical centers, it seems unwarranted to dismiss them. However, evidence exists that favors the continuance of *beta*-adrenergic blockers until anesthesia and operation. In fact, this evidence argues for the prophylactic

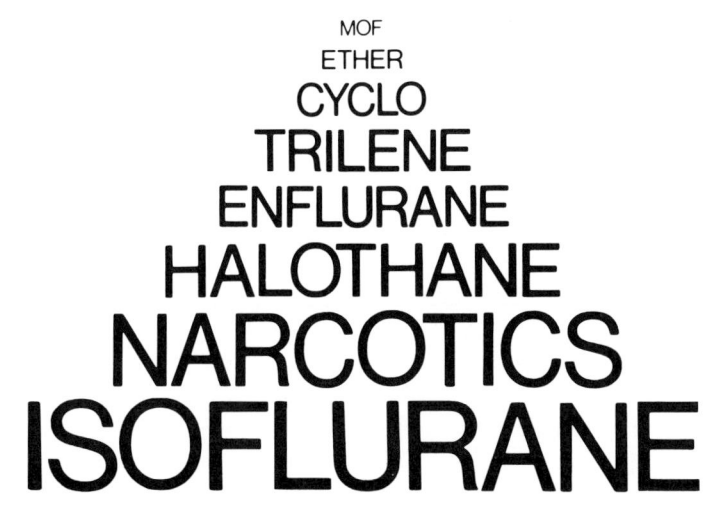

MOF
ETHER
CYCLO
TRILENE
ENFLURANE
HALOTHANE
NARCOTICS
ISOFLURANE

Fig. 9–13. Pyramid denoting the spectrum of compatibility of the combination of various anesthetic agents and *beta* blockade. See text for detail.

administration of *beta*-blockers prior to anesthesia in some instances, as well as their continuance throughout the entire postoperative period. The most compelling argument is the evidence that the discontinuance of *beta*-adrenergic blocking agents in patients who require these drugs for the control of severe angina is associated with an unacceptably high incidence of acute life-threatening, or even fatal, complications (Fig. 9–14).

In one carefully controlled study[4] (see Table 9–6), such complications, including two deaths, were observed in 6 of 20 patients. Increased severity of angina pectoris was observed in an additional four. Those patients who had the most severe angina pectoris were the ones who experienced the greatest difficulty. Many other studies confirm these data.[42,43] For example, a recent prospective, controlled study by Ponten and colleagues[45] demonstrated that discontinuation of *beta* blockade causes a substantial incidence of cardiovascular complications in noncardiac surgical patients with coronary artery disease. Withdrawal over four days was associated with a higher incidence of dysrhythmias, angina pectoris and ECG signs of myocardial ischemia. Continuing treatment is also safer prior to coronary artery surgery.[46] Lastly, recent experiments have dealt with the hypothesis that *beta*-adrenergic blockade might reverse ischemic regional dysfunction associated with anesthetic. In independent investigations, oxprenolol, a *beta*-adrenergic blocker with ISA, was administered after regional dysfunction had been induced by either 2% halothane[44] or 3.3% enflurane.[37b] Since oxprenolol is a partial agonist, heart rate and arterial pressure were not substantially modified. Similarly, indices of contractility (LV dP/dt, aortic blood acceleration, LV peak power) were slightly enhanced rather than depressed. Thus, an overall reduction of myocardial oxygen demand is unlikely to have taken place with these changes in the major determinants of myocardial oxygen demand.

Although regional function was unchanged in those regions supplied by a normal coronary artery, function was markedly improved in the area supplied by a narrowed coronary artery (Fig. 9–15). Systolic shortening was increased, post-systolic shortening decreased and "work" increased with, if anything, a small decrease in end-diastolic length. Experiments have not been performed to determine whether this improvement was due to the ISA or to the *beta* blockade per se. Potential mechanisms include improved collateral blood flow, protection of ATP stores, alterations of substrate metabolism, protection of the microvasculature against the effects of ischemia, or stabilization of cardiac lysosomal enzymes. The subject is sufficiently important to warrant further research.

Two pieces of information modify to a minor degree the recommendation to continue *beta*-blockers throughout the perioperative period. Wechsler, in a double-blind, controlled study, reported that patients receiving 320 to 480 mg propranolol per day had an increased incidence of requiring postoperative inotropic support.[48] Interestingly, no increased cardiac morbidity was noted by Wechsler in patients who required such support. The only question one might raise about this study is whether those patients who required such large doses of *beta*-blockers constituted a group at higher risk for requiring postoperative support.

The Johns Hopkins Cardiac Surgical Unit noted a higher incidence of postoperative hypertension in patients receiving preoperative *beta*-blockers,[49] and a linear ($r = 0.7$) correlation between postoperative serum propranolol levels and nitroprusside dose to maintain mean blood pressure between 80 and 90 mm Hg.[50] They administered supplemental propranolol postoperatively in order to achieve sufficiently high propranolol concentration in enough patients to establish the concentration dependence. This phenomenon appears to be due to *beta*-2 receptor blockade, and emphasizes

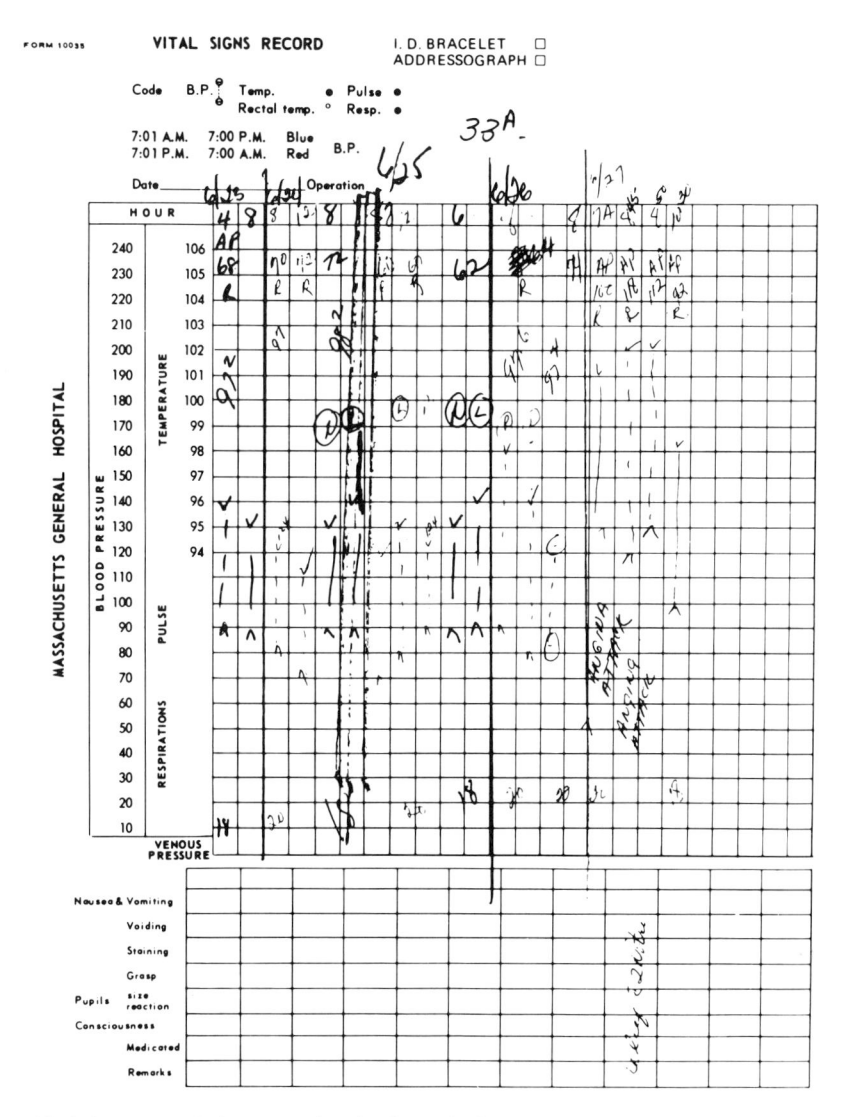

Fig. 9–14. Vital signs record demonstrating the hazard of preoperative discontinuance of propranolol in a patient with severe coronary artery disease. The last dose of propranolol was administered at 10 P.M. 6/25. Less than 36 hours later, the blood pressure had risen from a steady value of 130/90 to 200/130, and the heart rate from the low 60's to a maximum of 118 beats/min. These changes were associated with angina pectoris and severe (up to 6 mm) depression of the ST segment in the precordial leads.

the desirability of absolute receptor specific blockade. It is of note that both these studies were performed in cardiac surgical patients. Wechsler's 400 mg propranolol per day pales by contrast to the multiple *gram* per day dosage reported by Prys-Roberts in patients with renal hypertension undergoing noncardiac surgery.[51] In these patients, there was little evidence of an adverse response despite these massive doses.

In summary, we can draw several conclusions with confidence. The hazard of withdrawal, even when performed gradually, far outweighs that of continuation in surgical patients with a valid indication for *beta*-adrenergic blockade. It is possible that tapering the dose to the equivalent of 360

Table 9-6
Complications Associated with Acute Cessation of Propranolol in 20 Patients Receiving it for Symptoms of Coronary Artery Disease

Fatalities	2
(Sudden death .... 1)	
(Fatal myocardial infarction .... 1)	
Acute life-threatening events	4
(Unstable angina pectoris .... 3)	
(Ventricular tachycardia .... 1)	
Increased severity of angina pectoris	4

(Data from Miller, R.R., et al.: Propranolol-withdrawal rebound phenomenon. N. Engl. J. Med., 293:416, 1975.)

EFFECT OF OXPRENOLOL ON REGIONAL FUNCTION

Before oxprenolol ——————
After oxprenolol − − − − − −

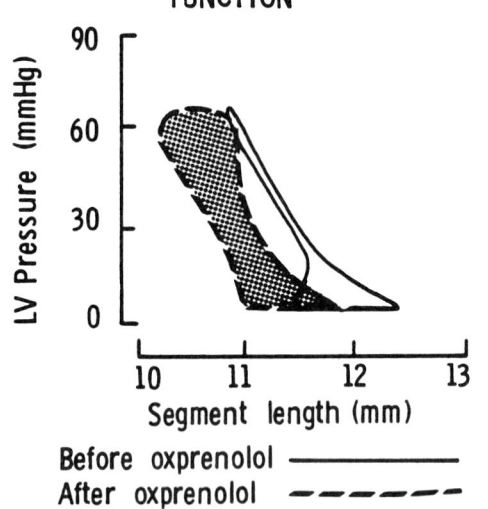

Fig. 9–15. Regional myocardial function, estimated by the instantaneous relationship between left ventricular pressure and segment length, is severely depressed by halothane in myocardium supplied by a critically narrowed left anterior descending coronary artery. The area inside the pressure-length loop, proportional to regional work, is small. After oxprenolol (0.3 mg·kg⁻¹ IV), end-diastolic length is shorter and the area inside the pressure-length loop is greatly increased, indicating improved function.[28a]

mg or less propranolol per day may prevent the need for postoperative inotropic support in cardiac surgical patients. Modern inhalation anesthetics are well tolerated in the presence of *beta* blockade, and are not associated with "mysterious" interactions accounting for untoward circulatory events. Selective *beta* receptor blockade, though desirable, is hard to achieve reliably. It is therefore reasonable to assume some peripheral blockade despite administration of a cardioselective drug. Lastly, there is experimental evidence to suggest that *beta*-adrenergic blockers may enhance performance of acutely ischemic myocardium, associated with anesthetic administration in regions supplied by a narrowed coronary artery. This enhancement occurs in the absence of changes in hemodynamic measurements. This is not predictable with *beta*-blockers that do not possess ISA.

REFERENCES

1. Jorfeldt, L., et al.: Propranolol in ether anesthesia. Acta Anaesthesiol. Scand., 11:159, 1967.
2. Viljoen, J.F., Estafanous, F.G., and Kellner, G.A.: Propranolol and cardiac surgery. J. Thorac. Cardiovasc. Surg., 64:826, 1972.
3. Kaplan, J.A., et al.: Propranolol and cardiac surgery: A problem for the anesthesiologist? Anesth. Analg. (Cleve.), 54:571, 1975.
4. Miller, R.R., et al.: Propranolol-withdrawal rebound phenomenon. N. Engl. J. Med., 293:416, 1975.
5. Prys-Roberts, C., et al.: Studies of anaesthesia in relation to hypertension. V.: Adrenergic *beta*-receptor blockade. Br. J. Anaesth., 45:671, 1973.
6. Lefkowitz, R.J.: *Beta*-adrenergic receptors: recognition and regulation. N. Engl. J. Med., 295:323, 1976.
7. Boudoulas, H., et al.: Hypersensitivity to adrenergic stimulation after propranolol withdrawal in normal subjects. Ann. Intern. Med., 87:433, 1977.
8. Ahlquist, R.P.: A study of the adrenotropic receptors. Am. J. Physiol., 153:586, 1948.
9. Lands, A.M., et al.: Differentiation of receptor systems activated by sympathomimetic amines. Nature, 214:597, 1967.
10. Dreyer, A.C., and Offermeier, J.: Indications for the existence of two types of cardiac *beta*-adrenergic receptors. Pharmacol. Res. Commun., 7:151, 1975.
11. Boudoulas, H., et al.: Differential time course of inotropic and chronotropic blockade after oral propranolol. Cardiovasc. Med., 2:511, 1977.
12. Frishman, W.H.: β-Adrenoreceptor antagonists: New drugs and new indications. N. Engl. J. Med., 305:500, 1981.

13. Hollifield, J.W., et al.: Proposed mechanisms of propranolol's antihypertensive effect in essential hypertension. N. Engl. J. Med., *295*:68, 1976.
14. Holland, O.B., and Kaplan, N.M.: Propranolol in the treatment of hypertension. N. Engl. J. Med., *294*:930, 1976.
16. Coltart, D.J., and Shand, D.G.: Plasma propranolol levels in the quantitative assessment of *beta*-adrenergic blockade in man. Br. Med. J., *3*:731, 1970.
17. Faulkner, S.L., et al.: Time required for complete recovery from chronic propranolol therapy. N. Engl. J. Med., *289*:607, 1973.
19. James, I.M., et al.: Effect of oxprenolol on stagefright in musicians. Lancet, *2*:952, 1977.
20. Stenson, R.E., et al.: Hypertrophic subaortic stenosis. Clinical and hemodynamic effects of longterm propranolol therapy. Am. J. Cardiol., *31*:763, 1973.
21. Zacest, R., Gilmore, E., and Koch-Weser, J.: Treatment of essential hypertension with combined vasodilation and *beta*-adrenergic blockade. N. Engl. J. Med., *286*:617, 1972.
22. Berk, J.L., et al.: The treatment of shock with *beta*-adrenergic blockade. Arch. Surg., *104*:46, 1972.
24. Pitt, B., and Ross, R.S.: *Beta* adrenergic blockade in cardiovascular therapy. Mod. Concepts Cardiovasc. Dis., *38*:47, 1969.
25. Braunwald, E.: The determinants of myocardial oxygen consumption. Physiologist, *12*:65, 1969.
26. Aronow, W.S.: The medical treatment of angina pectoris. VI. Propranolol as an antianginal drug. Am. Heart. J., *84*:706, 1972.
27. McGregor, M.: Drugs for the treatment of angina. In Internationaal Encyclopedia of Pharmacology and Therapeutics. Edited by L. Lasagna. Oxford, Pergamon, 1966, Vol. II, Section 6.
28. Reul, G., et al.: Protective effect of propranolol on the hypertrophied heart during cardiopulmonary bypass. J. Thorac. Cardiovasc. Surg., *68*:283, 1974.
28a. Foëx, P., et al.: Beta-adrenergic blockade and anesthesia. In The clinical impact of beta-adrenergic blockade. Burley, D.M. and Birdwood, G.F.B., editors. Horsham, England, CIBA Laboratories, 1980, pp. 75–96.
28b. Sum, C.Y., et al.: Kinetics of esmolol, an ultrashort-acting blocker, and of its major metabolite. Clin. Pharmacol. Ther., *34*:427, 1983.
29. Bernecker, C., and Roetscher, I.: The *beta*-blocking effect of practolol in asthmatics. Lancet, *2*:662, 1970.
30. Jorfeldt, L., et al.: Cardiovascular effects of *beta*-receptor blocking drugs during halothane anaesthesia in man. Acta Anesthesiol. Scand., *14*:35, 1970.
31. Philbin, D.M., and Lowenstein, E.: Lack of *beta*-adrenergic activity of isoflurane in the dog: A comparison of circulatory effects of halothane and isoflurane after propranolol administration. Br. J. Anaesth., *48*:1165, 1976.
32. Horan, B.F., et al.: Haemodynamic responses to isoflurane anaesthesia and hypovolaemia in the dog, and their modification by propranolol. Br. J. Anaesth., *49*:1179, 1977.
33. Merin, R.G., and Tonnesen, A.S.: The effect of *beta*-adrenergic blockade on myocardial haemodynamics and metabolism during light halothane anaesthesia. Can. Anaesth. Soc. J., *16*:336, 1969.
34. Roberts, J.G., et al.: Haemodynamic interactions of high-dose propranolol protreatment and anaesthesia in the dog. I: Halothane dose-response studies. Br. J. Anaesth., *48*:315, 1976.
35. Kopriva, C.J., Brown, A.C.D., and Pappas, G.: Hemodynamics during general anesthesia in patients receiving propranolol. Anesthesiology, *48*:28, 1978.
36. Slogoff, S., et al.: Failure of general anesthesia to potentiate propranolol activity. Anesthesiology, *47*:504, 1977.
37. Horan, B.F., et al.: Haemodynamic responses to enflurane anaesthesia and hypovolaemia in the dog, and their modification by propranolol. Br. J. Anaesth., *49*:1189, 1977.
37a. Horan, B.F., et al.: Haemodynamic responses to enflurane anaesthesia and hypovolemia in the dog and their modification by propranolol. Br. J. Anaesth., *49*:1189, 1977.
37b. Cutfield, G.R., et al.: The effects of oxprenolol on myocardial function during enflurane anesthesia. Br. J. Anaesth., *53*:668, 1981.
38. Roberts, J.G., et al.: Haemodynamic interactions of high-dose propranolol pretreatment and anaesthesia in the dog. III: the effects of haemorrhage during halothane and trichloroethylene anaesthesia. Br. J. Anaesth., *48*:411, 1976.
39. Saner, C.A., et al.: Methoxyflurane and practolol: a dangerous combination? Br. J. Anaesth., *47*:1025, 1975.
40. Philbin, D.M., and Lowenstein, E.: Lack of *beta* adrenergic activity of isoflurane in the dog: A comparison of circulatory effects of halothane and isoflurane after propranolol administration. Br. J. Anaesth., *48*:1165, 1976.
41. Slome, R.: Withdrawal of propranolol and myocardial infarction. Lancet, *1*:156, 1973.
42. Mizgala, H.F., and Counsell, J.: Acute coronary syndromes following abrupt cessation of oral propranolol therapy. Can. Med. Assoc. J., *114*:1123, 1976.
43. Jones, E.L., et al.: Propranolol therapy in patients undergoing myocardial revascularization. Am. J. Cardiol., *38*:697, 1976.
44. Foëx, P., et al.: The interactions between β-blockers and anaesthetics. Experimental observations. Acta Anaesth. Scand. Supplement, *76*:38, 1982.
45. Pontén, J., Biber, B., Bjurö, T., and Henriksson, B-Å, and Hjalmarson, Å: Withdrawal—a preoperative problem in general surgery. Acta Anaesth. Scand. Supplement, *76*:32, 1982.
46. Oka, Y., Frishman, W., Becker, R.M., et al.: Appraisal and reappraisal of cardiac therapy. Am. Heart J., *99*:255, 1980.
47. Cutfield, G.R., et al.: Myocardial function and critical constriction of the left anterior descending coronary artery: protective effect of oxprenolol. Br. J. Anaesth., *53*:189p, 1981a.
48. Wechsler, A.S.: Assessment of prospectively randomized patients receiving propranolol therapy before coronary bypass operation. Ann. Thorac. Surg., *30*:128, 1980.
49. Whelton, P.K., Flaherty, J.T., MacAllister, N.P.,

Watkins, L., Potter, A., Johnson, D., Russell, R.P., and Walker, W.G.: Hypertension following coronary artery bypass surgery. Hypertension, 2:291, 1980.
50. Bolling, S.F., Flaherty, J.T., Potter, A.M., et al.: Propranolol-induced postoperative hypertension following coronary artery bypass grafting. J. Thorac. Cardiovasc. Surg., 87:112, 1984.
51. Prys-Roberts, C.: Interactions of anaesthesia and high preoperative doses of β-receptor antagonists. Acta Anaesth. Scand. Supplement, 76:47, 1982.

Supported in part by NHLBI SCOR grant HL23591.

|10|

CALCIUM-CHANNEL BLOCKERS AND OTHER VASODILATING ANTIANGINAL AGENTS

PATRICIA A. KAPUR

The addition of calcium-channel blockers to our therapeutic efforts has widened the scope of antianginal therapy and is a welcome addition to the therapeutic options for myocardial ischemia, i.e., the nitroglycerin family of drugs and the *beta*-blockers. This chapter will discuss calcium-channel blockers and the nitroglycerin compounds. Several of the presently available calcium-channel blockers possess conduction interfering properties at clinical concentrations and manifest antidysrhythmic effects as well.

CALCIUM-CHANNEL BLOCKERS

The term "calcium-channel blockers" as commonly used refers to a group of drugs which interfere with some aspect of the functioning of the slow calcium channel of excitable cell membranes. Unlike chelating agents, these drugs are not true calcium antagonists, they are rather a subgroup of a broad class of drugs which are called calcium entry blockers and which share the ability to modulate contractile and other intracellular processes by interfering with calcium influx across the cell membrane.[1]

The slow calcium-channel blockers are the first of this large group to be widely recognized. However, it is important to remember that there are multiple sites of possible interference with the effects of extracellular calcium influx (Table 10–1). These include (1) the voltage dependent slow calcium channel; (2) receptor activated calcium channels triggered by norepinephrine, serotonin, histamine, prostaglandins, etc.; (3) passive membrane diffusion channels for calcium; (4) membrane storage sites for calcium; and (5) secondary effects of such drugs on intracellular organelles that sequester calcium.[2] None of the currently available calcium-channel blockers is specific for one type of calcium channel. In addition to effects on various types of cal-

Table 10–1
Sites for Alteration of Calcium Homeostasis in Cardiovascular Cells

Slow calcium channel: requires depolarization, "voltage sensitive"
Receptor-activated calcium channels: requires cell membrane receptor interaction with appropriate agonist (e.g. norepinephrine)
Passive diffusion channels: depends on ionic gradient, limited significance
Membrane storage sites for calcium: displaceable calcium pool
Intracellular calcium storage organelles (e.g. sarcoplasmic reticulum, mitochondria): secondary effects of calcium channel blocking drugs

cium channels, calcium-channel blockers may also affect sodium or potassium fluxes, which contributes to their net clinical effects.

The slow channel inhibitors verapamil, nifedipine, and diltiazem are widely prescribed for the treatment of vasospastic and obstructive angina pectoris. Verapamil is also used to treat slow calcium-channel sensitive dysrhythmias. The pharmacodynamic profiles of these drugs also offer therapeutic possibilities for the treatment of hypertension, hypertrophic obstructive cardiomyopathy, peripheral and cerebral vasospastic disease, and for myocardial protection. Thus, anesthesia practitioners will be called upon to care for patients on chronic oral therapy with these drugs as well as encounter a variety of intraoperative indications for their administration. A thorough understanding of their pharmacology and interactions with agents used during anesthesia is essential for their safe and effective use.

CASE REPORT

A 70-year-old, 75-kg man, was diagnosed as having a gas gangrene wound infection of his left leg 2 days after undergoing a below the knee amputation and 20 days after undergoing a failed left ilio-femoral bypass graft procedure. His medical history included insulin-dependent diabetes mellitus and a cerebrovascular accident 2 years previously. He did not have a history of heart failure. At 8:30 P.M. he came to the operating room for an emergency above the knee amputation. Upon arrival in the operating room, his blood pressure was 150/90 and heart rate was 90. Preoperative serum glucose was 240 mg·dl^{-1}, serum potassium was 4.8 mEq·L^{-1}, and arterial blood gases with spontaneous respirations and oxygen by face mask were pH 7.46, PO$_2$ 100 mm Hg, PCO$_2$ 27 mm Hg and base excess −3.4 mEq·L^{-1}. The patient received thiopental 250 mg; succinylcholine 100 mg; followed by tracheal intubation and controlled ventilation (F$_I$O$_2$ = 1.0). Enflurane was titrated to control systolic blood pressure between 130 and 160 mm Hg. A total of 6 mg of pancuronium was administered during the remainder of the procedure. When the surgeons began to actively manipulate the ischemic extremity, the heart rate then soared to 160 from 100 beats per min; systolic blood pressure dropped to 75 mm Hg; and the electrocardiogram showed a supraventricular tachycardia. Verapamil (2.5 mg IV) transiently abolished the dysrhythmia with an improvement in blood pressure. There were, however, three more episodes of the dysrhythmia during the next 15 minutes which responded to verapamil 2.5, 5, and 5 mg, by intravenous bolus, while the systolic blood pressure gradually decreased again to 90 mm Hg. The enflurane was temporarily turned off and calcium chloride, 1 g in divided doses, was administered. The systolic pressure then rose to 140 mm Hg.

Laboratory results from the time of extremity manipulations showed arterial pH 7.30, PO$_2$ 127 mm Hg, PCO$_2$ 32 mm Hg, base excess −9.6 mEq·L^{-1}, and potassium 5 mEq·L^{-1}. Bicarbonate, 44 mEq, was also administered. Dysrhythmias ceased after the amputation was completed. The systolic blood pressure remained between 130 and 150 mm Hg. At 10:45 P.M., the patient was transferred to the recovery room in stable condition.

This case report illustrates an unanticipated indication for acute verapamil administration during anesthesia for a high-risk patient with known occlusive vascular disease. Paroxysmal supraventricular tachydysrhythmias are generally reentrant in nature and are converted to sinus rhythm with a high degree of efficacy by verapamil.[3] However, the patient was receiving an inhalation anesthetic, had an unknown electrolyte status, and was suffering from cardiovascular depression secondary to the acidosis and release of ischemic metabolites from his gangrenous leg. Depressant cardiovascular effects of the calcium-channel blockers are additive with inhalational anesthetics and verapamil is less well tolerated in the presence of myocardial dysfunction. Titration of small intravenous increments of verapamil was accompanied by calcium administration to allow dysrhythmia control without further compromise of blood pressure. Upon removal of the ischemic leg, there were no further recurrences of the dysrhythmia.

Consequences of Slow Channel Inhibition

The morphology of the action potential of myocardial cells is dependent upon membrane fluxes of Na$^+$, Ca^{++}, and K$^+$ that occur when the appropriate voltage conditions are met in the course of the depolarization and repolarization of such cells.[4] The membrane channels which are permeable to these ions differ in their rates of activation. At a membrane potential of −60 to −70 mV, relatively rapidly activated membrane channels assume favorable configurations, allowing the inward passage of sodium ions, which results in the rapid upstroke (Phase 0) of the action potential of normal atrial and ventricular myocardial cells (Fig. 10–1a). At −30 to −40 mV, more slowly activated membrane channels "open," which are permeable to calcium ions. In the normal myocardium, this calcium current contributes to the action potential plateau (Phase 2). Sinoatrial and proximal atrioventricular tissues lack fast sodium channels, and hence generate action potentials with slower, calcium channel dependent upstrokes (Fig. 10–1b). If fast sodium channels are inactivated by hyperkalemia or ischemia, normal myocardium can become slow channel dependent for its activation.

While local anesthetics inhibit the fast sodium channel, the slow calcium channel is affected by a diverse group of compounds that includes verapamil, nifedipine, and diltiazem, as well as a number of other drugs under development. Structurally dissimilar, rather than acting as classic competitive inhibitors, these drugs may affect various functional aspects of the slow channel. For example, verapamil slows the recovery kinetics of the slow channel after activation, while nifedipine interferes with the passage of calcium through the channel.[4] Different pharmacodynamic actions may also result because different cardiovascular tissues may possess varying proportions of the different calcium entry mechanisms, and channel configurations (ease of drug access) and channel kinetics may also vary at different tissue sites.[5] Both diltiazem and the dextro isomer of racemic verapamil have fast channel blocking properties.[4] The currently available slow calcium-channel blockers also possess inhibitory effects at receptor activated calcium channels.[1]

The main cardiovascular effects induced by a decrease in slow channel calcium influx include (1) interference with the generation of an action potential in the SA node, the AV node, and other cells that may be slow-channel dependent, (2) a decrease in myocardial contractility secondary to the reduced influx of calcium per se, and (3) vascular relaxation secondary to reduced calcium influx into vascular smooth muscle cells. The latter two effects result because the amount of calcium passing inward through the channels is presumed to trigger the release of proportional amounts of calcium from internal stores. This released calcium acts through troponin and calmodulin mechanisms in cardiac and vascular smooth muscle, respectively, to enhance the cross linking and subsequent contraction of the actin and myosin strands.[6] A reduced trigger amount would

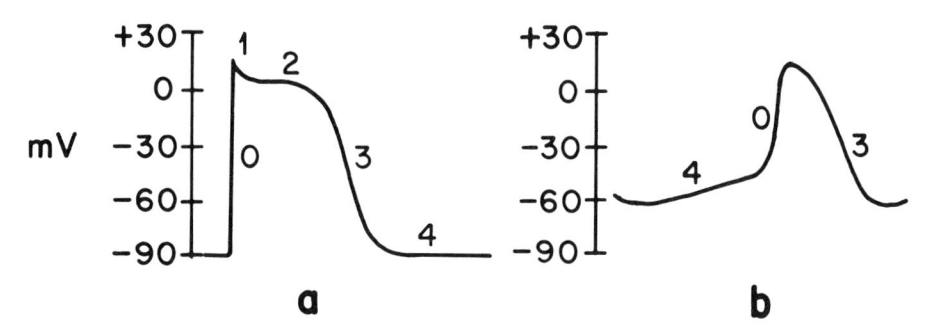

Fig. 10–1. (a) Myocardial cell action potential with fast sodium channel dependent upstroke (phase 0); (b) sinoatrial node action potential with less rapid phase 0 depolarization resulting from slow calcium-channel activation. The vertical numeric scale represents transmembrane potential in millivolts. (By permission of Kapur, P.A.: Cardiovascular pharmacology: beta receptor blockers and slow calcium channel inhibitors. Semin. Anesth., 1:196, 1982.)

reduce the amount of calcium released from internal stores and would thus impair contractility.

In subjects with intact autonomic nervous systems, the direct cardiovascular depressant effects of slow channel blockers are subject to modification by autonomically mediated homeostatic reflexes, although with varying degrees of compensation. Some drugs such as nifedipine usually exhibit no depressant effects on conduction in normal subjects, and its administration frequently results in a net reflex tachycardia.[4] Thus nifedipine is unsuitable as an antidysrhythmic agent. Diltiazem, a good coronary though a poor peripheral vasodilator, often induces bradycardia and a delay in atrioventricular conduction. Verapamil may delay conduction in normal subjects. Because of its ability to slow AV nodal conduction, verapamil is effective for the converting of re-entrant paroxysmal supraventricular tachydysrhythmias to sinus rhythm, and can decrease the ventricular rate in atrial fibrillation and flutter.[3] Differences in the clinical profiles of the three drugs are shown in Table 10–2, from which it is apparent that the drugs are not homogeneous in their clinical effects. Different results may occur if one is substituted for another.

In autonomically intact subjects nifedipine and diltiazem seldom interfere with myocardial function. The myocardial depressant effects of verapamil have been correlated with the degree of pre-existing myocardial dysfunction.[7] The electrophysiologic and hemodynamic depressant effects of these drugs are generally related to their plasma levels. The antidysrhythmic effects of verapamil are evident at lower plasma levels, while the hemodynamic effects require a higher plasma level.[8,9]

Reversal of Slow Channel Inhibition

To understand how to antagonize some of the undesired effects of slow calcium-channel inhibitors, it is important to realize that the number of membrane channels in the responsive state and likely to allow the influx of calcium is not static. The availability of these channels is modulated by the level of *beta*-1 stimulation via cyclic-AMP as a second messenger.[4]

To reverse undesired effects on contractility it is necessary to increase the influx of calcium. This can be done either by (1) increasing the gradient for calcium across the channels that remain open by administering ionized calcium or (2) increasing the number of open channels at the same ionic gradient, by administering a *beta*-1 agonist. However, to reverse undesired conduction interference by a slow channel inhibitor, i.e., to improve the voltage dependent characteristics of cardiac cells, it appears that the number of channels available for depolarization has to be increased, which can be accomplished by increasing intracellular cyclic AMP with a *beta*-1 agonist (e.g., isoproterenol, dopamine, epinephrine, etc.).

Thus, in order to antagonize hypotension, calcium or a *beta*-1 agonist would be appropriate therapies, while for an undesired AV block or bradycardia, a *beta*-1 agonist will be more appropriate. Part of the choice in either case will depend upon the clinical circumstances, since the effects of the calcium-channel blocker are plasma level related. Calcium may be more appropriate to antagonize transient hypotension induced by the rapid intravenous admin-

Table 10–2
Relative Net Cardiovascular Effects of Calcium Channel Blockers

	Nifedipine	Verapamil	Diltiazem
Vascular smooth muscle relaxation	+ +	+	+
Decreased myocardial contractility	−	+	−
Conduction interference	−	+ +	+

istration of a slow calcium-channel blocker. If the hypotensive effect is intermediate in duration, either repeated calcium administration or an infusion of dopamine, for example, would be chosen. In the case of a drug overdose, a *beta*-1 agonist infusion would most appropriately counteract persistent hypotension. If conduction effects such as 1° or 2° heart block are observed in an otherwise stable patient, they may be tolerated and will wane as drug levels fall. If the untoward conduction effects are severe and are compromising the status of the patient, a *beta*-1 agonist must be used. In cases of drug overdose, a temporary pacemaker may be required until the drug is substantially eliminated.

It must be emphasized that verapamil interferes with intracardiac conduction at lower plasma levels than required for depression of myocardial contractility or for vasodilation. Therefore, the PR interval of the EKG should be carefully monitored. Prolongation of the PR intervals is likely if sufficient verapamil is used to produce vasodilation, for example. On the other hand, if the desired antidysrhythmic effects are accompanied by a decreased blood pressure, calcium can restore normotension without interference with antidysrhythmic efficacy.[10]

Effects of Interference with Reflex Compensation

As previously discussed, autonomically mediated compensatory reflexes counteract and lessen the direct depressant effects of calcium-channel blockers in normal subjects. Therefore, patients who have autonomic dysfunction, whether on a physiologic, an anatomic, or a pharmacologic basis, may have interference with such compensatory reflexes and be at greater risk to experience the direct depressant effects of calcium-channel blockers (Fig. 10–2). Severe combined depressant effects have been described following the concomitant intravenous administration of verapamil and *beta* antagonists. The combination of oral verapamil or nifedipine with oral *beta* antagonists for the chronic treatment of angina pectoris often results in improved angina control, but has on occasion, resulted in additive depressant effects. The latter variability of results depends partly upon the extent of individual pre-existing ventricular dysfunction.[11]

Patients with sick sinus syndrome are particularly at risk to develop impaired sinoatrial function and may require artificial pacing if calcium-channel-blocker therapy is indicated. Care should also be taken in patients affected by other forms of autonomic dysfunction as well (Shy-Drager syndrome).

Interactions in Distribution and Metabolism

Protein Binding. Verapamil, nifedipine, and diltiazem are 80 to 90% protein bound.[12] An increase in the "free" fraction of these drugs may result if they are displaced from plasma proteins by other drugs with high protein binding such as lidocaine, propranolol, diazepam, or aspirin.

Hepatic Dysfunction. Prolonged elimination of verapamil has been demonstrated in patients with liver disease or with conditions that alter hepatic blood flow.[13] Altered verapamil pharmacokinetics may be encountered if surgical or anesthetic conditions compromise hepatic perfusion. In an animal model, similar verapamil infusion rates resulted in much higher verapamil plasma levels during halothane anesthesia compared to plasma levels achieved when the animals were in the awake state.[14]

Interactions with Cardioactive Agents

Cardiac Glycosides. The effects of digoxin and verapamil are additive in the control of ventricular rate in patients with atrial fibrillation, since digoxin alone often fails to prevent the excessive ventricular rates that may occur during exercise when sympathetic responses are enhanced and

```
         SLOW CALCIUM CHANNEL BLOCKADE
              +  /           \  +
                /             \
               ↙               ↘
      VASODILATION       MYOCARDIAL DEPRESSION
              ↖  \  +        ↗
             -  \\          /  -
                 ↘         /
           AUTONOMIC REFLEX ACTIVATION
                       ↑
                       | -
                       |
              AUTONOMIC DYSFUNCTION
                 BETA BLOCKADE
```

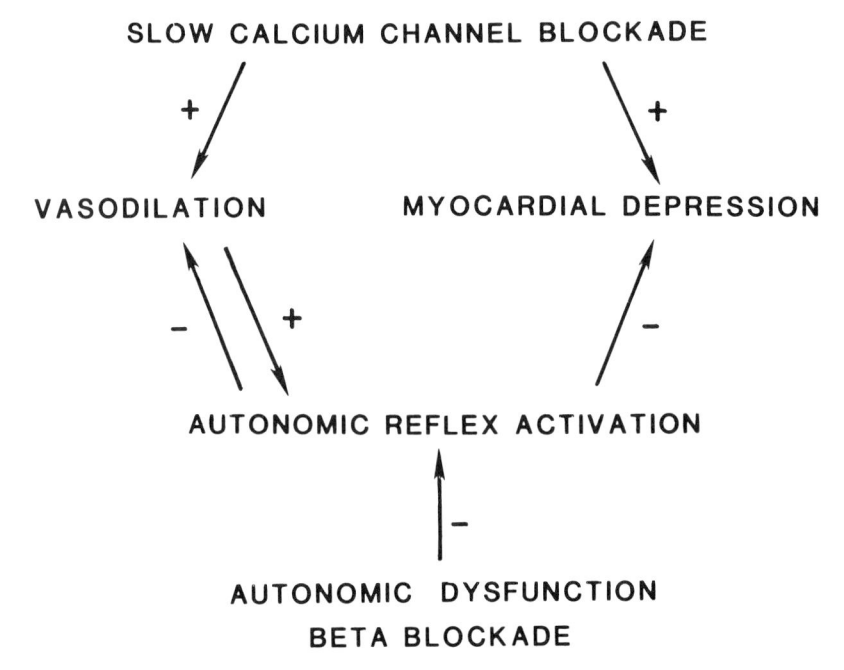

Fig. 10–2. Schematic diagram of the compensatory interaction of the autonomic nervous system with the direct hemodynamic depressant effects of the slow calcium-channel blockers, + = causes; − = opposes. Interference with reflex compensation may unmask the direct depressant effects of the drugs.

vagal tone decreased. However, the administration of verapamil during digoxin therapy raises the serum digoxin concentration by decreasing its renal clearance and may require a reduction of the digoxin maintenance dose.[15]

Theophylline. Because of the role of cyclic AMP as a second messenger to increase the number of available slow channels, phosphodiesterase inhibitors, which interfere with the degradation of cyclic AMP, can also oppose the effects of calcium-channel blockers on hemodynamics as well as on intracardiac conduction. Conversely it has been shown that verapamil is effective in suppressing aminophylline-toxic dysrhythmias.[16]

Potassium. In addition to the fact that calcium and potassium act as physiologic antagonists, verapamil does affect membrane potassium currents. An animal study has suggested greater cardiovascular impairment with the combination of hyperkalemia and verapamil compared with hyperkalemia alone, as judged by the depression of cardiac index and the incidence of AV block. The same amount of administered potassium resulted in higher extracellular potassium concentrations in verapamil pre-treated animals.[17]

Interactions with Anesthetic Agents and Adjuvants

CASE REPORT

A 44-year-old, 80-kg man was scheduled for elective triple vessel coronary artery bypass surgery. His usual medications were nifedipine (30 mg 3 times daily), propranolol (80 mg every 6 hours), isosorbide dinitrate (80 mg every 6 hours) and nitroglycerin ointment (1" every 6 hours). On these medications, his baseline blood pressure was 140/90 mm Hg with a mean arterial pressure (MAP) of 105, and a heart rate of 64 beats per minute. Cardiac output was 6.4 L·min^{-1}, systemic vascular resistance (SVR) was 1250 dynes·s·cm^{-5}, pulmonary capillary wedge pressure was 10 mm Hg, and the pulmonary artery diastolic (PAD) pressure was 11 mm Hg. His anesthetic before cardiopulmonary bypass consisted of fentanyl 50 μg·kg^{-1}, diazepam 10 mg, and pancuronium 10 mg, with supplemental isoflurane to control blood pressure. Revascularization required an aortic cross clamp time of 39 minutes with 76 minutes of cardiopulmonary bypass, that was terminated without difficulty. Blood pressure was 128/78, cardiac output was 4.5 L·min⁻¹, SVR was 1620 dynes·s·cm⁻⁵, and PAD was 8 mm Hg. Supplemental fentanyl and diazepam were then given. Approximately 15 minutes after termination of cardiopulmonary bypass the patient had an episode of hypotension (50–70/20–30 mm Hg) associated with elevation of the ST segment of the EKG that was resistant to rapid injections of phenylephrine, as well as to infusion of dopamine and isoproterenol. Nifedipine 10 mg was withdrawn from a capsule and administered sublingually, the blood pressure increased to 90/60 mm Hg and the ST segment changes resolved. However, after nifedipine, with a MAP of 70, the cardiac output was still only 4.6 L·min⁻¹, though SVR was then 1200 dynes·s·cm⁻⁵. However, PAD was 3 mm Hg and the hemoglobin level was 8 mg·dl⁻¹. Infusion of 2 units of packed red blood cells, each diluted with 200 ml of normal saline solution, raised the PAD to 12 mm Hg and the blood pressure to 118/75, at which time a repeat cardiac output was 5.9 L·min⁻¹. The chest was closed and the patient was transferred to the intensive care unit on a nitroglycerin infusion. The postoperative course was uneventful.

This case illustrates a patient on chronic nifedipine therapy coming for a high-risk operation who developed an intraoperative indication for nifedipine administration. The addition of nifedipine to a high-dose narcotic technique may result in additional systemic vasodilation, and possible reduction in cardiac output if the patient's intravascular volume is low. In the case reported, the low PAD after nifedipine administration was easily optimized with appropriate fluid therapy, in which packed red blood cells were included to correct a low hemoglobin level. Thus, the patient benefitted from the afterload reduction caused by nifedipine, in addition to relief of his coronary vasospasm.

This episode of postcardiopulmonary bypass hypotension resistant to inotropic therapy is similar to other reports of coronary vasospasm after coronary revascularization.[18] Coronary vasospasm has also been associated with withdrawal of nifedipine.[19] Perhaps the coronary vasospasm was related to decreased effective drug levels of nifedipine in the patient because of the dilution and exposure to light that occurred during cardiopulmonary bypass. Nifedipine is photosensitive and is rapidly inactivated by exposure to light. The episode resolved after sublingual administration of nifedipine, which is consistent with the known efficacy of nifedipine for treatment of coronary vasospasm-induced ischemia, whether or not associated with a revascularization procedure.[20,21] Inotropic drugs are ineffective in these situations because they increase the work of the heart without relieving the vasospasm, and thus may worsen the myocardial insult.

Inhalation Anesthetics. In general, the cardiovascular depressant effects of inhalation anesthetics and calcium-channel blockers are additive. Verapamil can further slow intracardiac conduction and depress myocardial contractility,[22,23] while nifedipine remains largely a vasodilator at commonly used clinical concentrations of these drugs and the inhalation agents.[24] Lower doses than those recommended for awake patients should be titrated to the desired effect. Avoidance of high peak plasma verapamil levels will reduce the likelihood of hemodynamic depression if verapamil is used for an antidysrhythmic indication.[22] Nitrous oxide allowed better reflex compensation than halothane when verapamil was given in a porcine model.[25] Similarly, hemodynamic changes were less when nifedipine was given during morphine-nitrous oxide compared with halothane anesthesia in an animal model, presumably because of better reflex preservation by morphine-nitrous oxide.[26]

Narcotic Anesthesia. When administered during low dose narcotic anesthesia, calcium-channel blockers showed predictable effects on vascular tone and intracardiac conduction. In one preliminary report, the administration of sublingual nifedipine during high dose fentanyl anesthesia in man induced moderate though clinically tolerable hypotension.[27] Verapamil appears to be well tolerated during high dose morphine[28] and fentanyl[29] anesthesia in patients with good left ventricular function if vital signs are stable.

Chronic Administration and Anesthesia. Calcium-channel blockers have therapeutic benefits for patients in whom anesthesia is planned, including coronary vasodilation, antidysrhythmic effects, and myocardial protection, while their abrupt withdrawal has been associated with exacerbation of vasospastic angina pectoris (e.g., nifedipine).[19] In addition to the probable additive effects with inhalation agents, high dose narcotic anesthesia in combination with calcium-channel blockers may induce a higher degree of vasodilation. Thus the volume status should be carefully assessed and maintained when patients on chronic calcium blocker therapy are anesthetized, and pressor drugs kept available for instances in which compensatory volume replacement is contraindicated or impractical.

Muscle Relaxants. The interactions of calcium-channel blockers with muscle relaxants has not been well defined. *In vitro* and *in vivo* studies have indicated that calcium-channel blockers may reduce the margin of safety at the neuromuscular junction.[30,31] This may include a pre-junctional effect, since skeletal muscle relies little on extracellular calcium for normal contraction. Whether these observations are clinically relevant remains to be determined, although in one animal study anticholinesterase reversal of pancuronium was equally effective despite greater initial twitch depression in the presence of verapamil.[32]

Malignant Hyperpyrexia. Calcium-channel blockers have been suggested as adjuvants to dantrolene in the treatment of this disorder. Dantrolene, however, has been associated with greater cardiac depression and hyperkalemia in the presence of verapamil in animal models.[33,34] Given the multiplicity of calcium-channel blockers, perhaps another drug of this class could be used.

Effects on Organ Perfusion Relevant to Anesthesia.

Cerebral Blood Flow. Calcium channel inhibitors improve cerebral perfusion after anoxic insults by preventing cerebral artery spasm. They are cerebral vasodilators under normoxic conditions as well, and have been associated with deleterious rises in intracranial pressure and decreased cerebral perfusion pressure in patients with intracranial mass lesions.[35]

Pulmonary Blood Flow. These agents are potential pulmonary vasodilators and have been proposed for the treatment of pulmonary hypertension. Nifedipine has been associated with increased shunt fraction during anesthesia[36] and care should be taken in the presence of abnormal ventilation-perfusion relationships.

Renal Function. Verapamil pretreatment has been reported to preserve renal blood flow better during halothane-induced hypotension compared with saline-solution-treated animals.[37] Verapamil has also been reported to attenuate post-ischemic renal failure in an animal model.[38]

Other Physiologic Effects

Bronchospasm resulting from mediator release in subjects with reactive airways is inhibited by nifedipine[39] or verapamil.[40] This may be important for patients in whom treatment of a cardiovascular disorder with a *beta* antagonist would provoke bronchoconstriction.

Platelet adhesion is inhibited by diltiazem, nifedipine and verapamil.[41] Whether surgical bleeding is significantly affected at therapeutic plasma levels of these drugs is unknown.

NITROGLYCERIN COMPOUNDS

The other vasodilating antianginal drugs in clinical use today are the nitroglycerin group of drugs. Preparations are available for oral (nitroglycerin, isosorbide dinitrate, pentaerythritol tetranitrate), topical (nitroglycerin ointment or gel), and intravenous (nitroglycerin) administration. In addition to the chronic therapy of angina pectoris, indications for the acute administration of a nitroglycerin preparation frequently arise in the perioperative and intraoperative period.

Controversy exists over the mechanism of angina relief by these agents, primarily whether the beneficial effects are a result of coronary or systemic vasodilation. Depending upon the relevance of other variables, four fundamental pharmacodynamic actions of nitroglycerin interact and may predominate according to the circumstances: (a) the reduction of systolic pressure by nitrates can significantly reduce oxygen demand if reflex tachycardia is avoided; (b) venous pooling resulting from nitrate-induced reductions in venous tone, especially when ventricular diastolic pressure has previously been elevated, can induce beneficial effects on the oxygen supply and demand relationship; (c) relaxation of normal or increased vascular smooth muscle tone in large coronary arteries by nitroglycerin is beneficial in the presence of atherosclerotic narrowing or coronary spasm; (d) myocardial areas dependent upon a collateral blood supply may benefit from dilation of those collaterals or the conduit vessels from which they arise by nitroglycerin therapy.[42]

While nitroprusside is also known to be a coronary vasodilator, its propensity to dilate small resistance arterioles improves coronary perfusion of non-ischemic areas at the expense of ischemic zones, a so-called coronary steal.[43] The would-be beneficial effects of nitroprusside induced hypotension are countered by reflex tachycardia with a consequent increase in myocardial oxygen demand.

Anesthetic Implications of Nitroglycerin Therapy

Chronic Therapy. Patients may be on chronic therapy with oral or topical nitroglycerin preparations for the control of obstructive or vasospastic angina pectoris, or they may come to surgery with intravenous nitroglycerin for the control of unstable or intractable angina pectoris or for control of pre-load and after-load conditions after an acute myocardial infarction. In any of these situations, the patient should be maintained on his nitroglycerin therapy up until the time of surgery. Patients with critical coronary lesions may be changed from oral/topical therapy to intravenous nitroglycerin prior to anesthesia to assure accurate and timely control of the nitroglycerin dosage during the anesthetic period.

The anesthetic plan should incorporate the assumption that the patient may be relatively vasodilated and the volume status of the patient must be carefully observed when vasodilating anesthetic techniques are employed. Temporary adjustments of the nitroglycerin infusion rate may help control undesirable additive effects on peripheral vascular resistance, especially during anesthetic induction.

Intraoperative Use. The intraoperative use of nitroglycerin is well established.[44] Current indications include intraoperative myocardial ischemia, systemic hypertension, elevated pulmonary arterial pressures, treatment of acute ventricular dysfunction, and treatment of coronary artery spasm. Since nitroglycerin adheres to a variety of plastic products,[45] prior flushing of intravenous infusion sets has been recommended in addition to titration of the administered dose to the desired clinical effect. The large surface area of cardiopulmonary bypass systems may similarly absorb this drug and necessitate dosage adjustments if nitroglycerin is indicated during cardiopulmonary bypass.

Nitroglycerin affects the neuromuscular blockade produced by pancuronium by increasing both the intensity and the duration of the blockade.[46] No effect was observed, however, with succinylcholine, d-tubocurarine, or gallamine.[47]

Effects on Organ Blood Flow Relevant to Anesthesia

Cerebral Blood Flow. Nitroglycerin-induced hypotension results in cerebral as well as coronary and systemic vasodilation and may increase intracranial pressure.[48] These effects were still evident in the presence of 0.5% and 1.0% end-tidal concentrations of halothane in an animal model in which the baseline intracranial pressure was within normal limits.[49] The bolus administration of nitroglycerin was much more likely to result in elevated intracranial pressure than was continuous infusion in animals with experimental intracranial hypertension during 1.0% end-tidal concentrations of halothane.[50]

Pulmonary Blood Flow. Nitroglycerin administration may also result in dilation of the pulmonary vasculature and has been shown to increase intrapulmonary shunting and interfere with hypoxic pulmonary vasoconstriction.[51,52] Increased inspired oxygen concentrations may be indicated if nitroglycerin infusions are administered during anesthesia.

Other Physiologic Interactions

Methemoglobinemia has been of serious concern only in the rare patient who has received either a nitroglycerin overdose or an inordinately large clinical dose of nitroglycerin over a prolonged period of time. Patients have been successfully treated with methylene blue (2 mg·kg^{-1}). An infusion rate of less than 7 µg·kg^{-1}·min^{-1} may be an upper limit for the long-term administration of intravenous nitroglycerin.[53]

Platelet aggregation is inhibited by nitroglycerin, though to a lesser extent than by sodium nitroprusside at similar concentrations.[54] The implications for surgical bleeding are presently unclear.

REFERENCES

1. Vanhoutte, P.M.: Calcium-entry blockers and vascular smooth muscle. Circulation, 65(Suppl 1):I–11, 1982.
2. Winquest, R.J., Webb, R.C., and Bohr, D.F.: Calcium antagonism is no rose. Federation Proceedings, 40:2852, 1981.
3. Waxman, H.L., Myerburg, R.J., Appel, R., et al.: Verapamil for control of ventricular rate in paroxysmal supraventricular tachycardia and atrial fibrillation or flutter. Ann. Intern. Med., 94:1, 1981.
4. Antman, E.M., Stone, P.H., Muller, J.E., et al.: Calcium channel blocking agents in the treatment of cardiovascular disorders. Part I: Basic and clinical electrophysiologic effects. Ann. Intern. Med., 93:875, 1980.
5. Van Neuten, J.M., and Vanhoutte, P.M.: Calcium entry blockers and vascular smooth muscle heterogeneity. Federation Proceedings, 40:2862, 1981.
6. Braunwald, E.: Mechanism of action of calcium-channel-blocking agents. N. Engl. J. Med., 307:1618, 1982.
7. Chew, C.Y.C., Hecht, H.S., Collett, J.T., et al.: Influence of severity of ventricular dysfunction on hemodynamic responses to intravenously administered verapamil in ischemic heart disease. Am. J. Cardiol., 47:917, 1981.
8. Kapur, P.A., and Flacke, W.E.: Lack of correlation of verapamil plasma level with cumulative protective effects against halothane-epinephrine ventricular arrhythmias. J. Cardiovasc. Pharmacol., 4:652, 1982.
9. Danilo, P., Hordof, A.J., Reder, R.J., and Rosen, M.R.: Effects of verapamil on electrophysiologic properties of blood superfused cardiac Purkinje fibers. J. Pharmacol. Exp. Ther., 213:222, 1980.
10. Weiss, A.T., Lewis, B.S., Halon, D.A., et al.: The use of calcium with verapamil in the management of supraventricular tachyarrhythmias. Int. J. Cardiol., 4:275, 1983.
11. Packer, M., Leon, M.B., Bonow, R.O., et al.: Hemodynamic and clinical effects of combined verapamil and propranolol therapy in angina pectoris. Am. J. Cardiol., 50:903, 1982.
12. Henry, P.D.: Comparative pharmacology of calcium antagonists: nifedipine, verapamil and diltiazem. Am. J. Cardiol., 46:1047, 1980.
13. Woodcock, B.G., Rietbrock, I., Vohringer, H.F., et al.: Verapamil disposition in liver disease and intensive-care patients: kinetics, clearance, and apparent blood flow relationships. Clin. Pharmacol. Ther., 29:27, 1981.
14. Rogers, K., Chelly, J., Merin, R.G., et al.: Verapamil-halothane interaction in the chronically instrumented dog. Anesth. Analg., 63:268, 1984.
15. Klein, H.O., and Kaplinsky, E.: Verapamil and digoxin: their respective effects on atrial fibrillation and their interaction. Am. J. Cardiol., 50:894, 1982.
16. Friesen, R.M., and Bonet, J.F.: The antiarrhythmic effects of verapamil and propranolol in aminophylline toxic dogs. Can. Anaesth. Soc. J., 30:124, 1983.
17. Nugent, M., Tinker, J.H., and Moyer, T.P.: Verapamil worsens rate of development and hemodynamic effects of acute hyperkalemia in halothane-anesthetized dogs: Effects of calcium therapy. Anesthesiology, 60:435, 1982.
18. Buxton, A.E., Goldberg, S., Harken, A., et al.: Coronary-artery spasm immediately after myocardial revascularization. N. Engl. J. Med., 304:1249, 1981.
19. Schick, E.C., Liang, C., Heupler, F.A., et al.: Ran-

domized withdrawal from nifedipine: placebo-controlled study in patients with coronary artery spasm. Am. Heart J., 104:690, 1982.
20. Antman, E., Muller, J., Goldberg, S., et al.: Nifedipine therapy for coronary-artery spasm. N. Engl. J. Med., 302:1269, 1980.
21. Kopf, G.S., Riba, A., and Zito, R.: Intraoperative use of nifedipine for hemodynamic collapse due to coronary artery spasm following myocardial revascularization. Ann. Thor. Surg., 34:457, 1982.
22. Kapur, P.A., and Flacke, W.E.: Epinephrine-induced arrhythmias and cardiovascular function after verapamil during halothane anesthesia in the dog. Anesthesiology, 55:218, 1981.
23. Kates, R.A., Kaplan, J.A., Guyton, R.A., et al.: Hemodynamic interactions of verapamil and isoflurane. Anesthesiology, 59:132, 1983.
24. Tosone, S.R., Reves, J.G., Kissin, I., et al.: Hemodynamic responses to nifedipine in dogs anesthetized with halothane. Anesth. Analg., 62:903, 1983.
25. Norfleet, E.A., Heath, K.R., Kopp,V.J., et al.: Verapamil—different cardiovascular responses during N$_2$O analgesia and halothane anesthesia. Anesthesiology, 57:A75, 1982.
26. Springman, S.R., Redon, D., and Rusy, B.F.: The effect of nifedipine on the circulation during morphine-N$_2$O and halothane anesthesia in dogs. Anesth. Analg., 62:284, 1983.
27. Nussmeier, N.A., Curling, P.E., Murphy, D.A., et al.: Nifedipine: cardiovascular effects after sublingual administration during fentanyl-pancuronium anesthesia in man. Anesthesiology, 59:A34, 1983.
28. Kates, R.A., and Kaplan, J.A.: Cardiovascular responses to verapamil during coronary artery bypass graft surgery. Anesth. Analg., 62:821, 1983.
29. Kapur, P.A., Norel, E.J., Cohen, G.R., et al.: Verapamil administration after high dose fentanyl with or without chronic nifedipine therapy in man. Anesth. Analg., 63:231, 1984.
30. Bikhazi, G.B., Leung, I., and Foldes, F.F.: Ca-channel blockers increase potency of neuromuscular blocking agents in vivo. Anesthesiology, 59:A29, 1983.
31. Durant, N.N., Nguyen, N., Briscoe, J.R., et al.: Potentiation of neuromuscular blockade by verapamil. Anesthesiology, 60:298, 1984.
32. Carpenter, R.L., and Mulroy, M.F.: Edrophonium antagonizes combined verapamil-pancuronium neuromuscular blockade. Anesthesiology, 59:A272, 1983.
33. Durbin, C.G., Fisher, N.A., and Lynch, C.: Cardiovascular effects in dogs of intravenous dantrolene alone and in the presence of verapamil. Anesthesiology, 59:A227, 1983.
34. Saltzman, L.S., Kates, R.A., Corke, B.C., et al.: Hyperkalemia and cardiovascular collapse after dantrolene and verapamil administration in swine. Anesth. Analg., 63:272, 1984.
35. Lynch, C., and Bedford, R.F.: Adverse effect of verapamil on ICP in patients with brain tumors. Anesthesiology, 59:A392, 1983.
36. Casthely, P.A., Villanueva, R., and Schneider, A.: Shunting during hypotension with nifedipine. Anesthesiology, 59:A510, 1983.
37. Hantler, C.B., Felbeck, P.G., Tait, A.R., et al.: Renal vascular interactions between halothane and verapamil. Anesthesiology, 59:A45, 1983.
38. Wait, R.B., White, G., and Davis, J.H.: Beneficial effects of verapamil on postischemic renal failure. Surgery, 94:276, 1983.
39. Brugman, T., Darnel, M., and Hirshman, C.A.: Nifedipine aerosol attenuates airway constriction in dogs with hyperreactive airways. Am. Rev. Resp. Dis., 127:14, 1983.
40. Patel, K.: Calcium antagonists in exercise-induced asthma. Br. Med. J., 282:932, 1981.
41. Kiyomoto, A., Sasaki, Y., Odawara, A., et al.: Inhibition of platelet aggregation by diltiazem: comparison with verapamil and nifedipine and inhibitory potencies of diltiazem metabolites. Circ. Res., 52 (Suppl I):I–115, 1983.
42. McGregor, M.: The nitrates and myocardial ischemia. Circulation, 66:689, 1982.
43. Mann, T., Cohen, P.F., Holman, B.L., et al.: Effect of nitroprusside on regional myocardial blood flow in coronary artery disease: Results in 25 patients and comparison with nitroglycerin. Circulation, 57:732–737, 1978.
44. Kaplan, J.A., Dunbar, R.W., and Jones, E.L.: Nitroglycerin infusion during coronary artery surgery. Anesthesiology, 45:11, 1976.
45. Baaske, D., et al.: Nitroglycerin compatibility with intravenous fluid filters, containers and administration sets. Am. J. Hosp. Pharm., 37:201, 1980.
46. Glisson, S.N., El-Etr, A.A., and Lum, R.: Prolongation of pancuronium-induced neuromuscular blockade by intravenous infusion of nitroglycerin. Anesthesiology, 51:47, 1979.
47. Glisson, S.N., Sanches, M.M., El-Etr, A.A., et al.: Nitroglycerin and the neuromuscular blockade produced by gallamine, succinylcholine, d-tubocurarine and pancuronium. Anesth. Analg., 59:117, 1980.
48. Ghani, G.A., Sung, Y.F., Wernstein, M.S., Tindall, F.T., Fleischer, A.S.: Effects of intravenous nitroglycerin on the intracranial pressure and volume-pressure response. J. Neurosurg., 58:562, 1983.
49. Scuderi, P.E., and Stullken, E.H.: Technique of administration alters intracranial pressure response to nitroglycerin but not to nitroprusside. Anesthesiology, 57:A311, 1982.
50. Prough, D.S., Stullken, E.H., and Scuderi, P.E.: Technique of administration alters increases in intracranial hypertension produced by nitroglycerin but not by nitroprusside. Anesthesiology, 59:A353, 1983.
51. Casthely, P.A., Lear, S., Cottrell, J.E., et al.: Intrapulmonary shunting during induced hypotension. Anesth. Analg., 61:231, 1982.
52. D'Oliveria, M., Sykes, M.K., Chakrabarti, M.K., et al.: Depression of hypoxic pulmonary vasoconstriction by nitroprusside and nitroglycerine. Br. J. Anaesth., 53:11, 1981.
53. Gibson, G.R., Hunter, J.R., Raabe, D.S., et al.: Methemoglobinemia produced by high-dose in-

travenous nitroglycerin. Ann. Intern. Med., 96:615, 1982.
54. Allen, F.B., Gerson, J.R., and Davey, F.R.: Platelet inhibition by nitroprusside and nitroglycerin. Anesthesiology, 51:S75, 1979.
55. Kapur, P.A.: Cardiovascular pharmacology: beta receptor blockers and slow calcium channel inhibitors. Seminars in Anesthesia, 1:196, 1982.

11

ANTIHYPERTENSIVES AND ALPHA BLOCKERS

ROBERT K. STOELTING

An estimated 20 to 25 million Americans suffer from essential hypertension. There is a convincing body of evidence that shows that the pharmacologic treatment of hypertension decreases both the morbidity and mortality associated with this disease. Drugs that selectively impair sympathetic nervous system functions are frequently chosen as antihypertensives for the ambulatory treatment of essential hypertension. Antihypertensives may act on the central nervous system, autonomic ganglia, postganglionic nerve endings, *alpha* adrenergic receptors, *beta*-adrenergic receptors or directly on vascular smooth muscle (Table 11–1).

As with all potent drugs, the rational use of antihypertensives requires an understanding of their fundamental mechanism of action. Furthermore, a knowledge of the anatomy and physiology of the peripheral autonomic nervous system is needed for the safe anesthetic management of patients receiving antihypertensives.

CASE REPORT

A 65-year-old, 85-kg man was admitted to the hospital with the diagnosis of an abdominal aortic aneurysm. The patient's current medications included a thiazide diuretic, *alpha*-methyldopa 1,000 mg/day, and hydralazine 80 mg/day for the treatment of essential hypertension. An unknown drug prescribed for the treatment of "depression" had not been taken for the past 4 weeks.

Preoperative laboratory measurements included:
Hemoglobin 15 g/dl
Sodium 145 mEq/L
Potassium 3.9 mEq/L
Creatinine 0.8 mg/dl
Serum glutamic oxaloacetic transaminase—slightly elevated
Total bilirubin 0.8 mg/dl
Prothrombin time 100%
Plasma thromboplastin time—normal

The patient's supine blood pressure was 140/85 mm Hg, and his heart rate was 56 beats/min. The electrocardiogram showed sinus bradycardia and left ventricular hypertrophy.

During the preoperative visit, the patient complained of back pain, tiredness, and a "dizzy feeling" on arising in the morning. Pending a satisfactory type and cross-match for ten units of whole blood, the operation was scheduled for the next morning.

Among the problems that this patient presented to the anesthesiologist were hypertension and the therapy for this condition.

ANATOMY AND PHYSIOLOGY OF THE PERIPHERAL AUTONOMIC NERVOUS SYSTEM

The peripheral autonomic nervous system consists of sympathetic and parasympathetic divisions (Fig. 11–1). Preganglionic fibers from both divisions synapse in autonomic ganglia. Adrenergic postganglionic fibers release norepinephrine as the neurotransmitter at adrenoceptive *(alpha* and *beta)* receptors. *Alpha-1, beta-1* and *beta-2* receptors are postsynaptic while *alpha-2*

Table 11-1
Antihypertensives Used for Ambulatory Treatment of Essential Hypertension

Classification	Generic Name	Trade Name	Oral Dose for Maintenance
Central sympatholytics	reserpine	Serpasil	0.1 to 0.5 mg/day
	methyldopa	Aldomet	250 to 3000 mg/day
	clonidine	Catapres	0.2 to 2.4 mg/day
Peripheral sympatholytics	guanethidine	Ismelin	10 to 300 mg/day
	guanabenz	Wytensin	8 to 32 mg/day
Alpha-adrenergic antagonists	prazosin	Minipress	3 to 20 mg/day
Combined alpha and beta-adrenergic antagonists	labetalol	Normodyne Trandate	500 to 1000 mg/day
Peripheral vasodilators	hydralazine	Apresoline	40 to 300 mg/day
	minoxidil	Loniten	5 to 40 mg/day
Converting enzyme inhibitors	captopril	Capoten	100 to 450 mg/day
Monoamine oxidase inhibitors	pargyline	Eutonyl	10 to 150 mg/day

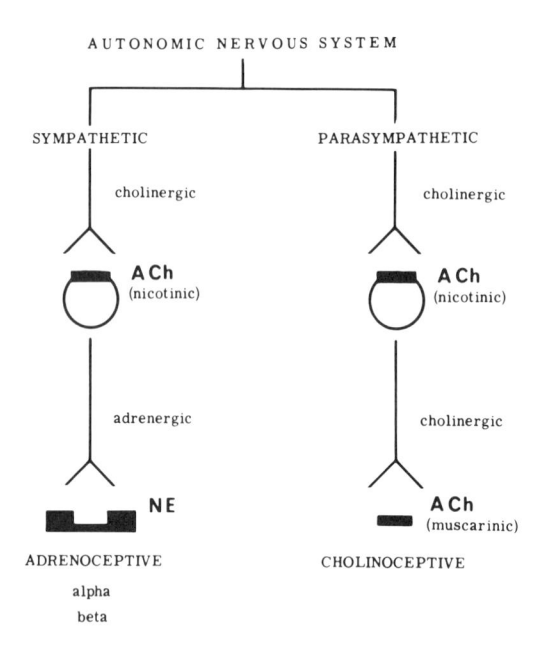

Fig. 11-1. A schematic diagram of the peripheral autonomic nervous system and its neurotransmitters, norepinephrine (NE) and acetylcholine (ACh).

receptors are presynaptic. *Alpha-1* receptors are located in peripheral vessels, and their stimulation produces vasoconstriction. *Alpha-2* receptors provide a negative feedback mechanism that modulates the release of norepinephrine. For example, stimulation of *alpha-2* receptors reduces the release of norepinephrine. Conversely, inhibition of *alpha-2* receptors allows the steady release of norepinephrine from the postganglionic nerve ending. *Beta-1* receptors are present mainly in the heart, and their stimulation increases heart rate and myocardial contractility. Vasodilation and bronchodilation result from stimulation of *beta-2* receptors. Preganglionic and postganglionic fibers that release acetylcholine are termed cholinergic and the corresponding receptors cholinoceptive. These receptors are divided further into nicotinic (autonomic ganglia and neuromuscular junction) and muscarinic (heart, airways, gastrointestinal tract, genitourinary system). The sympathetic is the most important autonomic segment with which antihypertensive agents are likely to interact.

INTERACTIONS OF ANTIHYPERTENSIVE DRUGS WITH ANESTHETICS

A properly functioning autonomic nervous system permits adaptation to sudden environmental changes (temperature, posture, light). Since antihypertensives interfere with normal autonomic nervous system functioning and since many anesthetic agents depend on a functioning sympathetic system to compensate for their inherent cardiovascular depressant properties, the question whether to discontinue these drugs preoperatively has been posed. The overwhelming evidence, however, is to continue therapy with antihypertensives throughout the preoperative period whenever these drugs are necessary to keep the blood pressure within the normal range. Specifically, a controlled study has demonstrated a greater incidence of precipitous blood pressure decline in untreated hypertensive patients than in those treated with reserpine.[3] Furthermore, ephedrine (15 to 50 mg) was found to be uniformly effective in raising systemic blood pressure in all patients requiring antihypertensive therapy. In addition, Prys-Roberts et al. have reported that treated or untreated hypertensive patients often develop hypotension accompanied by electrocardiographic evidence of myocardial ischemia during anesthesia.[4] In the same study, hypertensive patients who were rendered normotensive by pharmacologic means were indistinguishable from untreated normotensive patients. Finally, hypertensive patients, with or without antihypertensive therapy, are more likely to show marked fluctuations of blood pressure during anesthesia.

Hence, a good understanding of the mechanism of antihypertensive agents, rather than the abrupt discontinuation of therapy, is the essential prerequisite for the proper peri-anesthetic management of the hypertensive patient.

Specific concerns during anesthesia for the patient receiving antihypertensive therapy have been reviewed by Dingle.[5]

Attenuated Sympathetic Nervous System Activity

The impairment of circulatory homeostasis during anesthesia is secondary to the decrease of sympathetic tone induced by antihypertensive drugs on cardial function and peripheral vascular tone. Orthostatic hypotension is one of the inevitable consequences of sympathetic inhibition. Sudden hypotension may be the consequence of diminished peripheral vascular tone during hemorrhage, positive pressure ventilation of the lungs, sudden change in body position or vasodilation produced by anesthetics. When sympathetic tone is diminished, the blood pressure is likely to vary directly with blood volume. Even a minor blood loss may be followed by a disproportionate decrease in blood pressure. This is the consequence of a decrease in venous return secondary to inadequate vasoconstrictor reflexes. Similarly, peripheral vasoconstriction is necessary to insure an adequate venous return during positive pressure ventilation. Reduced cardiac sympathetic activity can decrease myocardial contractility, and facilitate the onset of pulmonary edema following vigorous inflation of the lungs. Reduced renal perfusion pressure will promote a compensatory fluid retention with expansion of the extracellular fluid volume.

Preoperative evaluation of sympathetic nervous system function would be particularly valuable in patients receiving antihypertensive medication. Unfortunately, no test reliably identifies those patients whose neurovascular instability poses an anesthetic risk. Orthostatic hypotension is the most commonly recognized abnormality of sympathetic nervous system dysfunction. Indeed, mild reductions in blood pressure on assuming the standing position may characterize the main pharmacologic effect of some antihypertensive agents. Positive intrathoracic pressure (Valsalva maneuver) provides the most useful index of autonomic nervous system function. This is not a practical clinical test, however, since a continuous recording of intra-arterial blood pressure is necessary for its correct interpretation. A normal Valsalva response requires intact baroreceptors, vasomotor center, sympathetic and parasympathetic nervous system activity and responsive receptors. With an intact autonomic nervous system, a baroreceptor-mediated vasoconstriction and heart rate increase occur during the decrease in blood pressure produced by positive intrathoracic pressure. Following the release of positive pressure, the heart rate slows in response to the blood pressure overshoot produced by the increased venous return. Impairment of sympathetic nervous system function is evidenced by an unchanged heart rate during positive intrathoracic pressure and absence of a blood pressure overshoot when positive pressure is released.

Modification of Response to Sympathomimetics

The response to a sympathomimetic (drug vasopressor) in the presence of antihypertenisve therapy depends on the mechanism of action of both classes of drugs. To evoke a response, the sympathomimetic must activate an *alpha* receptor directly (direct-acting drug) or stimulate norepinephrine release which in turn activates the *alpha* receptor (indirect-acting drug). Many sympathomimetics exert a combination of direct and indirect effects, with one usually predominating. Antihypertensives that deplete norepinephrine or that act on peripheral vascular smooth muscle decrease sensitivity to predominately indirect-acting sympathomimetics such as ephedrine (Table 11–2).[6] In contrast, sympathetic nervous system blockers, which deprives the *alpha* receptor of tonic impulses, results in increased sensitivity to norepinephrine and direct-acting sympathomimetics such as phenylephrine.

Parasympathetic Nervous System Predominance

The selective impairment of sympathetic nervous system activity favors an increase in parasympathetic activity (nasal stuffiness, bradycardia, increased gastric hydrogen ion secretion, diarrhea). Bradycardia may limit the cardiac contribution to circulatory homeostasis and obscure signs of anesthetic depth, hypovolemia or hypoventilation. Severe bradycardia could occur in combination with drugs that are administered during anesthesia and that normally increase vagal activity, such as anticholinesterases used to antagonize nondepolarizing neuromuscular blockade.

Sedation

Drugs that deplete central catecholamine stores have been shown in animal studies to reduce halothane anesthetic requirements (MAC) (Table 11–2).[6] Conceivably, an overdose of a potent inhaled anesthetic would be more likely if this drug was administered in the usual concentration. The doses of antihypertensives administered that reduce MAC in experimental animals far exceed the usual doses administered to patients (Tables 11–1 and 11–2).[6] Nevertheless, clinical observations that stimulated these animal studies, suggest that patients receiving certain antihypertensives need smaller amounts of both inhaled and injected anesthetics.[6]

PHARMACOLOGY OF ANTIHYPERTENSIVES

This section reviews the pharmacology and associated adverse effects of antihypertensives currently used to treat ambulatory essential hypertension (Table 11–3).[7-9] Similar discussions of other (beta-adrenergic blockers, diuretics) drugs also commonly used in the ambulatory treatment of essential hypertension are found in Chapters 7 and 11.

Central Sympatholytics

Reserpine (Serpasil). Reserpine is seldom used today for treatment of essential hypertension having been replaced by newer drugs. There is no generally accepted view as to the predominant mechanism of hypotension induced by reserpine, a mixture of central and peripheral mechanisms, although actions are usually invoked to ex-

Table 11-2
Effects of Antihypertensives on Canine Halothane Anesthetic Requirements (MAC) and Responses to Intravenous Ephedrine (0.5 mg/kg).

	MAC Decrease (Percent)	Systolic Blood Pressure Increase (mm Hg) in Response to Ephedrine Control	After Drug
reserpine (0.2 mg/kg/day)	14 ± 5†	74 ± 20	33 ± 5
methyldopa (50 mg/kg/day)	16 ± 5	86 ± 14	30 ± 10
guanethidine (15 mg/kg/day	1 ± 0.9	78 ± 21	19 ± 7

† = standard deviation; 5 animals in each group
Data from Miller, R.D., Way, E.L., and Eger, E.I.: The effects of alpha-methyldopa, reserpine, guanethidine and iproniazid on minimum alveolar anesthetic requirement (MAC). Anesthesiology, 29:1153, 1969.

plain it. Peripherally, reserpine prevents norepinephrine storage in the terminal vesicle but not in the nerve ending. This leaves the neurotransmitter unprotected against oxidation by interaxonal monoamine oxidase. The net effect is a gradual neurotransmitter depletion as storage granules deplete their contents spontaneously or in response to nerve stimulation. This results in a dose-dependent impairment of sympathetic nervous system function. Complete neurotransmitter depletion seems unlikely in man as the drug's toxicity limits the total adult reserpine dose to about 0.5 mg/day.

The side effect most frequently encountered is psychic depression, which seems to be due to depletion of 5-hydroxytryptamine and catecholamines from the central nervous system. Tricyclic antidepressants do not alleviate this depression and may interfere with effective blood pressure control. Sedation that accompanies reserpine therapy is associated with a reduced anesthetic requirement (Table 11–2).[6] Parasympathetic predominance manifests itself as nasal stuffiness, xerostomia, bradycardia and hyperchlorhydria.

The pharmacologic denervation induced by reserpine modifies the response to sympathomimetics. There may be increased sensitivity of the heart and smooth muscle to stimulation produced by direct-acting sympathomimetics. In contrast, drugs that act by releasing norepinephrine are less effective, since neurotransmitter stores are depleted. Ephedrine, which depends on both indirect and direct mechanisms for its pressor response, is less effective in animals treated with reserpine.[10] The reser-

Table 11-3
Comparison of Adverse Effects of Antihypertensives

	Reserpine	Methyldopa	Clonidine	Guanethidine	Prazosin	Hydralazine
psychic depression	+ + + +	+ +	+ +	0	+	+
orthostatic hypotension	+ +	+ + +	+ +	+ + + +	+ + +	+ +
sedation	+ + + +	+ + + +	+ + + +	0	+ +	+
sexual dysfunction	+ + +	+ + + +	+ + +	+ + + +	+ +	+ +
sodium retention	+ + +	+ + + +	+ + + +	+ + + +	+ + +	+ + + +
antihypertensive withdrawal syndrome	0	+	+ + +	0	0	+ +

0 = absent, + = very rare; + + = rare; + + + = occasional; + + + + = frequent
Data from Husserl, F.E., and Messerli, F.H.: Adverse effects of antihypertensive drugs. Drugs, 22:188, 1981.

pine doses (0.2 to 2 mg/kg) administered in these animal studies, however, exceed the maximum clinical dose used in man. Indeed, ephedrine is effective in increasing the blood pressure in reserpine-treated patients. This presumably indicates incomplete catecholamine depletion.[3]

In addition to the problems presented by the choice of the proper sympathomimetic agent during anesthesia, the reserpine-treated patient is theoretically more susceptible to neurovascular instability induced by anesthetic drugs with resulting hypotension, position change or hemorrhage. Nevertheless, circulatory responses to anesthetic drugs in man are not seriously altered by prior reserpine treatment.[11] Orthostatic hypotension is rare, suggesting that reflex constrictor responses of capacitance vessels are not completely inhibited.

Methyldopa (alpha-methyldopa, Aldomet). Methyldopa is a methyl-substituted amino acid acting as a precursor for a methylated catecholamine analog which displaces and competes with endogenous catecholamines in the nervous system. The antihypertensive effect is mainly due to accumulation of methylated catecholamine analogs in vasoactive centers of the central nervous system which interfere with the synthesis and physiologic actions of norepinephrine and other vasoactive catecholamines.[12] This accumulation of methylated catecholamines results in reduced sympathetic outflow from the central nervous system leading to a decrease in systemic vascular resistance. The resulting decline in blood pressure is associated with minimal changes in cardiac output.[13]

A less important mechanism of action of methyldopa is its effect as a pseudo-transmitter. It is speculated that the drug is first converted to *alpha*-methyldopamine by DOPA decarboxylase. *Alpha*-methyldopamine enters the storage vesicle and is converted by dopamine *beta*-oxidase to *alpha*-methylnorepinephrine, which has a weaker neurotransmitter action than norepinephrine. As a result, the release of *alpha*-methylnorepinephrine in response to nerve stimulation evokes a diminished vasoconstrictor response.

Parasympathetic predominance may be manifested as bradycardia. Orthostatic hypotension is seldom serious. Sedation, although usually milder than reserpine, occurs after prolonged therapy and is consistent with the reduced anesthetic requirements detected in the experimental animals (Table 11–2).[6] Although the pressor responses to ephedrine are diminished in animals, this is seldom the case in man (Table 11–2).[6]

Methyldopa is a logical choice in patients with renal disease, since the drug maintains or increases renal blood flow. The blood pressure reduction evoked by methyldopa, however, is exaggerated and prolonged in patients with renal failure.[9] This effect may be due to the accumulation of vasoactive metabolites that cannot be excreted by the uremic kidney.

About 20 to 30% of patients receiving methyldopa will develop a positive direct Coomb's test within 6 to 12 months of therapy.[9] This can be attributed to an IgG antibody specific for the Rh locus and will only rarely result in hemolytic anemia. A positive test without hemolysis does not require discontinuation of methyldopa. When hemolysis is present, however, difficulty in cross-matching may be encountered, and the drug must be discontinued.

A nonspecific flu-like syndrome that may progress to hepatitis is associated with elevations of serum transaminase enzymes.[9] For this reason, all patients receiving methyldopa should be subjected to periodic transaminase determinations. This determination is particularly appropriate before elective surgery. If abnormalities in liver function are detected, methyldopa should be discontinued. Furthermore, it is not advisable in general to use methyldopa in patients with known liver disease.[9]

Methyldopa is chemically similar to catecholamines and is known to interfere with the colorimetric determination of urinary catecholamines. Therefore, false-positive tests for pheochromocytoma may result when urinary catecholamines, but not vanillymandelic acid, are measured.

Patients treated with methyldopa may manifest severe hypertensive episodes upon receiving propranolol.[14] It is presumed that propranolol blocks the vasodilating effects of *alpha*-methylnorepinephrine revealing thus the *alpha*-stimulating component of this methyldopa metabolite. The pressor response resembles that seen with norepinephrine. The anesthesiologist should consider this hazard when contemplating the intraoperative administration of propranolol to a patient treated with methyldopa.

Another consideration is dementia, reported in patients treated first with methyldopa and subsequently with the butyrophenone, haloperidol.[15] This dementia may be caused by the ability of both drugs to block CNS dopamine receptors. This suggests caution in the use of Innovar, since this drug combination contains another butyrophenone, droperidol.

Clonidine (Catapres). Clonidine is an *alpha*-adrenergic receptor agonist that selectively stimulates postsynaptic receptors in the depressor area of the vasomotor center of the medulla oblongata and hypothalamus.[16,17] Stimulation of these *alpha* receptors diminishes efferent sympathetic outflow from the central nervous system with consequent peripheral vasodilation and concomitant increase in vagal activity. The predictable reduction in blood pressure and heart rate is not accompanied by a significant change in cardiac output. Plasma renin activity and urinary excretion of aldosterone and catecholamines are decreased.

Clonidine is almost completely absorbed after oral administration. Serious adverse side effects are uncommon (good clinical tolerance of the drug is almost 90%). There is little or no tendency to tachyphylaxis or orthostatic hypotension. Sexual dysfunction is less frequent than with methyldopa or guanethidine. This drug may be safely administered to patients with congestive heart failure, coronary artery disease, chronic obstructive airway disease, renal insufficiency and diabetes mellitus. As such, clonidine is one of the most versatile and effective drugs available for the ambulatory treatment of essential hypertension.

Sedation and xerostomia are the most common adverse effects associated with clonidine therapy. In view of the sedative effects of clonidine, it is not surprising that central nervous system depressants, such as barbiturates, may cause excessive drowsiness particularly during the initial phase of treatment.[9] Reductions in the requirements for volatile anesthetics are suggested by the documented reduction for MAC in experimental animals pretreated with clonidine.[18] Conversely, tricyclic antidepressants may interfere with the hypotensive action of clonidine.[9] Butyrophenones could behave in a similar manner and induce an abrupt antagonism of clonidine's hypotensive actions if droperidol is administered during anesthesia. This potential adverse drug interaction, however, remains undocumented and purely theoretical. Additional side effects include sinus bradycardia and high-grade atrioventricular heart block which seems to be more common in patients with pre-existing cardiac conduction defects or in those taking digitalis.

The most important adverse effect of clonidine is rebound hypertension with evidence of excess sympathetic activity when this drug is abruptly discontinued. This response has been designated as the antihypertensive withdrawal syndrome.[9] The hypothetical mechanism for this rebound hypertension is an abrupt increase in systemic vascular resistance due to the sudden release of catecholamines. The discontinuation of clonidine has been associated with the development of hypertension before the induction of anesthesia, as well as in the early postoperative period.[19,20] Cessation of clonidine treatment may be more serious in patients who continue to receive *beta*-adrenergic blockers. Presumably, the *beta*-adrenergic blocker antagonizes the vasodilating component of *beta* stimulation leaving *alpha* receptor-mediated vasoconstriction unopposed in the presence of elevated circulating concentrations of endogenous catecholamines.[9]

Rebound hypertension following abrupt discontinuation of antihypertensive therapy is not unique to clonidine.[9] Indeed, rebound hypertension of this type has also been observed following sudden cessation of treatment with reserpine, methyldopa, guanethidine, guanabenz, propranolol and metoprolol. Antihypertensives whose mechanism of action is independent of central and peripheral sympathetic activity (e.g., direct vasodilators, converting enzyme inhibitors) do not appear to provoke this antihypertensive rebound syndrome.[9] Finally, controlled prospective studies in patients receiving less than 1.2 mg/day of clonidine have not documented the occurrence of rebound hypertension when the drug is abruptly discontinued.[9]

Regardless of the drug used to treat essential hypertension, the important criterion is the avoidance of abrupt discontinuation of therapy. The dose of clonidine or any other antihypertensive should be tapered slowly over 4 to 5 days to avoid rebound hypertension. Continuation of clonidine throughout the perioperative period, however, is difficult, since a parenteral form of this drug is not available. Therefore, consideration should be given to replacing clonidine before elective surgery with an alternative antihypertensive.

Clonidine has been shown to be effective in suppressing the signs and symptoms of opiate withdrawal.[21] It is presumed that clonidine replaces opiate-mediated inhibition with *alpha*-2 mediated inhibition of central nervous system sympathetic activity.

Peripheral Sympatholytics

Guanethidine (Ismelin). Guanethidine acts selectively on the peripheral sympathetic nervous system to depress postganglionic sympathetic function. This selective action occurs because guanethidine uses the same uptake mechanism that transports norepinephrine into the postganglionic sympathetic nerve ending. Once it has gained access to storage vesicles, guanethidine causes norepinephrine release by a direct action (e.g., depletes intraneuronal norepinephrine stores) and also inhibits the depolarization induced by nerve stimulation. Decreased sympathetic responses at *alpha* and *beta* receptors result in decreaed venous return and cardiac output and consequent hypotension.

Decreased peripheral sympathetic responsiveness is also responsible for orthostatic hypotension that occurs to a varying degree in about one-third of all patients treated with guanethidine. This complication and the frequent occurrence of impotence limits the clinical usefulness of this drug.

Guanethidine lowers cardiac output, renal blood flow and secondarily, glomerular filtration rate. Therefore, renal function should be carefully monitored throughout treatment with guanethidine. Intestinal cramping, diarrhea and sinus bradycardia reflect an increase in vagal tone.

Guanethidine, like reserpine and methyldopa, sensitizes receptors to catecholamines and direct-acting sympathomimetics. Therefore, the use of guanethidine in a patient with a pheochromocytoma is not appropriate. In contrast, the patient's response to indirect-acting drugs is impaired. Unlike reserpine and methyldopa, guanethidine does not enter the central nervous system. This means that psychic depression, sedation and reduction of anesthetic requirements do not occur (Table 11–2).[6]

The hypotensive actions of guanethidine

may be impaired in patients receiving drugs that block norepinephrine uptake, since guanethidine depends on this mechanism for its adrenergic axonal uptake. Indeed, tricyclic antidepressants can trigger a hypertensive response in patients previously controlled with guanethidine.[22] Since tricyclic antidepressants block the uptake of norepinephrine, it is assumed that guanethidine's access to the nerve ending is also prevented. Other blockers of norepinephrine uptake include ephedrine (present in over-the-counter cold remedies), ketamine, cocaine, *alpha*-adrenergic blockers and possibly pancuronium.

Guanabenz (Wytensin). Guanabenz possesses a peripheral guanethidine-like adrenergic blocking action while blocking central sympathetic outflow. This central effect is chiefly responsible for its antihypertensive actions. Orthostatic hypotension, impotence and diarrhea are rare. The most common adverse side effects are similar to those caused by the centrally acting antihypertensive agents and consist of xerostomia, mild psychic depression and sedation.

Alpha-Adrenergic Antagonists

Prazosin (Minipress). This agent is an orally active antihypertensive that reduces blood pressure by producing peripheral vasodilation due to selective competitive blockade of postsynaptic *alpha*-1 vascular receptors.[23] This selective *alpha*-1 blockade results in balanced venous and arterial dilation similar to that produced by nitroprusside. Peripheral vasodilation not only lowers blood pressure, but also improves left ventricular stroke volume in patients with congestive heart failure. The fact that this drug is entirely metabolized in the liver allows its use in patients with renal failure without dose adjustment. Other uses of prazosin include treatment of peripheral vasospasm associated with Raynaud's phenomenon and as an antidysrhythmic. Indeed, in animals pretreated with prazosin, the dose of epinephrine necessary to induce cardiac ventricular dysrhythmias during halothane anesthesia is greatly increased.[24] This suggests a role for *alpha*-1 postsynaptic myocardial receptors in the induction of halothane dysrhythmias. Failure of prazosin to block significantly presynaptic *alpha*-2 receptors means that the normal *alpha*-1 mediated negative feedback mechanism that inhibits the release of norepinephrine remains intact. The hypotensive effect of prazosin is not accompanied by an increase in heart rate, levels of endogenous catecholamines or plasma renin activity. Failure to alter plasma renin activity is consistent with the hypothesis that *alpha*-2 receptors normally inhibit renin release.

The major adverse effect of prazosin is an acute syndrome associated with the first dose of the drug ("first dose phenomenon") which is characterized by transient fainting episodes and rarely syncope. In most instances, this response is due to acute orthostatic hypotension secondary to sudden peripheral vasodilation. The incidence and magnitude of this first dose phenomenon may be increased by pre-existing intravascular fluid volume depletion. Finally, indomethacin, a known prostaglandin inhibitor, can attenuate or block the antihypertensive effect of prazosin.[23]

Phenoxybenzamine (Diabenzyline) and Phentolamine (Regitine). Phenoxybenzamine and phentolamine are nonselective competitive antagonists at presynaptic *alpha*-2 and postsynaptic *alpha*-1 receptors. *Alpha*-1 blockade reduces systemic vascular resistance and the blood pressure fall which is associated with profound orthostatic hypotension. Conversely, inhibition of the negative feedback mechanism for the release of norepinephrine due to *alpha*-2 blockade results in elevation of the circulating concentrations of catecholamines. This response plus the reflex sympathetic stimulation due to reductions in blood pressure induces as tachycardia and increased myocardial contractility. Impotence is a predictable adverse effect of *alpha*-adrenergic blockade.

Prevention or treatment of hypertensive crises induced by release of endogenous (pheochromocytoma) or exogenous catecholamines is the most frequent indication for *alpha*-adrenergic blockade. These drugs have no clinical value in the ambulatory treatment of essential hypertension.

Combined Alpha and Beta Adrenergic Antagonists

Labetalol (Normodyne, Trandate). This is the prototype of a new class of antihypertensives that competitively blocks both peripheral *alpha* and *beta* receptors.[25] Specifically, labetalol is a selective *alpha*-1 antagonist and a nonselective *beta* antagonist. The degree of *alpha* blockade induced by labetalol is about one-half that produced by phentolamine, while its *beta* blockade is about one-fourth that of propranolol. In humans the ratio of *alpha* to *beta* blockade is approximately 7 to 1.

The combination of *alpha* and *beta* blockade results in a predictable decrease in blood pressure and systemic vascular resistance, while heart rate and cardiac output are minimally altered. The absence of significant heart rate or cardiac output changes distinguishes this drug from *beta*-blockers commonly employed to treat hypertension.

Labetalol, administered orally or intravenously, induces an abrupt decrease in systemic arterial pressure. This drug has been used to lower pressure in patients with pheochromocytoma and to treat hypertensive episodes following coronary artery bypass surgery.[26] This drug has also been used to induce controlled hypotension.

Orthostatic hypotension is the major adverse effect of labetalol. This complication is dose-related and seems to be accentuated by concomitant diuretic therapy. Sedation and sexual dysfunction have also been described in the hypertension clinic.

Peripheral Vasodilators

Hydralazine (Apresoline). Hydralazine presumably interferes with calcium transport in metarterioles and lowers blood pressure by direct vasodilation. Since baroceptor activity is unimpeded, reflex tachycardia and vasoconstriction are likely to antagonize the direct vasodilating actions of the drug. This reflex stimulation is prevented by combining hydralazine with a *beta*-adrenergic blocker. Concomitant use of diuretic therapy prevents the sodium retention characteristic of hydralazine and potentiates its antihypertensive effect. In the anesthetized patient, exaggerated hypotension could reflect the additive effects of vasodilating anesthetics.

Orthostatic hypotension is not a problem with hydralazine since cardiovascular reflexes and sympathetic nervous system function are not altered. Because it either maintains or increases renal blood flow, hydralazine is a logical choice for patients with renal disease.

In some patients, a lupus-like syndrome develops after several months of therapy with hydralazine. Typically, this syndrome occurs in patients treated for more than 6 months and manifess itself mainly in patients who are genetically slow-acetylators. Other adverse effects include a pyridoxine-responsive neuropathy, impotence, depression and possible hydralazine-induced hepatitis.[9] Although not documented clinically, it is theoretically possible that hydrazine-containing compounds, such as hydralazine, may result in enhanced defluorination of volatile anesthetics, such as enflurane.[27]

Minoxidil (Loniten). Minoxidil is an orally effective antihypertensive that reduces blood pressure by direct vascular smooth muscle relaxation.[28] This drug acts predominately on arterioles and has little effect on venous capacitance vessels. As it occurs with most peripheral vasodilators, minoxidil produces reflex sympathetic stimulation which increases the plasma concentration of norepinephrine and plasma renin activity. This reflex stimulation manifests itself with tachycardia, increased stroke volume and cardiac output, and sodium and fluid retention. For these reasons, minoxidil is usually administered in combination with a *beta*-blocker and a diuretic. This drug is particularly useful in the treatment of patients with severe and refractory hypertension.

Reversible hypertrichosis is a harmless but unpleasant side effect which appears to some degree in nearly all patients treated for more than 1 month.[9] Typically, this new hair growth appears on the lower face, forehead and upper arms. Pulmonary hypertension associated with minoxidil is probably due to fluid retention rather than to a unique effect of this drug on pulmonary vasculature. This drug has been associated with pericardial effusions particularly in patients with severe impairment of renal function. Changes in the T wave on the electrocardiogram during the first 2 weeks of therapy have been observed. These changes are usually not associated with symptoms or elevations of cardiac enzymes.

Converting Enzyme Inhibitors

Captopril (Capoten). Captopril is an orally active inhibitor of angiotensin-converting enzyme. This enzyme[29] is necessary for the conversion of inactive angiotensin I to the powerful vasoconstrictor, angiotensin II. As such, this drug lowers blood pressure by decreasing systemic vascular resistance. Typically, there is no concomitant change in heart rate or cardiac output. Captopril is used for the treatment of hypertension associated with a documented increased plasma renin activity.

Adverse side effects from treatment with captopril are rare. The most common is rash sometimes accompanied by fever and joint discomfort.[9] Disturbance in taste and the presence of xerostomia occur less frequently. More serious but rare reactions include proteinuria, renal failure and agranulocytosis. Serum potassium concentrations may increase particularly if the patient is treated with oral potassium supplements or potassium-sparing diuretics. Finally, indomethacin, a known inhibitor of prostaglandins, attenuates the ability of captopril to reduce plasma renin activity and arterial blood pressure.[9]

Monoamine Oxidase Inhibitors

Monoamine oxidase inhibitors are rarely used for the ambulatory treatment of essential hypertension, having been replaced by less toxic drugs. For example, adverse side effects of pargyline include postural hypotension, sodium retention, increased appetite, urinary retention and impotence. Undesirable drug interactions may ensue because tyramine is no longer inactivated by monoamine oxidase enzyme in the gastrointestinal tract. Hypertensive crises may accompany the ingestion of tyramine-containing foods (e.g., cheese, beer, wine, chicken liver). Slowed or altered metabolism may be responsible for atypical responses to narcotics, particularly meperidine (hyperthermia, excessive depression of ventilation).[9] Likewise, prolonged and excessive sedation may accompany barbiturate administration.

The probable mechanism of action of monoamine oxidase inhibitors is the production of a false neurotransmitter, octopamine. Octopamine produces less *alpha* stimulation and vasoconstriction than norepinephrine.

Since monoamine oxidase inhibitors prevent the oxidative deamination of norepinephrine, the blood pressure response to indirect-acting sympathomimetics such as ephedrine (even in cold remedies) may be exaggerated. This response reflects the increased availability of neurotransmitter, since its biochemical disposition is blocked, while the endogenous synthesis of norepinephrine continues unimpeded.

Pargyline is the only monoamine oxidase inhibitor available for the control of blood pressure. This drug should be discontinued at least 2 weeks prior to the administration of any elective anesthetic or surgery. The substitution of other antihypertensives must be performed cautiously. For example, reserpine and guanethidine may stimulate norepinephrine release and cause a hypertensive crisis in the presence of a residual pargyline effect.

TREATMENT OF HYPERTENSIVE CRISES

The drugs of choice for the management of intraoperative or postoperative hypertension are nitroprusside (Nipride), trimethaphan (Arfonad) or diazoxide (Hyperstat).

Nitroprusside

Nitroprusside provides rapid control of blood pressure, but its great potency requires careful dose titration, preferably with an infusion pump. During anesthesia, an infusion rate of 0.5 to 5 μg/kg/min is usually adequate. The lower doses are indicated in the presence of potent inhaled anesthetics. Since nitroprusside has no effect on the myocardium or the autonomic nervous system, cardiac output is usually maintained or even increased when blood pressure is lowered. Cyanide toxicity should be suspected in any patient who is resistant (e.g., requires greater than 10 μg/kg/min) or who develops tachyphylaxis or metabolic acidosis. Nitroprusside should be immediately discontinued in such patients and appropriate cyanide antagonists should be employed if hypotension or metabolic acidosis persists.

Trimethaphan

Trimethaphan is a ganglionic blocking drug that acts rapidly. Its action is so brief that it must be administered by continuous intravenous infusion. As with nitroprusside, constant blood pressure monitoring is necessary. Because trimethaphan relaxes capacitance vessels and blocks sympathetic reflexes, it lowers blood pressure by arteriolar vasodilation as well as diminishes cardiac output. The ensuing reflex tachycardia may offset reductions in blood pressure and contribute to occasional resistance to the hypotensive effects of this drug. Histamine release secondary to trimethaphan administration makes this drug inappropriate in patients with pheochromocytoma. Large doses of trimethaphan may potentiate nondepolarizing neuromuscular blockers by an unknown mechanism.[30]

Diazoxide

Diazoxide is a nondiuretic thiazide derivative that has been used for the management of postoperative hypertension.[31] This drug reduces systolic and diastolic blood pressure by a direct relaxant action on arteriolar smooth muscle. It has no significant effect on sympathetic reflexes, hence the decrease in systemic vascular resistance is concomitant to baroreceptor-mediated increase in heart rate and cardiac output.

A single intravenous injection of diazoxide of 2.5 to 5 mg/kg over 10 to 20 seconds rapidly lowers blood pressure to an acceptable level in 2 to 5 minutes without the need for constant monitoring. Since at least 90% of the drug is bound to protein, slow injection may not permit sufficient free drug to reduce blood pressure appropriately. Blood pressure gradually returns to control levels over the next 12 hours. The absence of a sedative effect allows the physician to evaluate the patient's mental status. Although excessive hypotension is unlikely, it is not possible to adjust the dose of the drug to the patient's response. This is a distinct disadvantage versus nitroprusside. It must be remembered that the response to diazoxide is accentuated in patients who are receiving *beta*-blockers, since the baroreceptor-mediated sympathetic responses to hypotension are blocked. When used in toxemic patients, diazoxide acts as a powerful uterine relaxant, but contractions may be re-established with oxytocin. Diazoxide inhibits the release of insulin from the pancreas, but hypoglycemia is not a contraindication to its limited use. Stimulation of catecholamine release prohibits the use of this drug in patients with pheochromocytoma.

REFERENCES

1. Coakley, C.A., Alpert, S., and Boling, J.S.: Circulatory responses during anesthesia of patients on rauwolfia therapy. J.A.M.A., 161:1143, 1956.
2. Crandell, D.L.: The anesthetic hazards in patients on antihypertensive therapy. J.A.M.A., 179:495, 1962.
3. Katz, R.L., Weintraub, H.D., and Papper, E.M.: Anesthesia, surgery and rauwolfia. Anesthesiology, 25:142, 1964.
4. Prys-Roberts, C., Meloche, R., Foëx, P.: Studies of anesthesia in relation to hypertension I: Cardiovascular responses to treated and untreated patients. Br. J. Anaesth., 43:122, 1971.
5. Dingle, H.R.: Antihypertensive drugs and anaesthesia. Anesthesia, 21:151, 1966.
6. Miller, R.D., Way, W.L., Eger, E.I. II: The effects of alpha-methyldopa, reserpine, guanethidine and iproniazid on minimum alveolar anesthetic requirement (MAC). Anesthesiology, 29:1153, 1969.
7. Melmon, K.L.: The clinical pharmacology of commonly used antihypertensive drugs. In: Cardiovascular Drug Therapy. Edited by K.L. Melmon. Philadelphia, F.A. Davis Co., 1974.
8. Gottlieb, T.R., Chidsey, C.A.: The clinician's guide to pharmacology of antihypertensive agents. Geriatrics, 31:99, 1976.
9. Husserl, F.E., and Messerli, F.H.: Adverse effects of antihypertensive drugs. Drugs, 22:188, 1981.
10. Eger, E.I. II, and Hamilton, W.K.: The effect of reserpine on the action of various vasopressors. Anesthesiology, 20:641, 1959.
11. Bagwell, E.E., and Woods, E.F.: Influence of reserpine on the cardiovascular responses to cyclopropane anesthesia. Fed. Proc., 22:186, 1963.
12. Myhre, E., Rugstad, H.E., and Hansen, T.: Clinical pharmacokinetics of methyldopa. Clin. Pharmacokinetics, 7:221, 1982.
13. Dollery, C.T., Harrington, M., and Hodge, J.V.: Haemodynamic studies with methyldopa: Effect on cardiac output and response to pressor amines. Br. Heart J., 25:670, 1963.
14. Nies, A.S., and Shand, D.G.: Hypertensive response to propranolol in a patient treated with methyldopa—a proposed mechanism. Clin. Pharmacol. Ther., 14:823, 1973.
15. Thornton, W.E.: Dementia induced by methyldopa with haloperidol. N. Engl. J. Med., 294:1122, 1976.
16. VanZwieten, P.A.: The central action of antihypertensive drugs mediated via central alpha receptors. J. Pharm. Pharmacol., 25:89, 1973.
17. Houston, M.C.: Clonidine hydrochloride. South. Med. J., 75:713, 1982.
18. Bloor, B.C., Flacke, W.E., and Randall, F.: Clonidine potentiation of halothane anesthesia and reversal. Anesthesiology, 53:S16, 1980.
19. Bruce, D.L., Croley, T.E., and Lee, J.S.: Preoperative clonidine withdrawal syndrome. Anesthesiology, 5:90, 1979.
20. Brodsky, J.B., and Bravo, J.J.: Acute postoperative clonidine withdrawal syndrome. Anesthesiology, 44:519, 1976.
21. Gold, M.S., Pottash, A.C., Sweeney, D.R., and Kleber, H.D.: Opiate withdrawal using clonidine. A safe, effective and rapid nonopiate treatment. J.A.M.A., 241:343, 1980.
22. Kosman, M.E.: Evaluation of a new antihypertensive agent. Prazosin hydrochloride (Minipress). J.A.M.A., 238:157, 1977.
23. Colucci, W.S.: Alpha-adrenergic receptor blockade with prazosin. Considerations of hypertension, heart failure, and potential new applications. Ann. Intern. Med., 97:67, 1982.
24. Maze, M., and Smith, C.M.: Identification of receptor mechanism mediating epinephrine-induced arrhythmias during halothane anesthesia in the dog. Anesthesiology, 59:322, 1983.
25. Wallin, J.D., and O'Neill, W.M.: Labetalol. Current research and therapeutic status. Arch. Intern. Med. 143:485, 1983.
26. Morel, D.R., Forster, A., and Suter, P.M.: I.V. labetalol in the treatment of hypertension following coronary-artery surgery. Br. J. Anaesth., 54:1191, 1982.
27. Mazze, R.I., Woodruff, R.E., and Heerdt, M.E.: Isoniazid-induced enflurane defluorination in humans. Anesthesiology, 57:5, 1982.
28. Campese, V.M.: Minoxidil: A review of its pharmacological properties and therapeutic use. Drugs, 22:257, 1982.
29. Vidt, D.G., Bravo, E.L., and Fouad, F.M.: Captopril. N. Engl. J. Med., 306:214, 1982.
30. Wilson, S.L., Miller, R.M., Wright, C., and Hasse, D.: Prolonged neuromuscular blockade associated with trimethaphan: A case report. Anesth. Analg., 55:353, 1976.
31. Wester, J.K.: Diazoxide. N. Engl. J. Med., 294:1271, 1976.

12

CHOLINERGIC AND ANTICHOLINERGIC AGENTS

WERNER E. FLACKE and JOAN W. FLACKE

CASE REPORT

A 38-year-old, 60-kg nurse underwent a cholecystectomy. Except for gallbladder disease, her past history was essentially negative. The only item of note was a history of severe bronchial asthma as a child. The frequency of attacks had decreased with age, and the last asthmatic episode had been more than ten years earlier. The patient had received general anesthesia at age 15 for an appendectomy, apparently without incident, but no anesthetics since that time.

Anesthesia was induced with intravenous thiopental and maintained uneventfully with nitrous oxide, 60% in oxygen, intravenous meperidine, and pancuronium for muscle relaxation. Near the conclusion of the operation, the patient was given atropine, 1 mg intravenously followed by neostigmine, 2.5 mg intravenously. Good reversal of neuromuscular block (as ascertained by nerve stimulation and by measurement of inspiratory force) was obtained. The patient's chest was clear, and there was no bradycardia. The patient was allowed to breathe spontaneously, and an additional dose of thiopental (50 mg) was given to keep her asleep for the placement of skin sutures. Approximately 10 minutes after the neostigmine had been given, nitrous oxide was discontinued and replaced by 100% O_2. The patient awoke and promptly developed severe bronchospasm with a prolonged expiratory phase and little air entry bilaterally. Her heart rate fell from 85 to less than 60 per minute. The endotracheal tube was removed immediately, which resulted in sufficient improvement such that it was possible to ventilate her with oxygen by mask. Neither intravenous aminophylline (300 mg) nor another dose of atropine (2 mg) relieved the bronchospasm, although they did abolish the bradycardia. The patient was taken to the recovery room, treated with manually assisted ventilation by mask and oxygen, 100%, and with Vaponefrin mist inhalation. She gradually improved over the next hour.

Comment. The crux of this case is the abnormal sensitivity of the patient's airway musculature to bronchoconstrictor agents (acetylcholine) and the endogenous vagal nervous activity depending on the state of consciousness. The dose of atropine given prior to neostigmine was sufficient to prevent early vagal effects on the heart and bronchial smooth musculature. When atropine was given, the patient was still anesthetized and apparently had a low vagal tone. However, the buildup with time of acetylcholine (ACh) at the cholinergic receptors and the sudden increase in vagal activity and ACh release associated with awakening overcame the antagonistic effect of the previously effective dose of atropine and resulted in bradycardia and bronchospasm. The additional 2 mg of atropine might have been sufficient to alleviate this, but by now other bronchospastic humoral agents may have been maintaining the bronchoconstriction. Airway smooth muscle in sensitive patients is much more responsive not only to acetylcholine but also to other bronchospastic agonists, such as histamine and slow-reacting substance.

This chapter discusses the interactions of cholinergic and anticholinergic agents, with emphasis on their pharmacology and their use in anesthesia.

MORPHOLOGY, BIOCHEMISTRY, AND PHYSIOLOGY

Acetylcholine was the first chemical identified as a neurohumoral transmitter by the classic experiments of Otto Loewi, who demonstrated that the effects of vagal nerve stimulation on the frog heart could be transferred to a second heart by the bathing fluid of the first heart taken during the stimulation.[1]

Loewi's demonstration was in a postganglionic parasympathetic system, but Sir Henry Dale had recognized earlier the similarity between the effects of ACh and the responses to stimulation of different peripheral nerves.[2] Within 15 years of Loewi's experiment, the transmitter role of ACh was firmly established at all preganglionic autonomic nerve endings, parasympathetic postganglionic nerve endings, and the terminals of motor nerves (neuromuscular junction). Somewhat later, convincing evidence was added that ACh is a transmitter also in the central nervous system.[3] It is further known that ACh can stimulate sensory nerve endings, but this effect probably has no physiologic significance. Moreover, not all tissues that possess receptors for and therefore respond to ACh have cholinergic innervation (for example, vascular smooth muscle).

Sir Henry Dale also posited that different effects of ACh could be mimicked or blocked by different drugs: *muscarine* and atropine at postganglionic parasympathetic effector sites, *nicotine* at autonomic ganglia and at the neuromuscular junction. These observations have led to the classification of "muscarinic" and "nicotinic" cholinergic systems. Nicotinic effects can be further subdivided because *hexamethonium* and related agents block ganglionic effects relatively selectively, whereas *curare*-type drugs do the same at the neuromuscular junction.

Synthesis of ACh in all cholinergic nerve endings is catalyzed by choline acetylase in the presence of coenzyme A. ACh is then stored in the nerve terminals and is inactive until released into the extracellular space or synaptic junction during nerve activity. (Reid Hunt of Harvard Medical School early recognized the high potency of ACh, which he had synthetized from choline extracted from the adrenal medulla, but he rejected the idea of a biological role of ACh because it was "much too toxic" to exist in the body. This shows how difficult it was to conceive of storage of a chemical in the body in such a way that it was inactive or "nontoxic," but so that it could be released as a free or active compound.) Free ACh is rapidly hydrolyzed by cholinesterases, which are among the most widely distributed enzymes in the body and occur both in solution and bound to tissue components. Thus free ACh, that is ACh in a nonstorage condition, has a brief lifetime and is present only during nerve activity near the terminals of cholinergic nerves.

For the physiologic functions of ACh, or of any transmitter, morphologic as well as biochemical factors are important. The synaptic gap, the distance from the site of release to the site of the receptors on postsynaptic or effector cell membranes, differs greatly. At the neuromuscular junction the gap is about 400 to 500 Å wide; in autonomic ganglia and in the central nervous system (CNS) gaps of only 50 to 150 Å occur; at postganglionic parasympathetic junctions (for example, in the heart, in smooth muscle tissues in the airways, or in the intestine) the distance from the site of release to the receptor sites may be 10,000 Å or more. The transmitter must diffuse to the receptor sites, and the time required is determined by the distance. The time varies from one millisecond or less at the neuromuscular junction or in autonomic ganglia to several hundred milliseconds or more in the case of some parasympathetic postganglionic junctions.

The size of the synaptic (or junctional) gap also determines the importance of the hydrolyzing enzymes for terminating the carbachol, and bethanechol are less rapidly hydrolyzed, and therefore their effects are longer lasting. Although they can be given subcutaneously or even by mouth, their importance and their use is limited.

Pilocarpine is a plant-derived alkaloid with muscarinic activity; it is used widely in the treatment of glaucoma by topical administration. Although systemic effects can occur with overdosage or with special sensitivity, the ophthalmic use of pilocarpine is one of the few examples of successfully sustained localized drug application, and toxicity is not common.

A common characteristic of the systemic effects of the muscarinic cholinomimetic agents is that they affect homeostatically controlled systems, such as heart rate and blood pressure, less than they affect functions that lack such compensatory mechanisms, such as bronchial constriction and airway secretions, salivation, sweating, and cardiac impulse conduction. All the last effects are antagonized easily by small doses of any anticholinergic drug.

Of much greater importance than the foregoing directly produced muscarinic cholinomimetic effects are those produced indirectly as a result of the inhibition of cholinesterases. Anticholinesterase drugs are used routinely in anesthesia to reverse nondepolarizing neuromuscular block. They are also used in the treatment of myasthenia gravis[24] and glaucoma. Furthermore, since organophosphate anticholinesterase agents are widely encountered in the environment as household and agricultural pesticides, exposure to such agents can be encountered.

Among anticholinesterase drugs one must distinguish between those that do and those that do not enter the CNS. The anticholinesterase drugs used for their effects on neuromuscular transmission are carbamic acid esters and quaternary ammonium compounds. They do not pass the blood-brain barrier to any significant extent. To reach their site of action, the compounds used as pesticides must have high lipid solubility, and all of these agents do have CNS effects. Most of the pesticide anticholinesterase agents are organophosphates. In contrast to the carbamates, these agents are not competitive, surmountable inhibitors of cholinesterase; rather they are nonsurmountable and, for practical purposes, irreversible enzyme inhibitors. Thus their effect is much longer lasting and is cumulative. Fortunately, the only members of this group in medicinal use are the eyedrops echothiophate and isofluorophate. Theoretically the functional consequences of cholinesterase inhibition should parallel the degree of inhibition, and measurement of plasma cholinesterase or, even better, of red cell cholinesterase, should be an important diagnostic and predictive tool. However, this has not proved to be the case, as the symptomatology caused by anticholinesterase inhibitors does not seem to correlate well with the degree of enzyme inhibition.[25]

One factor that may explain this discrepancy in part is that the consequence of the inhibition of cholinesterase depends not only on the dose of the inhibitor and the magnitude of the biochemical effect, but especially on the magnitude of the nerve activity, that is, on the amount of ACh being released at the time of enzyme inhibition. For example, there may be no parasympathomimetic effects resulting from an anticholinesterase drug when parasympathetic nerve activity is low or absent. For a given dose in a given system, the effect of an anticholinesterase drug is proportional to the magnitude of parasympathetic nerve activity.

Organophosphate eyedrops can be important clinically. Patients may be careless about the amount of eyedrops they use. Absorption is variable, but often considerable. The only safe way to avoid an interaction is to elicit from the patient a careful and detailed history of taking these drugs. Since inhibition is long-term, agents such as succinylcholine that require cholinesterase to terminate their action should be avoided for 2 to 3 weeks after the cessation of therapy with these organophosphate eyedrops.

Cholinolytic Agents

Nicotinic. This group of drugs, which acts on autonomic ganglia, produces a nondepolarizing ganglionic block. Hexamethonium, pentolinium, trimethaphan, and chlorisondamine are examples of such drugs. These agents were the first to be used in the treatment of hypertension, but they produce block of impulse transmission in all ganglia, sympathetic and parasympathetic, with little selectivity. Hence their side effects are global and severe: fully effective doses produce almost complete pharmacologic autonomic denervation. For this reason, they have been replaced by more selective agents for the treatment of chronic hypertension. In anesthesia, they have a limited application for deliberate, controlled, short-lasting hypotension. Ganglion blocking drugs have been advocated also for the acute treatment of congestive heart failure, since they lower arterial pressure and thus reduce the load on the failing heart.

The overriding characteristic of ganglion blocking drugs is their lack of selectivity. Ganglion block implies the interruption of sympathetic and parasympathetic efferent pathways, with the consequent paralysis of autonomic functions, from tear production to cessation of intestinal motility. Such a condition requires special care on the part of the anesthetist to substitute for the missing "protective" effect of the autonomic system. Fortunately, however, complete ganglionic block is unnecessary for the foregoing uses of ganglionic blocking drugs in anesthesia.

It is not surprising that ganglion blocking activity is a side effect of some of the nondepolarizing neuromuscular blocking drugs in view of the close pharmacologic relationship between the two classes of agents. Among the neuromuscular blocking drugs presently in use, d-tubocurarine is the most potent ganglionic blocker and the margin between neuromuscular blocking doses and doses that have autonomic side effects is so large with vecuronium and atracurium that such side effects may be expected only with massive overdoses. Several inhalation anesthetic agents also inhibit nicotinic ganglionic transmission to some degree in commonly used concentrations.[26] The clinical significance of this phenomenon has not been determined. In addition, it has been established that impulse transmission through some autonomic ganglia is not fully blocked by nicotinic blocking drugs, and that the remaining transmission is sensitive to small doses of atropine-type agents; that is, it is muscarinic in nature.[27,28] Again, the clinical relevance of these findings has not been established.

Muscarinic. The pharmacology of the cholinolytic, antimuscarinic drugs, often somewhat inaccurately called "anticholinergic" or "atropine-like," is too well known to be repeated here except for some special points.[29-32] Several, if not all, of these agents are not "pure" antagonists. Atropine and scopolamine in small doses produce bradycardia and, perhaps, slowing of AV impulse conduction. These effects were earlier attributed to a central vagal stimulating effect after IV administration at a time when the concentration in the periphery was too small to produce vagal blockade.[33,34] Homatropine, which combines a weak peripheral blocking effect with a potent central stimulation, causes the most pronounced dose-related bradycardia.[35] However, methylatropine, the quaternary congener of atropine, does not enter the CNS easily, yet still produces bradycardia.[36] Bradycardia from these drugs has been seen even after bilateral vagotomy. Thus, although a central component cannot be excluded, these cholinolytics must have a peripheral site of action. This is further supported by the observation that both salivation and pupillary accommodation are initially stimulated before being paralyzed.[32] These phenomena may be due to a partial agonist effect of the antagonists.

A distinction must be made between the antagonistic effect of these drugs against circulating cholinomimetic agents (including ACh, if it should "spill over" during massive anticholinesterase poisoning) and the usual effect of blocking parasympathetic nerve activity. The former situation is relatively simple, involves more or less equilibrated agonist (generally of low concentrations), and is sensitive to small doses of antimuscarinic drugs. However, when the agonist is released from nerve endings, a situation more commonly encountered in the operating room, it may be much more concentrated in time and in space. Whereas block of low-magnitude nerve activity, associated with small and transient concentrations of transmitter, can be achieved with relatively small doses of antagonist, the same doses may not block a massive burst of nerve activity, which results in high and more prolonged transmitter concentrations. The situation is aggravated by the inhibition of cholinesterase and by the consequent potentiation of parasympathetic nerve activity. These conditions can be demonstrated in the experimental animal, and the case report deals with an analogous clinical situation.

The recent observations of the interaction of sympathetic and parasympathetic nerve activity in the periphery may give a new dimension to the understanding of the effects of anticholinergic agents. These observations imply that such effects involve not only the antagonism of parasympathetic activity directly on effector systems, but also an indirect effect resulting from a block of the inhibition or attenuation of release of the sympathetic transmitter, norepinephrine, in organs or systems with dual, antagonistic innervation. This effect of atropine on the release of norepinephrine during simultaneous stimulation of sympathetic and vagal nerves has indeed been observed in the heart,[19,20] and this phenomenon may shed a new light on clinical observations of a "sympathomimetic" effect of atropine. However, more work is required in order to clarify the situation both in animals and in man.

There are variations in sensitivity of different effector systems to anticholinergic drugs and differences among different agents in relative potency.[30,32] The effects on salivary secretion and, probably, airway secretion—which have, however, not been measured—and on sweating are the most sensitive. These occur in man with drug doses that have little or no cardiac vagolytic action.[30,31] Atropine is a more potent agent in blocking cardiac vagal effects than scopolamine, whereas scopolamine is more potent as an antisialogogue.[32] As expected, both these alkaloids have more marked central and ocular effects than do the quaternary ammonium antimuscarinic agents. The central effects are discussed separately in this chapter.

CLINICAL USE OF CHOLINERGIC DRUGS IN ANESTHESIA

Two main types of drugs that affect the parasympathetic nervous system are used in anesthesia:

1. antimuscarinic anticholinergic agents (atropine-like)
   a. for premedication
   b. as protection against the muscarinic consequences of cholinesterase inhibition
2. anticholinesterase agents to improve transmission after nondepolarizing neuromuscular blocking drugs

We shall first consider the use of atropine-like drugs for premedication, the most controversial question.

Antimuscarinic Anticholinergic Agents

Historically, atropine was introduced to protect the heart from vagal influences during chloroform anesthesia, and to prevent excessive secretions during diethyl ether anesthesia. Since these agents are no longer used in this country, the question has been asked whether the routine use of anticholinergic drugs prior to anesthesia is justified.[37–39]

Eger[30] concluded over 20 years ago that belladonna drugs should "not be given by rote" and Gravenstein and Anton have written:[40] "Anticholinergic drugs often can be omitted from premedication. A healthy young woman coming for a minor operative procedure, such as dilatation and curettage, does not require premedication with an anticholinergic drug if thiopental and nitrous oxide are used as exclusive anesthetics." This is a cautious statement from researchers known for their careful and extensive work in this area. Yet the statement has been criticized on the basis of a study of 150 patients who underwent minor gynecologic procedures during which thiopental and nitrous oxide were used primarily, although some patients received enflurane, halothane, or fentanyl as well.[38]

The patients were divided into two groups: One group received 25 mg of hydroxyzine hydrochloride intramuscularly as premedication and the other received the same dose of hydroxyzine plus 0.2 mg glycopyrrolate intramuscularly (time interval between injection and induction not stated). The patients were evaluated on a double-blind basis as having "satisfactory" or "unsatisfactory" premedication. Of the group that received no glycopyrrolate, 35.9% were judged unsatisfactory, as compared with 19.4% of the group that had received the anticholinergic agent. The difference was statistically significant. When the results were broken down further, the difference was significant only in the group that had not undergone intubation (13.6% unsatisfactory with glycopyrrolate versus 27.4% without). The incidence of "unsatisfactory" was much higher among the patients who had been intubated (42.9% after glycopyrrolate versus 66.7% without the anticholinergic agent), but the difference between the groups with or without premedication was not significant. The authors concluded that the dose had been insufficient for intubation. No information on the effects of the drug on cardiovascular functions was given.

The most recent report we have found was not based on a controlled, randomized procedure. Eleven anesthetists were asked to report the following on patients who had been anesthetized during a period of one year: (1) whether "secretions constituted a problem during or after anesthesia, if anticholinergic premedication was omitted;" (2) the nature of the problem if there had been one; and (3) whether an anticholinergic drug was given and with what result.[39] Answers for 404 patients were evaluated, 244 of whom had not received an anticholinergic drug for premedication, and 160 of whom had been given either 0.6 mg atropine or 0.4 mg scopolamine intramuscularly one hour before the induction of anesthesia. The trachea was intubated in 56% of the patients with premedication and in 85% of those without. Among the patients not premedicated with an anticholinergic agent, there were 13% who had "problem secretions," as opposed to 3.75% of the premedicated patients. Of the patients reported to have had troublesome secretions, 16% were given atropine during the operation "with success." Hence, only in 2% of the nonpremedicated group did the amount of secretions prompt the anesthetist to administer an anticholinergic agent. The authors concluded that this incidence of troublesome secretions did not warrant the routine administration of anticholinergic drugs before general anesthesia.

This study can also be criticized, and it seems appropriate to pursue this question more vigorously. Yet we are still impressed by the results just quoted, for they seem to be based on sound reasoning and valid observations, even though they were the product of experiments not conducted under double-blind conditions.

What are the risks and benefits of premedication with an antimuscarinic anticholinergic agent with regard to secretions? The benefit is a lower incidence of secretions in amounts considered sufficiently serious to warrant action in the form of the intraoperative injection of an anticholinergic drug. Secretions are serious if they hinder ventilation, and deterioration of blood gases (when it is possible to determine their levels rapidly) is the best evidence of this. The risks are secondary to inhibition of secretions with the potential for inspissation of mucus, breakdown of ciliary function, and possibly obstruction of small airways.[40,41] It would be of interest to compare postanesthetic pulmonary complications with and without anticholinergic medication. In this connection, it may be remembered that anticholinergic drugs have been all but abandoned in the routine treatment of bronchial asthma.[31]

The second important question concerns the possible risks and benefits resulting from the cardiac effects of antimuscarinic drugs. Given the complex physiology of the parasympathetic cardiac innervation and the equally complex pharmacology of antimuscarinic agents, the answer is not easy.

Until recently, no studies had evaluated the preventive use of anticholinergic drugs with respect to cardiac functions as thoroughly as those that evaluated the effects of these drugs on secretions. Observations showed a high incidence of both dysrhythmias and tachycardia when atropine was given *during* anesthesia. These studies indicated that the effects of anticholinergic drugs were most severe (a) under conditions when sympathetic tone could be assumed to be high, and (b) in the presence of a general anesthetic agent known to sensitize the heart towards catecholamines. This was the case on the one hand with light levels of anesthesia, especially during painful surgical procedures such as oral surgery, and on the other with agents such as diethyl ether, cyclopropane, and halothane.[42-44]

One study was designed as a double-blind procedure to investigate the effect of atropine on the bradycardia seen with a second dose of succinylcholine injected 5 minutes after the first dose under halothane-nitrous oxide anesthesia, a situation associated with strong vagal activity.[45] Two episodes of extreme bradycardia prompted the investigators to break the code (these had occurred in patients who had not received atropine) and to continue without the group that had not received atropine. However, preoperative atropine blocked the vagal manifestations only when present in such concentrations that extreme tachycardia was a by-product. The investigators felt that this was too high a price to pay.

Another team of investigators compared groups that were given atropine and groups that were not with random allocations also under halothane-nitrous oxide anesthesia.[46] There was no significant difference in the incidence of dysrhythmias between the two groups when the patients had not undergone intubation, although the dysrhythmias in one group were clustered during and after the injection of atropine. With endotracheal intubation, the incidence of dysrhythmias was higher in the atropine group and was associated mainly with the intubation.

These observations, involving systematic and lengthy ECG (electrocardiogram) monitoring, did show that the incidence of cardiac dysrhythmias under the conditions chosen was high, but the authors made the point that dysrhythmias, even those of ventricular origin, rarely progress to ventricular fibrillation. This corresponds to common experience, but it is not proven. The authors again emphasized the price of anticholinergic medication in the form of tachycardia and suggested that this consequence could cause myocardial jeopardy, especially in the presence of coronary artery disease.

In this discussion we have paid little attention to the fact that the conditions predisposing to dysrhythmias are well known: a high level of sympathetic/adrenergic activity, the presence of a general anesthetic known to sensitize the heart, and the presence of hypercapnia and hypoxia.[54] Whereas the studies discussed were conducted under circumstances that are probably common today, there were no special efforts made to reduce the foregoing factors. It is known that the incidence of dysrhythmias, even when atropine is injected during the anesthesia, is lower with thiopental-nitrous oxide anesthesia, neurolept anesthesia, and enflurane.[42,47] It is further possible to reduce sympathetic/adrenergic influences by the use of *beta*-adrenergic blocking drugs. No systematic explorations of the effects of anticholinergic agents under such conditions have been presented.

It seems significant that the majority of investigators who have done experimental work on these questions, who have considered the problems carefully, and who may be assumed to have a degree of expertise have advised against the *routine* use of anticholinergic drugs for premedication. They conclude that an anticholinergic drug may be given during anesthesia when there is a specific indication for it, such as in the presence of bradycardia or when situations known to cause vagal reflex activity can be anticipated (for example, with a second dose of succinylcholine), and in patients known to be prone to bradycardic dysrhythmias. In these patients it is, of course, important to avoid the special risk factors discussed and to give the anticholinergic drug under conditions associated with a low incidence of dysrhythmias.

Anticholinesterase Agents

The situation is different when an anticholinesterase drug has to be given to improve neuromuscular transmission. The most severe dysrhythmias ever reported occurred in patients during cyclopropane anesthesia, when 0.8 mg of atropine was given after severe bradycardia, and marked inhibition of AV (atrioventricular) conduction occurred following deliberate injection of 0.8 to 2.0 mg neostigmine.[48] Intermittent AV block was reported in one subject without anesthesia during another series when neostigmine was given prior to atropine.[49]

Soon after the introduction of curare into clinical medicine, several sudden deaths were reported following the injection of neostigmine-atropine.[50-52] These catastrophic events were attributed to the simultaneous injection of the two drugs.[53] In retrospect, the patients were probably underventilated at the time when the mixture of anticholinesterase-anticholinergic was given. The role of hypercapnia and hypoxia in the pathogenesis of cardiac dysrhythmias was not appreciated until later, and methods for monitoring blood gases did not become more widely available until later. It has since been shown many times that the simultaneous injection of anticholinesterase and anticholinergic drug leads first to transient tachycardia and only much later to bradycardia.[54-61]

This does not mean that the common practice of giving a fixed dose combination of anticholinesterase-anticholinergic is unequivocally endorsed. On the contrary, the practice contradicts pharmacologic rationale, and the issue should not be decided on a statistical basis. The rate of onset and the ultimate magnitude of cholinergic (muscarinic) effects depend on the magnitude of existing parasympathetic tone, as does the dose of the anticholinergic drug required. If for any reason the patient's vagal tone is exceptionally high during the injection of the anticholinesterase drug, a severe bradycardia may develop. If such a possibility is anticipated, the anticholinergic drug should be given prior to the enzyme inhibitor. The action of atropine on the so-called lower esophageal sphincter has come under more scrutiny. The risk of regurgitation is related to the pressure differential between intragastric pressure and pressure within the area of the lower esophageal sphincter. Atropine—and all other cholinolytic drugs examined—reduced the latter for a prolonged period of time. The routine use of atropine has been questioned especially in obstetric anesthesia.

The consequences of the changes produced by both types of cholinergic drugs are well known in principle: bradycardia and slowing or block of AV-conduction may permit the emergence of secondary, ectopic pacemakers and hence cardiac dysrhythmias.[62] An effective dose of an antimuscarinic agent can certainly block any reflex or drug-induced bradycardia (for example, from succinylcholine, halothane, narcotic analgesic, or anticholinesterase drugs), but only in doses that cause marked tachycardia.[30,63] The bradycardic effect of the atropine-like drugs themselves cannot be forgotten. On the other hand, tachycardia and the increase in cardiac output and, at times, arterial blood pressure represent an additional load on the heart, and increase the myocardial oxygen requirement.[64] This situation is hazardous in patients with coronary artery disease or with mitral stenosis. Furthermore, the resulting shift toward sympathetic/adrenergic prevalence may increase the probability of cardiac dysrhythmias, and is especially dangerous in the presence of anesthetic agents known to sensitize the myocardium to catecholamines.[54]

Additional reasons for the conservative use of anticholinergic antimuscarinic drugs emerge from recent observations of a potentially beneficial effect of vagal activity on the heart and the evidence that parasympathetic activity regulates the release of sympathetic transmitter.[7-22]

We conclude that there is not sufficient evidence at this time to permit a full evaluation of the risks and benefits of the use of antimuscarinic, anticholinergic drugs for preanesthetic medication. With regard to secretions, such premedication is at least not mandatory, but the cardiac consequences are less clear-cut. The intravenous administration of an anticholinergic drug during anesthesia, which may become necessary, is definitely hazardous with anesthetic agents like cyclopropane and under light anesthesia during painful procedures, somewhat less hazardous with halothane, and considerably less during thiopental-nitrous oxide or neurolept anesthesia. A higher dose of atropine, given rapidly intravenously, seems to be less hazardous than a smaller one.[47]

The other effects of the antimuscarinic drugs—on body temperature, on pupillary constriction and hence intraocular pressure, and on micturition—are minor by comparison.[30-32,66,67] Atropine in clinical doses does not prevent the effects of neostigmine on intestinal motility.[65]

THE SO-CALLED CENTRAL ANTICHOLINERGIC SYNDROME

Of the many putative neurotransmitters in the mammalian central nervous system, acetylcholine (ACh) is the best documented. It is its muscarinic and not its nicotinic activity that is mainly involved. Evidence for this conclusion is based importantly on the effects of pharmacologic agents.[3,68] All anticholinesterase agents and antimuscarinic antagonists of ACh that pass the blood-brain barrier affect central nervous system functions. Biochemical studies have shown abundant acetylcholine receptors of the muscarinic type in the mammalian brain.[69]

It has long been known that atropine and scopolamine, as well as plants and plant extracts containing the belladonna alkaloids (Table 12–1), can cause a typical CNS syndrome, which has been termed the "central anticholinergic syndrome."[70] Symptoms range from sedation, stupor, and unconsciousness to anxiety, restlessness, hyperactivity, disorientation, delirium, hallucinations, loss of recent memory, dysarthria, and ultimately, convulsions, and respiratory depression.[71] The difference between the effects of small doses of atropine and of scopolamine is well known.[30,31] Small doses of the latter (0.3 to 0.5 mg) given subcutaneously, but not orally, usually cause profound seda-

Table 12-1
Anticholinergic Antimuscarinic Agents

Belladonna alkaloids	atropine
	scopolamine
	homatropine
	cyclopentolate
Anticholinergic drugs for Parkinsonism	benztropine (Cogentin)
	biperiden (Akineton)
	ethopropazine (Parsidol)
	procyclidine (Kemadrin)
	trihexyphenidyl (Artane)
Some over-the-counter drugs	Asthma-Dor
	Compoz
	Sleep Eze
	Sominex
Plants containing anti-cholinergic alkaloids	Bittersweet (Solanum dulcamara)
	Deadly nightshade (Atropa belladonna)
	Potato leaves and sprouts (Solanum tuberosum)
	Jimson weed (Datura stramonium)
So-called antispasmodics (quaternary anticholinergics)	Methantheline (Banthine)
	Propantheline (Probanthie)

tion, whereas atropine, in doses up to 1 mg, has few CNS effects of clinical significance. The minimal dose causing somnolence was stated by Longo[71a] to be 2 mg although electroencephalographic changes were observed after lower doses. It is old clinical knowledge that the condition of the patient at the time when the drug is given can make a difference: patients who have suffered head trauma, or are in pain, or are in a state of excitement are likely to respond to scopolamine with delirium and violent motor activity. Atropine in doses as high as 200 mg has been used in psychiatry for "coma therapy" in physically healthy patients, although much smaller doses have been reported to have been fatal, especially in children.[72] Therefore, care must be used with this agent.

Physostigmine, which is a tertiary amine, completely reverses even the delirium produced by a large dose of atropine, whereas it is known that neostigmine and the other quaternary ammonium anticholinesterase agents have little or no CNS effect.[73] This is logical if one considers the different lipid solubilities of the tertiary and quaternary compounds. Patients who do not respond to physostigmine (after exclusion of hypoxia and preexisting psychotic illness) often respond to pain relief by a narcotic. Thus, pain may contribute to the postanesthetic anticholinergic delirium and may be the reason for apparent failure of reversal by physostigmine.[74a]

Anesthesia potentiates the CNS effects of the anticholinergic drugs. In one series of 1,727 patients, premedicated with up to 0.5 mg scopolamine and anesthetized with different anesthetics, 11.2% were diagnosed to have a "postoperative reaction" attributed to scopolamine.[74] Of these, 85.2% had prolonged somnolence, and 14.8% had delirium. Greene conducted several studies the results of which are summarized in her 1971 paper.[74a] In 1967 10.2% of 545 patients who had been pretreated with scopolamine developed postoperative delirium and in a repeat study in 1969, 8.2% of 619 patients did. In 1971 she reported her hospital's experience with the reversing effects of physostigmine which had been redetected in the meantime in her own hospital.[70] This time she included some patients who had received atropine (from 0.2 to 0.6 g) rather than scopolamine.

She wrote that "patients who had received atropine were indistinguishable from delirious patients who had received scopolamine." They also responded to physostigmine in the same way. She also describes one patient who had received scopolamine and was not delirious but unresponsive to (strong) stimuli for 2 hours postoperatively. Five minutes after receiving 0.8 mg physostigmine he was awake and rational.

Thus there are two different types of postoperative central anticholinergic conditions, one characterized by profound and prolonged somnolence, the other by excitement, delirium, and motor violence. This situation seems analogous to that in patients without anesthesia, where "paradoxical," that is, excitatory, reactions to scopolamine may also occur. That both types of reactions respond quickly to the injection of physostigmine is evidence that both conditions are causally related to anticholinergic medication.[74] So far, there is no precise information about the conditions that may determine which type of reaction occurs.

Anticholinergic, antimuscarinic activity is not restricted to agents so classified (see Table 12-1), but is seen with many drugs from antihistaminics to tricyclic antidepressants. Such agents are also often contained in drug combinations and in over-the-counter preparations, and may be present in "street drugs." A partial listing is given in Tables 12-1 and 12-2. It has been stated that more than 600 pharmaceutic preparations contain agents with central anticholinergic activity.[71] Thus patients may be exposed to such drugs without the knowledge of the physician. After prolonged use of some such preparations, residual concentrations may remain in the body for a long time without causing clear symptoms. For the anesthesiologist this means that the remaining activity of such agents may be additive to that of anticholinergic drugs administered before or during anesthesia.

Table 12-2
Drugs Possessing Anticholinergic Activity

Tricyclic antidepressants:
  Amitriptyline (Elavil)
  Desipramine (Norpramine, Pertofrane)
  Doxepin (Sinequan)
  Imipramine (Tofranyl, SK-Pramine)

Antipsychotic agents:
  Chlorpromazine
  Thioridazine (Mellaril)
  Haloperidol
  Droperidol

Antihistamine agents:
  Chlorpheniramine (Ornade)
  Diphenhydramine (Benadryl)
  Orphenidrine (Disipal)
  Promethazine (Phenergan)

Drugs not having anticholinergic activity but reported to have been antagonzied by physostigmine:
  Diazepam (Valium)
  Chlordiazepoxide (Librium)
  Lorazepam
  Glutethimide (Doriden)
  Narcotic analgesics

It has been reported that physostigmine has been used successfully to treat CNS depression from drugs with no known anticholinergic activity, such as diazepam.[75,76] It has also been claimed that physostigmine antagonizes the depressant effect of narcotic analgesics without reducing their analgesic activity.[77] These observations have led to the claim that physostigmine may be a nonspecific CNS stimulant or analeptic, independent of its anticholinesterase action. Although this could be so, there is no need to postulate it. An anticholinesterase agent "potentiates" cholinergic synaptic transmission or increases neuronal activity even if no receptor antagonist is present. There is evidence, for example, that anticholinesterase agents can improve transmission in situations where the defect is due to decreased release of transmitter.[78] An indirect effect on the function of central cholinergic neuronal systems is possible with many drugs.

The indications for the use of physostigmine differ widely from institution to institution and from one anesthesiologist to the next. Risks and benefits must be weighed as always, but little information on their magnitude is available in this case.

It seems from a survey of the literature that the risks of physostigmine administration are small, as long as the recommended dose is not exceeded, the indication is strictly established, and the many contraindications are heeded. The dose is 1 or 2 mg given slowly intravenously, with a possible second dose after 10 to 15 minutes, if the response to the first dose has been positive but insufficient. Physostigmine should only be given if there are signs of antimuscarinic medication in the periphery in addition to symptoms of the presence of a central anticholinergic syndrome. Relative contraindications and precautions are the same as for those anticholinesterase drugs that do not enter the CNS. If evidence of physostigmine overdosage is seen, the balance may be restored with a further dose of an anticholinergic drug, either scopolamine or atropine. If there are only symptoms of peripheral cholinergic preponderance, a quaternary ammonium anticholinergic (methylscopolamine, glycopyrrolate, methantheline, proprantheline) should be used. The duration of action of physostigmine is shorter than that of the anticholinergic agents involved; thus it may be necessary to repeat its injection if the symptoms alleviated by the first dose should recur.

An interesting drug that has been released here only recently, but has been available in Europe, is metoclopramide (Reglan). It stimulates gastric motility and hastens gastric emptying without affecting secretory activity. Metoclopramide's main pharmacologic property is a dopamine receptor antagonism. However, its effect is blocked by atropine (and narcotics); thus it is said to exert its functions by facilitating cholinergic transmission. It is used in anesthesia to promote gastric emptying and as an antiemetic agent, but its efficacy has not been firmly established. At any rate, it can be expected to promote gastric emptying prior to induction only in patients who have not received an anticholinergic or a narcotic.[79–81]

REFERENCES

1. Loewi, O.: Über humorale Übertragbarkeit der Herznerven Wirkung. Arch. Ges. Physiol., *189*:239, 1921.
2. Dale, H.H.: The action of certain esters and ethers of choline, and their relation to muscarine. J. Pharmacol Exp. Ther., *6*:147, 1914.
3. Koelle, G.B.: Neurohumoral transmission and the autonomic nervous system. *In* The Pharmacological Basis of Therapeutics. Edited by L.S. Goodman and A. Gilman. New York, Macmillan, 1975.
4. Haefely, W.: Electrophysiology of the adrenergic neuron. *In* Handbook of Experimental Pharmacology. Edited by H. Blaschko and E. Muscholl. Berlin, Springer-Verlag, 1972, Vol. 33.
5. Cannon, W.B.: Organization for physiological homeostasis. Physiol. Rev., *9*:399, 1929.
6. Higgins, C.B., Vatner, S.F., and Brunwald, E.: Parasympathetic control of the heart. Pharmacol. Rev., *25*:119, 1973.
7. Kent, K.M., et al.: Electrical stability of acutely ischemic myocardium: influences of heart rate and vagal stimulation. Circulation, *47*:291, 1973.
8. Kolman, B.S., Verrier, R.L., and Lown, B.: The effect of vagus nerve stimulation upon vulnerability of the canine ventricle. Circulation, *52*:578, 1975.
9. Kolman, B.S., Verrier, R.L., and Lown, B.: Effect of vagus nerve stimulation upon excitability of the canine ventricle. Am. J. Cardiol., *37*:1041, 1976.
10. Rabinowitz, S.H., Verrier, R.L., and Lown, B.: Muscarinic effects of vagosympathetic trunk stimulation on the repetitive extrasystole (RE) threshold. Circulation, *53*:622, 1976.
11. Lown, B., and Verrier, R.L.: Neural activity and ventricular fibrillation. N. Engl. J. Med., *294*:1165, 1976.
12. Cope, R.L.: Suppressive effect of carotid sinus on premature ventricular beats in certain instances. Am. J. Cardiol., *4*:314, 1959.
13. Lown, B., and Levine, S.A.: The carotid sinus: clinical value of its stimulation. Circulation, *23*:776, 1961.
14. Lorentzen, D.: Pacemaker-induced ventricular tachycardia: reversion to normal sinus rhythm by carotid sinus massage. J.A.M.A., *235*:282, 1976.
15. Waxman, M.B., et al.: Phenylephrine (Neosynephrine^R) terminated ventricular tachycardia. Circulation, *50*:656, 1974.
16. Weiss, T., Lattin, G.M., and Engelman, K.: Vagally mediated suppression of premature ventricular contractions in man. Am. Heart J., *89*:700, 1975.
17. Lown, B., et al.: Effect of a digitalis drug on ventricular premature beats (VPBs). N. Engl. J. Med., *296*:301, 1977.
18. Lown, B., et al.: Sleep and ventricular premature beats. Circulation, *48*:691, 1973.
19. Löffelholz, K., and Muscholl, E.: Muscarinic in-

hibition of the noradrenaline release evoked by postganglionic sympathetic nerve stimulation. Naunyn Schmiedebergs Arch. Pharmacol., 265:1, 1969.
20. Levy, M.N., and Blattberg, B.: Effect of vagal stimulation on the overflow of norepinephrine into the coronary sinus during cardiac sympathetic nerve stimulation in the dog. Circ. Res., 38:81, 1976.
21. Ehinger, B., Falck, B., and Sporrong, B.: Possible axo-axonal synapses between peripheral adrenergic and cholinergic nerve terminals. Z. Zellforsch., 107:508, 1970.
22. Kent, K.M., et al.: Cholinergic innervation of the canine and human ventricular conducting system: anatomic and electrophysiological correlation. Circulation, 50:948, 1974.
23. Kharkevich, D.A.: Ganglion-Blocking and Ganglion-Stimulating Agents. Oxford, Pergamon Press, 1967.
24. Flacke, W.E.: Drug therapy. Treatment of myasthenia gravis. N. Engl. J. Med., 288:27, 1973.
25. DeRoeth, A., Jr., et al.: Effect of phospholine iodide on blood cholinesterase levels of normal and glaucoma subjects. Am. J. Ophthalmol., 59:586, 1965.
26. Garfield, J.M., et al.: A pharmacological analysis of ganglionic actions of some general anesthetics. Anesthesiology, 29:79, 1968.
27. Trendelenburg, Y.: Some aspects of the pharmacology of autonomic ganglion cells. Ergebn. Physiol., 59:1, 1967.
28. Flacke, W.E., and Gillis, R.A.: Impulse transmission via nicotinic and muscarinic pathways in the stellate ganglion of the dog. J. Pharmacol. Exp. Ther., 163:266, 1968.
29. Innes, I.R., and Nickerson, M.: Atropine, scopolamine and related antimuscarinic drugs. In The Pharmacological Basis of Therapeutics. Edited by L.S. Goodman and A. Gilman. New York, Macmillan, 1975.
30. Eger, E.I., II: Atropine, scopolamine and related compounds. Anesthesiology, 23:365, 1962.
31. Andrews, I.C., and Belonsky, B.: Parasympatholytics. In Clinical Anesthesia. Pharmacology of Adjuvant Drugs. Vol. 10. Edited by H.L. Zander. Philadelphia, F.A. Davis, 1973.
32. Herxheimer, A.: A comparison of some atropine-like drugs in man, with particular reference to their end-organ specificity. Br. J. Pharmacol., 13:184, 1958.
33. Morton, H.J., and Thomas, E.T.: Effect of atropine on the heart rate. Lancet, 2:1313, 1958.
34. Gravenstein, J.S., Andersen, T.W., and DePadua, C.B.: Effects of atropine and scopolamine on the cardiovascular system in man. Anesthesiology, 25:123, 1964.
35. Hayes, A.H., Jr., and Katz, R.A.: Homatropine bradycardia in man. Clin. Pharmacol. Ther., 11:558, 1970.
36. Kottmeier, C.A., and Gravenstein, J.S.: The parasympathomimetic activity of atropine and atropine methylbromide. Anesthesiology, 29:1125, 1968.

37. Holt, A.T.: Premedication with atropine should not be routine. Lancet, 2:984, 1962.
38. Fabick, Y.S., and Smiler, B.G.: Is anticholinergic premedication necessary? Anesthesiology, 43:472, 1975.
39. Leighton, K.M., and Sanders, H.D.: Anticholinergic premedication. Can. Anaesth. Soc. J., 223:563, 1976.
40. Gravenstein, J.S., and Anton, A.H.: Premedication and drug interaction. Clin. Anesth., 3:199, 1969.
41. Annis, P., Landa, J., and Lichtiger, M.: Effects of atropine on velocity of tracheal mucus in anesthetized patients. Anesthesiology, 44:74, 1976.
42. Jones, R.E., Deutsch, S., and Turndorf, H.: Effects of atropine on cardiac rhythm in conscious and anesthetized man. Anesthesiology, 22:67, 1961.
43. Munchow, O.B., and Denson, J.S.: Modification by light cyclopropane and halothane anesthesia of the chronotropic effect of atropine in man. Anesth. Analg. (Cleve.), 44:782, 1965.
44. Bradshaw, E.G.: Dysrhythmia associated with oral surgery. Anaesthesia, 31:13, 1976.
45. Viby-Mogensen, J., et al.: Halothane anesthesia and suxamethonium I: The significance of preoperative atropine administration. Acta Anaesthesiol. Scand., 20:129, 1976.
46. Eikard, B., and Sorensen, B.: Arrhythmias during halothane anesthesia I.: The influence of atropine during induction with intubation. II. The influence of atropine. Acta Anaesthesiol. Scand., 20:296, 1976, and 21:245, 1977.
47. Carrow, D.J., et al.: Effects of large doses of intravenous atropine on heart rate and arterial pressure of anesthetized patients. Anesth. Analg. (Cleve.), 54:262, 1975.
48. Jacobson, E., and Adelman, M.H.: Electrocardiographic effects of intravenous administration of neostigmine and atropine during cyclopropane anesthesia. Anesthesiology, 15:407, 1954.
49. Fielder, D.L., et al.: Cardiovascular effects of atropine and neostigmine in man. Anesthesiology, 30:637, 1969.
50. MacIntosh, R.R.: Death following injection of neostigmine. Br. Med. J., 1:852, 1949.
51. Clutton-Brock, J.: Death following neostigmine. Br. Med. J., 1:1007, 1949.
52. Hill, M.: Death after neostigmine injection. Br. Med. J., 2:601, 1949.
53. Kemp, S.W., and Morton, H.J.V.: The effect of atropine and neostigmine on the pulse rates of anaeshetized patients. Anaesthesia, 17:170, 1962.
54. Katz, R.L., and Epstein, R.A.: The interaction of anesthetic agents and adrenergic drugs to produce cardiac arrhythmias. Anesthesiology, 29:763, 1968.
55. Kemp, S.W., and Morton, H.J.V.: Effect of atropine and neostigmine on the pulse rates of anesthetized patients. Anaesthesia, 17:170, 1962.
56. Baraka, A.: Safe reversal. 1. Atropine followed by neostigmine. An electrocardiographic study. 2. Atropine-neostigmine mixture. An electrocardiographic study. Br. J. Anaesth., 40:27 and 30, 1968.

57. Hannington-Kiff, J.G.: Timing of atropine and neostigmine in the reversal of muscle relaxants. Br. Med. J., 1:418, 1969.
58. Ovassapian, A.: Effect of administration of atropine and neostigmine in man. Anesth. Analg., 48:219, 1969.
59. Ramamurthy, S., Shaker, M.H., and Winnie, A.P.: Glycopyrrolate as a substitute for atropine in neostigmine reversal. Can. Anaesth. Soc. J., 19:399, 1972.
60. Ostheimer, G.W.: A comparison of glycopyrrolate and atropine during reversal of nondepolarizing neuromuscular block with neostigmine. Anesth. Analg. (Cleve.), 56:182, 1977.
61. Miller, R.D., et al.: Comparative times to peak effect and durations of action of neostigmine and pyridostigmine. Anesthesiology, 41:27, 1974.
62. Han, J., and Moe, G.K.: Nonuniform recovery of excitability in ventricular muscle. Circ. Res., 14:44, 1964.
63. Roco, A.G., and Vandam, L.D.: Changes in circulation consequent to manipulation during abdominal surgery. J.A.M.A., 164:14, 1957.
64. Knoebel, S.B., et al.: Atropine-induced cardioacceleration and myocardial blood flow in subjects with and without coronary artery disease. Am. J. Cardiol., 33:327, 1974.
65. Wilkins, J.L., et al.: Effects of neostigmine and atropine on motor activity of ileum, colon, and rectum of anaesthetized subjects. Br. Med. J., 1:793, 1970.
66. Schwartz, H., DeRoetth, A., Jr., and Papper, E.M.: Preanesthetic use of atropine and scopolamine in patient with glaucoma. J.A.M.A., 165:144, 1957.
67. Effects of systemic drugs with anticholinergic properties on glaucoma. Medical Letter, 16:28, 1974.
68. Feldberg, W.: Present views on the mode of action of acetylcholine in the central nervous system. Physiol. Rev., 25:596, 1945.
69. Snyder, S.H., et al.: Biochemical identification of the mammalian muscarinic cholinergic receptor. Fed. Proc., 34Z:1915, 1975.
70. Duvoisin, R.C., and Katz, R.L.: Reversal of central anticholinergic syndrome in man by physostigmine. J.A.M.A., 206:1963, 1968.
71. Granacher, R.P., and Baldessarini, R.J.: The usefulness of physostigmine in neurology and psychiatry. In Clinical Neuropharmacology. Edited by H.L. Klawans. New York, Raven Press, 1976.
71a. Longo, V.G.: Behavioral and electroencephalographic effects of atropine and related compounds. Pharmacol. Rev., 18:965, 1966.
72. Forrer, G.R., and Miller, J.J.: Atropine coma: a somatic therapy in psychiatry. Am. J. Psychiatry, 115:455, 1958.
73. Janson, P.A., Watt, B., and Hermos, J.A.: Success with physostigmine and failure with neostigmine in reversing toxicity. J.A.M.A., 237:2632, 1977.
74. Holzgrafe, R.E., Vondrell, J.J., and Mintz, S.M.: Reversal of postoperative reactions to scopolamine with physostigmine. Anesth. Analg. (Cleve.), 52:921, 1973.
74a. Greene, L.T.: Physostigmine treatment of anticholinergic depression in postoperative patients. Anesth. Analg., 50:222, 1971.
75. Larson, G.F., Hulbert, B.J., and Wingard, D.W.: Physostigmine reversal of diazepam-induced depression. Anesth. Analg. (Cleve.), 56:348, 1977.
76. DiLiberti, J., O'Brien, M.D., and Turner, T.: The use of physostigmine as an antidote in an accidental diazepam intoxication. J. Pediatr., 23:106, 1975.
77. El-Naggar, M., and El-Ganzouri, A.R.: Physostigmine. Its use in the management of postoperative mental aberrations. Anesthesiology Rev., 5:49, 1978.
78. Gillis, R.A., et al.: Actions of anticholinesterase agents upon ganglionic transmission in the dog. J. Pharmacol. Exp. Ther., 163:277, 1968.
79. Dundee, J.W., and Clarke, R.S.J.: The premedicant and antiemetic action of metoclopramide. Postgrad. Med. J., 48:34, 1973.
80. Schulze-Delrieu, K.: Metoclopramide. Gastroenterology 77:768, 1979.
81. Wyner, J., and Cohen, S.E.: Gastric volume in early pregnancy: Effect of metoclopramide. Anesthesiology 57:209, 1982.

|13|

HISTAMINE H₂ BLOCKERS

HENRY CASSON

CASE REPORT

Fine and Churchill[1] describe a 46-year-old man undergoing long-term hemodialysis. The patient required large doses of narcotics to control hip and leg pain. In June 1980 morphine sulfate, 10 mg each 3 hours for seven total doses was administered and caused no notable side effects. On September 9, 1980 oral administration of cimetidine 300 mg 3 times per day was started for treatment of a bleeding gastric ulcer. Four days later morphine sulfate, 15 mg each 4 hours, intramuscularly, was reinstituted for worsening hip pain. Shortly after the sixth such dose of morphine, the patient's respiratory rate decreased to 3/minute. This respiratory depression responded to naloxone 0.4 mg. Over the next 80 hours repeated episodes of muscular twitching and apnea required a total of 8 doses of naloxone.

Hemodialysis was performed twice during this period, with no immediate change in the clinical status of the patient. The patient recovered completely from this episode.

A month later cimetidine was restarted at the much lower dose of 150 mg, twice a day, prior to surgical revision of a leg stump. He received seven doses of pantopon (15 mg) (a mixture of opium alkaloids, about half as potent as morphine sulfate) every 3 to 6 hours preoperatively. After the last dose he became apneic, confused, and had diffuse muscle twitching. His symptoms responded to naloxone, of which he required four doses of 0.4 mg over the next 24 hours. He recovered fully. In commenting on this report, Fine and Churchill observed that the patient had severe side effects on two separate occasions with the same drug combination, and no side effects when either of the two drugs was given alone.

This case report, though incomplete in its detail, suggests that alterations in drug disposition by cimetidine may prove clinically significant.

Cimetidine is the first clinically successful competitive blocker of the histamine H₂ receptor. It has a substituted imidazole ring, with a marked structural similarity to histamine. Its success in the treatment of duodenal ulcer and peptic hyperchloridia disease has made it one of the most widely prescribed agents.[2] Its congener ranitidine[3] replaces the histamine-like imidazole ring with a furan structure. It is more potent, and appears to have fewer side effects, particularly fewer interactions with other drugs.

MODES OF INTERACTION[4]

Effects on Gastric pH

The decrease in gastric acidity could potentially alter the ionization of a weakly basic drug and decrease its uptake by the stomach mucosa. The only substance for which this mechanism has been demonstrated is ketoconazole,[5] an antibiotic. A weakly acidic substance might have increased uptake. This has been demonstrated for oral midazolam.[6] Ranitidine, by decreasing hydrochloric acid production, can raise gastric pH and share with cimetidine the ability to produce such effects on absorption of drugs.

Enzymatic Degradation of Drugs

This is the most important mechanism

of cimetidine-related drug interaction. Cimetidine binds to hepatic microsomal cytochrome P450. This enzyme is a mosaic of closely similar isoenzymes, with variable substrate specificities. Cimetidine, and to a far lesser extent ranitidine, binds to these enzymes and leads to their inhibition. Since the cytochrome P450 system is important in the degradation of many drugs, any inhibition may produce higher than predicted blood levels of the agent and hence toxicity. Drugs with predominant clearance by this mechanism and narrow therapeutic ranges are most likely to produce significant drug interaction.

Where toxicity is a result of a metabolic byproduct of the drug of interest, inhibition of metabolic breakdown has the potential to decrease toxicity. Studies in an animal model suggest that cimetidine, but not ranitidine, protects against halothane toxicity.

Liver Blood Flow

A drug subject to high clearance by the liver will show a great flow-dependent reduction of this process. It has been generally stated that total hepatic blood flow is significantly decreased by cimetidine or ranitidine,[8] although a recent review[4] questions this assumption. Drugs which would be expected to show decreased clearance by this mechanism include lidocaine, propranolol and morphine.

Interactions with Other Agents

Warfarin. A 25% decrease in clearance of this agent has led to clinically significant increases in the prothrombin time.[9]

Phenytoin. A decrease in the clearance of this agent resulted in increases of up to 33% in steady-state concentration, leading to toxic effects.[10]

Theophylline. Theophylline has a relatively low therapeutic ratio, and the institution of H$_2$ blocker therapy has produced toxic levels of the drug. The levels of this important drug are readily measurable, and therapy should be adjusted accordingly. Generally, decreases in dosage of ¼ or ⅓ are necessary in the presence of cimetidine.[11]

Benzodiazepines. Benzodiazepines which depend on hepatic microsomal enzymes for their degradation show an increase in plasma level after cimetidine treatment. This increases and prolongs sedation. The agents most commonly involved include diazepam and chlordiazepoxide. On the other hand oxazepam and lorozepam, which are glucuronated and excreted, are not affected.[12]

Morphine. Morphine is glucuronated in the liver, a pathway that is unaltered by cimetidine. Decreased liver blood flow may be the mechanism for the interaction described in the case report. The issue is somewhat obscured by the coexisting abnormalities, since cimetidine itself has CNS effects, and other disease states may alter the function of the blood-brain barrier.

Lidocaine. There have been reports suggesting[13] and denying[4] that lidocaine levels can be increased by concomitant cimetidine therapy.

Propranolol. There is a report of increased bradycardia following the combination of cimetidine and propranolol.[8]

To conclude this chapter, it would be well to summarize the differences between cimetidine and ranitidine. Ranitidine, unlike cimetidine, almost totally lacks the ability to bind to hepatic microsomal enzymes. In addition, it is more potent, and is used in lower doses. Interactions that occur by enzymatic inhibition have been almost nonexistent, and it is expected that this and other more effective congeners will supplant cimetidine. An injectable form of ranitidine is available.

REFERENCES

1. Fine, A., and Churchill, D.: (Letter) Canad. Med. Assoc. J., 124:1434, 1981.
2. Freston, J.W.: Cimetidine. Ann. Intern. Med., 97:573, 1982.
3. Zeldis, J.B., Friedman, L.S., and Isselbacher, K.J.: Ranitidine: A new H2 receptor antagonist. N. Engl. J. Med., 309:1368, 1983.

4. Powell, J.R., and Donn, K.H.: Histamine H2 antagonist drug interactions in perspective: Mechanistic concepts and clinical implications. Am. J. Med., 77:suppl 5B:57, 1984.
5. van der Meer, J.W.M., Keuning, J.J., et al.: The influence of gastric acidity on the bioavailability of ketoconazole. J. Antimicrob. Chemother., 6:552, 1980.
6. Elwood, R.J., Hildebrand, P.J., et al.: Influence of ranitidine on uptake of oral midazolam. Br. J. Anaesth., 55:241, 1983.
7. Plummer, J.L., Gower, A.J., et al.: Effects of cimetidine and ranitidine on halothane metabolism and hepatotoxicity in an animal model. Drug Metab. Dispos., 12:106, 1984.
8. Feely, J., Wilkinson, G.R., and Wood, A.J.J.: Reduction of liver blood flow and propranolol metabolism by cimetidine. N. Engl. J. Med., 304:692, 1981.
9. Silver, B.A., and Bell, W.R.: Cimetidine potentiation of the hypoprothrombinemic effect of warfarin. Ann. Intern. Med., 90:348, 1979.
10. Hetzel, D.J., Bochner, F., et al.: Cimetidine interaction with phenytoin. Br. Med. J., 282:1512, 1981.
11. Lofgren, R.P., and Gilbertson, R.A.: Cimetidine and theophylline. Ann. Intern. Med., 96:378, 1982.
12. Klotz, U., and Reimann, I.: Delayed clearance of diazepam due to cimetidine. N. Engl. J. Med., 302:1012, 1980.
13. Feely, J., Wilkinson, G.R., McAllister, C.V., et al.: Increased toxicity and reduced clearance of lignocaine by cimetidine. Ann. Intern. Med., 96:592, 1982.

|14|

DIGITALIS

JOHN L. ATLEE, III and BEN F. RUSY

Digitalis, one of the most commonly prescribed drugs in the United States, is important from both therapeutic and toxicologic viewpoints.[1] Digoxin is the most commonly used preparation, probably because of its short plasma half-life of 31 hours (oral) and 33 hours (intravenous), thus offering the advantage of achieving optimal digitalization and in managing suspected toxicity.[2] Digitoxin, which has a plasma half-life of 5 to 7 days, is usually only used for maintenance digitalization.

The digitalis glycosides have one of the lowest therapeutic indices in the pharmacopeia. Approximately 20% of the patients who take digitalis exhibit some type of toxic reaction.[3,4] The principal therapeutic effect of digitalis is an increase in contractile performance (positive inotropy) in patients with cardiac failure. Digitalis is also used to delay conduction (negative dromotropy) through the atrioventricular node and thus to decrease ventricular rate in patients with atrial flutter or fibrillation. The positive inotropic effect of digitalis is directly proportional to the dose used; that is, its dose response is linear.[5] A dose that borders on toxicity, however, may be necessary to induce cardiac slowing. Furthermore, the therapeutic ratio is dependent on the preexisting autonomic tone.[5]

The response to digitalis is influenced by a multiplicity of factors such as the nature and severity of the underlying heart disease, the patient's age, the status of renal function and electrolyte balance, the presence of noncardiac disease, and the sensitivity to other drugs taken concomitantly.[5a] The circumstances of anesthesia and surgery may precipitate digitalis toxicity in an otherwise normally digitalized patient or in a patient who is undergoing digitalization. Two case reports, based both on documented interactions and on our own experience, illustrate interactions that are likely to be significant to the practicing anesthesiologist.

CASE REPORT

A 68-year-old, 66-kg man with intermittent claudication was scheduled for an aortofemoral bypass operation. He had a 20-year history of essential hypertension. Two years before admission he had been admitted to another hospital for treatment of congestive heart failure and had responded promptly to digitalis and diuretics. Present therapy included digoxin 0.25 mg q.d. and hydrochlorothiazide 25 mg b.i.d. Laboratory values on admission were normal except: BUN (blood urea nitrogen) = 22 mg/dl, creatinine = 1.8 mg/dl, Na = 132 mEq/L, K = 3.4 mEq/L, Cl = 92 mEq/L. The serum digoxin level was 2.4 ng/ml. The ECG showed sinus rhythm (64 beats/min) and signs of left ventricular hypertrophy. Occasional unifocal premature ventricular beats were also noted. The chest roentgenogram showed mild cardiac enlargement, but was otherwise normal. Blood pressure readings before surgery had ranged from 135 to 160 mm Hg systolic and 86 to 105 mm Hg diastolic.

Preanesthetic medication consisted of scopolamine (hyoscine), 0.43 mg, and morphine, 8 mg IM (intramuscularly). The patient's blood pressure was 156/88 mm Hg and the pulse rate 64 beats/min on arrival in the operating room. Lines were inserted for monitoring arterial (radial artery) and central venous (internal jugular) pressure. While the patient breathed oxygen, 100%, the induction of anesthesia was accomplished with intravenous morphine sulfate, 20 mg, diazepam, 10 mg, and thiopental, 250 mg. Succinylcholine, 100 mg IV was used to facilitate laryngoscopy for the topical application of 4% lidocaine (160 mg) to the trachea and for endotracheal intubation. During this procedure, the patient's blood pressure rose to 180/110 mm Hg, and there were frequent multifocal ventricular premature beats. The elevated blood pressure and dysrhythmias responded to thiopental (100 mg) and sodium nitroprusside. After a paralyzing dose of pancuronium, 6.5 mg, the patient's ventilation was controlled with nitrous oxide-oxygen (F_{IO_2} = 0.40). Minute volume was 8.2 liters. An additional 10 mg of morphine was given prior to the surgical incision, which was made approximately 20 minutes following the institution of controlled ventilation. The patient's blood pressure was 140/90 mm Hg and his pulse rate was 84 beats/min immediately prior to the incision.

Soon after the surgical incision, the patient's blood pressure rose to 160/100 mm Hg and frequent multifocal ventricular premature beats were noted, followed by ventricular tri- and quadrigeminy. While the elevated pressure responded to sodium nitroprusside, the ventricular dysrhythmias failed to respond to two intravenous boluses of lidocaine (100 mg). Ventilation with 100% oxygen was begun, with no improvement in the dysrhythmia. Arterial blood gas and electrolyte determinations, performed shortly after the dysrhythmias first appeared, revealed the following: pH = 7.46, P_{O_2} = 161 mm Hg, P_{CO_2} = 25 mm Hg, Na = 134 mEq/L, and K = 2.8 mEq/L. Minute ventilation was immediately reduced to 5.6 L/min. Potassium chloride (20 mEq) and phenytoin (diphenylhydantoin) (100 mg, in divided doses) were then administered intravenously. Over the next 15 minutes, the premature beats became less numerous, then unifocal in origin, and finally disappeared. Nitrous oxide was reinstituted (F_{IO_2} = 0.40), and the surgeons continued with the operation. Arterial blood-gas analysis 30 minutes later showed: pH = 7.41, P_{O_2} = 138 mm Hg, P_{CO_2} = 38 mm Hg, Na = 132 mEq/L, and K = 3.7 mEq/L. The remainder of the anesthetic course was uneventful.

CASE REPORT

A 74-year-old man was scheduled for a total hip arthroplasty. Significant findings on admission included a long history of hypertension complicated two years prior to admission by congestive heart failure, which had been treated with digitalis and diuretics. The patient had remained symptom-free until nine months prior to admission, when he experienced palpitations caused by atrial fibrillation, which was electrically converted to sinus rhythm. Prophylactic therapy with quinidine was instituted to reduce the chances of recurrence of the dysrhythmia.

During the initial preoperative hospital evaluation five days before surgery, the patient again experienced atrial fibrillation. Because of palpitations and the impending operation, it was decided to convert the dysrhythmia electrically and to increase the quinidine dose (200 to 300 mg q.i.d.). These measures restored sinus rhythm. The patient was also taking digoxin (0.25 mg qd) and hydrochlorothiazide (25 mg b.i.d.). The day before the operation, the serum electrolytes were Na = 135 mEq/L and K = 3.6 mEq/L. The patient's serum digoxin level on the second day of hospitalization was 1.6 ng/ml. On the morning of the operation, the ECG showed sinus rhythm (rate = 72 beats/min) with infrequent (<2/min) monofocal premature ventricular beats. Other laboratory values were within normal limits.

Anesthesia was induced, while the patient breathed oxygen, with thiopental (total dose 350 mg IV) and succinylcholine (60 mg IV), and maintained with nitrous oxide (F_{IO_2} = 0.5) and halothane (0.5–1.5 inspired). Pancuronium, 3 mg, was used for muscle relaxation. Ventilation was controlled ($\dot{V}_E$ = 8.5 L/min).

The induction of anesthesia and the first hour of the operation were uneventful except for occasional (<6/min) premature ventricular beats. These gradually increased in frequency as the operation progressed, and by approximately two hours into the procedure the patient showed ventricular bigeminy (blood pressure 130/90 mm Hg). Digoxin toxicity was considered to be a cause, and a blood sample was drawn for a digoxin serum level determination (this was later reported as 2.6 ng/ml). An arterial blood sample showed pH = 7.44, P_{O_2} = 142 mm Hg, P_{CO_2} = 30 mm Hg, Na = 136 mEq/L, and K = 3.2 mEq/L. Initial therapy consisted of the reduction of the minute volume of ventilation (8.5 to 6.0 L/min), and the administration of potassium chloride (30 mEq) over the next 40 minutes. During this time, the ventricular bigeminy was resolved and the ventricular premature beats became less numerous. By the end of the operation (3½ hours duration), their frequency was between six and eight beats/min. Arterial blood-gas values one hour after the initiation of therapy showed pH = 7.38, P_{O_2} = 128 mm Hg, P_{CO_2} = 40 mm Hg, Na = 136 mEq/L, and K = 4.1 mEq/L. The subsequent anesthetic and operative course was uneventful. After the operation, quinidine was continued, but the maintenance digoxin dose was reduced to 0.125 mg q.d. The patient experienced no further episodes of atrial fibrillation during his 2½-week hospital stay.

These case reports illustrate both problems and solutions for interactions involving digitalis, interactions that are likely to be encountered by anesthetists, including (1) potentiation of digitalis toxicity by *hypokalemia*, (2) *impaired renal function*, which reduces the rate at which digoxin is cleared from the plasma, (3) interactions between quinidine, as well as other drugs, and digoxin that promote toxicity, and (4) the beneficial actions of *phenytoin (diphenylhydantoin)* and *potassium chloride* in reversing ventricular dysrhythmias caused by digitalis intoxication, and (5) the use of vasodilators to promote the renal excretion of digoxin.

Hypokalemia is a common cause of digitalis intoxication in otherwise normally digitalized patients. Hypokalemia is often secondary to the potassium-wasting effects of potent diuretics, including the benzothiadiazines, bumetanide furosemide, and ethacrynic acid, which are commonly administered along with digitalis. Adequate potassium replacement or the use of potassium-sparing agents (spironolactone, triamterene, or the amiloride-hydrochlorthiazide combination) in patients who take potent diuretics is particularly important to digitalized patients.[6] Magnesium deficiency attendant to diuretic-induced losses of this cation may also predispose a patient to digitalis intoxication.[6] The actual mechanism for diuretic-induced digitalis intoxication is the probable increase in myocardial binding of the digitalis glycosides in the presence of hypokalemia, and the possible interference with membrane adenosinetriphosphatase (ATP-ase—dependent on magnesium ions, and activated by sodium and potassium ions) in cases of hypomagnesemia.[7,8] Although the serum levels of potassium prior to the operations in the case reports (3.4 mEq/L in the first, and 3.6 mEq/L in the second case) were in the borderline hypokalemic range, these levels were acutely lowered to definite hypokalemic status (2.8 and 3.2 mEq/L respectively) during surgery. Acute hypokalemia in these patients was most likely related to hyperventilation: the resulting respiratory alkalosis caused a shift in potassium into the cell in exchange for hydrogen ion. Edwards et al. noted approximately 0.5 mEq/L decrements in serum potassium level for every 10 mm Hg decrease in arterial P_{CO_2} in mechanically hyperventilated patients during anesthesia.[9] Metabolic alkalosis can also cause hypokalemia secondary to hydrogen ion shifts.

Impaired renal function is a major cause of digitalis intoxication with short-acting digitalis glycosides (ouabain, deslanoside, digoxin) that depend on renal excretion for their elimination.[7] The longer-acting preparations, digitoxin and digitalis leaf, are metabolized in the liver, while their less active metabolites are eliminated by renal excretion.[7] Impaired renal function probably was partly responsible for the preoperative borderline toxic serum digoxin level of 2.5 ng/ml in the first patient.[10] The mildly elevated BUN and creatinine levels in this patient suggest impaired renal function. Arteriosclerosis or atherosclerosis, long-standing hypertension, and the patient's age may have been responsible for the diminished renal function. Although the digoxin serum level prior to operation was only on the borderline of toxicity, and there were no ECG manifestations, anorexia, nausea or vomiting, the hypokalemia secondary to mechanical hyperventilation and diuretic therapy probably precipitated acute cardiovascular toxicity (ventricular dysrhythmias) during the course of the operation.

Quinidine administered to patients receiving digoxin may lead to increased and potentially toxic digoxin concentrations.[1,11,11a,11b] The same interaction probably occurs with digitoxin.[11c] Quinine and verapamil can also increase digoxin levels; disopyramide and procainamide do not.[11d] Several mechanisms for the digoxin-quinidine interaction have been suggested, including (1) reduced renal clearance of digoxin, (2) increased digoxin bioavailability due to increased absorption, (3) reduction in the apparent volume of distribution for digoxin, and (4) displacement of digoxin from tissue binding sites, particularly skeletal muscle.[5a,11e] In addition to quinidine and certain other antidysrhythmic agents, diazepam may also increase digoxin levels by decreasing its renal excretion, possibly secondary to increased plasma protein binding.[11f] Diazepam was used as an anesthetic adjunct in our first case and may have contributed, with hypokalemia, to digitalis toxicity and the precipitation of ventricular dysrhythmias. The quinidine-digitalis and diazepam-digitalis interaction, as well as the analogous interaction between digitalis and other similarly metabolized benzodiazepines, deserves further study in view of the fact that diazepam is often used as a preanesthetic medicant or as an adjunct to anesthesia.

Phenytoin is almost exclusively for the specific treatment for digitalis-induced ventricular dysrhythmias, as is *potassium chloride* for digitalis toxicity related to hypokalemia.[12,14] Whereas lidocaine may also be effective in treating ventricular dysrhythmias due to digitalis, it failed in the first case report patient.[12-14] Thus phenytoin and potassium chloride were administered while ventilation was decreased. It is impossible to decide which was most effective. Each was indicated under the circumstances, since ventricular tachycardia and/or fibrillation could have resulted had the dysrhythmias remained untreated. The suggested dose of phenytoin is 100 mg intravenously every 5 minutes until a therapeutic response is observed or until adverse effects are encountered.[1] The rate of intravenous injection should not exceed 50 mg/min. Usually about 700 mg is required; rarely are doses greater than 1000 mg needed.[1] For intravenous lidocaine, a loading dose of 2 to 3 mg/kg followed by a maintenance infusion of 20 to 30 µg/kg/minute (1.0 g lidocaine in 250 ml of normal saline solution), or 100 mg every 3 to 5 minutes are used.[13]

Vasodilator therapy with sodium nitroprusside or hydralazine can allegedly increase the renal clearance of digoxin by 50% in patients with chronic congestive heart failure.[11g] While it is unlikely that short-term intensive vasodilator therapy, achieved with sodium nitroprusside in our first case report, could have lowered significantly a borderline elevated digoxin level, it is possible that prolonged nitroprusside administration is beneficial. This finding may be very important in the postoperative patient, since prolonged vasodilator therapy may increase the required maintenance dose of digoxin.

PHARMACOLOGY OF DIGITALIS

Inotropic Effect: Mechanism of Action

Cardiac glycosides act directly on the heart to increase the force of contraction. Although the exact mechanism is unknown, the most likely subcellular system involved is Na^+, K^+-ATPase, an enzymatic ion transport system located in the cardiac cell membrane and often referred to as the sodium pump. Evidence for the involvement of this system is that Na^+, K^+-ATPase is inhibited by low concentrations of digitalis, whereas other subcellular systems are either not affected, or are affected only by high concentrations.[15] The rationale for this proposed mechanism of action is based on the premise that the inhibition of sodium pump activity by digitalis ultimately increases the concentration of myoplasmic ionized calcium, which is, in turn, responsible for the increase in the force of myocardial contraction.[16-22]

During the depolarization of a cardiac contractile cell, calcium ions flow inward across the cell membrane. The associated movement of charge produces a current (the slow inward calcium current) that accounts for the plateau of the cardiac action potential.[23,24] The amount of calcium that enters the cell in this way during each systole is not sufficient to activate contraction appreciably, but it does trigger the release of additional Ca^{++} from intracellular storage sites and could ultimately flood the cell with calcium, were it not for the existence of a mechanism for the extrusion of this divalent ion.[21,23,25,34] The extrusion mechanism involves a carrier-mediated exchange of 1 Ca^{++} for 2 Na^+; these ions compete for carrier sites on both sides of the membrane. Energy for outward calcium transport comes presumably from the coupled inward transport of Na^+ that flows down a concentration gradient provided originally by Na^+,K^+-ATPase sodium pump activity. Since calcium and sodium compete with one another for transport, any intervention that increases intracellular Na^+ causes fewer sites to be occupied by Ca^{++} for outward transport. Consequently, the myoplasmic concentrations of Ca^{++} increase until the ion can again compete successfully for enough transport sites to insure that its outward transport matches the inward flux. The increase in myoplasmic Ca^{++} concentration thus achieved leads to the sequestration of increased amounts of ion in the sarcoplasmic reticulum. This leads to an increased release of Ca^{++} from transport sites during depolarization and to an increase in contractile power. By inhibiting the sodium pump, digitalis induces an accumulation of Na^+ in the myocardial cell which will make more Ca^{++} available for contraction. This induces a sustained positive inotropic effect.[16,17,26,27]

Consideration of the process of cardiac contraction and of the steps leading to its activation reveals that there are numerous ways to produce a positive inotropic effect. Some of the mechanisms proposed, including the one described for digitalis, are outlined in Table 14-1.

Cardiac Electrophysiologic Effects

The normal transmembrane resting potential of cardiac cells (-80 to -90 mV intracellular with respect to extracellular) depends on sodium and potassium gradients that in turn depend on the integrity of the sodium-potassium activated pump mechanism (Na^+, K^+-ATPase) previously discussed. There is general agreement that the toxic effects of digitalis on the generation and conduction of cardiac impulses result from inhibition of the pump mechanism, although the mechanisms for the therapeutic and inotropic effects of digitalis are not fully understood.[1,14] Inhibition of the Na^+,K^+-ATPase pump mechanism leads to the accumulation of intracellular sodium and to a corresponding reduction in intracellular potassium.[1] This direct effect of digitalis on the heart is complicated by indirect or neurally mediated effects (see the section of this chapter entitled "Autonomic Actions").[1]

The electrical excitability of both the atrium and the ventricle in the intact dog heart is increased by lower doses of digitalis, but decreased by higher doses.[1,32] The increased excitability is largely due to the decreased diastolic intracellular negativity.[1] The atrium may be rendered inexcitable by doses that do not prevent propagated idioventricular impulses, although the specialized atrial conducting pathways are believed to be more resistant to such impulses than atrial muscle.[1] Purkinje fibers gradually become inexcitable at higher concentrations of digitalis, but ventricular muscle fibers are more resistant.[1] Thus resistance to digitalis-induced excitability increases progressively from the atria to the ventricles.[1] Similarly, conduction velocity within the atria and ventricles is increased by low, and decreased by toxic, doses of digitalis. Conduction through the atrioventricular node is slowed by both vagal and extravagal actions of digitalis (see "Autonomic Actions").[1,33,34]

Digitalis exerts different effects on the refractory periods of the various cardiac tissues.[1] It shortens the atrial refractory period and prolongs the functional refractory period of the atrioventricular node under conditions that permit reflex vagal activity. In the absence of vagal activity, digitalis prolongs the atrial refractory period and the magnitude of increase in nodal refractoriness is reduced. Digitalis shortens the ventricular refractory period (apparent in man as a reduced Q-T interval). This shortening effect is independent of vagal innervation.

The effects of digitalis on automaticity and on the ability of some cardiac cells to

Table 14–1
Summary of Mechanisms for Positive Inotropy

Subcellular Component	Proposed Mechanism for Positive Inotropy	Drugs Inducing Effect
1. Troponin	CAMP*, protein kinase-induced phosphorylation. Increased Ca++ affinity[28,29]	catecholamines xanthines
2. Myosin light chains	Phosphorylation[30]	
3. Sarcoplasmic reticulum	CAMP, protein kinase-induced phosphorylation. Increased storage and release of Ca++ [27]	catecholamines xanthines
4. Sarcolemma	(a) CAMP, protein kinase-induced phosphorylation.[27] Increased Ca++ influx (slow inward current)[23]	catecholamines xanthines
	(b) Non-CAMP dependent increased Ca++ influx[31]	positive rate staircase (treppe)
	(c) Na+, K+-ATPase inhibition[17]	digitalis glycosides

*Cyclic adenosinemonophosphate

undergo spontaneous depolarization are complex because it appears that two forms of automaticity are involved.[1,18–20] The first and better understood of the two mechanisms, namely spontaneous diastolic (phase 4) depolarization, is enhanced by digitalis at low extracellular concentrations of potassium (<4.0 mEq/L), especially in the ventricles.[1] The second and more recently described mechanism, namely delayed afterdepolarizations, is seen at higher extracellular potassium concentrations (> 4.0 mEq/L).[1] If these reach threshold, a spontaneous action potential is generated. Delayed afterpotentials are also a toxic manifestation of digitalis and, under these circumstances, they are enhanced by low levels of potassium and high levels of calcium.[35–37] At present, the clinical differentiation between these two forms of automaticity is often impossible.

These two mechanisms of automaticity are described in more detail in Chapter 12. Of particular interest to anesthesiologists is the ability of halothane to antagonize digitalis-enhanced phase 4 automaticity.[38] Cyclopropane enhances whereas pentobarbital has little effect on this form of automaticity.[38] Fentanyl, droperidol, ketamine, diethyl ether, methoxyflurane, enflurane, and, to a lesser extent, fluroxene and isoflurane also protect against digitalis-enhanced phase 4 automaticity.[39,40] The effects of anesthetics on automaticity due to delayed afterpotentials have not been described. Toxic levels of digitalis may cause dysrhythmias by their effects on both automaticity and conduction.[1] In addition to actual heart block, alterations in conduction or refractoriness are also required to bring about dysrhythmias caused by reentry of excitation.[41]

Autonomic Actions

Three autonomic actions of digitalis have been documented in animal studies: vagomimetic actions; sensitization of baroreceptors; and, in large doses, sympathetic activation.[42] Therapeutic doses of digitalis enhance vagal tone, and, as a result, slow the sinus rate, slow atrioventricular conduction, decrease atrial ectopic pacemaker automaticity, and decrease the refractory period of atrial muscle.[42] Sensitization of the carotid baroreceptors by digitalis has several important therapeutic consequences:[43] (1) it may explain in part the vagomimetic actions of digitalis as outlined previously; (2) the decrease in cardiac sympathetic tone resulting from baroreceptor activation might contribute to the ability of digitalis to convert paroxysmal supraventricular tachycardias to sinus rhythm; and (3) it may explain the antidysrhythmic effect of therapeutic levels of digitalis in patients with ventricular dysrhythmias that are due in part to enhanced sympathetic tone.[42] The sympathomimetic action of digitalis is understood less fully.[42,44] Low doses inhibit sympathetic discharge because of baroreceptor sensitization.[42] In animal studies, however, large doses of digitalis excite the central nervous system and result in enhanced sympathetic tone and cardiac dysrhythmias.[42,45,46] The central stimulating effects of large doses of digitalis are not confined to the cardiac sympathetic nerves, but can be detected also in peripheral sympathetic and motor phrenic nerves.[42] The autonomic effects of digitalis have important implications for anesthesiologists. They are poorly understood, however, owing to the simultaneous use of many other drugs that also affect autonomic function.

Pharmacokinetics

The availability of reliable assays for measuring the level of digitalis in biologic fluids has contributed greatly to our understanding of the pharmacokinetics of the digitalis glycosides.[2,47–49] This knowledge is clinically valuable, as it enables the physician to manage digitalized patients more effectively and decreases the frequency of digitalis intoxication.

Digoxin, when given daily without an initial loading dose, accumulates until a steady state is reached within five to seven days.[50,51] This is due to a pattern of drug elimination that is characterized by the excretion of a percentage of the daily amount of the body stores instead of the excretion of a constant amount each day.[52] In patients with normal renal function, one-third of the total accumulated dose of digoxin is excreted daily.[52] Thus if 0.25 mg is absorbed daily, and one-third of this amount is excreted, the total accumulated dose after 24 hours will be 0.17 mg (0.28 mg at 2 days, 0.35 mg at 3 days). After 7 days, an approximate steady-state level (0.47 mg) will be reached, since the amounts of drug absorbed and excreted nearly balance each other. This is reflected by a plateau in the serum digoxin levels.

When the administration of digoxin is discontinued, the serum level declines as a function of its serum half-life (digoxin = 31 to 33 hours, digitoxin = 5 to 7 days).[2] The relation between serum half-life and steady-state drug accumulation in the body is: three half-lives = 90%, and five half-lives = 99% accumulation; thus approximately 7 days (digoxin) and 2 to 3 weeks (digitoxin) are required to achieve a plateau effect.[52]

The daily fluctuation between maximum and minimum serum levels depends also on the half-life of the drug used.[52] For example, if digoxin is given once daily, the variation will be approximately 33%; if given twice daily, it will be approximately 16%. For digitoxin given once daily, there will be a 10% variation in serum levels. This consideration is of practical importance when high doses of digitalis are required to control dysrhythmias (e.g., atrial fibrillation with cardiac decompensation).[52] Divided daily doses of digoxin allow one to achieve the high serum levels necessary to obtain the desired therapeutic effect and avoid toxicity. Little is gained, however, by administering digitoxin twice daily.

When a loading dose of digoxin is used for rapid digitalization, as is frequently the case in anesthetic practice for patients with heart failure or with supraventricular tachydysrhythmias, there is a greater risk of associated toxicity.[52,53] This risk is avoided if the loading dose is selected on the basis of the anticipated maintenance dose, and if it is given in divided doses.[52] Generally, the loading dose in patients with normal kidney function should be three times the anticipated maintenance dose.[52] Thus if the estimated maintenance digoxin dose is 0.25 mg daily, 0.75 mg given in divided doses during the first 24 hours will result in an accumulated body dose of 0.5 mg (33% excreted in the first 24 hours). This is approximately the same dose as that which accumulates in one week if 0.25 mg is given on a daily basis, as discussed. If 1.5 mg in divided doses is selected as the initial loading dose, 1.0 mg will accumulate by the end of 24 hours. If this is followed by 0.25-mg maintenance doses daily, the accumulated body dose will gradually be reduced by 50% to the steady-state level of 0.5 mg. We usually digitalize patients acutely in the operating room by administering digoxin, 0.5 mg intravenously, followed in eight hours by an additional 0.5 mg intravenously. An additional 0.25 to 0.50 mg can be given at 16 hours if required.

The serum half-lives for digoxin administered orally or intravenously are similar, but the serum levels reach a plateau sooner (2 to 4 as opposed to 5 to 6 hours) following intravenous administration.[2,48,49] Following intramuscular administration, the digoxin serum half-life is 38 hours; plateau serum levels are achieved in 10 to 12 hours.[2,48,49] The intramuscular route offers no advantage over other routes for achieving digitalization. We suspect that this is mainly due to the unpredictability of absorption following intramuscular injections.

The major determinant of the maintenance dose of digoxin and ouabain, serum half-life 21 hours,[7] is renal function.[52] Digoxin excretion is linearly related to glomerular filtration or creatinine clearance.[6,54] Jelliffe suggests that a reasonable approximation of the percentage of daily loss of digoxin is:[55]

$$\frac{\text{creatinine clearance (ml/min)}}{5} + 14$$

Since this value may not be readily available, an estimate based on the serum creatinine level (expressed as C) can be made:[55]

$$\text{creatinine clearance (men)} = \frac{100}{\text{serum creatinine (mg/100 ml)}} - 12$$

$$\text{creatinine clearance (women)} = \frac{80}{\text{serum creatinine (mg/100 ml)}} - 7$$

These expressions can be combined thus:[6]

$$\% \text{ daily loss (men)} = 11.6 + \frac{20}{C} \qquad \% \text{ daily loss (women)} = 12.6 + \frac{16}{C}$$

The rate of accumulation of digoxin in the body depends on the excretion of a certain percentage of the total body stores daily, which can be calculated as suggested, for patients with impaired renal function. Thus a man with a serum creatinine level of 2.4 mg/100 ml can be expected to excrete only 20% of his daily dose of digoxin. Using calculations similar to those used earlier for the 33% excretion of a 0.25-mg maintenance dose of digoxin, it can be determined that a steady-state level for accumulated digoxin (0.95 mg) will not be reached for 15 days. The digoxin serum half-life (and total accumulated dose) will approximately double as a result of impaired renal excretion. The serum half-life will increase to a maximum of 4.4 days in the absence of renal function.[6] A suggested rule of thumb is that the dose of digoxin should be reduced by 50% when the serum creatinine level is in the range of 3 to 5 mg/100 ml and by 75% in the absence of renal function.[52]

The frequent observation that digoxin is poorly tolerated in older patients is related both to reduced glomerular filtration with advancing age and to a decrease in muscle mass.[52,56] The major body store of digoxin is skeletal muscle, and a decrease in this reservoir results in increased serum and myocardial levels of the drug.[52] Little digoxin is accumulated in fat; therefore, the determinant of digoxin dose is lean body mass rather than total body weight.[7,52,57]

Toxicology and Indications for Obtaining Serum Levels

Cardiac toxicity can manifest itself by almost any rhythm of conduction disturbance.[1,14] There is little evidence that toxic amounts of digitalis have a direct, deleterious effect on the mechanical activity of the heart.[1] Extrasystoles, whether of ventricular or of atrial origin, are probably the most common. Ventricular extrasystoles frequently appear as coupled beats (bigeminy, trigeminy), but are not specific for digitalis.[1] Digitalis can cause marked sinus bradycardia and also induce complete SA block, both of which are more likely to occur in patients with preexisting sinus node disease.[1] Atrial dysrhythmias, including extrasystoles and paroxysmal and nonparoxysmal atrial tachycardias, can be induced by enhanced spontaneous phase 4 automaticity, delayed afterdepolarizations, or re-entry of excitation.[1] Paroxysmal atrial tachycardia with heart block is considered to be dangerous.[58,59] Digitalis toxicity at the AV junction manifests itself by the high level of the block and by the appearance of AV junctional dysrhythmias. The most typical disturbances appear as either escape beats or a nonparoxysmal AV junctional tachycardia.[1] While this latter dysrhythmia is almost always caused by digitalis, it may also be due to acute inferior wall infarction or carditis.[1] The development of AV block may be in part due to the indirect (vagal) effects of digitalis (hence, it can be occasionally reversed by atropine) or to a direct effect of digitalis on the AV node.[1] Ventricular tachycardia, which is frequently preceded by ventricular extrasystoles and which may lead to ventricular fibrillation, calls for the immediate cessation of digitalis therapy. There are no unequivocal electrocardiographic features that can distinguish dysrhythmias due to digitalis from those due to other causes.[14] Dysrhythmias that combine the features of increased automaticity of ectopic pacemakers with conduction defects suggest digitalis toxicity.[14] The treatment of digitalis-induced dysrhythmias includes the withholding of digitalis and the correction of associated factors (for example, hypokalemia related to diuretics or to other causes). Potassium chloride administered intravenously to produce a serum level close to the upper limits of the normal range may suppress digitalis-caused dysrhythmias.[1] Phenytoin, as discussed above, is often effective in treating both ventricular and supraventricular tachycardias caused by digitalis.[1,12-14] Lidocaine suppresses ventricular tachycardia, but is less effective than phenytoin against supraventricular dysrhythmias.[1] Although propranolol (1 to 3 mg IV) is effective in treating extrasystoles and tachycardia of both ventricular and supraventricular origin, its tendency to prolong nodal conduction limits its usefulness in the presence of atrioventricular block.[1] Electrical countershock should not be used to convert digitalis-induced dysrhythmias, since it may precipitate ventricular fibrillation.[1]

Other manifestations of digitalis toxicity include gastrointestinal and central nervous system effects.[1,14] Anorexia is often an early manifestation of toxicity, and was significantly correlated with serum glycoside levels in a prospective study.[60] Anorexia usually precedes nausea and vomiting, but vomiting may occur first, especially when large doses of digitalis are given rapidly.[1] Diarrhea and abdominal discomfort or pain may also be symptoms of toxicity.[1] In some cases, it may be difficult to relate gastrointestinal symptoms to digitalis since these symptoms may also be caused by cardiac failure or associated illnesses.[14] Central nervous system effects include headache, fatigue, malaise, drowsiness, neuralgic pain, disorientation, aphasia, confusion, delirium, hallucinations and convulsions.[1,14] Visual symptoms are not infrequent, and include scotomata, flickering, halos, and alterations in color perception.[1,14] These symptoms, when noted during the preanesthetic visit, should be considered valid evidence of digitalis toxicity.

A determination of digitalis level in the serum is necessary whenever there is a suspicion of digitalis toxicity or to determine the degree of digitalization.[10] An accurate estimate of the myocardial level of digoxin can be made only in the presence of a steady-state level of the drug (i.e., intake matches excretion).[10,61] The fundamental question that needs to be answered at first is whether the patient is taking digitalis. An affirmative reply to this question justifies the determination of its serum level irrespective of the presence of toxicity.[10] Each laboratory should establish its own limits of confidence and normal values for serum levels of digoxin. Levels between 0.5 and 2.5 ng/ml are usually considered to be therapeutic and those above 3.0 ng/ml to be definitely toxic, although there may be some overlap between 2.0 and 3.0 ng/ml.[10] Compared with adults, infants and children tolerate higher levels of digitalis without signs of toxicity; accordingly, the normal values for this age group should probably be revised upward about 1 ng/ml.[10] Whereas the determination of serum digitalis levels may be helpful in the management of toxicity, the diagnosis of toxicity is always based on clinical criteria, owing to the range of individual variation.[62] High serum levels of digoxin without a toxic reaction are often observed in atrial dysrhythmias (which can require large doses to control the ventricular response) and in renal failure with hyperkalemia.[10] Normal or low serum levels with a toxic reaction are common with hypokalemia, hypomagnesemia, recent myocardial infarction, myxedema, hypoxia, and in the presence of other radioisotopes that interfere with the digoxin assay.[10] Reduced gastrointestinal absorption of digoxin may require the administration of large oral doses to maintain optimal digitalization.[10] This may be the case with rapid transit syndromes, hyperthyroidism, intestinal malabsorption, or the concurrent administration of cholestyramine, antacids, or kaolin with pectin.[10]

FACTORS THAT AFFECT DIGITALIS TOXICITY

Some factors have already been alluded to or discussed in the preceding two sections. However, other factors that affect digitalis toxicity are presented in alphabetical order for the convenience of the reader.

Age. Infants and children have an increased tolerance to digitalis; the range of normal serum digoxin levels should be revised upward approximately 1.0 ng/ml from the normal range for adults (from <2.5 ng/ml to <3.5 ng/ml).[7,10] The reduction in glomerular filtration rate and the decrease in muscle mass with advancing age decrease the tolerance to digoxin; the former because of reduced renal excretion and the latter because skeletal muscle is the major body depository for digoxin.[52]

Amiodarone. Plasma digoxin concentrations after 3 days of amiodarone therapy rose by an average of 75% in 7 patients, 4 of whom developed symptoms suggestive of digitalis toxicity.[62a] Amiodarone, a promising, but at present investigational, antidysrhythmic in the United States, is discussed in more detail in Chapter 12.

Anesthetics. Halothane, enflurane, diethyl ether, methoxyflurane, ketamine, fentanyl droperidol, and, to a lesser extent, isoflurane and fluroxene protect against experimental ventricular dysrhythmias in digitalized dogs.[38–40] Cyclopropane enhances and pentobarbital has little effect on similar dysrhythmias in dogs.[38] Documentation of this interaction in humans is unavailable.

Amphotericin B. Hypokalemia, which may occur following amphotericin B therapy (fungal and protozoal infestations), may increase the potential for digitalis toxicity.[64a]

Antacids. The simultaneous administration of antacids that contain magnesium trisilicate, magnesium hydroxide, or aluminum hydroxide may decrease the gastrointestinal absorption of orally administered cardiac glycosides.[63,64] To help compensate for these medications, it is suggested that digoxin capsules, rather than tablets, be used and that serum digoxin levels be monitored.[64b]

Barbiturates. Phenobarbital may increase the metabolism of digitoxin by inducing hepatic microsomal enzymes.[65-67] Digitoxin is excreted partially by enzymatic conversion to digoxin and other breakdown products in the liver. The metabolic products are excreted in the urine. The clinical significance of this interaction is unknown, but patients taking digitoxin and phenobarbital, as well as other enzyme-inducing drugs, should be observed for underdigitalization.

Calcium. Parenteral calcium may precipitate fatal cardiac dysrhythmias in patients receiving digitalis therapy.[68] A lowering of the blood concentration of calcium in patients may help abolish cardiac dysrhythmias due to digitalis excess.[69] Additional documentation of calcium-digitalis interactions in humans is needed. Until such evidence is available, however, parenteral calcium should be given judiciously and with careful monitoring in digitalized patients.[6]

Cardioversion. The attempted electrical conversion of digitalis-induced dysrhythmias may precipitate ventricular fibrillation.[1] If electrical conversion cannot be avoided, one should start with low-energy discharges and gradually increase until the dysrhythmia is terminated or until there is evidence of further electrical instability.[6,14]

Cholestyramine. Digitoxin undergoes enterohepatic circulation, and agents that bind the drug within the intestinal lumen could decrease its half-life.[14,70] Steroid binding resins, including cholestyramine and colestipol, have been used effectively in man for this purpose.[71-73] Although digoxin has only a minimal enterohepatic circulation, cholestyramine interferes with its initial absorption from the gut.[14,74]

Diazepam. Diazepam was reported to increase serum digoxin levels, an effect not explained by other factors.[11f] In subsequent studies in human volunteers, a moderate increase in the digoxin plasma half-life was found in five of seven subjects, as well as a substantial reduction in urinary excretion of digoxin in all seven subjects. *In vitro* studies by these same investigators demonstrated a 15% increase in plasma protein binding of digoxin. Whether this interaction extends to other benzodiazepines is uncertain.

Diuretics. Potassium-wasting diuretics, including furosemide, the benzothiadiazides, and ethacrynic acid may cause acute or chronic hypokalemia and thus may precipitate digitalis toxicity. Adequate potassium replacement or the use of potassium-sparing agents (spironolactone, triamterene) in patients who are given such potent diuretics is particularly important for those who take digitalis.[9]

Erythromycin. In approximately 10% of digoxin-treated patients cardioinactive metabolites constitute 30 to 40% of the total urinary excretion of digoxin.[74a] This may, in some cases, increase the requirement of the drug for optimal digitalization. In one study in man, wide-spectrum antibiotic therapy with erythromycin and tetracycline reduced the ability of the liver to convert digoxin to cardioinactive metabolites. This observation implies that antibiotic therapy can precipitate digitalis toxicity in that percentage of patients in whom the liver converts digoxin into inactive metabolites.

Gastrointestinal Function. Unpredictable absorption of orally administered digitalis preparations may occur in patients with intestinal malabsorption or rapid transit syndromes.[75] Similarly, drugs that alter gastrointestinal motility also cause unpredictable absorption.[76]

Glucose Infusions. Large infusions of carbohydrate may cause an intracellular shift of potassium with a resultant decrease in serum levels of potassium.[66] The similar action of insulin to promote potassium uptake into cells is well known, and is mentioned here as a possible cause of hypokalemia and resultant digitalis toxicity.

Heparin. Animal studies indicate that digitalis preparations increase blood coagulability.[1] Most clinical studies indicate that digitalis has no effect either on coagulation or on heparin tolerance.[1]

Hydralazine. As stated above, vasodilator therapy with hydralazine and sodium nitroprusside can allegedly increase renal clearance of digoxin by 50% in patients with chronic congestive heart failure.[11g] This could lead to a decreased digoxin response when vasodilator therapy is used for prolonged periods of time.

Hypoxia. Hypoxia and disturbances of acid-base balance decrease a patient's tolerance to digitalis, and certainly contribute to problems in digitalizing patients with cor pulmonale or chronic lung disease.[6,7]

Kaolin-pectin. See antacids (above).

Lidocaine. This drug suppresses ventricular ectopy due to digitalis, but is less effective than phenytoin in the control of supraventricular dysrhythmias.[1,6,14]

Liver Disease. Patients with hepatic insufficiency metabolize and excrete digoxin in a normal fashion.[2] Digitoxin, however, is largely metabolized by the liver to digoxin and other by-products that are then excreted by the kidney.[1,7,44] Smaller doses of digitoxin may be required in patients with hepatic dysfunction.[2]

Magnesium. Hypomagnesemia may cause digitalis toxicity.[1,2,6,7] Magnesium may abolish digitalis-induced ventricular ectopy, but is rarely used for this purpose unless hypomagnesemia is also present.[76,77] Magnesium deficiency may or may not be associated with decreased intracellular potassium or with enhanced toxicity to digitalis.[78]

Nifedipine. It has been reported that steady-state plasma digoxin concentrations increased by approximately 45% in patients receiving nifedipine.[78a]

Nitroprusside. See hydralazine (above).

Obesity. One might anticipate a greater volume of distribution in obesity. This does not occur, however, since the concentration of digoxin is low in adipose tissue.[52] Serum digoxin levels and pharmacokinetics are the same before and after the loss of large amounts of adipose tissue in obese subjects, suggesting that lean body mass rather than total body weight should be used to calculate the dose of digoxin.[7,52,57]

Phenylbutazone. This drug enhances the metabolism of digitoxin, possibly through the induction of hepatic microsomal enzymes.[67,79] The known ability of phenylbutazone to induce sodium retention should also be considered carefully in patients who take digitalis.[67]

Phenytoin (Diphenylhydantoin). Phenytoin is a specific agent for the management of ventricular dysrhythmias caused by digitalis, and is frequently effective in supraventricular dysrhythmias as well.[1,12–14] Phenytoin can improve sinoatrial and atrioventricular block by increasing conduction prolonged by digitalis at these sites.[1,12,14,80] Although it has been reported that phenytoin may enhance digitalis-induced bradycardia or may decrease serum digitoxin levels, there is little evidence that these effects are clinically significant.[79,81]

Potassium. Hypokalemia frequently causes dysrhythmias in otherwise normally digitalized patients. Hypokalemia can be caused by excessive doses of digitalis or by the potassium-wasting effects of concomitant diuretic therapy. Potassium depletion may also result from corticosteroid therapy, malnutrition, or hemodialysis.[1] The administration of enough potassium to bring the serum limits to the upper limits of the normal range is indicated in the treatment of hypokalemia-induced digitalis dysrhythmias.[1] Monitoring of both potassium levels and the electrocardiogram is necessary, however, since too large or too rapid an increase in the serum level of potassium may intensify AV block and depress the automaticity of ventricular pacemakers.[1,82] The result may be complete AV block and cardiac arrest. Potassium is contraindicated if AV block is severe.

Propantheline. Propantheline, which decreases gastrointestinal motility, may delay the absorption of slowly dissolving types of digoxin.[83] The use of more rapidly dissolving preparations, for example, Lanoxin, can reduce the significance of this interaction.

Propranolol. This drug is useful in the treatment of some digitalis dysrhythmias due to supraventricular or ventricular ectopy.[1,14] It suppresses automaticity through its antiadrenergic action, whereas by virtue of its direct myocardial action it shortens the effective refractory period of atrial muscle, ventricular muscle, and Purkinje fibers, and slows the rate of depolarization and conduction velocity in these fibers.[14,84] Its tendency to increase atrioventricular nodal refractoriness limits its usefulness in situations where atrioventricular block is present.[1] Propranolol's negative inotropic effect may be deleterious in the presence of impaired myocardial function.

Quinidine. Quinidine administered to patients receiving digoxin may lead to potentially toxic digoxin concentrations[1,11,11a,11b]; the same probably applies to digitoxin.[11c] Possible mechanisms were discussed immediately following the case reports, above. The clinical course, electrocardiogram, and serum levels of digoxin should be monitored closely in patients who are receiving combined therapy with digoxin and quinidine.[11] Furthermore, quinidine and procainamide carry a substantial risk of cardiac toxicity that includes the depression of conduction, the potential for eliciting ventricular dysrhythmias, and decreased myocardial contractility.[14]

Renal Function. The route of excretion of digoxin and other shorter-acting digitalis preparations (ouabain, deslanoside) is primarily renal.[7] The fecal route accounts for a small fraction of the drug excreted.[52] Whereas in patients with renal failure there is a compensatory increase in fecal excretion, this is not an adequate alternative route of elimination.[85] Digitoxin and its metabolites are also excreted primarily by the kidney.[86,87] However, most of the drug is metabolized by the liver, and only 8% of the total dose is excreted in unchanged form.[52] Stool excretion of digitoxin is approximately 17% of the dose in the form of metabolites.[52] The metabolism of digitoxin is unique in that the fecal route is an alternative to the urinary route of excretion.[52] The blood levels are reported to be no higher in patients with impaired renal function who take digitoxin than in patients with normal function.[88] Patients with impaired renal function who take digoxin should be closely observed for signs of toxicity. The dose of digoxin should be adjusted based on measured or estimated creatinine clearances as discussed above in this chapter.

Reserpine. The likelihood of dysrhythmias, particularly in patients with atrial fibrillation, may be increased by the concurrent use of cardiac glycosides and reserpine or related rauwolfia alkaloids.[67,89,90] A true causal relationship has not been established, although the possibility of serious drug-related dysrhythmias should be considered when these drugs are used concomitantly.[67,90] The mechanism for this interaction is not known, but it may involve the central (neural) effects of digitalis and reserpine or the release of catecholamines by reserpine.[67,90]

Succinylcholine. Succinylcholine may cause ventricular dysrhythmias in fully digitalized patients.[67,91,92] The mechanism for this interaction is not established, but it may relate to the loss of intracellular potassium.[91,93] Tubocurarine has been recommended for the treatment of such dysrhythmias based on both clinical and experimental evidence.[91,93] One study did not demonstrate a statistically significant difference in the incidence of ventricular dysrhythmias following succinylcholine between digitalized and nondigitalized patients.[94] Until further information is available, succinylcholine should be used cautiously in fully digitalized patients. The possibility that this interaction might be prevented by a small (defasciculating) dose of a nondepolarizing relaxant is open to investigation.

Sympathomimetics. Sympathomimetics, especially those with significant *beta*-adrenergic activity (isoproterenol, epinephrine, norepinephrine), enhance automaticity, as do toxic doses of digitalis. The concomitant use of these drugs could at least theoretically increase the patient's propensity to dysrhythmias, although further clinical documentation of this interaction is needed.[67]

Tetracyclines. See erythromycin (above).

Thyroid Function. Thyroid disease affects digitalis sensitivity by two mechanisms.[2,6] Hyperthyroidism increases and hypothyroidism decreases the rate of renal excretion of ouabain and digoxin. In addition, the thyrotoxic heart is less sensitive to digitalis with respect to control of the ventricular rate in atrial flutter or fibrillation. The intrinsic sympathetic tone or concurrently administered drugs may be responsible for increased or diminished digitalis sensitivity in patients with disordered thyroid function.[6]

Verapamil. Verapamil may cause an increase in serum digoxin levels by reducing its renal clearance.[94a] This interaction warrants further investigation. In addition, both drugs can prolong AV nodal conduction time and could in combination or increase the level of AV block, even to the level of a complete block.

In summary, digitalis glycosides have one of the lowest therapeutic indices of all commonly used drugs. They are indicated in the treatment of heart failure (positive inotropic action) or atrial flutter or fibrillation (negative dromotropic action). The inotropic action is a linear function of the dose administered, whereas the dromotropic action may be observed only with nearly toxic doses of digitalis. During the preoperative visit, the anesthesiologist should attempt to assess the status of digitalization with the following questions: Is the patient digitalized? Has the desired therapeutic effect been achieved? Does the patient have symptoms or show signs of digitalis toxicity? Intraoperatively, the anesthesiologist should know how and when to digitalize patients. For this task, a familiarity with drug and other interactions involving digitalis will be helpful.

Concerning the status of digitalization, the need to observe the clinical effect is paramount. Serum levels of digitalis alone never establish the diagnosis of either a therapeutic or a toxic effect. A level of digitalis that is toxic for one patient may be therapeutic for another. For example, serum levels of digoxin in the lower toxic range (2.5 ng/ml for adults, 3.5 ng/ml for children) may be required for a therapeutic effect in more resistant cases of atrial flutter or fibrillation. Serum levels of digoxin below 0.5 ng/ml virtually eliminate the possibility of toxicity and usually call for more drug to achieve the desired effect. Therapeutic serum levels for digitoxin are approximately ten times higher than those for digoxin.

The toxicity of digitalis is manifested by cardiac, neural, and gastrointestinal disturbances. Cardiac toxicity is most important from the anesthesiologist's standpoint and includes almost every known form of rhythm disturbance. Life-threatening dysrhythmias are not uncommon. Cardiac toxic manifestations may be brought about by actual overdosage or by interactions with drugs or other factors. With the exception of succinylcholine-related dysrhythmias in digitalized patients, anesthetic or adjuvant drug interactions involving digitalis that are significant to anesthesiologists have not been well documented. The anesthesiologist must recognize, however, that disturbances of acid-base or electrolyte imbalance are the most common causes of digitalis toxicity in surgical patients. Hypokalemia secondary to diuretic therapy or related to metabolic or respiratory alkalosis should be monitored for in particular. Impaired renal function is also a common cause of digitalis toxicity, since it reduces the elimination of shorter-acting digitalis preparations.

Preoperatively and intraoperatively, digitalis is indicated for the treatment of heart failure and atrial flutter or fibrillation. In addition, digitalis is sometimes used as a prophylactic measure to reduce the risk of heart failure or the chance of supraventricular dysrhythmias attendant to cardiac or thoracic surgical procedures. The indications for prophylactic digitalization are not well established. In considering the low therapeutic index and the potential danger of some of the toxic effects of the digitalis glycosides, it is probably better to use these drugs only when a definite indication exists.

REFERENCES

1. Hoffman, B.F., and Bigger, J.T., Jr.: Digitalis and allied cardiac glycosides. In The Pharmacological Basis of Therapeutics. 6th Edition. Edited by A.G. Gilman, L.S. Goodman and A. Gilman. New York, Macmillan, 1980.
2. Doherty, J.E., and Kaul, J.J.: Clinical pharmacology of digitalis glycosides. Annu. Rev. Med., 26:159, 1975.
3. Rodensky, P.L., and Wasserman, F.: Observations on digitalis intoxication. Arch. Intern. Med., 108:171, 1961.
4. Smith, T.W., and Haber, E.: Digitalis. (Fourth of Four Parts). N. Engl. J. Med., 285:1125, 1973.
5. Kim, Y.I., Noble, R.J., and Zipes, D.P.: Dissociation of the inotropic effect of digitalis from its effect on atrioventricular conduction. Am. J. Cardiol., 36:359, 1975.
5a. AMA Division of Drugs: Agents used to treat congestive heart failure. In AMA Drug Evaluations. 5th Ed., Chicago, AMA, 1983.
6. Smith, T.W.: Digitalis glycosides. (Second of Two Parts). N. Engl. J. Med., 288:942, 1973.
7. Smith, T.W., and Haber, E.: Digitalis. (Third of Four Parts). N. Engl. J. Med., 289:1063, 1973.
8. Neff, M.S., et al.: Magnesium sulfate in digitalis toxicity. Am. J. Cardiol., 29:377, 1972.
9. Edwards, R., Winnie, A.P., and Ramamurphy, S.: Acute hypocapneic hypokalemia: An iatrogenic complication. Anesth. Analg. (Cleve.), 56:586, 1977.
10. Doherty, J.A.: How and when to use digitalis serum levels. J.A.M.A., 239:2594, 1978.
11. Leahey, E.B., et al.: Interaction between quinidine and digoxin. J.A.M.A., 240:533, 1978.
11a. Leahey, E.B., et al.: The effect of quinidine and other oral antiarrhythmic drugs on serum digoxin. Ann. Intern. Med., 92:605, 1980.
11b. Mungall, D.R., et al.: Effects of quinidine serum digoxin concentration. Ann. Intern. Med., 93:689, 1980.
11c. Garty, M., Sood, P., and Rollins, D.E.: Digitoxin elimination reduced quinidine therapy. Ann. Intern. Med., 94:35, 1981.
11d. Bussey, H.L.: The influence of quinidine and other agents on digitalis glycosides. Am. Heart J., 104:289, 1982.
11e. Aronson, J.K.: Cardiac glycosides and drugs used in dysrhythmias. In Side Effects of Drugs Annual 6. Amsterdam, Excerpta Medica, 1982.
11f. Castillo-Ferrando, J.R., Garcia, M., and Carmona, J.: Digoxin levels and diazepam. (Letter Lancet, 2:368, 1980).
11g. Cogan, J.J., et al.: Acute vasodilator therapy increases renal clearance of digoxin in patients with congestive heart failure. Circulation, 64:973, 1981.
12. Bigger, J.T., Jr., and Hoffman, B.F.: Antiarrhythmic drugs. In The Pharmacological Basis of Therapeutics. 6th Edition. Edited by A.B. Gilman, L.S. Goodman and A. Gilman. New York, Macmillan, 1980.
13. Bigger, J.T., Jr.: Arrhythmias and antiarrhythmic drugs. Adv. Intern. Med., 18:251, 1972.
14. Smith, T.W., and Haber, E.: Digitalis. (Fourth of Four Parts). N. Engl. J. Med., 289:1125, 1973.
15. Schwartz, A.: Newer aspects of cardiac glycoside action. Fed. Proc., 36:2207, 1977.
16. VanWinkle, W.G., and Schwartz, A.: Ions and Inotropy. Annu. Rev. Physiol., 38:247, 1976.
17. Langer, G.A.: Relationship between myocardial contractility and the effects of digitalis on ionic exchange. Fed. Proc., 36:2231, 1977.
18. Weber, A., and Murray, J.M.: Molecular control mechanisms in muscle contraction. Physiol. Rev., 53:612, 1973.
19. Lymn, R.W., and Taylor, E.W.: Mechanism of adenosine triphosphate hydrolysis by actomyosin. Biochemistry, 10:4617, 1971.
20. Ebashi, S.: Excitation-contraction coupling. Annu. Rev. Physiol., 38:293, 1976.
21. Fabiato, A., and Fabiato, F.: Calcium release from the sarcoplasmic reticulum. Circ. Res., 40:119, 1977.
22. Weber, A., and Winicur, S.: The role of calcium in the superprecipitation of actomyosin. J. Biol. Chem., 236:3198, 1961.
23. Reuter, H.: Exchange of calcium ions in the mammalian myocardium. Circ. Res., 34:599, 1974.

24. Reuter, H.: Divalent ions as charge carriers in excitable membranes. Prog. Biophys. Mol. Biol., 26:1, 1973.
25. Langer, G.A.: Ion fluxes in cardiac excitation and contraction and their relation to myocardial contractility. Physiol. Rev., 48:708, 1968.
26. Solaro, R.J., et al.: Calcium requirements for cardiac myofibrillar activation. Circ. Res., 34:525, 1974.
27. Dhalla, N.S., Ziegelhoffer, A., and Harrow, J.A.C.: Regulatory role of membrane systems in heart function. Can. J. Physiol. Pharmacol., 55:1211, 1977.
28. Reddy, Y.S., et al.: Phosphorylation of cardiac native tropomyosin and troponin. J. Mol. Cell Cardiol., 5:461, 1973.
29. Solaro, R.J., Moir, A.J., and Perry, S.V.: Phosphorylation of troponin I and inotropic effect of adrenalin. Nature, 262:615, 1976.
30. Reddy, Y.S., Pitts, B.J., and Schwartz, A.: Cyclic-AMP dependent and independent protein kinase phosphorylation of canine cardiac myosin light chains. J. Mol. Cell Cardiol., 9:501, 1977.
31. Endoh, M., et al.: Frequency dependence of cyclic AMP in mammalian myocardium. Nature, 261:716, 1976.
32. Mendez, D., and Mendez, R.: The action of cardiac glycosides on the excitability and conduction velocity of the mammalian atrium. J. Pharmacol. Exp. Ther., 121:402, 1957.
33. Watanabe, Y., and Dreifus, L.S.: Electrophysiologic effects of digitalis on A-V transmission. Am. J. Physiol., 211:1461, 1966.
34. Watanabe, Y., and Dreifus, L.S.: Interactions of lantoside-C and potassium on atrioventricular conduction in rabbits. Circ. Res., 27:931, 1970.
35. Ferrier, G.R.: Digitalis arrhythmias: Role of oscillatory afterpotentials. Prog. Cardiovasc. Dis., 19:459, 1977.
36. Cranefield, P.F.: Action potentials, afterpotentials, and arrhythmias. Circ. Res., 41:415, 1977.
37. Tsien, R.W.: Ionic mechanisms of pacemaker activity in cardiac Purkinje fibers. Fed. Proc., 37:2127, 1978.
38. Morrow, D.H., and Townley, N.T.: Anesthesia and digitalis toxicity: An experimental study. Anesth. Analg. (Cleve.), 43:510, 1964.
39. Ivankovich, A.D., et al.: The effects of ketamine and Innovar[R] anesthesia on digitalis tolerance in dogs. Anesth. Analg. (Cleve.), 54:106, 1975.
40. Ivankovich, A.D., et al.: The effect of enflurane, isoflurane, fluroxene, methoxyflurane, and diethyl ether anesthesia on ouabain tolerance in the dog. Anesth. Analg. (Cleve.), 55:360, 1976.
41. Moe, G.K.: Evidence for re-entry as a mechanism of cardiac arrhythmias. Rev. Physiol. Biochem. Pharmacol., 72:55, 1975.
42. Gillis, R.A., Pearle, D.L., and Levitt, B.: Digitalis: A neuroexcitatory drug. Circulation, 52:739, 1975.
43. Quest, J.A., and Billis, R.A.: Carotid sinus reflex changes produced by digitalis. J. Pharmacol. Exp. Ther., 177:650, 1971.
44. Smith, T.W., and Haber, E.: Digitalis. (First of Four Parts). N. Engl. J. Med., 289:945, 1973.
45. McLain, P.L.: Effects of cardiac glycosides on spontaneous efferent activity in vagus and sympathetic nerves of cats. Int. J. Neuropharmacol., 8:379, 1969.
46. Billis, R.A.: Cardiac sympathetic nerve activity: Changes induced by ouabain and propranolol. Science, 166:508, 1969.
47. Butler, V.P., Jr.: Assays of digitalis in the blood. Prog. Cardiovasc. Dis., 14:571, 1972.
48. Doherty, J.E.: The clinical pharmacology of digitalis glycosides: a review. Am. J. Med. Sci., 225:382, 1968.
49. Doherty, J.E.: Digitalis glycosides. Pharmacokinetics and their clinical implications. Ann. Intern. Med., 79:229, 1973.
50. Marcus, F.I., et al.: Administration of tritiated digoxin with and without a loading dose. Circulation, 34:865, 1966.
51. Marcus, F.I., et al.: The metabolic fate of tritiated digoxin in the dog: A comparison of digitalis administration with and without a loading dose. J. Pharmacol. Exp. Ther., 156:548, 1967.
52. Marcus, F.I.: Digitalis pharmacokinetics and metabolism. Am. J. Med., 58:452, 1975.
53. Ogilvie, R.F., and Ruedy, J.: An educational program in digitalis therapy. J.A.M.A., 222:50, 1972.
54. Bloom, P.M., Nelp, W.B., and Truell, S.H.: Relationship of the excretion of tritiated digoxin to renal function. Am. J. Med. Sci., 251:133, 1966.
55. Jelliffe, R.W.: Factors to consider in planning digoxin therapy. J. Chronic Dis., 24:407, 1971.
56. Ewy, G.A., et al.: Digoxin metabolism in the elderly. Circulation, 39:449, 1969.
57. Ewy, G.A., et al.: Digoxin metabolism in obesity. Circulation, 44:810, 1971.
58. Rios, J.C., Dziok, C.A., and Ali, N.A.: Digitalis induced arrhythmias: Recognition and management. In Arrhythmias. Guest edited by L.S. Dreifus. Philadelphia, F.A. Davis, 1970.
59. Lown, B., Wyatt, N.F., and Levine, H.D.: Paroxysmal atrial tachycardia with block. Circulation, 21:129, 1960.
60. Beller, G.A., et al.: Digitalis intoxication: Prospective clinical study with serum level correlations. N. Engl. J. Med., 284:989, 1971.
61. Doherty, J.A.: Digitalis serum level: Practical value. In Controversy in Cardiology. Edited by E. Cheung. New York, Springer-Verlag, 1976.
62. Noble, R.J., et al.: Limitations of serum digitalis levels. In Complex Electrocardiography 2. Edited by C. Fisch. Philadelphia, F.A. Davis, 1974.
62a. Moysey, J.O., et al.: Amiodarone increases plasma digoxin concentrations. Br. Med. J., 282:272, 1981.
63. Brown, D.D., and Juhl, R.P.: Decreased bioavailability of digoxin due to antacids and kaolin-pectin. N. Engl. J. Med., 295:1034, 1976.
64. Khalil, S.A.H.: The uptake of digoxin and digitoxin by some antacids. J. Pharm. Pharmacol., 26:961, 1974.
64a. United States Pharmacopeial Convention: Amphotericin B (Systemic). In Drug Information for the Health Care Provider. Rockville, Maryland, The United States Pharmacopeial Convention, Inc., 1983, pp. 61–62.
64b. Medical Letter. Table of Interactions. In The Med-

ical Letter Handbook of Drug Interactions. The Medical Letter, New Rochelle, New York, 1983, p. 51.
65. Jelliffe, R.W., and Blankenhorn, D.H.: Effect of phenobarbital on digitoxin metabolism. Clin. Res., 14:160, 1966.
66. Hansten, P.D.: Drug Interactions. 4th Edition. Philadelphia, Lea & Febiger, 1979.
67. Solomon, H.M., and Abrams, W.B.: Interactions between digitoxin and other drugs in man. Am. Heart J., 83:277, 1972.
68. Bower, J.O., and Mengle, H.A.K.: The additive effects of calcium and digitalis. J.A.M.A., 106:1151, 1936.
69. Jick, S., and Karsh, R.: The effect of calcium chelation on cardiac arrhythmias and conduction disturbances. Am. J. Cardiol., 4:287, 1959.
70. Okita, G.T., et al.: Metabolic fate of radioactive digitoxin in human subjects. J. Pharmacol. Exp. Ther., 115:371, 1955.
71. Caldwell, H.J., and Greenberger, N.J.: Interruption of the enterophepatic circulation of digitoxin by cholestyramine. I. Protection against lethal digitoxin intoxication. J. Clin. Invest., 50:2626, 1971.
72. Caldwell, J.H., and Bush, C.A.: Interruption of the enterohepatic circulation of digitoxin by cholestyramine. II. Effect on metabolic disposition of tritium-labeled digitoxin and cardiac systolic intervals in man. J. Clin. Invest., 50:2638, 1971.
73. Bazzano, G., and Bazzano, G.S.: Digitalis intoxication: treatment with a new steroid-binding resin. J.A.M.A., 220:828, 1972.
74. Doherty, J.E., et al.: Tritiated digoxin. XIV. Enterohepatic circulation, absorption, and excretion studies in human volunteers. Circulation, 42:867, 1970.
74a. Peters, U., Falk, L.C., and Kalman, S.M.: Digoxin metabolism in patients. Arch. Intern. Med., 138:1074, 1978.
74b. Lindenbaum, J., et al.: Inactivation of digoxin by the gut flora: reversal by antibiotic therapy. N. Engl. J. Med., 305:789, 1981.
75. Heizer, W.D., Smith, T.W., and Goldfinger, S.E.: Absorption of digoxin in patients with malabsorption syndromes. N. Engl. J. Med., 285:257, 1971.
76. Sodeman, W.A.: Diagnosis and treatment of digitalis toxicity. N. Engl. J. Med., 273:35, 93, 1965.
77. Peach, M.J.: Cations: calcium, magnesium, barium, lithium, and ammonium. In The Pharmacological Basis of Therapeutics. 5th Edition. Edited by L.S. Goodman and A. Gilman. New York, Macmillan, 1975.
78. Seller, R.H., et al.: Digitalis toxicity and hypomagnesemia. Am. Heart J., 79:57, 1970.
78a. Belz, G.G., Aust, P.E., and Munkes, R.: Digoxin plasma concentrations and nifedipine (Letter). Lancet, 1:844, 1981.
79. Solomon, H.M., et al.: Interactions between digitoxin and other drugs in vitro and in vivo. Ann. N.Y. Acad. Sci., 179:362, 1971.
80. Helfant, R.H., Scherlag, B.J., and Damato, A.N.: The electrophysiological properties of diphenylhydantoin sodium as compared to procainamide in the normal and digitalis/intoxicated heart. Circulation, 36:108, 1967.
81. Viukari, N.M.A., and Aho, K.: Digoxin-phenytoin interaction. Br. Med. J., 2:51, 1970.
82. Fisch, C., et al.: Potassium and the monophasic action potential, electrocardiogram, conduction and arrhythmias. Prog. Cardiovasc. Dis., 8:387, 1966.
83. Manninen, V., et al.: Altered absorption of digoxin in patients given propantheline and metoclopramide. Lancet, 1:398, 1973.
84. Davis, L.D., and Temte, J.V.: Effects of propranolol on the transmembrane potentials of ventricular muscle and Purkinje fibers of the dog. Circ. Res., 22:661, 1968.
85. Marcus, F.I., et al.: The metabolism of tritiated digoxin in renal insufficiency in dogs and man. J. Pharmacol. Exp. Ther., 152:372, 1966.
86. Lukas, D.S.: The pharmacokinetics and metabolism of digitoxin in men. In Symposium on Digitalis. Edited by O. Storstein. Oslo, Norway, Gyldendal Norsk Forlay, 1973.
87. Beermann, B., Hellstrom, K., and Rosen, K.: Fate of orally administered ^{3}H digitoxin in man with special reference to the absorption. Circulation, 43:852, 1971.
88. Rasmussen, K., et al.: Digitoxin kinetics in patients with impaired renal function. Clin. Pharmacol. Ther., 13:6, 1971.
89. Lown, B., et al.: Effect of digitalis in patients receiving reserpine. Circulation, 24:1185, 1961.
90. Ascione, F.J.: Digitalis-reserpine. In Evaluations of Drug Interactions. 2nd Edition. Washington, D.C., American Pharmaceutical Association, 1976.
91. Dowdy, E.G., and Fabian, L.W.: Ventricular arrhythmias induced by succinylcholine in digitalized patients. Anesth. Analg. (Cleve.), 42:501, 1963.
92. Smith, R.B., and Petrusack, J.: Succinylcholine, digitalis and hypercalcemia: A case report. Anesth. Analg. (Cleve.), 51:202, 1972.
93. Dowdy, E.G., Duggar, P.N., and Fabian, L.W.: Effect of neuromuscular blocking agents on isolated digitalized mammalian hearts. Anesth. Analg. (Cleve.), 44:608, 1965.
94. Perez, H.R.: Cardiac arrhythmias after succinylcholine. Anesth. Analg. (Cleve.), 49:33, 1970.
94a. Aronson, J.K.: Digitalis intoxication. Clin. Sci., 64:253, 1983.

|15|

INORGANIC CATIONS

ALDO N. CORBASCIO and N. TY SMITH

Inorganic cations (Ca^{++}, K^+, Na^+, Mg^+) are important therapeutic agents that are frequently employed in anesthesia. These agents serve many purposes, such as (1) replacement of loss (e.g., hypokalemia), (2) correction of electrolyte imbalances (e.g., acid-base disturbances), or (3) pharmacologic interventions (cardiac resuscitation). Anesthetists therefore avail themselves extensively of the pharmacodynamic properties of inorganic cations and could not function well without some knowledge of their effects and their propensity to interact with each other and other drugs. Perioperatively, cations are usually administered intravenously, either in bolus doses (e.g., calcium) or as infusions (e.g., potassium) to achieve particular effects or levels. Magnesium, as its sulfate, is the only ion that is injected intramuscularly.

CALCIUM

The example of calcium typifies the pharmacologic, as opposed to the replacement, uses of cations, and we shall review here its physiologic role, as well as some of its uses and indications. The pharmacologic role of calcium has not received the extensive treatment it deserves in most of our popular pharmacology textbooks. The reasons for this omission are unclear but probably arise from two causes: the lack of economic incentives related to a nonpatented agent, and inadequate perception of its worth by medical writers. Calcium ions are in fact used therapeutically in many different clinical situations and deserve more extensive discussion.

CASE REPORT

A 35-year-old, white male was admitted for the removal of a large chromaffine tumor (pheochromocytoma) located at the aortic bifurcation. His preoperative evaluation was essentially normal, except for a history of long-standing hypertension, headaches, tachycardia, episodes of flushing and collapse after alcohol ingestion. The patient had been managed during the previous 3 years with the following medications: Phenoxybenzamine 40 mg qd and propranolol 80 mg bid. This regimen maintained an almost normotensive state (140/90), with a resting heart rate of 80/m. All laboratory tests were normal except for an increase in the urinary output of catecholamine metabolites. Anesthesia was induced with thiopental and maintained with methoxyflurane.

Surgical excision of the tumor proved to be difficult owing to the size, location, and vascularity of the tumor. Hypertensive paroxysms during surgery were controlled with phentolamine 5 mg i.v. Tachydysrhythmia was managed with repeated propranolol 1 to 3 mg i.v. The removal of the tumor was followed by a persistent hypotension (70/40 mm Hg) unresponsive to norepinephrine or methoxamine. The hypotension and bradycardia persisted well into the recovery period. It was attributed to myocardial depression and persistent bradycardia induced by prolonged *beta*-blockade. The administration of calcium gluconate (20 mg 10% ml) induced a prompt reversal of the bradycardia and hypotension within 5 minutes. The patient recovered uneventfully.

This report occurred before the importance of preoperative adrenergic blockade and intraoperative volume maintenance was appreciated. Nevertheless, it does illustrate the ability of calcium to be effective when all else fails. This reliability stems in part from the involvement of Ca^{++} in many of the basic functions of the body. A particular prerequisite for a comprehensive understanding of calcium is a knowledge of the vital role that calcium plays in the cellular physiology of cardiac and vascular smooth muscle. This chapter discusses in detail some of the involvement of Ca^{++}, as well as its clinical uses.

Physiologic Role of Calcium

Calcium ions are ubiquitous in all body fluids. Ca^{++} appears to be the main intracellular messenger of a large number of essential physiologic processes. It plays a fundamental role in cellular excitability, muscle contraction, cardiac function, endocrine secretion and coagulation. Calcium ions (Ca^{++}) are essential to many biologic processes, such as excitation-contraction coupling, coupling of electrical activation to cellular secretion, neuronal excitability, hemostasis, and bone metabolism. An excess of calcium ions in the extracellular fluid decreases cellular excitability by increasing the depolarization threshold of biologic membranes. Conversely, a decrease of calcium in the extracellular environment leads to increased excitability and may even facilitate "ephaptic" (i.e., cross-wise) stimulation from surrounding cells or axons.

A steep gradient, up to 1:10,000, is actively maintained between intracellular (10^{-7m}) and extracellular (10^{-3m}) calcium ion concentrations. A transmembrane gradient exists also for monovalent cations such as Na^+ and K^+. Although this latter potential contributes substantially to the charge on the membrane, as well as to its bioelectrical activity, calcium ions are specifically required to activate intracellular processes such as contraction or exocytosis. There are at least 2 ionic pumps responsible for maintaining the high concentration gradient across the cell membrane. One is an ATP and Mg^{++} dependent pump identified in human red cells, neutrophils, neurons, and myocardium. The calcium carrier system has both a low-affinity, slow pumping mode and a high-affinity, rapid pumping mode. The mode change of this system is induced by a calcium binding protein called *calmodulin*. When calcium-activated calmodulin binds to the calcium carrier system, there is a great increase in the maximum velocity of calcium transport out of the cell. This ATP-dependent carrier system functions maximally when intracellular calcium levels rise, and adequate ATP is available. This unidirectional Ca^{++} pump differs from the sodium-potassium pump mentioned below because this is not an exchange system, and its ATP energy requirement is higher.

The cardiac cell membrane, or sarcolemma, can selectively transport Ca^{++} and other ions into the cell in a regulated fashion. It is an ion-impermeable lipid bilayer composed of phospholipid molecules that separate aqueous compartments. A widely accepted cell membrane model depicts membrane proteins grouped together as structural islands floating in a sea created by the lipid bilayer. This structure provides a barrier impermeable to many charged substances found in aqueous solutions. The membrane proteins are responsible for most of the biologic activities of the membranes. One function of these protein subunits is to provide a channel for the passage of various ionic substances across the hydrophobic lipid barrier. Relatively little is known about the actual structure of ion channels in the cell membrane, but since they are highly specific for a given ion species, it can be assumed that the aqueous "pore" within each channel is provided with a selectivity filter that limits the type of ion that can pass through that type of channel. Since ion channels can be open or shut, the channel also has voltage sensors—i.e., charged regions of the channel proteins that determine whether the channel "gates" are open or closed. Each type of ion moves through a highly selective ion channel. Separate channels for each ion have been postulated.

These voltage-sensitive ion channels can exist in three states—resting, activated, and inactivated. The transitions between the resting, activated, and inactivated states of the Na$^+$ gate are more rapid than those of the Ca^{++} gate by several orders of magnitude; hence the Na$^+$ channel is referred to as the *fast channel* and the Ca^{++} channel as the *slow channel*. The slow channels are 100 times more selective for Ca^{++} than Na$^+$ and therefore have also received the name "calcium channels."

When a propagated wave of depolarization approaches the membrane region containing the Ca^{++} channel, reduction of membrane potential (a decrease in the electronegativity in the cell interior) causes the activation gate to open, permitting Ca^{++} to cross the membrane and enter the cells. The gate closes when the interior of the cell has again become electronegative—i.e., when the resting level of the transmembrane potential has been restored. Since the movement of Ca^{++} through these channels is controlled by electrical potentials, they have been termed "voltage-dependent" channels.

An important feature of many, but not all, Ca^{++} channels is their sensitivity to control by sarcolemmal receptors. *Beta*-1 agonists in cardiac muscle and *alpha*-adrenergic agonists in vascular smooth muscle increase Ca^{++} influx via the slow inward current. This induces an increase in contractility, frequency, and conduction velocity in the heart (*beta*-receptor activation), while peripheral *alpha*-receptor activation causes vasoconstriction. Activation of adrenergic receptors does not appear to increase Ca^{++} influx by increasing the size of the Ca^{++} channels or the rates at which their gates open or close, but rather by the recruitment of additional active channels. Conversely, when endogenous adrenergic nervous activity is low or blocked by an adrenergic-receptor blocker, a certain proportion of the Ca^{++} channels are unable to open in response to a depolarizing stimulus. The channels acted upon by receptor-mediated events are termed "receptor-operated channels." Thus the upstroke phase of the slow action potential is determined by a slow Ca^{++}-dependent influx that is increased by Ca^{++}, *beta* sympathomimetics, or methylxanthine and inhibited by calcium antagonists, such as verapamil, nifedipine, or diltiazem.

The influx of Ca^{++} during depolarization triggers a further release of intracellular calcium stores, primarily from the sarcoplasmic reticulum but also from the mitochondria. This calcium raises the myoplasmic [Ca^{++}], allowing the initiation of the mechanical contractile process. By binding to tropin, Ca^{++} releases the inhibition of the troponin-tropomyosin complex on the actin filaments, enabling actin to activate myosin-ATPase. Thus, actin and myosin are able to slide over each other in an ATP-dependent process. This activation of contraction involves the formation of active crossbridges between these two elements. The maximum tension developed, which is an index of contractility and ATP utilization, depends upon the number of crosslinks that have been activated and is directly related to the amount of calcium available for interaction with the troponin-tropomyosin system. Therefore, the magnitude of the increase in intracellular calcium will determine energy expenditure and contractility of the myocardium. The amount of calcium influx during depolarization can be altered by pharmacologic interventions. In addition to the mechanisms outlined above, catecholamines increase the magnitude of the calcium current that traverses the opened slow channels by increasing intracellular cyclic (AMP) levels. This increases the rate of firing of the pacemaker cells (positive chronotropy) and the intensity of the contractile process (positive inotropy).

Phase 0 of the myocardial action potential arises from the rapid increase in the membrane conductance (permeability) for Na^+ resulting in turn in a fast inward current through the fast channels in the cell membrane. This current is dependent on the extracellular $[Na^+]$ and can be blocked selectively by tetrodotoxin and nonspecifically by the Type 1 antidysrhythmic agents, such as quinidine and procainamide or by local anesthetic agents.

When the cell has been depolarized from approximately -90 to $-40mV$, a second inward current related to Ca^{++} flux develops. This current subsequently contributes significantly to the plateau phase (Phase 2) of the cardiac action potential. Since the rates of activation and inactivation of this second inward current are several orders of magnitude slower than those of the fast inward current, it has been termed the "slow inward current." Thus, the conductance of the cell membrane for Ca^{++} increases less rapidly than its conductance for Na^+, and remains elevated for a much longer period.

Myoplasmic $[Ca^{++}]$ is controlled by at least seven known mechanisms.

(1) The first is the inward movement of Ca^{++} along its concentration gradient and across the sarcolemma—i.e., the electrogenic slow inward current through the slow Ca^{++} channels, discussed above.

(2) Since small quantities of Ca^{++} enter the cardiac cell with each contraction, there must be some mechanism for removal of Ca^{++} from the cell such that $[Ca^{++}]$ remains constantly in a steady state. There is now evidence for a bidirectional Na^+-Ca^{++} exchange system that mediates the movement of Ca^{++} across the sarcolemma. It moves one calcium ion from the cytosol into the interstitial fluid while it transiently moves three sodium ions into the cell. The energy required by this system for moving Ca^{++} out of the cell against a concentration gradient may be provided by the downhill movement of Na^+ into the cell along its electrochemical gradient. The direction of this exchange is dependent upon the relative concentrations of extracellular and intracellular Na^+ and Ca^{++}. When cardiac glycosides inhibit Na^+, K^+ ATPase, and thus the pump responsible for the Na^+-K^+ exchange, intracellular $[Na^+]$ is elevated. Hence, less Ca^{++} leaves the cell, inducing thus a marked positive inotropic effect.

(3) The sarcolemma possesses a Ca^{++} ATPase that extrudes Ca^{++} from the cell in an energy-requiring process.

(4) A Ca^{++}-stimulated magnesium ATPase in the membrane of the sarcoplasmic reticulum transports Ca^{++} into the lumen of the sarcoplasmic reticulum and sequesters it there in an energy-requiring process. When phospholamban, a protein associated with the sarcoplasmic reticulum, is phosphorylated by cyclic AMP (as a consequence of *beta*-adrenergic receptor activation), the uptake of Ca^{++} by the sarcoplasmic reticulum increases, accounting for the more rapid contraction and relaxation of cardiac muscle exposed to catecholamines.

(5) Ca^{++} can also be taken up and released by other intracellular structures, particularly the mitochondria and the internal layer of the sarcolemma. When intracellular $[Ca^{++}]$ rises, ATP generated by the mitochondria is involved in the uptake of Ca^{++} by these organelles; excess uptake of mitochondrial Ca^{++} in turn interferes with mitochondrial function.

(6) A variety of ionophores can effect the selective movement of Ca^{++} along its concentration gradient, directly across the sarcolemma—i.e., not through the slow channels.

(7) The buffering of Ca^{++} by intracellular proteins, such as calmodulin, troponin C, and myosin-phosphorylase light chains, is an important mechanism that regulates myoplasmic $[Ca^{++}]$.

Since normal cardiac contraction and relaxation are critically dependent on precisely timed modulations of myoplasmic $[Ca^{++}]$, abnormalities in any of the systems described above can affect myocardial performance.

Physiologic differences among skeletal, smooth and cardiac muscle depend partly upon the different availability of intracellular calcium stores in these tissues. Skeletal muscle shows the highest degree of specialization of its contractile mechanism, with a well developed and highly complex system of internal calcium release and reuptake (e.g., sarcoplasmic reticulum and mitochondria). Myocardial and smooth muscle cells do not possess such an elaborate machinery for internal calcium release, hence their activity is much more dependent on the concentration of ionized calcium in the extracellular fluid. One important physiologic consequence of this intracellular arrangement is the ability of skeletal muscle to maintain contraction even in the total absence of calcium, while myocardial or smooth muscle contraction fails as soon as the extracellular ionized calcium concentration declines below a certain critical level.

In summary, the contractile capacity of the heart is critically dependent on transmembrane conductivity and can be influenced by physiologic states or pharmacologic agents that affect membrane permeability to calcium ions. Calcium influx represents an essential component for the activation of contractility in the myocardial cell. The mechanism by which Ca^{++} triggers myocardial contraction envisages its uptake by troponin, a regulatory protein that modulates the interaction of actinomyosin filaments that induce shortening of myofibrillar elements.[1] The inotropic actions of *beta*-adrenergic agents depend partly on their ability to increase Ca^{++} fluxes across the depolarized myocardial membrane, which can in turn trigger the internal contractile mechanism. Conversely, drugs that impede the intracellular entry of calcium decrease myocardial contractility in a dose-dependent manner. A drug that increases the intracellular Ca^{++} concentration (e.g., digitalis) induces a dose-related increase in myocardial contractility.

With these premises, we can now consider some of the most important clinical applications of the pharmacodynamic action of calcium.

The total serum calcium concentration oscillates between 4.5 and 5.5 mEq/L. It is physiologically active only in the ionized form (4.5% of the total concentration), i.e., 2.0 to 2.5 mEq/L. The concentration of ionized calcium is critically dependent on arterial pH, being increased by acidosis and decreased by alkalosis. This occurs without any change in the total calcium concentration. Nonionized calcium is largely bound to serum albumin. When the plasma concentration of albumin declines, the concentration of total calcium is decreased. This is the most common cause of hypocalcemia. A serious functional hypocalcemia can be induced by hyperventilation. This is a common cause of muscle spasms, laryngospasm and tetanic manifestation in swimmers and infants. The response to nondepolarizing neuromuscular blocking agents can be potentiated by hypocalcemia.

We shall review the pharmacodynamic properties of calcium briefly here. The injection of calcium intravenously in doses within the clinical range 3 to 7 mg/kg produces a series of predictable cardiovascular responses that are partly due to (1) direct inotropic effect on the heart and musculotropic effect on the metarterioles and (2) liberation of endogenous catecholamines. The two fundamental responses attendant to the intravenous injection of calcium have been clarified by Lembeck.[2] They are:

1. An increase in myocardial inotropism, which is due to the intrinsic pharmacodynamic activity of calcium on the contractile mechanism of the heart.
2. A release of endogenous catecholamines (norepinephrine and epinephrine) with a marked increase in heart rate, mean arterial blood pres-

sure, ventricular contractility, contraction of the spleen and nictitating membrane (cat), and increased levels of catecholamines in adrenal venous blood. In this respect intravenous calcium behaves as an indirect sympathomimetic drug, analogous to metaraminol, for example.

The most common indications for calcium-ion therapy in anesthesia are:
1. To provide inotropic support for the failing myocardium in cardiac surgery. Calcium chloride is used routinely (200 to 500 mg IV bolus) to help reestablish blood pressure after cardiac bypass. It is also used to restore cardiac activity in asystole and to facilitate defibrillation. Its advantages are even more obvious in cases of electro-mechanical dissociation.
2. To antagonize hypotension and myocardial depression consequent to the rapid infusion of citrated blood (citrate toxicity).
3. To antagonize myocardial depression induced by an overdose of myocardial depressant drugs, such as lidocaine, procaine, halothane, *beta*-adrenergic blockers, or calcium-channel blockers.
4. To antagonize the hemodynamic depression caused by severe hyperkalemia (end-stage renal disease), as well as secondary hyperkalemia induced by verapamil overdose.
5. To antagonize severe hypotension and electro-mechanical dissociation (cardiovascular collapse, hyperkalemic arrest).
6. To stimulate ventricular automaticity in ventricular standstill.
7. To act as an adjuvant in the reversal of neuromuscular blockade induced by neomycin, streptomycin, gentamicin, kanamycin, or paromycin, especially when these antibiotics have been used in association with nondepolarizing neuromuscular blocking agents (see Chap. 24).
8. To counter anaphylactic shock in epinephrine-resistant patients or in patients who have been exposed to large doses of *beta*-adrenergic blockers and who are poorly responsive to epinephrine.[3]

The synergistic propensities of calcium ions with digitalis glycosides are well known. They are partly due to the summation of the inotropic actions of both drugs. Digitalis exerts its main inotropic effect by increasing myocardial intracellular Ca^{++} concentration by affecting its efflux from the myocardial cell during contraction. This is particularly evident if potassium depletion exists (e.g., administration of K-depleting diuretics). Potassium supplementation or i.v. administration in acute emergencies may restore the balance and antagonize digitalis toxicity. In these cases, if renal function is normal, a small intravenous dose of 2 to 5 mEq K^+ may be administered, provided there is no AV block. (K^+ prolongs the effective refractory period of junctional tissues.)

Calcium can sensitize the myocardium to the dysrhythmic actions of digitalis, partly because of its effect on the circulatory levels of catecholamines.

If K^+ is ineffective in controlling calcium-induced digitalis toxicity, phenytoin can be used to suppress ventricular tachycardias and supraventricular dysrhythmias. The usual dose is 100 mg intravenously repeated every 5 to 10 minutes until the abnormal rhythm is brought under control. Lidocaine can also be used to suppress ventricular tachycardia, although it is less effective than phenytoin against digitalis/calcium-induced supraventricular dysrhythmias. *Beta*-blockers can effectively antagonize digitalis-induced abnormal rhythms of ventricular and supraventricular origin.

Citrate Intoxication and Hyperkalemia

The hemodynamic picture of citrate intoxication and acute hypokalemia was described in the 1960s by Bunker, et al.[4] and by Corbascio and Smith.[5] It is characterized by hypotension, narrow pulse pressure, increased central pressure, decreased myocardial contractility and diminished tone of impedance vessels. Citrate intoxication is relatively infrequent owing to the liver's ability to metabolize citrate via the Krebs cycle. A serum level of ionized calcium below 0.5 mEq/L induces a serious depression of myocardial contractility, as well as coagulation problems.[4,6,7]

The rapid infusion of 500 ml of blood stored in acid-citrate-dextrose can induce a substantial lowering of serum ionized calcium. The serum Ca^{++} level tends to return rapidly to normal upon cessation of the infusion. In hypocapnic conditions, this self-correcting mechanism may fail, particularly in the presence of hyperkalemia (potassium may reach 32 mEq/L in stored blood), hypothermia, or liver disease.

Calcium replacement in suspected citrate intoxication should be guided by firm diagnostic criteria, such as diminished serum calcium levels, prolongation of the QT interval, or hyperkalemia > 6 mEq/L. In such cases replacement with calcium chloride is indicated.

Since calcium ions administered intravenously can act as secondary sympathomimetic amines, the theoretical possibility exists for a synergistic effect with tricyclic antidepressants (amitriptyline) or with monoamine oxidase inhibitors (phenelzine, tranylcypromine). These agents block norepinephrine uptake into nerve endings and may sensitize the myocardium to the dysrhythmic actions of endogenous catecholamines or induce drastic arterial pressure changes and precipitate a cerebrovascular accident.

Calcium ions used in anesthesia are administered exclusively by the intravenous route in the form of soluble salts such as the chloride, gluconate, or gluceptate. Calcium chloride can cause tissue sloughing if it is injected in tissues owing to the irritating properties of this salt. Since calcium chloride injection U.S.P. is also irritating when injected by vein, it should be well diluted. It is available in concentrations of 5 to 10% (0.68 to 1.36 mEq/Ca^{++}/ml). $CaCl_2$ contains four times more calcium by weight than Ca-gluconate (37% by weight versus 9% of the gluconate). Calcium gluconate injection U.S.P. is available in a 10% solution (0.45 mEq Ca^{2+}/ml). It delivers a lower concentration of calcium ions, but it is better tolerated and less irritating. Calcium gluceptate injection U.S.P. is a 23% solution (0.9 mEq Ca^{2+}/ml) that can be administered in doses of 5 to 20 ml (4.5 to 18 mEq). It is less irritating than the previous two salts and can be injected intramuscularly in a dose not exceeding 5 ml.

SODIUM

Sodium is the most prevalent ion in the extracellular fluid. Hence it is the main contributor to plasma osmotic pressure and a major factor in the tonicity of all other body fluids. Changes in total body sodium are concomitant with increments or decrements in total body water. Actually, sodium concentration (hypo- or hypernatremia) is generally the expression of changes in total body water rather than sodium deficits. Excessive sodium loss, however, can induce a deficit of this electrolyte (e.g., adrenal insufficiency, salt losing nephritis, or diuretic phase of renal failure). Sodium loss leads to a decrease in extracellular fluid volume and to dehydration. This type of dehydration differs from dehydration due to water loss because the hematocrit and the total serum protein concentrations are increased, while the sodium and chloride concentrations are unchanged. Loss of extracellular fluid induces hypotension with a reduction in glomerular filtration and an increase in serum creatinine. Any increase in total body sodium is generally due to excessive Na retention (e.g., hepatic cirrhosis or congestive heart failure). This induces an increase in extracellular fluid volume without an increase in serum sodium concentration. In these conditions, sodium is either unchanged or lower owing to inadequate water excretion by the kidney.

Hyponatremia with a decrease in plasma osmolarity not secondary to water retention or adrenal failure is seen in acute infections, e.g., pneumonia, and in certain types of lung carcinoma. In the latter case the hyponatremia is generally due to inappropriate secretion of antidiuretic hormone by the tumor tissue.

A sodium concentration above 145 mEq/L constitutes prima facie evidence of a total body water deficit. This situation is clinically rare, particularly in the presence of normal renal function, and occurs in such conditions as diabetes insipidus or tubular unresponsiveness to ADH. A similar picture is seen in hypercalcemia, hypokalemia, chronic nephritis or prolonged mechanical ventilation of the lungs with unhumidified air.

In these cases the administration of isotonic electrolyte free water is mandatory. Its administration should be gradual and guided by constant monitoring of blood pressure, urinary output and sodium concentration, because drastic changes in serum osmolarity can cause cerebral edema and irreversible brain damage.[8]

A decrease in intravascular fluid volume secondary to total body water deficit will exaggerate the hypotensive effects of anesthetics, particularly the hypotension induced by intravenous narcotics, tubocurarine or halothane. Positive pressure ventilation can magnify hypovolemic hypotension. The sensitivity to nondepolarizing neuromuscular blocking agents and barbiturates, which distribute themselves prevalently to the extracellular fluid, is likely to be increased as a consequence of the decreased volume of distribution of these drugs.

In contrast to hypernatremia, a reduction in total body sodium (> 130 mEq/L) is a common occurrence after surgery. The most common cause of hyponatremia is an increase in total body water rather than a deficiency of sodium. This distinction is important, because low serum sodium due to total body sodium deficit causes a decrease in extracellular fluid, in circulatory volume, and in cardiac output and an increase in hematocrit, while hyponatremia secondary to an increase in body water causes the opposite, i.e., an increase in extracellular fluid and in circulatory volume, as well as an increase in cardiac output if the heart is not in failure.

Excessive postoperative hemodilution may lead to failure of the intracellular pump mechanism (sick cell syndrome) with an increased accumulation of intracellular sodium at the expense of other intracellular ions, such as potassium, magnesium and calcium. Surgical hyponatremia is a common occurrence owing to the tendency to administer hypo-osmotic solutions. This is particularly true of the overhydration frequently incident to transurethral prostatic resection, in which large volumes of water are used for irrigation. Rapid absorption of hypo-osmotic fluid can lead to low values of serum sodium (< 120 mEq/L) and can induce generalized signs such as grand mal seizures, arterial hypotension, bradycardia, increased central venous pressure and pulmonary edema. This rapidly evolving syndrome requires the administration of hypertonic saline solution and loop diuretics. Surgical pain, the administration of barbiturates, intravenous narcotics, or halothane, combined with positive pressure ventilation, may induce retention of free water and liberation of *ADH*. Functional extracellular fluid volume may be reduced by "third-space" formation, which will also trigger ADH release.

Anesthesia may induce a profound depression of glomerular filtration rate (up to 70%) with decreased ability to excrete water, while the endogenous oxidation of fats and the breakdown of muscle tissue can add 500 ml of water per day to the excretory load. A clear distinction between sodium and water imbalance is often impossible in the average clinical situation, because the prime causative agent may be difficult to identify.

The fine homeostatic tuning between serum osmolarity, renal function and *ADH* secretion is profoundly deranged by surgical pain and anesthesia. Hence, it is common to observe natriuresis in spite of dilution hyponatremia following surgery. It seems that this paradoxical response is brought about by volume receptors that are sensitive to overall volume changes in circulatory volume rather than by changes in sodium and serum osmolarity.

POTASSIUM

Derangements of serum K^+ are common in medicine and anesthesia, and their correction is of paramount importance in the management of the surgical patient. The more common derangement of this ion is hypokalemia, which is usually defined as a serum K^+ concentration below 3.5 mEq/L. The changes in transmembrane potassium gradients have a profound effect on muscle tissues, with generalized muscle weakness, hypotension, and the onset of life-threatening dysrhythmias. Myocardial contractility and cardiac competence are generally depressed. The hypokalemic heart is sensitive to the dysrhythmogenic actions of digitalis or catecholamines and requires appropriate steps for immediate correction.

Hyperkalemia is defined as a serum potassium greater than 5.5 mEq/L. An increase in K^+ in serum, if not appropriately treated, can be rapidly fatal due to the effects of K^+ on the myocardial fiber and the specific conduction tissue of the heart. Severe disturbances in cardiac rhythm, including heart block and ventricular fibrillation, are likely to ensue. The heart is sensitized to the dysrhythmogenic action of halogenated anesthetics. The administration of large amounts of *beta*-adrenergic agents can acutely increase the blood levels of potassium to dangerous levels. The most commonly incriminated agent is succinylcholine, a depolarizing neuromuscular blocking agent that can induce a massive release of K^+ via activation of endogenous catecholamine stores in burned patients, in patients who have sustained spinal cord injuries, or in patients who have progressive neuromuscular diseases.[9]

Hyperkalemia is a latent threat in most patients with endstage renal disease. The cardiovascular actions of hyperkalemia can be antagonized with the prompt injection of calcium chloride, 10% in 1 ml increments, to antagonize the myocardial depression and muscular debility. This can be supplemented by the intravenous administration of glucose (50 g), regular insulin (20 μ), and sodium bicarbonate (100 mEq).

MAGNESIUM

Like potassium, magnesium is prevalently an intracellular cation. The average 70-kg adult has about 2000 mEq of magnesium in the body, of which approximately one-half resides in bone. Thus a normal extracellular concentration can conceal a serious intracellular depletion. The normal range of serum concentrations is 1.75 to 2.5 mEq/L, about one-third of which is bound to protein. Serum levels below 0.5 mEq/L are accompanied by serious neuromuscular manifestations of which tetany is the most evident manifestation.

Magnesium sulfate is still widely used for the treatment of the toxemia and eclampsia of pregnancy. Excess magnesium in the extracellular fluid induces a decrease in ACH release at the neuromuscular junction and decreases the endplate sensitivity to ACH, as well as the amplitude of the endplate miniature potential.

Both depolarizing and nondepolarizing

neuromuscular blocking agents are enhanced by excess magnesium. These depressant effects on neuromuscular transmission are antagonized by calcium.

When plasma magnesium concentration exceeds 10 mEq/L, deep tendon reflexes are abolished. Hypermagnesemia induces a profound depression of CNS function and is sometimes a factor in the late emergence from anesthesia.

In patients who have received magnesium sulfate, the requirements of succinylcholine are significantly decreased.[10] Interactions between magnesium and curare have also been described. Ghoneim and Long have shown in the isolated phrenic-diaphragm preparation of the rat that magnesium sulfate shifts the dose response curve of curare, decamethonium and succinylcholine to the left.[11] It appears that reduced liberation of acetylcholine from the motor nerve terminal is responsible for this potentiation, which is antagonized by calcium, an ion that increases acetylcholine release without any effect on end-plate sensitivity or the muscle membrane electrical threshold. Further discussion of magnesium can be found in Chapters 24 and 27.

REFERENCES

1. Fleckenstein, A.: Calcium antagonists in heart and smooth muscle. New York, John Wiley and Sons, Inc., 1983.
2. Lembeck, F., and Juan, H.: Are there therapeutic indications of intravenous injections of calcium gluconate? Arzneim. Forsch. (Drug Res.), 25:10, 1975.
3. Corbascio, A.N.: Propranolol. Clin. Pharmacol. Therap., 12:3, 1971.
4. Bunker, J.P., et al.: Hemodynamic effects of intravenously administered sodium citrate. N. Engl. J. Med., 266:372, 1962.
5. Corbascio, A.N., and Smith, N. Ty: Hemodynamic effects of experimental hypercitremia. Anesthesiology, 28:510, 1967.
6. Miller, R.D.: Complications of massive blood transfusions. Anesthesiology, 39:83, 1973.
7. Miller, R.D.: Blood, blood components, colloid, and autotransfusion therapy. In Miller, R.D. (ed). Anesthesia. New York, Churchill Livingstone, 1981.
8. Hypernatremia and brain damage. (Editorial) Lancet, 1:186, 1968.
9. Cooperman, L.H.: Succinylcholine-induced hyperkalemia in neuromuscular diseases. J.A.M.A., 213:1867, 1980.
10. Morris, R., and Giesecke, A.H.: Potentiation of muscle relaxant by magnesium sulfate therapy in toxemia of pregnancy. South. Med. J., 61:25, 1968.
11. Ghoneim, M.M., and Long, J.P.: The interaction of magnesium and other neuromuscular blocking agents. Anesthesiology, 32:23, 1970.

16

DIURETICS

ROBERT G. MERIN and R. DENNIS BASTRON

CASE REPORT

A 44-year-old man was admitted to the emergency department of a hospital with a complaint of vomiting blood. His past medical history included more than 15 years of alcohol abuse, documented hepatic cirrhosis for ten years, recurrent ascites and edema, and congestive heart failure of undetermined cause. Current medications included furosemide, 20 mg t.i.d., and digoxin, 0.25 mg q.d. The patient had been feeling poorly for several days and had been drinking heavily with little food or other fluid intake. However, he had taken his medications. Shortly after his arrival in the Emergency Room he vomited a large quantity of blood and lost consciousness. An anesthesiologist was summoned for resuscitation and intubated the trachea with considerable difficulty because of blood in the mouth and resistance by a semicomatose patient. Immediately after endotracheal intubation, the pulse became irregular and then absent. An electrocardiogram showed ventricular fibrillation. There was considerable difficulty in restoring an adequate rhythm. A serum potassium level was reported as 2.5 mEq/L. By means of judicious intravenous injection of potassium, volume replacement, alkalization, and ventilation, cardiac output was restored. The serum digoxin concentration was subsequently reported as 1.8 ng/ml.

Fortunately, the anesthesiologist is not often faced with such a patient. Most of us are aware of the hazards of hypokalemia in a patient taking potent diuretic drugs, and would not anesthetize this patient without knowing the level of serum potassium. Here, however, the combination of an emergency endotracheal intubation, hypokalemia (both from cirrhosis and from diuretic therapy), and digitalis produced ventricular irritability and fibrillation. Although other drug interactions that involve the use of diuretics may not be so dramatic, there is a potential for serious interaction between diuretics and other drugs administered to patients. We frequently anesthetize patients who are taking diuretic agents for the treatment of salt and water retention and for hypertension, and less frequently for disorders such as diabetes insipidus and hypercalcemia.[1-5] Moreover, we administer diuretic agents to surgical patients to reduce brain size or intracranial pressure;[6] to treat acute fluid overload;[2] and to prevent or to diagnose the cause of oliguria.[7-9] In order to understand the basis for interactions between diuretics and other drugs, it is necessary to understand the way in which the body and the kidney regulate water and electrolyte balance and to have a basic knowledge of the pharmacology of diuretic drugs.

OSMOTIC PRESSURE AND DISTRIBUTION OF WATER

Osmotic pressure depends solely on the number of particles in solution, not on their size or molecular weight. One gram molecular weight of a nondissociating compound is equivalent to one osmole. If the compound dissociates into two molecules (for example, NaCl), one gram molecular weight equals two osmoles. Body solutions average around 0.3 osmoles (300 milliosmoles) per kilogram of water.

Perhaps osmotic pressure is easier to understand if we consider the forces that regulate the movement of water across membranes. Passive movement of ions across membranes can be accomplished by establishing concentration gradients. Thus, if a 0.1 molar sodium chloride solution is separated from another 0.1 molar sodium chloride solution by a permeable membrane, the concentration (escaping tendency) of sodium from each solution will be equal, and no net exchange will occur. If, however, the solution on one side of the membrane is 1 molar, and the other side remains 0.1 molar, the sodium activity or escaping tendency in the concentrated solution will cause net flux of sodium into the more dilute solution (less activity) until the concentration gradient is abolished.

Pure water has a greater activity or escaping tendency for water than does a solution; that is, in a solution, water molecules are diluted and have less molecular activity. Movement of water across a membrane depends on two factors: water "activity" and hydrostatic pressure. If the water level is higher on one side of a membrane separating two chambers, the higher hydrostatic pressure will provide a driving force (gradient) down which water will flow until hydrostatic pressure is equal on both sides of the membrane and the gradient is abolished. At this point, the concentration and, therefore, the tendency of water molecules to escape is equal on both sides of the membrane. Assuming that the membrane is freely permeable to water but not to substance "X," if substance X is added to one side of the membrane, water activity on that side will decrease. This creates a gradient that will cause a net transfer of water into the chamber containing X. The flow of water will continue until the tendency of water molecules to escape into the solution "X-water" (osmotic pressure) is balanced by the hydrostatic pressure gradient. At this point net transfer of water will again be zero (Fig. 16–1). If the membrane is freely permeable to water and to

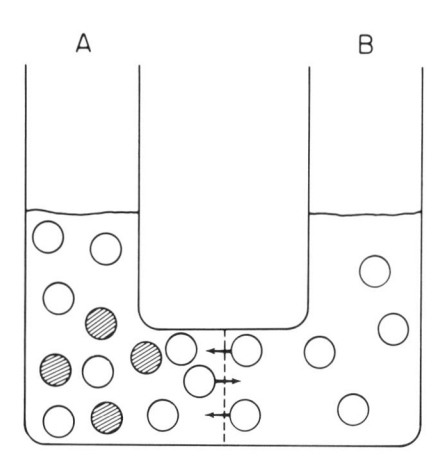

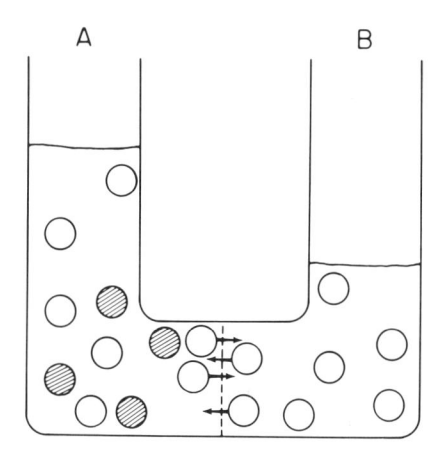

Fig. 16–1. Chambers A and B are separated by a membrane that is permeable to water but not to certain compounds. A nondiffusible compound, "X", (shaded circles) is added to chamber A. This decreases ("dilutes") the water (open circles) activity of A, i.e., it increases the osmotic pressure of A, causing a gradient for the water-escaping tendency from B to A. Thus, the net flux of water is from B to A (top figure). This continues until the escaping tendency for water from B to A is balanced by the hydrostatic pressure gradient tending to move water from A to B (bottom figure). Therefore, the oncotic pressure of a solution is equal to the hydrostatic pressure required to stop osmotic transfer of a solvent into a solution through a semipermeable membrane.

solute "Y", there will be concentration gradients for both water and Y that will rapidly disappear as Y equalizes on both sides of the membrane. In this instance, although solution Y has the colligative property of osmotic pressure, no actual pressure gradient exists across the membrane, and no net flux of water occurs.

Various water compartments in the body are separated by membranes that are freely permeable to water but are less permeable to certain compounds. These compounds are osmotically active and, along with hydrostatic pressure, determine the volume of each compartment. For example, intravascular water is separated from interstitial water by capillary endothelium. The capillary endothelium is readily permeable to small molecules (for example, water, sodium chloride, and mannitol) but is less permeable to larger molecules such as albumin. Albumin exerts osmotic pressure and draws water from interstitial fluid into the vascular bed. Interstitial water is separated from intracellular water by cell membranes that are relatively impermeable to such molecules as sodium and mannitol. Sodium and mannitol exert osmotic pressure in the extracellular space and draw intracellular water into that space. Some molecules, such as water, carbon dioxide, and hydrogen ion, easily pass through all membranes and therefore do not exert any osmotic pressures.

RENAL REGULATION OF WATER AND ELECTROLYTES

Although it is well known that juxtamedullary nephrons are essential to the formation of concentrated urine, the influence of shifts of blood flow between the cortex or medulla on salt metabolism is less certain.[10-12] Moreover, the primary actions of diuretics are on tubular function, even though some changes in renal blood flow may also occur. Therefore, this discussion focuses on diuretic actions on renal tubules (Fig. 16-2). Additionally, whereas simplified descriptions of tubular functions may not be accurate, they are useful functional models.

Urine formation begins with ultrafiltration of plasma by the glomeruli. Approximately 20% of total plasma flow is filtered and enters Bowman's capsule (capsula glomeruli) and the renal tubule. In the adult, this amounts to about 180 liters a day and contains large amounts of NaCl, $NaHCO_3$ and other essential compounds that must be reabsorbed, as well as various waste products that must be eliminated from the body.

Modification of the glomerular filtrate begins in the proximal convoluted tubule where approximately 60 to 80% of the filtrate is reabsorbed. The major fraction is reabsorbed down-gradients generated by active sodium transport. Sodium reabsorption in proximal tubules is isosmotic; that is, no concentration of urine occurs. The reabsorptive mechanism is designed to transport large volumes of salt and water against small gradients.

Sodium is actively transported out of proximal tubule cells into intercellular spaces (Fig. 16-3). This transport creates an electrical gradient that causes sodium to move from tubular fluid into the cell. Moreover, osmotic and electrochemical gradients are generated, causing water and chloride to move from tubular fluid to the intercellular space. Sodium chloride (followed by water) then diffuses either back into tubular fluid or into peritubular capillaries and is "reabsorbed." As in all other capillary beds, the amount of fluid that enters peritubular capillaries is influenced by Starling's forces. Therefore, an increase in capillary oncotic pressure favors reabsorption, whereas increased capillary hydrostatic pressure results in greater back-diffusion and less reabsorption.[13,14] Changes in oncotic pressure can occur with changes in filtration fraction and in systemic oncotic pressure.[15,16] Peritubular capillary hydrostatic pressure increases with renal perfusion pressure.[17] This may be partly respon-

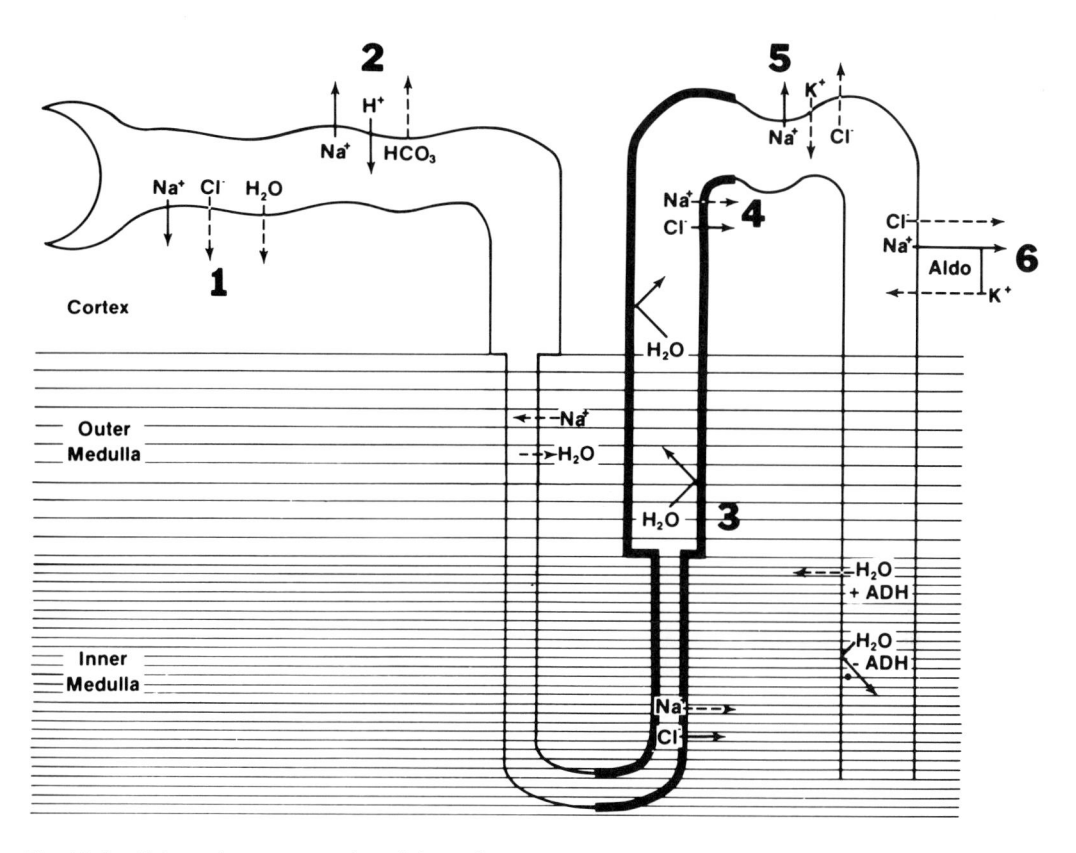

Fig. 16–2. Schematic representation of the major transport processes in the nephron. Solid arrows indicate active transport; dashed arrows indicate passive transport. Low permeability is shown as reflected arrows.

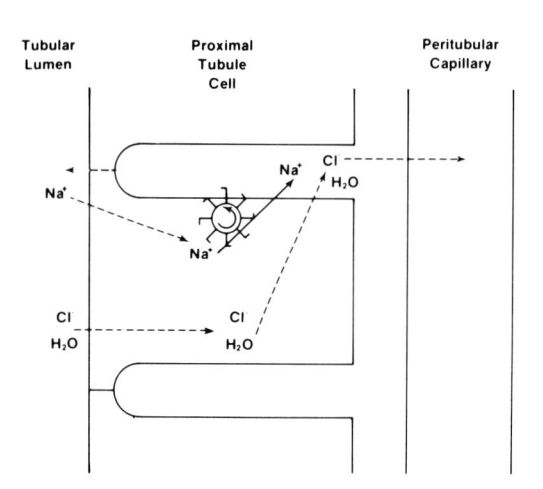

Fig. 16–3. Schematic representation of proximal tubule salt and water reabsorption.

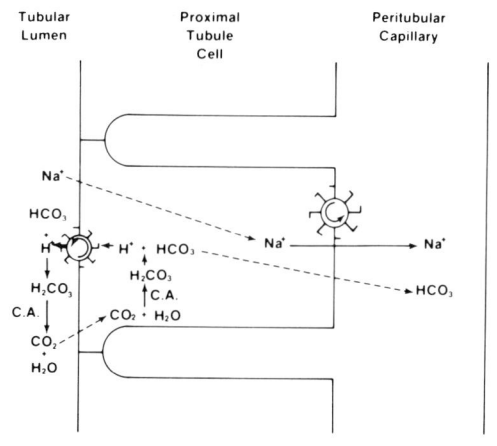

Fig. 16–4. Schematic representation of hydrogen ion secretion and bicarbonate reabsorption in the proximal tubule.

sible for the well-known phenomenon of pressure natriuresis.[18,19]

Another transport process in the proximal convoluted tubule results in the secretion of hydrogen ions and in the reabsorption of sodium bicarbonate ($NaHCO_3$). This mechanism depends on carbonic anhydrase in the brush (luminal) border (Fig. 16–4) and is designed to transport large amounts against small gradients. Sodium is actively pumped out of the cell into peritubular fluid. This creates a gradient that causes sodium to diffuse passively from tubular fluid into the cell. Intracellular hydrogen ions are actively transported into the tubular lumen.[20] The hydrogen combines with bicarbonate to form carbonic acid, which, in the presence of luminal carbonic anhydrase, is rapidly dehydrated to form carbon dioxide and water. The carbon dioxide diffuses into the cell where it rehydrates, in the presence of intracellular carbonic anhydrase, to form carbonic acid. This compound then dissociates into hydrogen ion, which is transported into the lumen, and bicarbonate, which diffuses down an electrochemical gradient into peritubular fluid.

The majority of phosphate reabsorption also occurs in proximal convoluted tubules. This is why phosphaturia has been used as an indicator of proximal tubular inhibition.[21]

Only a small portion of the filtered fluid enters the descending limb of Henle's loop. At this point the tubular fluid is still isosmotic, although its composition is considerably modified. The descending limb is permeable to water and relatively impermeable to salt.[22] Consequently, as the tubule descends into the hypertonic medullary tissue, water leaves the tubule to maintain osmotic equilibrium between tubular fluid and the interstitium. The thin ascending limb of Henle's loop is relatively impermeable to water but permeable to salt.[23] Sodium chloride passively diffuses from lumen to interstitium down a concentration gradient. This helps to maintain the high medullary interstitial osmolality and causes the concentration of tubular fluid to decrease gradually.

The thick portion of the ascending limb remains almost impermeable to water.[24,25] Chloride is actively transported out of the tubule followed passively by sodium.[24,25] Since water does not follow, this causes further reduction in tubular fluid osmolality until the fluid becomes hypotonic compared to both plasma and interstitium. The medullary portion contributes the active force for maintaining hypertonicity of medullary interstitium and therefore is the concentrating segment of the nephron. The cortical segment, which pumps chloride (and sodium), but not water, into the isotonic cortical interstitium, is the major diluting segment of the nephron.[26] (The difference in tonicity between hypertonic medullary interstitium and isotonic cortical interstitium is related to differences in blood-flow rates, the anatomic pattern of medullary circulation, and the recycling of urea. These factors are important in the concentrating mechanism but are not germane to this discussion.)

The distal convoluted tubule is also relatively impermeable to water.[27] Sodium is actively reabsorbed and potassium is passively secreted. The amount of potassium secretion is loosely related to distal sodium delivery; that is, urinary potassium secretion increases with increased distal sodium delivery and reabsorption.[28] Tubular fluid then enters the collecting duct where further sodium reabsorption and potassium secretion can occur. This process is modulated by mineralocorticoids.[27] Collecting-duct epithelium is permeable to water in the presence of antidiuretic hormone and relatively impermeable in its absence.[29] When water permeability is increased, osmotic equilibrium is attained between tubular fluid and the hypertonic medullary interstitium, and small volumes of concentrated urine are produced. In the absence of antidiuretic hormone, tubular fluid remains hypotonic and large volumes of dilute urine result.

There are other hormonal interactions besides those of antidiuretic hormone involved in the renal regulation of water and salt.[30] The stimulus for the release of the mineralocorticoid, aldosterone, on the distal tubule and collecting duct (increasing sodium reabsorption and potassium secretion) may be either direct or indirect. Catecholamines and antidiuretic hormone stimulate aldosterone secretion by the adrenal cortex. The major physiologic regulator of aldosterone secretion appears to be the renin-angiotensin system. Conditions associated with decreased fluid volumes or sodium content stimulate renin secretion. Renin is converted to a decapeptide, angiotensin I, that is subsequently converted to an octapeptide, angiotensin II. Angiotensin II is not only a potent vasoconstrictor, but also a potent stimulator of aldosterone secretion by the adrenal cortex. Aldosterone then increases sodium reabsorption by the distal tubule that results in volume expansion and decreased renin production. There is also an interplay between the renin-angiotensin system and the antidiuretic hormone system.[31] Prostaglandins may also be involved in renal salt and water homeostasis.[32] Prostaglandins E and possibly A are synthesized in the renal medulla and produce efferent arteriolar vasodilation, particularly in the inner cortical nephrons. This results in an increased glomerular filtration rate. A concomitant, but less well understood, effect on tubular mechanisms increases free water and osmolar clearance. Opposing this effect, sodium restriction in man increases plasma prostaglandin A, aldosterone, and plasma renin activity. Infusion of prostaglandin A also increases plasma renin activity and aldosterone. Thus, it appears that prostaglandins affect the regulation of salt and water homeostasis by the kidney.

SITES OF ACTION OF DIURETICS

Various methods have been employed to localize the sites of action of diuretics. These include clearances of sodium, chloride, bicarbonate, phosphate, and water; stop-flow techniques; and micropuncture, including the recently developed methods to perfuse isolated segments of renal tubules.[33] For an analysis of these methods the interested reader should consult the review by Goldberg.[34]

Osmotic Diuretics

Mannitol, a six-carbon sugar, is the prototype of osmotic diuretics and the most commonly used osmotic diuretic in clinical practice. It is distributed primarily in plasma and interstitial fluid. The initial effect of intravenous administration of mannitol is increased plasma osmolality. Intravascular and interstitial volumes then increase and intracellular volume decreases. The effects of mannitol in the kidney are complex. Increased blood volume may temporarily increase renal plasma flow. Moreover, mannitol may decrease resistance in the afferent arterioles, thereby increasing plasma flow and glomerular filtration.[35] In poorly perfused kidneys, this action on the afferent arteriole may be related to the suppression of renin release.[3] In addition, mannitol diuresis results in significant decreases in medullary interstitial osmolality, possibly secondary to increased medullary blood flow.[37,38]

Renal tubular effects of mannitol are related to its poor reabsorption. Under usual circumstances, sodium is actively reabsorbed by the proximal tubule, and water and chloride follow passively. The sodium transport mechanism is capable of transporting large amounts of sodium but can do so only against a small electrochemical gradient. The presence of a nonreabsorbable compound such as mannitol decreases water reabsorption (Fig. 16–5). Since sodium reabsorption continues in excess of water reabsorption, tubular sodium concentration decreases, eventually to a level where net transport of sodium is zero.[39] Net sodium transport is also decreased in the proximal convoluted tubule secondary

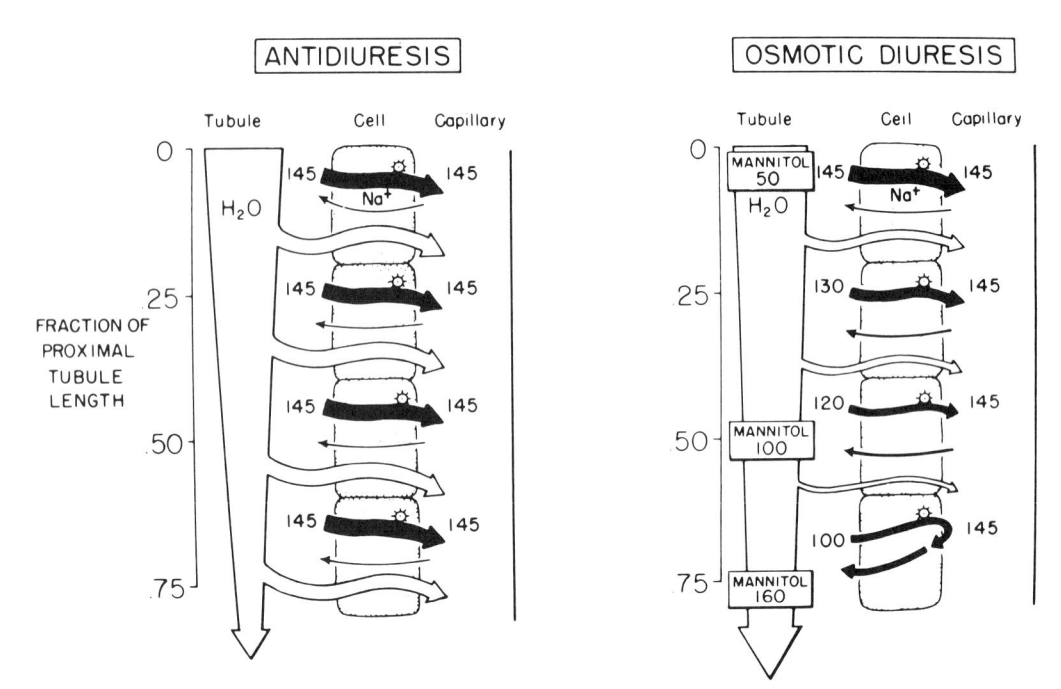

Fig. 16–5. Schematic representation of sodium and water reabsorption in the proximal tubule during antidiuresis and osmotic diuresis. During antidiuresis, the concentration of sodium in the tubular fluid does not change; during osmotic diuresis, the presence of mannitol in the filtrate (50 mmoles per liter) reduces water reabsorption. Thus tubular-fluid sodium concentration falls progressively as sodium reabsorption proceeds.(From Gennari, F.J., and Kassier, J.P.: Osmotic diuresis. N. Engl. J. Med., 291:715, 1974.)

to decreased oncotic pressure in peritubular capillaries.[40]

An even greater effect of hypertonic mannitol on salt transport occurs in the loop of Henle. This results from a combination of the intratubular osmotic effect and the washout of the high medullary interstitial osmolality.[41] Decreased salt and water reabsorption by the loop of Henle is probably the major component of the action of mannitol and other osmotic diuretics.

Other clinically useful osmotic diuretics include urea and glycerol. Anesthesiologists should also be aware that glucose in the urine (that is, filtered glucose load that exceeds glucose reabsorptive capacity) can produce an osmotic diuresis. Moreover, contrast material used for angiography may cause osmotic diuresis if given in high doses or if injected directly into a renal artery.[39]

Osmotic diuretics are used most commonly to "protect" the kidneys against acute renal failure (for example, in transfusion reactions or in high renal risk surgical patients), to evaluate the cause of oliguria, and to reduce intracranial pressure.[6-9] Mannitol may be useful in the treatment of myocardial ischemia by decreasing cellular edema.[42]

One predictable side effect of osmotic diuretics is increased extracellular fluid volume, which may be disastrous in patients with impending pulmonary edema. If large doses of osmotic diuretics are administered to a patient who is unable to excrete them, severe plasma hyperosmolality may ensue. If a brisk diuresis does occur, it may cause severe electrolyte disturbances and loss of water.

Acid-forming Salts

Ammonium chloride is the most commonly used acidifying salt. The administration of ammonium chloride results in hyperchloremic metabolic acidosis. With increased chloride delivery to the tubules, less chloride is reabsorbed and therefore less is excreted along with an equivalent amount of cation (sodium and potassium) and water. Over a period of 1 or 2 days, renal compensatory processes against acidosis result in the excretion of chloride with ammonium ion, and the diuretic effect is lost. Thus the usefulness of acidifying salts as sole diuretics is limited. They are used most commonly to compensate for alkalosis produced by other diuretics. Severe acidosis may occur in patients whose renal function is impaired. The use of ammonium chloride is contraindicated in patients with hepatic failure.[43]

Carbonic Anhydrase Inhibitors

Acetazolamide produces noncompetitive inhibition of carbonic anhydrase. Renal effects of acetazolamide include decreased glomerular filtration rate and urinary loss of bicarbonate, phosphate, and potassium that results in hypokalemic metabolic acidosis.[44-46] As acidosis becomes more pronounced, the effectiveness of acetazolamide is diminished. Phosphaturia and fractional excretion of bicarbonate exceeding 20% of the filtered load suggest that the primary site of action is the proximal tubule,[29] although distal delivery of excess bicarbonate is responsible for urinary potassium loss.[47] In high doses, acetazolamide may cause drowsiness and paresthesias and may disorient patients with cirrhosis.[43]

Acetazolamide is used to reduce intraocular pressure, to alkalinize the urine, and to treat edema, periodic paralysis, and convulsive disorders.[43] Sulfamylon, used to treat burns, is also a carbonic anhydrase inhibitor.[48]

Mercurial Diuretics

Mercurial diuretics are the oldest potent diuretics. They appear to affect proximal tubular transport mechanisms, but their major action is to interfere with chloride transport in the thick ascending limb of the loop of Henle.[49] Distal tubular effects are variable; if potassium secretion is high (for example, in a potassium-loaded patient), it is reduced, whereas in cases of potassium depletion where excretion is initially low, potassium losses are augmented.[50,51] With the repeated administration of mercurial diuretics, a hypochloremic alkalosis eventually develops. When this occurs, these agents become less effective.[52]

Mercurial diuretics are used primarily to treat edema. General side effects, related to chloride loss in excess of sodium loss, are fluid deficits and metabolic alkalosis. Toxic effects include mercury poisoning, bone marrow depression, and, rarely, fatal dysrhythmias.[43]

Thiazides

Thiazides appear to decrease glomerular filtration rate even in the absence of decreased blood volume.[34] These drugs are secreted by proximal tubules as organic acids.[53] Probenecid, a competitive inhibitor of organic acid transport, can block the effect of minimal doses of thiazides but not that of large doses.[34] This suggests that the tubular fluid concentration of drug is an important determinant of activity. The proximal tubular effects of thiazides are variable and related to the degree of carbonic anhydrase inhibition caused by different compounds.[54] The main site of action is in the cortical diluting segment, where chloride transport is inhibited.[55,56] This inhibition results in diluting effects and in increased distal delivery of salt and water. Increased distal delivery of sodium augments potassium secretion.

Thus the consequences of prolonged thiazide administration include increased urinary losses of water, sodium, chloride, potassium, and some loss of bicarbonate. These losses can cause hypochloremic, hypokalemic metabolic alkalosis. In addition, thiazide administration may cause hyperuricemia, bone marrow depression, and dermatitis with photosensitivity.[43] Thiazide diuretics are used to treat edema, hypertension, and diabetes insipidus.[2]

Loop Diuretics

Ethacrynic acid and furosemide are the most potent diuretics available. Although chemically different, their actions are similar, except that furosemide is a mild inhibitor of carbonic anhydrase. Both drugs are protein-bound and are secreted into the proximal tubules by organic acid transport.[57,58] In low doses, furosemide inhibits proximal reabsorption of bicarbonate.[59] In high doses, both drugs appear to decrease proximal reabsorption of sodium. A new loop diuretic, Bumetanide, has recently been approved for use in the United States. Except for increased potency (40×) and oral bioavailability (80%), the drug appears to produce effects which are indistinguishable from furosemide.[59a]

The major effect of these agents is to inhibit active chloride transport along the length of the ascending limb of the loop of Henle.[60,61] Far smaller concentrations are effective on the luminal side of the tubular membrane than on the capillary side. Consequently, any interference in tubular secretion of the drugs could affect the diuretic response. Tubular action interferes with both concentrating and diluting capacities and results in the excretion of an almost isotonic urine. Recent evidence suggests that the action of furosemide and ethacrynic acid may be involved with renal prostaglandins. Administration of the potent inhibitor of prostaglandin synthesis, indomethacin, has resulted in an inhibited increase in renal blood flow produced by both drugs.[62,63] Consequently, the increase may be a result of prostaglandin effect on renal arterioles. Indomethacin also decreases the natriuretic effect of furosemide in man.[64,65] Since this effect was not seen in dogs, the interaction is not certain. The increased distal delivery of salt and water increases potassium secretion.[66,67]

These renal effects may result in the contraction of extracellular fluid volume, and hypochloremic, hypokalemic metabolic alkalosis. Other effects include hyperuricemia, deafness, and hepatic dysfunction.[68,69] These drugs are used primarily to treat fluid retention and oliguria.

Ethacrynic acid and furosemide can cause severe electrolyte disturbances if replacement therapy is not carefully carried out.

Potassium-sparing Diuretics

Included in this group of distally acting drugs are spironolactone, triamterene, and amiloride. Although the effect of these drugs is mild natriuresis and decreased potassium excretion, each agent acts differently.[34] Spironolactone is an aldosterone antagonist and is effective only when aldosterone is present and affects potassium secretion.[70] Triamterene and amiloride block potassium secretion unrelated to aldosterone.[71,72]

Potassium-sparing diuretics are used as a second drug, along with more proximal-acting diuretics, in treating refractory edema with potassium loss. Hyperkalemia may result from the use of these diuretics.

Figure 16–6 provides a summary of the site of various diuretics.

DIURETIC-DRUG INTERACTION

Drug interaction with diuretics can be divided into two categories: the first group is related to the desired effect of the diuretic therapy, that is, the increased excretion of salt and water. The potent diuretics interfere with normal salt and water regulation. Consequently, patients may develop both volume and electrolyte abnormalities that may change pharmacologic response to other drugs. The second group of drug interactions involves specific and subtle effects of the diuretic drugs. In most cases undesirable side effects are involved, although sometimes the combination may be advantageous (for example, in antihypertensive therapy).

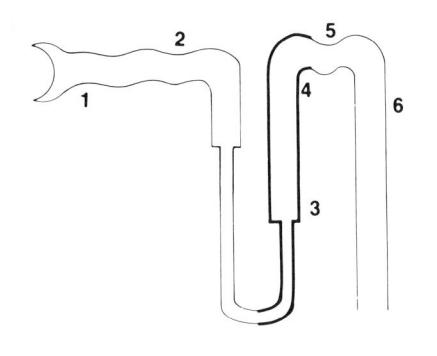

	Site					
Diuretic	1	2	3	4	5	6
Mannitol	(+)		+	(+)	(+)	
Acetazolamide		+			(+)	
Mercurial Diuretics	(+)		+	(+)		(+)
Thiazide Diuretics		(+)		+	(+)	
Ethacrynic acid	(+)		+	(+)	(+)	
Furosemide	(+)	(+)	+	(+)	(+)	
Spironolactone						+
Triamterene					+	
Amiloride					+	

+ = major (+) = minor actions

Fig. 16–6. Sites of action of diuretics.

Interactions From the Deranged Salt and Water Regulation

Digitalis. The following case report illustrates the interaction between digitalis and diuretics in combination with a high intake of potassium.

CASE REPORT

A 75-year-old man was admitted to a hospital emergency department with an incarcerated left inguinal hernia. In addition to a painful inguinal mass, he also complained of shortness of breath and reported episodes of fainting. The patient was known to have chronic rheumatic valvular disease involving the aortic and mitral valves. He had been seen regularly as an outpatient and had been in stable condition and adequately compensated until the day of admission. He had been treated with a low-sodium diet, digoxin, and spironolactone (Aldactone), 100 mg daily. On admission, the patient appeared lethargic and weak. His breathing was labored. His systemic arterial blood pressure was 90 mm Hg systolic and his radial pulse was faint and regular at a rate of 12 to 15 beats per minute. The patient's jugular venous pressure was moderately elevated and basilar crepitant rales were heard bilaterally. The cardiac apical impulse was displaced to the left anterior axillary line and down to the sixth intercostal space. Murmurs of aortic and mitral regurgitation were heard. The patient's extremities were free of edema. There was a firm tender mass in the left inguinal region, bowel sounds were hypoactive, and the abdomen was soft but slightly tender. The electrocardiogram taken on admission demonstrated atrial arrest with an idioventricular rhythm at a rate of 12 per minute. Laboratory determinations were as follows: Serum potassium, 7.8 mEq/L; serum sodium, 119 mEq/L; BUN, 57 mg/100 ml; creatinine, 1.8 mg/100 ml. A transvenous right ventricular endocardial pacing electrode was inserted immediately after the electrocardiogram was taken and capture was effected at a pacemaker output of 0.6 milliamperes. Immediate improvement in the patient's hemodynamic and clinical status was observed as soon as his heart rate was restored to 70 beats per minute. After premedication with diazepam (Valium), 10 mg, the patient was taken to the operating room, where a hyperbaric spinal anaesthetic was administered using tetracaine, 10 mg. After an analgesic level to the sixth thoracic dermatome was achieved, an uneventful herniorrhaphy was accomplished. The patient was taken to the surgical intensive care unit for hyperkalemia where a potassium-exchange resin lowered his serum potassium level to normal value within 24 hours. The patient's heart then resumed its previous rhythm, which had been a chronic atrial tachycardia and AV dissociation with a junctional rhythm and a ventricular rate of 70 beats per minute. The patient's sudden clinical deterioration and the development of severe hyperkalemia were puzzling until his wife told us that he had been liberally using a commercially available salt substitute for several days prior to admission. This salt substitute was composed predominantely of potassium salts, particularly potassium chloride.

In the case report that introduced this chapter, the combination of cirrhosis, diuretics, alcoholism, and digitalis produced cardiovascular collapse as a result of *hypo*kalemia. Here the combination of diuretics, digitalis, and high potassium intake resulted in cardiovascular collapse due to *hyper*kalemia. The latter case emphasizes the importance of knowing what type of diuretic the patient is taking. The potassium-sparing diuretics are used to prevent hypokalemia and, hence, digitalis toxicity in patients who take both digitalis and diuretics. However, digitalis may prevent skeletal muscle from serving as the normal sink for potassium. Tissue hypoxia from congestive heart failure may actually mobilize potassium from body stores. Thus it is possible, particularly with an increased potassium intake, that the effect on serum potassium opposite from that desired may occur.[73] In this case a temporary transvenous pacemaker produced an acceptable cardiovascular system for the emergency operation. However, this may not always be the case.

CASE REPORT

A 76-year-old woman was admitted to the hospital with the chief complaints of weakness and syncope. One year before, she had been subjected to the insertion of a permanent demand pacemaker because of "sick sinus" syndrome and second degree AV block. During the next year, the patient developed shortness of breath and orthopnea, and she was placed on furosemide 10 mg t.i.d. with supplemental enteric-coated potassium chloride. Her symptoms of congestive heart failure progressed over the next several months and she was placed on digoxin. Shortly after this, five days prior to hospital admission, her diuretic therapy was changed to Dyazide (hydrochlorothiazide and triamterene). The patient continued to take potassium chloride. On examination, her pulse was found to be slow and she complained of weakness. An electrocardiogram showed regular pacemaker spikes at a constant rate, but most of the impulses failed to stimulate the ventricles that were contracting independently at a rate of approximately 30 beats per minute. Her serum potassium level was 6.9 mEq/L; sodium level, 135 mEq/L; chloride level 101 mEq/L; and BUN 135 mg/100 ml. The patient was admitted to the medical intensive care unit where the hyperkalemia was treated with sodium bicarbonate, glucose, and insulin. Triamterene was discontinued. Within 48 hours, the serum potassium concentration had declined to 4.6 mEq/L. Pacemaker capture was maintained after the drug therapy was discontinued; the atrial rhythm reverted to fibrillation with marked atrioventricular block.[74]

Thus there are times when the effect of hyperkalemia on normal cardiac rhythm may not respond to artificial pacing because of a change in the pacing threshold. This is a particular problem in the case of a permanently implanted pacemaker where current strength cannot be adjusted. These three case reports indicate that the interaction of diuretics and digitalis may produce severe alterations in cardiac function from more than one mechanism. Careful attention to electrolyte status, especially potassium, is mandatory in these patients.

The problem must be corrected before anesthesia and operation are performed, if abnormalities are detected.

Anesthetics. Evidence for the interactions between anesthetics and diuretics is theoretical and anecdotal. Certainly, patients whose fluid volume has been depleted by overzealous diuretic therapy will be prime candidates for cardiovascular collapse when potent anesthetics that cardiodepress, vasodilate, and adrenergically block are administered. Similarly, substantial sympathetic blockade from a regional anesthetic will be poorly tolerated. Although there is experimental evidence to suggest that some general anesthetics protect the heart from the dysrhythmias of digitalis intoxication, there have been no clinical reports.[75,76] Most anesthesiologists can recall a case with cardiac complications (hypotension, dysrhythmia), when a patient with unknown hypokalemia was anesthetized. As documented with digitalis, the other extreme can be just as dangerous, since hyperkalemia can also result in cardiovascular collapse.[77] The obvious conclusion is that one should carefully assess the state of hydration and electrolyte balance in patients who take diuretics on a regular basis before administering an anesthetic. Judicious correction of an imbalance of either condition may require considerable time, particularly in a patient with a compromised cardiovascular system.

Neuromuscular Blocking Drugs. As in the case of anesthetics, the fluid-depleted patient may respond with exaggerated hypotension to a large dose of d-tubocurare. However, the important interactions between neuromuscular blocking drugs and diuretics involve the potassium ion again. Theoretically, the hypokalemic patient may have reduced skeletal muscle function.[78] Consequently, great care is advised in administering neuromuscular blocking drugs to these patients. The patient with hyperkalemia may be an even greater risk. The administration of succinylcholine to patients with renal failure and a high serum potassium has been associated with dangerous dysrhythmias and with cardiac arrest.[79] Because of this, the risk to the patient who is receiving the potassium-sparing diuretics (spironolactone and triamterene) and whose potassium intake is above normal may be especially high. Again, it is the responsibility of the anesthesiologist to ascertain the fluid and electrolyte (particularly potassium) status of patients taking diuretics before giving a neuromuscular blocking drug. In hyperkalemic patients, succinylcholine is best avoided. In patients with hypokalemia, nondepolarizing neuromuscular blockers should be carefully titrated.

Specific Interactions: Beneficial Effects

Diuretic-Antihypertensive Drugs. Because the thiazides are mildly antihypertensive, probably by means of direct vasodilating activity, smaller doses of more potent antihypertensives such as reserpine, guanethidine, *alpha*-methyldopa, minoxidil, and clonidine are often effective.[80] Conversely, the usual doses of these drugs may cause unwanted hypotension. The decrease in intravascular volume produced by potent diuretics may trigger reflex tachycardia, which can be effectively prevented by small doses of the *beta*-adrenergic blocking drug propranolol.[81]

Specific Interactions: Modification of Dose Effect

Furosemide-Anticonvulsant Therapy. The diuretic response to oral and intravenous furosemide is blunted in patients with seizure disorders who are taking phenytoin (diphenylhydantoin) and phenobarbital.[82] This may be due to the stimulation of membrane transport of sodium by these drugs.

Furosemide-Indomethacin. The prostaglandin synthetase inhibitor, indomethacin, appears to decrease the diuretic response of patients to furosemide.[65,66] This decrease is probably related to the role of the intrarenal prostaglandins in sodium and water regulation discussed previously.

Spironolactone-Acetylsalicylic Acid (Aspirin). Aspirin decreases the diuretic response to spironolactone by a mechanism that is unknown at this time.[83]

Furosemide-d-Tubocurarine. Furosemide given after d-tubocurarine enhanced the neuromuscular blockade produced in three patients with chronic renal failure.[84] *In-vitro* and intact animal experiments suggest that the interaction may be at the motor-nerve terminal, but the significance for patients with normal renal function is not established (see Chap. 23).

Diuretics-Lithium. The loop diuretics (furosemide and ethacrynic acid) decrease the tubular reabsorption of sodium and conversely increase the tubular reabsorption of lithium.[85] Consequently, serum levels of lithium increase and acute toxicity may be produced if the dosage is not reduced (see Chap. 19).

Spironolactone-Digitalis. Spironolactone appears to decrease the serum half-life of digitoxin and to increase the excretion of its metabolites, probably through enzyme induction.[86] On the other hand, spironolactone has been shown to decrease renal excretion and to increase the plasma levels of digoxin.[87] A recent study confirmed the action of spironolactone to decrease digoxin excretion and increase plasma levels.[87a] Triamterene had no appreciable interaction, but amiloride increased digoxin excretion and lowered plasma levels. Furosemide does not affect the pharmacokinetics of digoxin in man.[88]

Ethacrynic Acid-Warfarin. Both enhancement of and interference with the anticoagulant effect of warfarin have been reported with ethacrynic acid.[89,90] Therefore, careful monitoring of the clotting status of a patient is necessary when diuretics and Coumadin are administered concurrently.

Thiazide Diuretics—Chlorpropamide. The thiazide diuretics possess a weak diabetogenic action (most potent in the hypotensive agent diazoxide, which is not a diuretic). Consequently, diabetes, particularly in those patients who control the disease by diet alone or by oral hypoglycemic drugs, may be exacerbated by the initiation of diuretic therapy.[91]

Thiazide Diuretics—Probenecid. Thiazide diuretics cause the retention of uric acid and can cause a flare-up of gouty arthritis even in patients taking probenecid.[92] In addition, the effects of anesthesia and surgery may also decrease uric acid excretion.[93] Consequently, patients with gout must be carefully followed if diuretics and anesthetics are being used.

Specific Interactions: Toxic Effects

Ethacrynic Acid and Aminoglycoside Antibiotics. Both ethacrynic acid and aminoglycoside antibiotics can cause deafness with prolonged high-dose therapy. The combination in lower doses of each drug has also resulted in this complication.[94] This is particularly likely to happen to patients with renal failure.

Furosemide-Cephalosporin. The renal toxicity of cephalosporin may be enhanced by simultaneous furosemide administration.[95]

CLINICAL IMPLICATIONS OF DIURETIC-DRUG INTERACTIONS

Deranged Salt and Water Regulation

Clearly, the interactions most important for the anesthesiologist between diuretics and other drugs involve the predictable effect of diuresis on salt and water homeostasis.

The state of the circulating blood volume of all patients who take diuretics regularly and who are scheduled for anesthesia and operations should be carefully evaluated. Although isotopic measurements are ideal, obviously, this is impractical. Clinically, the most important signs are the response of the blood pressure and heart rate to maneuvers that decrease venous return, such as rapid change from the supine to the upright position or a Valsalva maneuver. A decrease in blood pressure of more than 15% and/or an increase in heart rate of more than 25% should arouse suspicion. A decrease in skin turgor or in ocular tension is a good indicator in children, but if present, indicates significant hypovolemia.[96] "Furrowing" of the tongue also suggests a decrease in extracellular fluid volume. A valuable sign of adequate circulating blood volume is an increase in the volume of urine with a fluid challenge. Laboratory indications of hemoconcentration (increased hematocrit, BUN, sodium, chloride) may corroborate the suspicion of hypovolemia. Low central or pulmonary artery occluded ("wedge") pressure are valuable confirmatory signs.

In patients without significant cardiac or renal disease, fluid deficits can usually be easily corrected overnight by the infusion of electrolyte solutions appropriate to the patient's status. However, most patients who take diuretics on a regular basis will have cardiac or renal disease. For elective surgery, a day or two of careful replacement, using blood and *urinary* electrolyte measurements as a guide, may be necessary. Urinary electrolyte measurement indicates the kidney's response to the body deficit (or surplus) and helps to guide replacement therapy. Patients who are scheduled for emergency operations will need faster correction. This may be safely accomplished by careful monitoring of blood pressure, heart rate, urine output, and at least central venous pressure, but preferably pulmonary artery occluded pressure. For both anesthetic and neuromuscular blocking drug use, an adequate circulating blood volume is essential.

A second important aspect of the derangement of homeostasis is the state of body potassium.

CASE REPORT

A 46-year-old obese woman was admitted to the hospital with a history of fat intolerance and episodic cramping epigastric pain. An oral cholecystogram showed poor visualization and small radiolucent stones. She had been taking "water pills" for several years because of ankle edema, but was told that her heart was "O.K." She was admitted for cholecystectomy and possible common duct exploration. At the time of the preanesthetic visit, no blood had been taken for electrolyte determination. Aside from obesity (weight–84 kg, height–160 cm) and mild hypertension, the patient's history and physical examination were unremarkable. Properly, the anesthesiologist insisted on knowing the serum electrolyte concentration. On arrival in the operating room the next morning, he was informed that the electrolytes were: Na 132 mEq/L, Cl 98 mEq/L, K 2.8 mEq/L, CO_2 23 mEq/L. An SMA–12 was within normal limits. The surgeon was anxious to proceed with the operation and cited possible common duct obstruction as the reason.

Hypokalemia is more common than hyperkalemia in chronic diuretic therapy. Although hypokalemia can cause renal concentrating defects, its effects on nerve and muscle activity are more important to the anesthesiologist. These include: paralytic ileus, severe weakness or flaccid paralysis, hypotension, atrial and ventricular dysrhythmias, and potentiation of digitalis toxicity.[97] Serum potassium levels are not reliable indicators of total body potassium. Nevertheless, serum potassium concentration is the only clinical indicator of potassium stores. It has been claimed that a serum potassium concentration of 3 mEq/L implies a 200 to 400 mEq deficit and that below 3 mEq/L, each 1 mEq/L decrease in serum potassium indicates an additional 200 to 400 mEq loss.[98,99] Therefore, in the patient discussed in this last case report, one should suspect a potassium deficit of at least 200 mEq. There is little scientific basis for setting a lowest acceptable level of serum potassium. We believe that it is reasonable, however, until proven otherwise, to suggest a minimum level of 3.0 mEq/L in patients who are not digitalized and of 3.5 mEq/L in patients who are.

Elective operations and anesthesia should be delayed until acceptable potassium levels are attained by oral potassium chloride replacement and/or by the addition of potassium-sparing diuretics to the therapeutic regimen. In the case of an emergency operation, intravenous potassium chloride can be administered. In our patient, the operation was not an emergency. Without evidence of bile duct obstruction (normal SMA-12), it is prudent to proceed cautiously with potassium replacement. The rate of replacement should not exceed 40 mEq/hr, and the concentration should not exceed 40 mEq/L unless continuous electrocardiographic monitoring is performed. Hyperkalemia can result if the potassium-containing solution is infused too rapidly or if potassium chloride is added to solutions in flexible plastic bags without careful mixing.[100,101] Consequently, at least five hours of intravenous potassium therapy would be necessary to bring the patient back in balance. One must be careful to avoid respiratory or metabolic alkalosis in hypokalemic patients, so as to prevent the intracellular movement of potassium and the further decrease in extracellular potassium. Glucose, insulin, and bicarbonate solutions, even if they contain potassium, can drive potassium intracellularly and can potentiate hypokalemia. Therefore these solutions must be administered with caution.[102] There is considerable evidence that the sympathetic nervous system also regulates the extra-intracellular potassium ratio. Beta-2 agonism causes increased muscle uptake of potassium with a resultant decrease in serum potassium.[102a] Beta-adrenergic blocking drugs can decrease intracellular potassium by blocking this effect.[102b] This potentiation can be especially hazardous if the patient is digitalized.

Recently, considerable debate about the importance of diuretic induced hypokalemia has surfaced.[102c] Harrington, et al. could find little evidence to support the common practice of administering supplemental potassium with chronic diuretic therapy except for those patients with congestive heart failure, refractory edema or low sodium diets.[102d] Dyckner and Wester reported that hypomagnesemia was a more important factor in producing cardiac dysrhythmias than hypokalemia in a group of patients with either congestive heart failure or hypertension being treated with diuretics.[102e] In abstract form only, Vitez and colleagues found no correlation between serum potassium levels and perioperative dysrhythmias (24-hour Holter monitoring) in 38 normokalemic, 25 moderately hypokalemic (3.4 to 3.0 mEq/L) and 10 severely hypokalemic (<3.0 mEq/L) surgical patients.[102f] On the other hand, Hollifield and Slaton reported a definite relationship between hypokalemia and dysrhythmias in hypertensive patients treated with hydrochlorthiazide. In addition, higher diuretic doses decrease serum potassium more and produce more dysrhythmias.[102g] Poole-Wilson was disturbed by the nihilist attitude toward hypokalemia and advocated the use of potassium sparing diuretics and beta-adrenergic blocking drugs together with chronic administration of diuretics.[102h] Except for the unpublished study of Vitez, et al., however, none of these reports addressed the problem of preparing the patient on chronic diuretic therapy with hypokalemia for surgery. Until definitive work on that subject appears, we still hold to our recommendations as noted in the preceding section.

Hyperkalemia can cause ascending muscular weakness, myocardial conduction defects, ventricular dysrhythmias, and ileus.[103] Elective operations and anesthesia should not be performed on a patient who is hyperkalemic, but rather should be delayed until normal serum potassium levels can be obtained by appropriate means. In a patient with normal renal function, this can usually be accomplished by decreasing the potassium intake and/or by withholding potassium-sparing diuretics. In patients with renal failure, it may be necessary to use ion exchange resins, peritoneal- or hemodialysis, or some of the regimens outlined in the next paragraph.

Hyperkalemic patients admitted to a hospital for an emergency operation must be treated more aggressively. Serum potassium levels can be lowered by the intravenous administration of 10% calcium gluconate, 20 or 30 ml; by the correction of any existing metabolic acidosis with sodium bicarbonate; or by the administration of a combination of regular insulin, 15 units, with glucose, 50 grams. There is insufficient information pertaining to a safe upper limit for serum potassium levels. A review of anesthetics in 33 patients with chronic renal failure described cardiac arrests in two patients in whom preoperative potassium levels had been greater than 5.5 mEq/L.[77] On this basis, 5.5 mEq/L serum potassium was recommended as the highest acceptable level. One should remember that acidosis, depolarizing muscle relaxants, and certain sympathomimetic amines can increase serum potassium slightly.[79,104]

Untoward effects of digitalis, anesthetics, and neuromuscular blocking drugs are minimized by careful attention to potassium balance in patients who take diuretic drugs.

Types of Interactions

In general, the awareness that there are drug interactions between diuretics and the drugs mentioned under this category is the most important factor. Puzzling preoperative symptoms in patients (for example, disorientation from lithium toxicity) can be explained. Poor control of diabetes or gout might be anticipated. Patients who take anticoagulants should be carefully evaluated prior to anesthesia and operation regardless of the drugs that they take, but poor control is more understandable in patients taking diuretics. The hypertensive patient who is subject to combined drug therapy may be more sensitive to cardiodepressant anesthetics. It is important to be certain that these patients are adequately hydrated.

Some specific interactions are important in the intraoperative management of patients. Larger doses of a diuretic may be necessary for acute effects in patients taking anticonvulsant or anti-inflammatory (aspirin, indomethacin) agents. Careful attention to the degree of neuromuscular blockade is necessary when diuretics are given, at least in patients with renal failure. Finally, the toxicity of aminoglycoside antibiotics may be increased, and perhaps another drug should be substituted if the patient is receiving or needs to receive a diuretic.

As in most phases of the practice of anesthesiology, knowledge of the pharmacology and physiology involved in each case will allow physicians to provide optimal management of their patients.

REFERENCES

1. Frazier, H.S., and Yager, H.: The clinical use of diuretics. N. Engl. J. Med., *288*:246, 455, 1973.
2. Gifford, R.W.: A guide to the practical use of diuretics. J.A.M.A., *235*:1890, 1976.
3. Martinez-Maldonado, M., Eknoyan, G., and Suki, W.N.: Diuretics in nonedematous states. Arch. Intern. Med., *131*:797, 1973.
4. Early, L.E., and Orloff, J.: The mechanism of antidiuresis associated with the administration of hydrochlorothiazide to patients with vasopressin-resistant diabetes insipidus. J. Clin. Invest., *41*:1988, 1962.
5. Suki, W.N., et al.: Acute treatment of hypercalcemia with furosemide. N. Engl. J. Med., *283*:836, 1970.
6. Michenfelder, J.C., Gronert, G.A., and Rehder, K.: Neuroanesthesia. Anesthesiology, *30*:65, 1969.
7. Barry, K.G., et al.: Mannitol infusion II: The prevention of acute renal failure during resection of an aneurysm of the abdominal aorta. N. Engl. J. Med., *264*:967, 1961.
8. Barry, K.G.: Post-traumatic renal shutdown in humans: its prevention and treatment by the intravenous infusion of mannitol. Milit. Med., *128*:224, 1963.
9. Franklin, S.S., and Maxwell, M.H.: Acute renal failure. In Clinical Disorders of Fluid and Electrolyte Metabolism. Edited by M.H. Maxwell and C. R. Kleeman. New York, McGraw-Hill, 1972.
10. O'Dell, R., and Schmidt-Nielsen, B.: Concentrating ability and kidney structure. Fed. Proc., *19*:366, 1960.
11. Barger, A.C.: Renal hemodynamic factors in congestive heart failure. Ann. N.Y. Acad. Sci., *139*:276, 1966.
12. Stein, J.H.: The renal circulation. In The Kidney. Edited by B.M. Brenner and F.C. Rector, Jr. Philadelphia, W.B. Saunders, 1976.
13. Daugharty, T.M., et al.: Interrelationship of physical factors affecting sodium reabsorption in the dog. Am. J. Physiol., *215*:1442, 1968.
14. Grandchamp, A., and Boulpaep, E.L.: Pressure control of sodium reabsorption and intracellular backflux across proximal kidney tubule. J. Clin. Invest., *54*:69, 1974.
15. Brenner, B.M., et al.: Quantitative importance of changes in postglomerular colloid osmotic pressure in mediating glomerulotubular balance in the rat. J. Clin. Invest., *52*:190, 1973.
16. Martino, J.A., and Earley, L.E.: Demonstration of role of physical factors as determinants of natriuretic response to volume expansion. J. Clin. Invest., *46*:1963, 1967.
17. DiBona, G.F., Kaloyanides, G.J., and Bastron, R.D.: Effect of increased perfusion pressure on proximal tubular re-absorption in an isolated kidney. Proc. Soc. Exp. Biol. Med., *143*:830, 1973.
18. Starling, E.H., and Verney, E.B.: The secretion of urine as studied in the isolated kidney. Proc. R. Soc. Lond. [Biol.], *97*:321, 1925.
19. Martino, J.A., and Earley, L.E.: Relationship between intrarenal hydrostatic pressure and hemodynamically induced changes in sodium excretion. Circ. Res., *23*:371, 1968.
20. Rector, F.C., Jr., Carter, N.W., and Seldin, D.W.: The mechanism of bicarbonate reabsorption in the proximal and distal tubules of the kidney. J. Clin. Invest., *44*:278, 1965.
21. Strickler, J.C., et al.: Micropuncture study in inorganic phosphate excretion in the rat. J. Clin. Invest., *43*:1596, 1964.
22. Kokko, J.P.: Sodium chloride and water transport in the descending limb of Henle. J. Clin. Invest., *49*:1838, 1970.
23. Imai, M., and Kokko, J.P.: Sodium chloride, urea and water transport in thin ascending limb of Henle. Generation of osmotic gradients by passive diffusion of solutes. J. Clin. Invest., *53*:393, 1974.
24. Burg, M.B., et al.: Furosemide effect on isolated perfused tubules. Am. J. Physiol., *225*:119, 1973.
25. Rocha, A.S., and Kokko, J.P.: Sodium chloride and water transport in the medullary thick ascending limb of Henle. Evidence for active chloride transport. J. Clin. Invest., *52*:612, 1973.
26. Burg, M.B.: Renal chloride transport and diuretics (Editorial). Circulation, *53*:587, 1976.
27. Gross, J.B., Imai, M., and Kokko, J.P.: A functional comparison of the cortical collecting tubule and the distal convoluted tubule. J. Clin. Invest., *55*:1284, 1975.
28. Giesbisch, G.: Functional organization of proximal and distal tubular electrolyte transport. Nephron, *6*:260, 1969.
29. Gottschalk, C.W.: Micropuncture studies of tubular function in the mammalian kidney. Physiologist, *4*:35, 1961.
30. Papper, S.: Sodium and water: an overview. Am. J. Med. Sci., *272*:43, 1976.
31. Schrier, R.W., and Berl, T.: Nonosmolar factors affecting renal water excretion. N. Engl. J. Med., *292*:81, 1975.
32. Lee, J.B., Patek, R.V., and Mookerjee, B.K.: Renal prostaglandins and the regulation of blood pressure and sodium and water homeostasis. Am. J. Med., *60*:798, 1976.
33. Burg, M.B., et al.: Preparation and study of frag-

ments of single rabbit nephrons. Am. J. Physiol., 210:1293, 1966.
34. Goldberg, M.: The renal physiology of diuretics. In Renal Physiology. Handbook of Physiology, Section 8. Edited by J. Orloff and R.W. Berliner. Washington, D.C., American Physiological Society, 1973.
35. Flores, J., et al.: The role of cell swelling in ischemic renal damage and the protective effect of hypertonic solute. J. Clin. Invest., 51:118, 1972.
36. Morris, C.R., et al.: Restoration and maintenance of glomerular filtration by mannitol during hypoperfusion of the kidney. J. Clin. Invest., 51:1555, 1972.
37. Goldberg, M., and Ramirez, M.A.: Effects of saline and mannitol diuresis on the renal concentrating mechanisms in dogs: alterations in renal tissue solutes and water. Clin. Sci., 32:475, 1967.
38. Thurau, K.: Renal hemodynamics. Am. J. Med., 36:698, 1964.
39. Gennari, F.J., and Kassirer, J.P.: Osmotic diuresis. N. Engl. J. Med., 291:714, 1974.
40. Blantz, R.C.: Effect of mannitol on glomerular ultrafiltration in the hydropenic rat. J. Clin. Invest., 54:1135, 1974.
41. Seely, J.F., and Dirks, J.H.: Micropuncture study of hypertonic mannitol diuresis in the proximal and distal tubule of dog kidney. J. Clin. Invest., 48:2330, 1969.
42. Willerson, J.T., et al.: Influence of hypertonic mannitol on ventricular performance and coronary blood flow in patients. Circulation, 51:1095, 1975.
43. Mudge, G.H.: Drugs affecting renal function and electrolyte metabolism. In The Pharmacological Basis of Therapeutics. Edited by L.S. Goodman and A. Gilman. New York, Macmillan, 1975.
44. Rosin, J.M., et al.: Acetazolamide in studying sodium reabsorption in diluting segment. Am. J. Physiol., 219:1731, 1970.
45. Maren, T.H.: Pharmacological and renal effects of Diamox (6063), new carbonic anhydrase inhibitor. Trans. N.Y. Acad. Sci., 15:53, 1953.
46. Maren, T.H.: Carbonic anhydrase: chemistry, physiology and inhibition. Physiol. Rev., 46:597, 1967.
47. Malnic, G., Klose, R.M., and Giebisch, G.: Micropuncture study of distal tubular potassium and sodium transfer in rat kidney. Am. J. Physiol., 211:529, 1966.
48. White, M.G., and Asch, M.J.: Acid-base effects of topical mafenide acetate in the burned patient. N. Engl. J. Med., 284:1281, 1971.
49. Burg, M.B., and Green, N.L.: Effect of mersalyl on the thick ascending limb of Henle's loop. Kidney Int., 4:245, 1973.
50. Goldstein, M.H., et al.: Effect of meralluride on solute and water excretion in hydrated man: comments on site of action. J. Clin. Invest., 40:731, 1961.
51. Orloff, J., and Davidson, D.G.: The mechanism of potassium secretion in the chicken. J. Clin. Invest., 38:21, 1959.
52. Levy, R.I., Weiner, I.M., and Mudge, G.H.: The effects of acid-base balance on diuresis produced by organic and inorganic mercurials. J. Clin. Invest., 37:1016, 1958.
53. Kessler, R.H., Hierholzer, H., and Guard, K.S.: Localization of action of chlorothiazide in the nephron of the dog. Am. J. Physiol., 46:1346, 1959.
54. Holzgreve, H.: The pattern of inhibition of proximal tubular reabsorption by diuretics. In Renal Transport and Diuretics. Edited by K. Thurae and H. Jahrmarker. Heidelberg, Springer/Verlag, 1969.
55. Earley, L.E., Kahn, M., and Orloff, J.: The effects of infusions of chlorothiazide on urinary dilution and concentration in the dog. J. Clin. Invest., 40:857, 1961.
56. Suki, W., Rector, F.C., Jr., and Seldin, D.W.: The site of action of furosemide and other sulfonamide diuretics in the dog. J. Clin. Invest., 44:1458, 1965.
57. Beyer, H.K., et al.: Renotropic characteristics of ethacrynic acid: a phenoxyacetic saluretic-diuretic agent. J. Pharmacol. Exp. Ther., 147:1, 1965.
58. Hook, J.B., and Williamson, H.E.: Influence of probenecid and alterations of acid-base balance on the saluretic activity of furosemide. J. Pharmacol. Exp. Ther., 149:404, 1965.
59. Puschett, I.B., and Goldberg, M.: The acute effects of furosemide on acid and electrolyte excretion in man. J. Lab. Clin. Med., 71:666, 1968.
59a. Brater, D.C., et al.: Bumetamide and furosemide. Clin. Pharmacol. Ther., 34:207, 1983.
60. Burg, M., et al.: Furosemide effect on isolated perfused tubules. Am. J. Physiol., 225:119, 1973.
61. Burg, M., and Green, N.: Effect of ethacrynic acid on the thick ascending limb of Henle's loop. Kidney Int., 4:301, 1973.
62. Williamson, H.E., et al.: Inhibition of ethacrynic acid induced increase in renal blood flow by indomethcin. Prostaglandins, 8:297, 1974.
63. Williamson, H.E., et al.: Furosemide induced release of prostaglandin E to increase renal blood flow. Proc. Soc. Exp. Biol. Med., 150, 1975.
64. Frolich, J., et al.: Effect of indomethacin on furosemide stimulated renin and sodium excretion. Circulation (Suppl. 2), 52:75, 1975.
65. Patak, R., et al.: Antagonism of the effects of furosemide by indomethacin in normal and hypertensive man. Prostaglandins, 10:649, 1975.
66. Bailie, M.D., Crosslan, K., and Hook, J.B.: Natriuretic effects of furosemide after inhibition of prostaglandin synthetase. J. Pharmacol. Exp. Ther., 199:469, 1976.
67. Durate, C.G., Chomety, F., and Giebisch, E.: Effect of amiloride, ouabain and furosemide on distal tubular function in the rat. Am. J. Physiol., 221:632, 1971.
68. Quick, C.A., and Hoppe, W.: Permanent deafness associated with furosemide administration. Ann. Otol. Rhinol. Laryngol., 84:94, 1975.
69. Mitchell, J.R., et al.: Hepatic necrosis caused by furosemide. Nature, 251:508, 1974.
70. Liddle, G.W.: Aldosterone antagonists and triamterene. Ann. N.Y. Acad. Sci., 139:466, 1966.

71. Baba, W.I., et al.: Pharmacological effects in animals and normal human subjects of the diuretic amiloride hydrochloride. Clin. Pharmacol. Ther., 9:318, 1968.
72. Baba, W.I., Tudhope, G.R., and Wilson, G.M.: Site and mechanism of action of the diuretic triamterene. Clin. Sci., 27:181, 1964.
73. Sobel, B.E.: Valvular heart disease, hyperkalemia and death. Am. J. Med., 62:743, 1977.
74. O'Rielly, M.V., Murnaghan, D.P., and Williams, M.B.: Transvenous pacemaker failure induced by hyperkalemia. J.A.M.A., 228:336, 1974.
75. Morrow, D.H., Knapp, D.E., and Logic, J.R.: Anesthesia and digitalis toxicity V: Effect of the vagus on ouabain-induced ventricular automaticity during halothane. Anesth. Analg. (Cleve.), 49:23, 1970.
76. Logic, J.R., and Morrow, D.H.: Effect of halothane on ventricular automaticity. Anesthesiology, 36:107, 1972.
77. Hampers, C.L., et al.: Major surgery in patients on maintenance hemodialysis. Am. J. Surg., 115:747, 1968.
78. Feldman, S.A.: Muscle Relaxants. London, W.B. Saunders, 1973.
79. Koide, M., and Waud, B.E.: Serum potassium concentration after succinylcholine in patients with renal failure. Anesthesiology, 36:142, 1972.
80. Ascione, F.J.: Guanethidine-hydrochorothiazide. In Evaluation of Drug Interactions. 2nd Edition. Washington, D.C., American Pharmaceutical Association, 1976.
81. Lorimer, A.R., et al.: Beta-adrenoreceptor blockade in hypertension. Am. J. Med., 60:877, 1976.
82. Ahmad, S.: Renal insensitivity to furosemide caused by chronic anti-convulsant therapy. Br. Med. J., 3:657, 1975.
83. Ascione, F.J.: Spironolactone-aspirin. In Evaluations of Drug Interactions. 2nd Edition. Washington, D.C., American Pharmaceutical Association, 1976.
84. Miller, R.D., Sohn, Y.J., and Matteo, R.S.: Enhancement of d-tubocurarine neuromuscular blockade by diuretics in man. Anesthesiology, 45:442, 1976.
85. Ascione, F.J.: Lithium carbonate-chlorothiazide. In Evaluations of Drug Interactions. 2nd Edition. Washington, D.C., American Pharmaceutical Association, 1976.
86. Wirth, K.E., et al.: Metabolism of digitoxin in man and its modification by spironolactone. Eur. J. Clin. Pharmacol., 9:345, 1976.
87. Steiness, E.: Renal tubular secretion of digoxin. Circulation, 50:103, 1974.
87a.Waldorff, S., et al.: Interaction between digoxin and potassium sparing diuretics. Clin. Pharmacol. Ther., 33:418, 1983.
88. Malcolm, A.D., et al.: Digoxin kinetics during furosemide administration. Clin. Pharmacol. Ther., 21:567, 1977.
89. Koch-Weser, J., and Sellers, E.M.: Drug interactions with coumarin anticoagulants. Part I. N. Engl. J. Med., 285:487, 1971.
90. Koch-Weser, J., and Sellers, E.M.: Drug interactions with coumarin anticoagulants. Part II. N. Engl. J. Med., 285:547, 1971.
91. Ascione, F.J.: Chlorpropamide-hydrochlorothiazide. In Evaluations of Drug Interactions. 2nd Edition. Washington, D.C., American Pharmaceutical Association, 1976.
92. Ascione, F.J.: Probenecid-chlorothiazide. In Evaluations of Drug Interactions. 2nd Edition. Washington, D.C., American Pharmaceutical Association, 1976.
93. Samuelson, P.N., et al.: Toxicity following methoxyflurane anaesthesia. IV. The role of obesity and the effect of low dose anaesthesia on fluoride metabolism and renal function. Can. Anaesth. Soc. J., 23:465, 1976.
94. Ascione, F.J.: Kanamycin-ethacrynic acid. In Evaluations of Drug Interactions. 2nd Edition. Washington, D.C., American Pharmaceutical Association, 1976.
95. Dodds, M.G., and Foorb, R.D.: Enhancement by potent diuretics of renal tubular necrosis induced by cephaloridine. Br. J. Pharmacol., 49:277, 1970.
96. Berry, F.A.: Pediatric fluid and electrolyte therapy. Regional Refresher Courses in Anesthesiology, 3:1, 1975.
97. Lindeman, R.D.: Hypokalemia: causes, consequences and correction. N. Engl. J. Med., 272:5, 1976.
98. Huth, E.J., Squires, R.D., and Elkington, J.R.: Experimental potassium depletion in normal human subjects. II. Renal and hormonal factors in the development of extracellular alkalosis during depletion. J. Clin. Invest., 38:1149, 1959.
99. Schribner, B.H., and Burnell, J.M.: Interpretation of the serum potassium concentration. Metabolism, 5:468, 1956.
100. Chambers, D.G.: Dangers of rapid infusion of potassium. Med. J. Aust., 2:945, 1973.
101. Williams, R.H.P.: Potassium overdosage: A potential hazard of non-rigid parenteral fluid containers. Br. Med. J., 1:714, 1973.
102. Kunin, A.S., Surawicz, B., and Sims, E.A.H.: Decrease in serum potassium concentrations and appearance of cardiac arrhythmias during infusion of potassium with glucose in potassium-depleted patients. N. Engl. J. Med., 266:228, 1962.
102a.Epstein, F.H., and Rosa, R.M.: Adrenergic control of serum potassium. N. Engl. J. Med., 309:1450, 1983.
102b.Steiness, E.: Negative potassium balance during beta-blocker therapy of hypertension. Clin. Pharmacol. Ther., 31:691, 1982.
102c.Kolata, G.: Should Hypertensives take potassium? Science, 218:361, 1983.
102d.Harrington, J.T., et al.: Our national obsession with potassium. Am. J. Med., 73:155, 1982.
102e.Dyckner, T., and Wester, P.O.: Ventricular extra systoles and intracellular electrolytes before and after potassium and magnesium infusions on patients on diuretic therapy. Am. Heart. J., 97:12, 1979.
102f.Vitez, T.S., Soper, L.E., and Soper, P.C.: Chronic hypokalemia does not increase anes-

thetics dysrhythmias. Anesth. Analg., *61*:221, 1982 (Abs.).
102g. Hollifield, J.W., and Slaton, P.E.: Thiazide diuretics, hypokalemia and cardiac arrhythmias. Acta Med. Scand. (Suppl. 647):*67*, 1981.
102h. Poole-Wilson, P.A.: Hypokalemia induced by thiazide diuretics in the therapy of hypertension: A cause for concern not nihilism. Postgrad. Med. J., *59* (Suppl.3):137, 1983.
103. Whang, R.: Hyperkalemia: Diagnosis and treatment. Am. J. Med. Sci., *272*:19, 1976.
104. Smith, N.T., and Corbascio, A.N.: The use and misuse of pressor agents. Anesthesiology, *33*:58, 1970.

17

ANTIDYSRHYTHMIC AGENTS

JOHN L. ATLEE, III

Anesthesiologists are frequently required to administer anesthesia to patients receiving antidysrhythmic therapy. Moreover, in patients with possible concurrent cardiovascular, pulmonary, renal, or metabolic disease, the development of dysrhythmias during anesthesia is likely. Indeed, cardiac dysrhythmias have been reported to occur in as many as 61.7% of anesthetized patients.[1] The majority of these dysrhythmias, however, are not sufficiently serious to require pharmacologic or electrical conversion. Dysrhythmias require treatment only when (1) they cannot be corrected promptly by removing the precipitating cause, (2) hemodynamic function or myocardial oxygen supply is seriously compromised, and (3) the nature of the disturbance predisposes the patient to life-threatening rhythm disturbances such as ventricular tachycardia or fibrillation. Whether a patient to be anesthetized is receiving antidysrhythmic drug therapy, or whether this therapy is required during the course of anesthesia, the potential for an adverse drug interaction exists. This is not surprising, since anesthetics and adjuvant drugs have profound and, also, diverse effects on cardiac function.

Three types of adverse anesthetic-antidysrhythmic drug interactions are likely to be encountered clinically:

1. Hemodynamic effects: The cardiovascular side effects of antidysrhythmic drugs, which are usually depressant, augment that depression from anesthetics; for example, verapamil and propranolol each enhance the negative inotropic effects of anesthetics.
2. Altered antidysrhythmic effects: The expected antidysrhythmic action of a specific drug is altered by anesthetic or adjuvant drugs with the abolition of response or by precipitation of a more serious cardiac irregularity; for example, initial catecholamine release by bretylium tosylate could enhance the sensitizing action of anesthetics.
3. Extracardiac effects: Antidysrhythmic drugs possess pharmacologic actions that may modify those of anesthetics or adjuncts; for example, potentiation of neuromuscular blockade.

ELECTROPHYSIOLOGY OF CARDIAC DYSRHYTHMIAS

Cardiac dysrhythmias result from abnormalities in impulse initiation, propagation, or both.[2] Impulse initiation, or automaticity, is a property of specialized fibers located within the sinoatrial node, the atrioventricular node, and the His-Purkinje system. These fibers differ from ordinary atrial and ventricular muscle fibers in their ability to undergo spontaneous, diastolic depolarization. Characteristic cardiac action potentials for different heart fi-

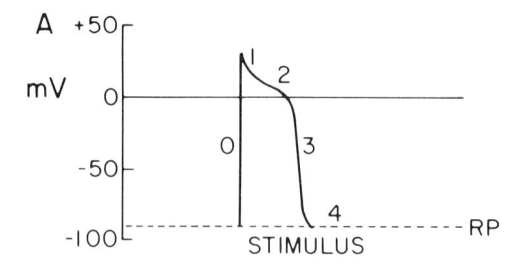

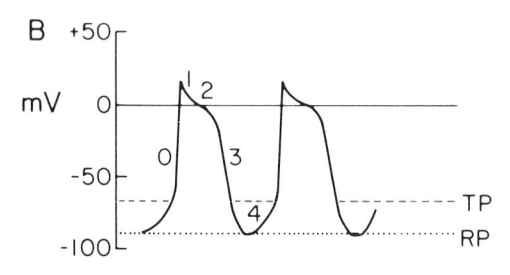

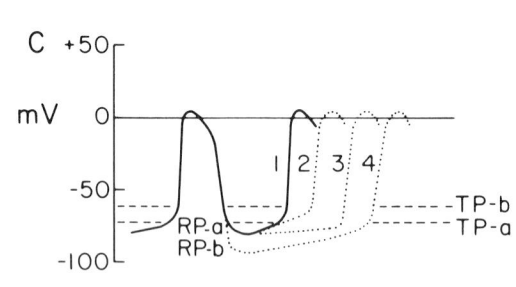

Fig. 17-1. Schematic diagrams of action potentials recorded from ventricular muscle (Panel A), Purkinje (Panel B), and SA nodal (Panel C) fibers. RP = resting transmembrane potential level. TP = threshold potential. See text for discussion.

bers are schematically shown in Figure 17-1. A resting ventricular muscle fiber (Panel A) normally has a transmembrane potential of approximately −90 millivolts inside with respect to outside. On arrival of a propagated action potential or on application of an external electrical stimulus, the fiber is rapidly depolarized (phase 0). The transmembrane potential polarity is reversed, becoming approximately +30 millivolts inside because of the rapid influx of sodium ions accompanied by a slower inward movement of calcium ions. Subsequently, the fiber repolarizes, rapidly at first (phase 1), then more gradually (phase 2 or plateau), and once again rapidly (phase 3). Repolarization is associated with an outward movement of potassium ions that restores the negative intracellular potential. Active extrusion of sodium ions from within the cell against an electrochemical gradient takes place during the quiescent phase (phase 4) before the arrival of the next stimulus or propagated impulse.

The events outlined in the previous paragraph are different from those occurring in a Purkinje fiber that exhibits automaticity (Fig. 17-1, Panel B). These fibers, as well as those found within the sinus or atrioventricular nodes (Fig. 17-1, Panel C), can undergo spontaneous, diastolic (phase 4) depolarization. When phase 4 depolarization reaches a critical level of threshold potential, rapid (phase 0) depolarization follows. The remaining electrophysiologic events are similar to those outlined for a ventricular muscle fiber. Different fiber types (Fig. 17-1, Panels A, B, and C) vary with respect to the amount of overshoot or final positivity reached during phase 0. A critical level of overshoot must occur for the action potential to be propagated.

The ionic mechanism for spontaneous phase 4 depolarization (normal automaticity) must take into account a net gain in intracellular positive charges during diastole.[2a] How this gain is achieved differs according to fiber type.[2a,3] For *Purkinje fibers*, there may be a decrease in an outward potassium current (I_{k_2} or pacemaker current) while a constant background current carried by sodium moves intracellularly, and then a slow inward current carried by sodium depolarizes the cell to threshold.[3a] The pacemaker current (I_{k_2}) differs from two other currents carried by potassium: I_{k_1}, involved in maintaining the resting transmembrane potential; and I_{x_1}, the repolarization current.[2a] Alternatively, it has been proposed that spontaneous phase 4 depolarization in Purkinje fibers results primarily from activation of an inward sodium current (I_f), a special pacemaker current, rather than from inactivation of the outward Ik$_2$ current.[3b] This pacemaker current (I$_F$) is blocked by tetrodotoxin, lidocaine and quinidine, but not procainamide.[3c] Spontaneous phase 4 depolarization in the *SA node* appears to result from the varying degress of inactivation of a time-dependent potassium current (Ik, or Ix), activation of a pacemaker current (I$_F$), and progressive activation of the slow inward current (Isi).[2a] The decrease in the outward potassium current (Ik$_2$), increase in sodium influx via the pacemaker current (I$_F$), and calcium influx via the slow inward current gradually depolarize the cell to membrane potentials at which the slow inward current is fully activated, giving rise to the upstroke (phase 1) of the action potential.[3d]

The rate at which pacemaker cells discharge is determined by the slope of phase 4 depolarization and by the values of transmembrane resting and threshold potential (Fig. 17–1, Panel C). The normal rate of discharge (condition 1) is slowed by raising the threshold potential (TP-a to TP-b, condition 2), by decreasing the slope of phase 4 (condition 3), or by lowering the resting membrane potential (RP-a to RP-b, condition 4). Epinephrine augments automaticity by increasing the slope of phase 4; however, this is accompanied by a small increase in resting membrane potential that limits this effect.[3] Acetylcholine, on the other hand, decreases automaticity by simultaneously increasing (hyperpolarizing) the resting membrane potential and reducing the rate of phase 4 depolarization.[3] Halothane slows the heart by reducing spontaneous phase 4 depolarization and by increasing the threshold potential.[5]

Abnormal automaticity may arise from cells that have reduced maximum diastolic potentials, often in the range of −50 to −60 millivolts.[2a] This type of abnormal automaticity has been found in Purkinje fibers removed from dogs subjected to myocardial infarction,[5a] in rat myocardium damaged by epinephrine,[5b] in atrial tissue from diseased human hearts,[5c] and in ventricular myocardial tissue from patients undergoing aneurysmectomy and endocardial resection for recurrent ventricular tachydysrhythmias.[5d,5e] The rate of spontaneous abnormal automatic discharge increases with progressive depolarization, but decreases with hyperpolarization.[2a] Perhaps partial depolarization and failure to reach normal maximum diastolic potential can induce automatic discharge in most if not all cardiac fibers.[5f] The ionic mechanisms responsible for abnormal automaticity from cells with reduced levels of maximum diastolic potential are not known, and probably not the same under each of the circumstances noted above.[2a] Oscillatory activity may develop in cells both before and after full repolarization.[2a,5b] Oscillations with a variety of contours have been observed[5e] and may represent another cause of automatic activity.[2a] Their relation to clinical dysrhythmias as well as their ionic causes and distinction from other types of depolarization (see below) are uncertain at present.[2a]

While *triggered activity* is a form of disordered impulse formation, it is to be distinguished from abnormal automaticity since the latter is consequent to a preceding impulse or series of impulses, without an interval of electrical quiescence.[2a] Technically, triggered activity is not an automatic (self-generating) mechanism; automaticity (both normal and abnormal) is, since it does not require prior stimulation and since there is not electrical quiescence in the absence of stimulation.[2a] Triggered activity is initiated by impulses variously referred to as low-amplitude potentials, transient depolarizations, or oscillatory afterpotentials.[6] These depolarizations may occur before or after full repolarizations of the fiber and are best termed early or late afterdepolarizations, respectively.[7] They may arise from cells exhibiting high (Purkinje fibers) or low (mitral valve) diastolic membrane potentials.[2a] Afterdepolarizations that reach threshold potential may trigger another one and induce a self-perpetuating rhythm.[2a] Early afterdepolarizations may be precipitated by an abrupt reduction in extracellular potassium,[2a] by high concentrations of catecholamines,[2a] and by some antidysrhythmic drugs.[5f] They may also be found in myocardium damaged by catecholamines[5b] or in myocardium removed from patients with ventricular dysrhythmias.[2a,5e] Delayed afterdepolarizations and triggered activity have been demonstrated in Purkinje fibers,[6,7a] specialized atrial fibers[8] and ventricular muscle fibers[6,9] exposed to digitalis preparations. Fibers in human mitral valve superfused with norepinephrine exhibit the capacity for sustained triggered rhythmic activity.[9a] As verapamil suppresses triggered activity in these preparations, it is possible that the slow inward current plays a role in its genesis.[2a] Dysrhythmias *(in vivo)* possibly due to triggered activity have been reported in the dog[9b] and in humans.[9c,9d,9e] However, at the present state of knowledge it is difficult to prove that triggered activity is a clinically operational mechanism for dysrhythmia, even though it is tempting to ascribe to it certain atrial tachycardias that might originate in the coronary sinus, dysrhythmias due to digitalis, or dysrhythmias in patients with mitral valve prolapse. Finally, the ionic basis responsible for delayed afterdepolarizations and triggering is not clear and may be diverse.[2a] Both the slow inward current (Isi) and a sodium inward current are thought to be involved.[2a]

Altered impulse propagation or conduction is the other possible dysrhythmia mechanism, which is necessary for dysrhythmias caused by reentry of excitation.[2] Reentry occurs when there is an imbalance between conduction and refractoriness in cardiac tissues. Reentry is illustrated schematically in Figure 17–2. With the exception of occasional premature extrasystoles and parasystole, almost all clinical dysrhythmias have at some time been ascribed for reentry of excitation.[10]

The mechanisms invoked as the cause for a particular dysrhythmia, be they phase 4 automaticity, abnormal automaticity, triggered activity, or reentry of excitation, will determine the type of therapy employed. Unfortunately, the mechanism at work in the anesthetic and nonanesthetic environments may not be the same. Anesthetic-related dysrhythmias have usually been ascribed to abnormal pacemaker activity; that is, the dominant (sinus node) pacemaker is suppressed with the emergence of latent pacemakers within the atrioventricular junctional tissues or below.[5,11,12] This applies particularly to ventricular dysrhythmias caused by catecholamine sensitization. This mechanism, however, has been challenged by the proponents of reentry.[13–15] It is certain that anesthetic agents have effects on specialized atrioventricular conduction and refractoriness.[16,16a,17] These effects may be related causally to reentry of excitation.[18] Furthermore, anesthetic effects on conduction are altered by those of adjuvant drugs, including antidysrhythmics, used during anesthesia.[19–21]

In summary, although much is known about the electrophysiology of cardiac dysrhythmias and the drugs used to treat these disturbances in the nonanesthetic setting, comparable information is lacking for anesthetic-related dysrhythmias. More knowledge of how anesthetic agents and adjuvant drugs cause dysrhythmias, as well as of potential adverse interactions between anesthetic and antidysrhythmic drugs, is required. This is because rational treatment for any dysrhythmia demands that one take a causal approach based on sound physiologic and pharmacologic concepts.

CLASSIFICATION OF ANTIDYSRHYTHMIC DRUGS

Currently available antidysrhythmic drugs may be classified into four discrete categories.[22,22a,22b] This categorization, while not universally accepted,[22a,22aa] is

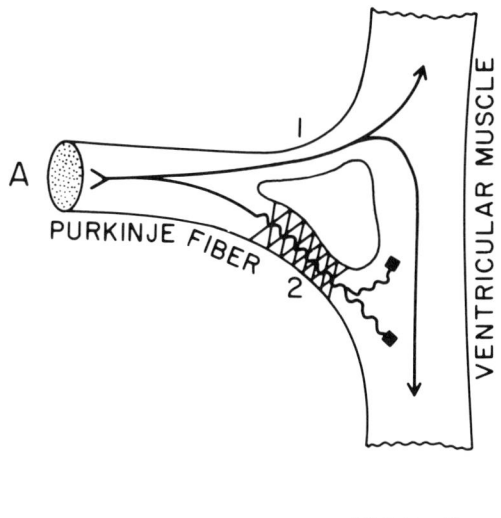

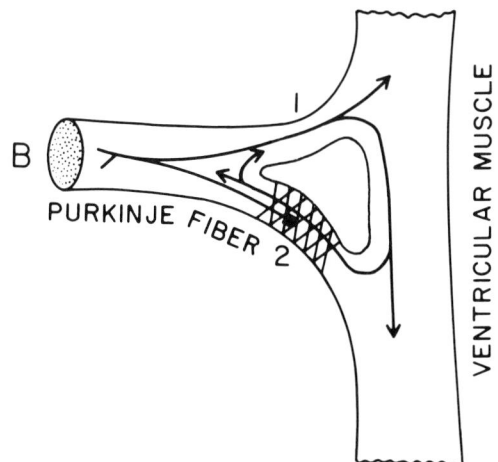

Fig. 17-2. Schematic representation of branching Purkinje fiber terminating on a ventricular muscle fiber; model for reentry of excitation. Reentry is prevented in Panel A, but permitted in Panel B. In Panels A and B, the impulse arriving from above conducts normally through branch 1 and excites the ventricular muscle fiber. The impulse in branch 2, however, fails to conduct normally. This may happen when the fibers are subject to hypoxia, stretch, catecholamines, digitalis excess, electrolyte imbalances, or possibly, anesthetics. In Panel A, the impulse *propagates slowly* through branch 2 to excite the ventricular fiber, which is now refractory following previous excitation by the impulse conducted through branch 1. In Panel A, reentry is not possible because the impulse traveling through branch 1 cannot be conducted antidromically through branch 2, and the impulse traveling orthodromically and slowly through branch 2 cannot excite the ventricular fiber. Reentry of excitation is possible in Panel B where the orthodromically conducted impulse is *blocked* in branch 2. The impulse conducted through branch 1 excites the ventricular fiber and returns antidromically through branch 2, which is no longer absolutely refractory. The impulse traveling back through branch 2 excites the more proximal portions of the Purkinje fiber and returns via branch 1 to reexcite the ventricular fiber resulting in a return extrasystole. If the reentry circuit is maintained, a series of extrasystoles or tachycardia results. Reentry is abolished if another impulse from above reaches branch 1 before the return extrasystole coming back up branch 2. Whereas the reentrant circuit discussed above involves the ventricular muscle-Purkinje fiber junction, the potential for reentry exists anywhere in the heart.

based on the observation that virtually all known antidysrhythmic drugs have one dominant electrophysiologic effect on the myocardial cell, albeit one which may be modulated by the drug's subsidiary myocardial actions and extracardiac effects.[22a] Antidysrhythmic drugs are classified according to their dominant, *in vitro* electrophysiologic action[22a,22c,22d,22e] in Table 17-1. Their effects on the electrocardiogram and atrioventricular conduction intervals[22aa] and extracardiac actions[22a] are summarized in Table 17-2.

Class I. Antidysrhythmic drugs in this class, in general, are potent local anesthetics with similar depressant effects on the myocardial membrane (block inward flux of sodium during phase 0), such that much lower concentrations to produce comparable physiologic changes require much lower concentrations in myocardial fibers than in nerves.[22f] The dominant electrophysiologic property of this class of drugs has been related to their ability to reduce the maximal rate of depolarization (Vmax, phase 0) in cardiac muscle.[22a] In clinically relevant concentrations, the changes in rate of depolarization are associated with an increase in the threshold of excitability, a depression in conduction velocity, and a marked prolongation in the effective refractory period.[22a] These alterations, which occur without a significant change either in the resting transmembrane potential or in the action potential duration, are invariably associated with the

Table 17-1
Electrophysiologic Actions

Class	Agent	Depression of the Fast Response	Effect on Action Potential Duration	Sympatholytic Effect	Depression of the Slow Response
I	Quinidine	+ + + +	Prolong +	+[1]	0
	Procainamide	+ + + +	Prolong +	0	0
	Lidocaine	+ + + +	Shorten +	0	0
	Phenytoin	+ + + +	Shorten +	0	0
	Disopyramide	+ + + +	Prolong +	0	0
	Aprindine	+ + + +	0	0	+
	Mexiletine	+ + + +	0	0	0
	Tocainide	+ + + +	0	0	0
II	Propranolol	+	Shorten +	+ + + +[2]	0
III	Bretylium	Increases phase 4	Prolong + + + +	+[3]	0
	Amiodarone	Decreases phase 4 only	Prolong + + + +	+[4]	0
IV	Verapamil	Phase 4 only	Prolong phases 1 and 2	+[1]	+ + + +

Key: + + + + = principal electrophysiologic action; + = subsidiary electrophysiologic action; 0 = no effect at presumed therapeutic plasma levels; 1 = noncompetitive antagonism; 2 = competitive antagonism; 3 = neuronal blockade; 4 = noncompetitive blockade.

inhibition of spontaneous phase 4 depolarization in automatic fibers.[22a] However, this effect on pacemaker cells is usually seen with concentrations of the drug much lower than those which influence conduction velocity or the electrical threshold of excitability.[22a] By depressing spontaneous phase 4 depolarization, Class I antidysrhythmic drugs control dysrhythmias due to enhanced automaticity. By increasing the threshold of excitability, depressing conduction velocity and prolonging the effective refractory period, Class I drugs are likely to be effective in aborting reentrant tachydysrhythmias.

Class II. The rationale for classifying *beta*-adrenergic blocking drugs as Class II antidysrhythmics stems from the observation that hyperactivity of the sympathetic nervous system has been shown to be a significant factor in the genesis of certain cardiac dysrhythmias.[22g] Indeed, a decreased availability of the sympathetic transmitter is antidysrhythmic,[22g] while sympathetic blockade, whether achieved presynaptically by adrenergic neuron blocking

Table 17-2
Electrocardiographic (ECG), Atrioventricular (AV) Conduction and Principal Extracardiac Effects of Antidysrhythmic Drugs

Class	Drug	Rate	(ECG Intervals) P-R	QRS	Q-T	(A-V Conduction) A-H	H-V	Extracardiac
I	Quinidine	0 ↑	↓ 0 ↑	↑	↑	↓ 0 ↑	0 ↑	Anticholinergic; vasodilation
	Procainamide	0	0 ↑	↑	↑	0 ↑	0 ↑	Vasodilation
	Lidocaine	0	0	0	0	0 ↓	0 ↓	Local anesthetic
	Phenytoin	0	0	0	0 ↓	0 ↓	0	Anticonvulsant
	Disopyramide	0 ↑	0	0 ↑	0 ↑	0	0 ↑	Anticholinergic
	Aprindine	↓	↑	↑	0 ↑	↑	↑	Anticonvulsant
	Mexiletine	0	0	0	0	0 ↑	0 ↑	Anticonvulsant
	Tocainide	0 ↓	0	0	0 ↓	0 ↑	0	Local anesthetic
II	Propranolol	↓	0 ↑	0	0 ↓	0 ↑	0	Insignificant
III	Bretylium	0 ↓	0 ↑	0	0 ↑	ND	ND	Hypotension
	Amiodarone	↓	0 ↑	0	↑	↑	0	Coronary vasodilation
IV	Verapamil	0 ↓	↑	0	0	↑	0	Coronary vasodilation

Key: ↑ = increase; 0 = no change; ↓ = decrease; ND = no data available
Abbreviations: A-H = AV nodal conduction time; H-V = His-Purkinje conduction time

drugs[22l,22i] or by competition at the receptor site by specific *beta*-adrenergic blocking compounds, lowers the incidence of clinical and experimental dysrhythmias.[22a] The widest experience has been obtained with *beta*-adrenergic blocking drugs which, soon after their introduction, were found to be potent local anesthetics on nerve[22j] with comparable effects on cardiac muscle.[22f,22k] While controversy has existed as to the relative contribution of the *beta*-adrenergic blocking and local anesthetic properties of Class II drugs to their antidysrhythmic action, it now seems reasonably clear, at least for therapeutic concentrations, that these drugs act largely and perhaps exclusively via *beta*-adrenergic blockade, and that the associated local anesthetic properties evident at high concentrations are largely irrelevant in the control of cardiac dysrhythmias.[22g,22l] The principal electrophysiologic effect on heart muscle at clinical concentrations is depression of spontaneous phase 4 depolarization.[22a]

Class III. The justification for attributing an independent antidysrhythmic mechanism to drugs which prolong the duration of the action potential as their principal electrophysiologic action stems from the observation that atrial dysrhythmias are common in thyrotoxicosis and relatively rare in hypothyroidism.[22a] Additionally, in experimentally induced thyrotoxicosis in rabbits, atrial action potential durations were markedly abbreviated, and, in hypothyroidism they were significantly and homogeneously prolonged.[22m] A situation analagous to the effects of hypothyroidism on cardiac intracellular potentials was later found with the chronic administration of the antianginal drug amiodarone, which prolonged action potential duration in atrial as well as ventricular muscle. Amiodarone has since been found to be a potent clinical antidysrhythmic drug.[22o,22p,22q,22r] It has no local anesthetic actions on the cardiac membrane, and in experimental studies has been shown to have an extremely weak Class I action.[22n] Similarly, the drug does not exhibit beta-adrenergic blocking properties, although it possesses a mild noncompetitive inhibitory effect on sympathetic stimulation.[22s] Therefore, the antidysrhythmic actions of amiodarone were attributed to its property of prolonging the action potential duration with the consequent lengthening of the absolute refractory period.[22n] Bretylium tosylate, which is also included in this class, prolongs the action potential duration in both ventricular and Purkinje fibers but has no electrophysiologic effects on atrial muscle.[23,24] Thus it is effective in treating ventricular, but not supraventricular, dysrhythmias.[22,22h,22i]

Class IV. A number of experimental studies have indicated the potential significance of the slow response in the genesis of sudden onset (e.g., paroxysmal) cardiac dysrhythmias.[22a,25] It is known that with depression of the fast response, a marked reduction in conduction velocity may occur in association with the emergence of the slow response, and action potentials with pacemaker activity may also arise entirely on the basis of the slow response.[25] Thus, the presence of the slow response may lead to the initiation of dysrhythmias both on the basis of reentry of excitation as well as abnormal automaticity. Experimentally the slow response is effectively suppressed by the calcium-channel blocker, verapamil,[25] which has potent antidysrhythmic actions both in the experimental animal[22c] and in humans, particularly in the presence of supraventricular tachydysrhythmias.[25a,25b,25c] Verapamil generally has not been effective in the treatment of recurrent ventricular tachydysrhythmias.[25d] Data from animal studies suggest its potential clinical usefulness in reducing or preventing ventricular dysrhythmias due to acute myocardial infarction.[2a,25e]

The following two case reports, the first from this institution and the second extracted from the literature,[26] involve the hemodynamic effects, antidysrhythmic actions, or extracardiac effects of antidysrhythmic drugs and anesthetic agents.

INTERACTIONS INVOLVING HEMODYNAMIC AND ANTIDYSRHYTHMIC EFFECTS

CASE REPORT

A 62-year-old man underwent elective four-vessel coronary revascularization. His medical history included 5 years of episodic anginal attacks, which were relieved by nitroglycerin and rest, and a 15-pack-year history of smoking. No other coronary risk factors, such as obesity or hypertension, were evident.

Two weeks before hospital admission the patient had had an episode of severe anginal pain, associated with dizziness and diaphoresis, for which he was admitted to the coronary care unit. The initial diagnosis of acute myocardial infarction was not substantiated. He underwent cardiac catheterization on the fifth hospital day. His systemic, pulmonary, and right- and left-sided filling pressures were normal, as was his cardiac index. The patient had diffuse, high grade, occlusive disease involving both the left and right coronary arteries and their major branches. The proximal left anterior descending artery, the distal portions of which filled from collaterals, was 100% occluded. An operation was scheduled for the following week.

Digoxin (250 μg/day, orally) was started 3 days prior to the operation with nitroglycerin continued sublingually as needed. The patient's blood chemistries and serum electrolytes were all normal the day before the operation. Premedication consisted of scopolamine (hyoscine), 0.43 mg, and morphine, 10 mg IM (intramuscularly).

When the patient arrived in the operating room, his arterial blood pressure (Riva-Rocci) was 126/70 mm Hg and his heart rate was 83 beats/min. The ECG (II) showed sinus rhythm (Fig. 17–3A). Peripheral and central venous catheters were placed and percutaneous radial artery cannulation was performed to monitor direct arterial pressure and to sample blood gases and electrolytes. Anesthesia was induced with thiopental (250 mg, IV [intravenously]) followed by halothane (0.5 to 2.0%, inspired) and nitrous oxide (50%). Following anesthetic induction, pancuronium (8 mg, IV) was given. A supraventricular tachycardia (150 to 160 beats/min, Fig. 17–3B) appeared within 3 minutes. This was associated with a decrease in arterial pressure to 80/50 mm Hg. Arterial blood gases drawn at this time revealed: Po_2 = 220 mm Hg, Pco_2 = 33 mm Hg, pH = 7.40, serum K^+ = 3.4 mEq/L (preanesthetic induction value = 4.6 mEq/L). Halothane was discontinued and edrophonium was administered (10 mg, IV), but these maneuvers failed to abolish the tachycardia (Fig. 17–3C). Lidocaine (200 mg, IV) was administered next, also without success (Fig. 17–3D), and this in turn was followed by propranolol (1.5 mg IV, divided doses over 2 minutes). Five minutes after the administration of propranolol, the patient's ventricular rate had slowed substantially (Fig. 17–3E), and he appeared to be experiencing atrial flutter with varying degrees of atrioventricular block. His arterial blood pressure was 150/80 mm Hg. Approximately 15 minutes after the administration of pancuronium, the patient still was not sufficiently relaxed to allow endotracheal intubation. Peripheral nerve stimulation demonstrated well-sustained tetanus without post-tetanic facilitation or twitch

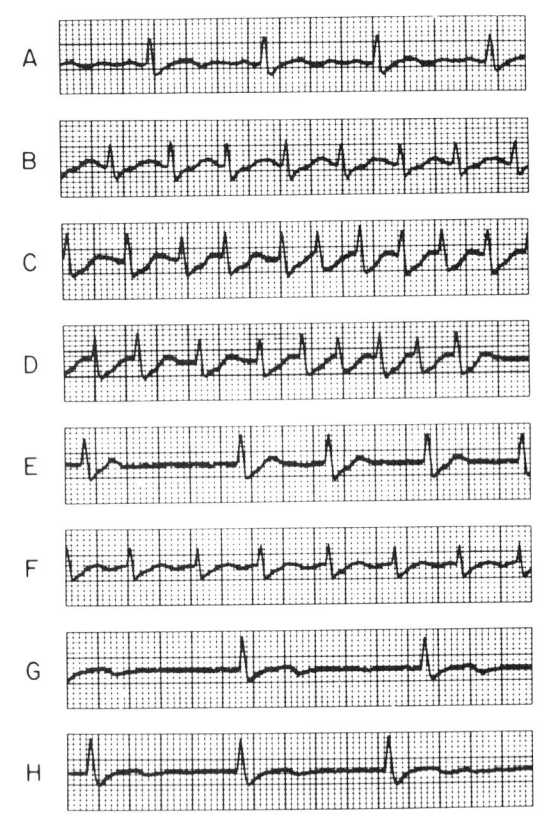

Fig. 17–3. ECG (II) recordings (25 mm/sec) from patient described in first case report. Panel A—sinus rhythm before induction of anesthesia. Panel B—supraventricular tachycardia following first dose of pancuronium. Panel C—supraventricular tachycardia after edrophonium 10 mg, IV. Panel D—supraventricular tachycardia after lidocaine 200 mg, IV. Panel E—atrial flutter, varying degrees of atrioventricular block, after propranolol 1.5 mg, IV. Panel F—supraventricular tachycardia following second dose of pancuronium. Panel G—sinus bradycardia prior to third dose of pancuronium. Panel H—junctional bradycardia following third dose of pancuronium.

suppression. Halothane was reinstituted, and a second dose of pancuronium (8 mg, IV) was administered. The patient then appeared to be relaxed, and his trachea was intubated successfully. However, the tachycardia reappeared (Fig. 17–3F), accompanied by a decrease in arterial blood pressure. Sinus rhythm (Fig. 17–3G) was restored within 15 minutes after an additional dose of propranolol (0.5 mg, IV). This rhythm persisted for the next 2½ hours, during which time the patient's blood pressure was stable (range 120 to 140 mm Hg systolic). Two minutes after the second dose of pancuronium, the patient's serum potassium was 2.6 mEq/L, and 10 minutes later it was 4.1 mEq/L. Concomitant arterial blood gas analyses revealed a mild, compensated metabolic acidosis (pH = 7.41, P_{CO_2} = 33 and 35 mm Hg at both sampling intervals). A third dose of pancuronium (7 mg, IV) immediately before cardiopulmonary bypass resulted in a junctional bradycardia (Fig. 17-3H). This lasted approximately 2 minutes and was accompanied by a small, transient decrease (0.5 mEq/L) in serum potassium level. The remainder of the patient's surgical and anesthetic course was uneventful, as was his postoperative course. He was discharged from the hospital on the fourteenth postoperative day.

This case illustrates the dilemma faced by the clinician when confronted with a serious cardiac dysrhythmia. Several possible drug interactions could have caused the hemodynamic alterations and rhythm disturbances encountered. Digitalis, halothane, and pancuronium could have caused the dysrhythmias. The prophylactic administration of digitalis has been recommended in patients undergoing aortocoronary bypass surgery, since prophylactic digitalization was found to lower the incidence of postoperative supraventricular tachycardia.[27] Our experience supports this practice. However, an increase in supraventricular dysrhythmias was found in coronary bypass surgery patients given prophylactic digitalis.[27a] Furthermore, Morrison and Killip found that patients developed evidence of digitalis toxicity at much lower serum digoxin levels following open heart surgery.[27b] Experimental studies indicate that digoxin has no effect on electrically stimulated supraventricular dysrhythmias in normo- or hypocapnic, halothane-anesthetized dogs.[27c] From the above, it is uncertain whether an interaction between halothane and digoxin could explain the supraventricular dysrhythmia seen in the patient described in the Case Report. An interaction among halothane, pancuronium, and digitalis is certainly possible, but unproven. Several reports taken together indicate that both supraventricular and ventricular dysrhythmias are more likely when halothane and pancuronium are used in association than with other volatile anesthetics.[28-30] Since this association is not proven, it awaits further clinical verification.

Acute hypokalemia in the patient in our case report appeared to be temporally related to the administration of pancuronium. However, the administration of pancuronium or of other nondepolarizing muscle relaxants is not believed to be associated with significant acute alterations in serum potassium. Regardless of cause, the hypokalemia noted in this patient could have precipitated digitalis toxicity in an otherwise nontoxic patient. Acute hypocapnia produced by mechanical ventilation may be associated with a concomitant fall in serum potassium level, although this did not appear to be so in our patient. It is well known that acutely induced hypokalemia potentiates digitalis toxicity. Hypokalemia also augments the neuromuscular effects of pancuronium.[31,32] Whether it alters the cardiac electrophysiologic effects of pancuronium or of halothane is unknown.

The treatment of the supraventricular tachycardia in this patient deserves comment. Because of known coronary and presumed carotid atherosclerosis, carotid massage was not attempted, since this maneuver might have caused embolization of atherosclerotic plaques. Maneuvers that increase parasympathetic tone, such as anticholinesterase therapy, or *alpha*-adrenergic vasopressors, have been recommended.[33,34] Vasopressors were not chosen for this patient because of the potential danger of hypertension with a tachycardia. In addition to contractile force development, heart rate and blood pressure are determinants of myocardial oxygen consumption. This patient's myocardial oxygen supply appeared to be seriously compromised. Because the patient did not respond to edrophonium, a longer acting anticholinesterase drug (for example, neostigmine) was not given. Despite the lack of effect in our case, edrophonium is often effective in treating supraventricular tachycardia. It alters the refractoriness of supraventricular conducting pathways under parasympathetic control. Presumably, this makes conduction more homogeneous and reduces the likelihood of reentry. Whatever the reason for the lack of an edrophonium effect in our patient (it could be argued that an additional 10 mg should have been given), the choice of this drug was logical. Verapamil, not available at the time of this case report, would have been indicated therapy for this patient following failure of vagal maneuvers.

Intravenous lidocaine was also ineffective. I have noted occasionally that sinus rhythm is restored after the administration of lidocaine (2 to 3 mg/kg body weight, IV) in apparent cases of supraventricular tachycardia during halothane or enflurane anesthesia. Whereas lidocaine is generally considered to be ineffective in supraventricular dysrhythmias, its beneficial effect during anesthesia may relate to an action of lidocaine that promotes less temporal dispersion of refractoriness in reentry loops responsible for supraventricular dysrhythmias. Its effects on supraventricular excitability during inhalation anesthesia have not been tested. It is also possible that the apparent effectiveness of lidocaine in treating some supraventricular tachycardias is spurious. Supraventricular tachycardia associated with aberrant ventricular conduction is easily mistaken for ventricular tachycardia, and lidocaine is the drug preferred in the treatment of the latter. I do not advocate the use of lidocaine as a first choice for the treatment of supraventricular tachycardias. Indeed, it may cause alarming ventricular acceleration during atrial flutter, and has been reported to cause SA nodal arrest when used with quinidine.[35,36] However, when a presumed supraventricular tachycardia associated with aberrant ventricular conduction fails to convert following cholinergic interventions, the possibility that the dysrhythmia is of ventricular origin must be considered. Lidocaine should be tried under these circumstances.

Propranolol is recommended for the treatment of supraventricular tachydysrhythmias.[22aa] It was used in the patient in our case report to prolong atrioventricular nodal conduction and thereby to slow the ventricular response to the supraventricular tachycardia. In addition to reducing myocardial oxygen demand, the slower ventricular rate can improve hemodynamics by allowing an improvement in ventricular filling as well as an increase in coronary blood flow due to an increase in diastolic minute time. Such an effect can also be expected from digitalis, which slows atrioventricular nodal conduction as well. In this patient, however, one cannot be certain that the dysrhythmia was not the direct result of acute digitalis intoxication brought about by sudden changes in the serum potassium level. The use of additional digitalis, therefore, seemed inadvisable under the circumstances. Propranolol had the desired effect of reducing the ventricular rate (Fig. 17–3E), and of restoring blood pressure to more acceptable levels (systolic range 120 to 140 mm Hg). Furthermore, this intervention revealed the underlying mechanism, namely atrial flutter, as evidenced by the small, regular undulations in the baseline (Fig. 17–3E). The additional dose of propranolol (0.5 mg) used to treat the episode of supraventricular tachycardia (Fig. 17–3F) after the second dose of pancuronium also slowed the ventricular rate, and shortly thereafter it restored sinus rhythm (Fig. 17–3G). This response could be attributed to a direct membrane-stabilizing effect of propranolol, or to the hemodynamic improvement and return of serum potassium to more physiologic levels.

It has been reported that succinylcholine is effective in abolishing supraventricular dysrhythmias during anesthesia.[37] In retrospect this might have been the best treatment after the first attack of tachycardia. Succinylcholine would have controlled the tachycardia either by a direct myocardial or postganglionic sympathetic stimulating effect, or by simultaneously increasing the serum potassium level and providing adequate muscle relaxation for endotracheal intubation.[38–40] As for the use of additional pancuronium, it can be argued that this was improper and that metocurine, 4:1 metocurine-pancuronium, or d-tubocurarine, agents unlikely to precipitate tachycardia,[40a] should have been administered.

The case report illustrates the complexities of treating dysrhythmias during anesthesia. These complexities arise because we are poorly informed of the type of interactions involved. In dysrhythmic patients, there is little assurance that the remedy will not be worse than the disease.

INTERACTIONS INVOLVING EXTRACARDIAC EFFECTS

The main noncardiac interactions of this kind involve the well-known potentiation of a nondepolarizing neuromuscular blockade by antidysrhythmic drugs. A clinical example is quinidine. The following case report was extracted from the literature:[26]

CASE REPORT

A 71-year-old man was scheduled for a cholecystectomy following an episode of acute cholecystitis. He had had a myocardial infarction 10 years before. Three weeks prior to admission, an operation under general anesthesia for a hip fracture was performed without problems. The patient was taking oral quinidine (200 mg, q.i.d.) for ventricular premature beats, which included runs of quadrigeminy and trigeminy noted on a preoperative ECG. Sinus rhythm had been restored by quinidine therapy by the time of the operation.

Anesthesia was induced with cyclopropane and maintained with nitrous oxide supplemented by meperidine (160 mg) and by tubocurarine (36 mg). Several episodes of intraoperative hypotension responded well to the administration of intravenous fluids and plasma protein fraction. Ephedrine sulfate (total dose 100 mg IV and 45 mg IM) was also administered. At the conclusion of a 160-minute procedure, the neuromuscular block was reversed with atropine, 1.4 mg, and neostigmine, 3.5 mg.

The patient's condition for the first hour in the recovery room was stable. He then received 300 mg of quinidine IM. Shortly thereafter (approximately 20 minutes), the patient appeared mildly cyanotic and was breathing shallowly. Oxygen therapy by mask was started and the patient received an additional 1.0 mg of neostigmine and 0.4 mg of atropine. He did not respond and his condition further deteriorated to apnea. Nasal tracheal intubation was performed and controlled ventilation with oxygen was started. The patient's condition worsened, complicated by severe hypotension and ventricular dysrhythmias. The former did not respond to fluids and ephedrine. An acceptable level of blood pressure (100 mm Hg systolic) was achieved with a metaraminol drip. Neuromuscular function failed to improve in response to edrophonium 10 mg, IV. Controlled ventilation was continued for approximately six hours, at which time the patient was able to breathe spontaneously and the endotracheal tube was removed. Dysrhythmias were still present at this time, but neuromuscular function was normal.

The following morning the patient was mildly cyanotic and dyspneic. The nasotracheal tube was reinserted and intermittent positive pressure breathing (IPPB) was started, with resultant clinical improvement. An ECG at this time showed normal sinus rhythm with ST-T wave changes probably due either to quinidine or to residual myocardial ischemia. The remainder of the patient's postoperative course was uneventful.

In this patient the neuromuscular block probably became reestablished after the administration of quinidine in the recovery room. Quinidine and many other antidysrhythmic drugs including lidocaine, procainamide, phenytoin and propranolol, enhance the neuromuscular block produced by d-tubocurarine.[41,42]

The interaction between neuromuscular blocking and antidysrhythmic drugs may become manifest under another circumstance. It is not unusual for the clinician to administer a small, "defasciculating" dose of pancuronium or of d-tubocurarine prior to the administration of succinylcholine. This is a common practice in minor or outpatient surgical procedures requiring endotracheal intubation such as dental extractions and laparoscopies. Many of these patients have negative medical histories, but still frequently have diastolic pressures between 85 and 95 mm Hg and systolic pressures between 130 and 140 mm Hg. Endotracheal intubation following the induction of anesthesia (thiopental, succinylcholine) in these borderline-hypertensive patients is frequently associated with hypertension, where systolic pressures in some cases reach 200 mm Hg or more. Hypertension of this magnitude is often associated with ventricular dysrhythmias, including multifocal extrasystoles. Based on experimental evidence gathered by C. Prys-Roberts et al., it is not an uncommon practice to administer a small dose of intravenous propranolol (1.0 to 2.0 mg) 10 minutes before the induction of anesthesia in borderline hypertensive patients.[43] This effectively obtunds the hypertensive response to laryngoscopy and surgical stimulation. On several occasions, however, I have seen patients become weak and acutely dyspneic following a "defasciculating" dose of pancuronium (1.0 mg) given 5 to 10 minutes after the propranolol. The same response has been observed with "defasciculating" doses of d-tubocurarine or metocurine. The most reasonable explanation for this occurrence is the potentiation of nondepolarizing neuromuscular block by propranolol.

ANTIDYSRHYTHMIC DRUGS

In the following section, those drug actions of interest to anesthesiologists, aside from the cardiac electrophysiologic effects discussed earlier, with the greatest potential for causing interactions are discussed for each antidysrhythmic agent.

Quinidine

Quinidine depresses myocardial automaticity, conduction, and contractility. Large doses may produce hypotension by reducing peripheral resistance through the mechanism of *alpha*-adrenergic blockade.[22aa] In addition, quinidine has a significant anticholinergic effect which, in addition to reflex sympathetic stimulation resulting from *alpha*-adrenergic blockade, may increase sinus node discharge rate and improve atrioventricular nodal conduction.[22aa] This is a disadvantage when quinidine is used to treat supraventricular tachydysrhythmias: it enhances the conductivity of the atrioventricular node and prolongs the atrial effective refractory period. Unfortunately, these effects are contrary to what is needed to treat supraventricular tachycardia. Quinidine is most effective in the treatment of atrial flutter or fibrillation and of other supraventricular dysrhythmias. It has rarely been used in the long-term treatment of ventricular dysrhythmias since the advent of other drugs that are both less toxic and at least as effective (for example, procainamide, phenytoin). Quinidine and propranolol administered together in reduced doses appear to be more effective than high doses of either drug alone in converting supraventricular tachydysrhythmias to sinus rhythm.[44,45]

Anesthetists must be cautious in their approach to patients who take quinidine, not only because of quinidine's neuromuscular blocking actions mentioned earlier, but also because of its depressant effects on the circulation. Thus quinidine administered parenterally to patients who are deeply anesthetized with halothane or enflurane might cause additional circulatory depression. Also, vasodilators should be used cautiously by patients receiving quinidine. More appropriate and effective measures are available for the treatment of cardiac dysrhythmias including, in addition to drugs, direct current (DC) cardioversion in more refractory cases.

Drugs that induce hepatic enzyme production, such as phenytoin and phenobarbital, may shorten the duration of quinidine's action and reduce its serum concentration for a given dose by increasing its rate of elimination.[22aa] Quinidine may elevate serum digoxin[43c] and digitoxin concentrations[43d] by decreasing the clearance, volume of distribution, and affinity of tissue receptors for digoxin.[43e]

Procainamide

Procainamide has a myocardial depressant action similar to that of quinidine. However, it has less of an anticholinergic action than either quinidine or procainamide[43b] and more of a local anesthetic effect than quinidine.[22aa] It does not produce alpha-adrenergic blockade, but may result in peripheral vasodilation via a mild ganglionic blocking action that impairs cardiovascular reflexes.[43b] Following intravenous administration, its cardiac depressant and vasodilating properties may be dangerous to patients whose circulation is already compromised, particularly those on potent inhalation anesthetics or receiving vasodilation therapy. Both procainamide and quinidine should not be administered to patients with advanced atrioventricular conduction block, and should be administered only cautiously to patients with partial block.[43f] In patients who have a complete block with dependence on a junctional or idioventricular pacemaker, procainamide may suppress the pacemaker and cause asystole. Furthermore, an incomplete block can progress to a complete one with consequent asystole. Anesthetics may enhance this adverse effect.[16,18] The problem of producing asystole, however, is less serious today because most patients with symptomatic atrioventricular conduction block benefit from pacemaker therapy. Procainamide may be used to convert atrial fibrillation of recent onset to sinus rhythm.[43g] As with quinidine, prior treatment with digitalis, propranolol or verapamil is recommended to prevent acceleration of the ventricular response following procainamide therapy.[22aa] Finally, procainamide or quinidine may be used in conjunction with ventricular pacing in patients with the sick sinus syndrome clinically manifested as the bradycardia-tachycardia syndrome.[46] These drugs may be used when retrograde activation of the atria during ventricular pacing fails to effectively suppress ectopic atrial rhythms.

Lidocaine

Lidocaine is an effective, safe, and rapidly acting drug for the treatment of ventricular dysrhythmias and is well suited for intraoperative use. Clinically significant adverse hemodynamic effects are rarely noted unless left ventricular function is severely impaired. It is the drug preferred for most ventricular dysrhythmias that occur during anesthesia, except perhaps for those caused by digitalis excess where phenytoin is indicated (see the section on phenytoin). Lidocaine is not recommended for the treatment of supraventricular dysrhythmias, except when aberrant conduction is present and when confusion exists as to the diagnosis of ventricular tachycardia (see discussion following first case report).[43f] This drug has accelerated the ventricular response during atrial flutter and has caused sinus arrest when used in conjunction with quinidine.[35,36] As noted earlier, in relation to the first case report, lidocaine may restore sinus rhythm in apparent cases of supraventricular tachycardia during anesthesia with either enflurane or halothane. This beneficial effect could be spurious, or it could be attributed to an undiagnosed ventricular tachycardia. Furthermore, lidocaine may have different cardiac electrophysiologic effects in the presence of potent volatile anesthetic agents, effects that are responsible for its apparent usefulness in some cases of supraventricular tachycardia.[19] Until more information is available, however, lidocaine should be used cautiously in the treatment of supraventricular tachydysrhythmias during anesthesia. Cholinergic maneuvers, verapamil, propranolol, or digitalis are preferred to lidocaine. Finally, lidocaine may cause seizures. To achieve a therapeutic (antidysrhythmic) effect and to avoid seizures, the initial intravenous dose of lidocaine should not exceed 2 to 3 mg/kg body weight. A maintenance infusion of lidocaine (1.0 g in 250 ml normal saline solution) can be administered at the rate of 20 to 30 µg/kg body weight per minute.

Phenytoin (Diphenylhydantoin)

Phenytoin, or diphenylhydantoin, shares many of the cardiac electrophysiologic properties of lidocaine.[22aa] It is effective in suppressing digitalis-induced atrial and ventricular dysrhythmias in man.[22aa,46a] Lidocaine is not as effective as phenytoin in this regard.[43f] Procainamide is also effective against ventricular dysrhythmias. It differs from phenytoin in that atrioventricular conduction is further impaired by procainamide, whereas phenytoin has minimal effects on conduction.[22aa] Sinus discharge rate is minimally affected by phenytoin.[22aa] Phenytoin is of little use in treating atrial flutter or fibrillation, but it is effective in some cases of paroxysmal supraventricular tachycardia, particularly when associated with digitalis toxicity.[48] Therapeutic levels of phenytoin can be attained by the slow administration of 50 to 100 mg doses IV every 10 to 15 minutes until a therapeutic response is observed or until a maximum dose of 10 to 15 mg/kg of body weight has been given.[48-50]

Disopyramide

Disopyramide, a Class I antidysrhythmic agent, is approved in the United States by the oral route only for the treatment of ventricular dysrhythmias. Hence it cannot be used in the management of dysrhythmias encountered during anesthesia, but may be encountered in patients coming to surgery. Its efficacy is comparable with quinidine and procainamide against a similar spectrum of dysrhythmias.[22aa] Disopyramide however has disturbing side effects, including cardiovascular depression (particularly in patients with impaired left ventricular function[50a]) and ventricular tachydysrhythmia provocation (commonly associated with disopyramide-related QT prolongation, which may present itself as a peculiar type of ventricular tachycardia called torsades de pointes[50b,50c,50d]). The drug also has bothersome anticholinergic properties.[22aa] Disopyramide can, in high doses, slow the rate of sinus discharge[50e] and significantly depress sinus activity in patients with sinus node dysfunction.[22aa] It has variable effects on AV nodal conduction and prolongs His-Purkinje conduction.[22aa] In view of the above actions, the potential for additive myocardial depression and impairment of AV conduction with potent volatile inhalation agents should be expected in patients pretreated with disopyramide. Finally, disopyramide, as other Class I antidysrhythmics, can potentiate nondepolarizing neuromuscular blockade.

Propranolol

The principal use of propranolol in treating cardiac dysrhythmias is to control the ventricular rate in patients with supraventricular tachycardia. Dysrhythmias related to catecholamine excess (anesthetic sensitization, thyrotoxicosis, pheochromocytoma) often respond well to propranolol. Its *beta*-blocking as opposed to its quinidine-like action causes prolongation of atrioventricular nodal conduction and its refractory period. The *beta*-blocking action of propranolol sets it apart from other antidysrhythmic drugs that either do not affect or improve atrioventricular conduction and accelerate the ventricular rate.[22aa] Its main drawback in anesthetic practice resides in its myocardial depressant effects, which may be augmented by the presence of anesthetic agents. Thus propranolol should be given in small doses (that is, up to 3.0 mg IV in 0.5-mg increments). The desired effect is slowing of the ventricular rate sufficient to improve the cardiac output. Extreme caution should be exercised in the presence of atrioventricular block. Finally, based on experimental evidence, propranolol is expected to augment the slowing of conduction produced by halothane or enflurane.[16]

Bretylium Tosylate

Bretylium is selectively concentrated in sympathetic ganglia and their postganglionic adrenergic nerve terminals. After an initial norepinephrine discharge, it prevents further release from sympathetic nerve terminals. This is accomplished without depressing pre- or postganglionic sympathetic nerve conduction, impairing conduction across sympathetic ganglia, depleting the adrenergic stores of norepinephrine, or decreasing the responsiveness of adrenergic receptors.[50f] During chronic bretylium treatment, the *beta*-adrenergic responses to circulatory catecholamines are increased.[22aa] This has implications for the anesthetist who may consider vasopressor therapy. Furthermore, initial catecholamine release may aggravate some dysrhythmias, such as those caused by digitalis excess,[50g] and may increase the sensitizing action of anesthetics. Bretylium does not depress myocardial contractility[50f] and, after an increase in blood pressure, may cause significant hypotension by blocking the efferent limb of the baroreceptor reflex.[22aa] It apparently does not potentiate the effects of neuromuscular blocking drugs. Bretylium is currently recommended only for life-threatening ventricular dysrhythmias not responsive to lidocaine, quinidine, procainamide, or disopyramide and is not indicated for dysrhythmias due to digitalis excess. It can be given intravenously in doses of 5 to 10 mg/kg body weight administered slowly over 10 to 20 minutes. This dose may be repeated in 1 to 2 hours if the dysrhythmia persists, provided that 30 mg/kg in 24 hours are not exceeded.

Verapamil

By blocking the slow inward current, verapamil exhibits electrophysiologic effects quite different from those of other antidysrhythmic drugs (Table 17–1). It has a negative inotropic action and causes marked vasodilation in both the coronary and peripheral vascular beds.[22aa,50h] Verapamil prolongs AV nodal conduction time[50i] without affecting infranodal conduction, and minimally affecting the sinus rate of discharge (Table 17–2). The hemodynamic and AV conduction depressant effects of verapamil are likely to be magnified by potent inhalation anesthetics and *beta*-adrenergic blockers. Whether verapamil potentiates nondepolarizing neuromuscular blockade is unknown. Intravenous verapamil is the drug of choice for terminating sustained paroxysmal supraventricular tachycardias that do not respond to simple vagal maneuvers.[22aa] It should be tried prior to treatment with vasopressors, pacing, direct current cardioversion or digitalis.[22aa] Verapamil is also indicated to decrease the ventricular response over the AV node in the presence of atrial flutter or fibrillation,[50j,50k] and may convert a small number of episodes, particularly those of recent onset, to sinus rhythm.[22aa] Quinidine, however, appears to be more effective than verapamil in restoring sinus rhythm in patients with chronic atrial fibrillation.[50] Verapamil is administered intravenously in a dose of 5 to 10 mg over 1 to 2 minutes. This may be repeated in 20 to 30 minutes.

New Antidysrhythmic Drugs

Amiodarone. Amiodarone is a benzofuran derivative introduced almost 20 years ago as a peripheral vascular and coronary vasodilator. It also possesses a broad spectrum of antidysrhythmic action.[22o,22p,22q,22r] Clinically, it may slow sinus activity and prolong AV nodal conduction time.[22aa] It is useful for suppressing supraventricular and ventricular tachydysrhythmias.[22r,50m,50n,50o] Whether potent inhalation anesthetics augment the vasodilator or negative chronotropic and dromotropic effects of amiodarone is not known. Amiodarone may be associated with neuromuscular disturbances, particularly at high doses, but its interactions with neuromuscular blocking drugs are not known.

Aprindine. Aprindine exerts prominent local anesthetic (Class I) effects in higher concentrations, and possesses slow-channel blocking properties as well.[22aa] It appears effective against both supraventricular and ventricular tachydysrhythmias, and it prolongs conduction time and refractoriness in both the AV node and accessory pathways in patients who have the reciprocating tachycardia of Wolff-Parkinson-White syndrome.[50p] Its potential for interactions with anesthetics is unknown. Since it is a Class I antidysrhythmic, it would be expected to potentiate non-depolarizing neuromuscular blockers.

Mexiletine. Mexiletine, a local anesthetic with anticonvulsant properties, is similar to lidocaine in its electrophysiologic actions.[22aa] It has the advantage over lidocaine of reliable oral abosorption. Its effects on the sinus rate of discharge and AV nodal conduction time are variable,[50q] as are those of lidocaine. It is most effective in ventricular dysrhythmias.[22aa] Cardiovascular side effects, which appear at dose levels slightly higher than therapeutic, include hypotension, bradycardia and exacerbation of dysrhythmias.[50r] Mexiletine is likely (Class I antidysrhythmic) to potentiate neuromuscular blocking drugs.

Tocainide. Tocainide is an orally effective primary amine analog of lidocaine with similar electrophysiologic effects.[22aa] It can reduce the frequency of ventricular premature beats but apparently is not as effective in preventing recurrent ventricular tachycardia-ventricular fibrillation.[22a] The response to lidocaine may be helpful in predicting the chances of failure with tocainide: if lidocaine fails to suppress a ventricular dysrhythmia, tocainide has about an 85% chance of failing.[22aa] Adverse effects for tocainide are dose-related, and similar to those of lidocaine.[22aa] The drug may potentiate nondepolarizing neuromuscular blockade.

In conclusion, cardiac dysrhythmias occur frequently during anesthesia and thus concern the anesthetist. They warrant treatment when impaired hemodynamics compromise tissue perfusion, when there is an unfavorable ratio between myocardial oxygen supply and demand, or when the dysrhythmia is likely to predispose the patient to ventricular tachycardia or fibrillation. Treatment in most cases simply involves the removal of the precipitating cause, which frequently is hypoxia, inadequate ventilation, or an electrolyte imbalance. In many patients, however, the precipitating cause is not readily apparent; or, as in the case of digitalis intoxication, it is not easily removed. Antidysrhythmic agents themselves, when used improperly, may cause or further aggravate existing dysrhythmias. Increasing evidence suggests that anesthetic agents may alter the pharmacologic properties of commonly used antidysrhythmic agents. Further research is needed to elucidate the mechanisms and frequency of anesthetic-antidysrhythmic drug interactions. In the meantime, a cautious approach to the problem is advised. An increased understanding on the part of clinicians of dysrhythmia mechanisms and of the pharmacology of antidysrhythmic drugs could decrease the incidence of adverse interactions or could direct their proper management. In addition, careful monitoring and selection of drugs, or the use of smaller doses, are recommended.

REFERENCES

1. Kuner, J., et al.: Cardiac arrhythmias during anesthesia. Dis. Chest, 52:580, 1967.
2. Cranefield, P.F., Wit, A.L., and Hoffman, B.F.: Genesis of cardiac arrhythmias. Circulation, 47:190, 1973.
2a. Zipes, D.P.: Genesis of cardiac arrhythmias: Electrophysiological considerations. In Heart Disease. Braunwald, E., (ed.), Philadelphia, W.B. Saunders Co., 1984, p. 605.
3. Noble, D.: The Initiation of the Heartbeat. Oxford, Clarendon Press, 1975.
3a. Vassalle, M.: Cardiac automaticity and its control. In Excitation and Neural Control of the Heart. Levy, M.N., and Vassalle, M., (eds.), Bethesda, American Physiological Society, 1982.
3b. DiFrancesco, D.: A new interpretation of the pacemaker current in calf Purkinje fibers. J. Physiol. (Lond.), 314:359, 1981.
3c. Carmeliet, E., and Saikawa, T.: Shortening of the action potential and reduction of pacemaker activity by lidocaine, quinidine and procainamide in sheep cardiac Purkinje fibers. An effect on Na or K currents? Circ. Res., 50:257, 1982.
3d. Brown, H.F.: Electrophysiology of the sinoatrial node. Physiol. Rev., 62:505, 1982.
4. Noble, D., and Tsien, R.W.: The kinetics and rec-

tifier properties of the slow potassium current in cardiac Purkinje fibers. J. Physiol. (Lond.), 195:185, 1968.
5. Reynolds, A.K., Chiz, J.F., and Pasquet, A.F.: Halothane and methoxyflurane: A comparison of their effects on cardiac pacemaker fibers. Anesthesiology, 33:602, 1970.
5a. Friedman, P.L., Stewart, J.R., and Wit, A.L.: Spontaneous and induced cardiac arrhythmias in subendocardial Purkinje fibers surviving extensive myocardial infarction in dogs. Circ. Res., 22:612, 1973.
5b. Gilmour, R.F., Jr., and Zipes, D.P.: Electrophysiological characteristics of rodent myocardium damaged by adrenaline. Cardiovasc. Res., 14:582, 1980.
5c. Ten Eick, R.E., and Singer, D.H.: Electrophysiological properties of diseased human atrium. I. Low diastolic potential and altered cellular response to potassium. Circ. Res., 44:545, 1979.
5d. Spear, J.F., Horowitz, L.N., and Moore, E.N.: The slow response in human ventricle. Zipes, D.P., et al. (eds.): The Slow Inward Current and Cardiac Arrhythmias. The Hague, Martinus Nijhoff, 1980, p. 309.
5e. Singer, D.H., Baumgarten, C.M., and Ten Eick, R.E.: Cellular electrophysiology of ventricular and other dysrhythmias. Studies on diseased and ischemic heart. Prog. Cardiovasc. Res., 49:1, 1981.
5f. Hoffmann, B.F., and Rosen, M.R.: Cellular mechanisms for cardiac arrhythmias. Circ. Res., 49:1, 1981.
6. Ferrier, G.R.: Digitalis arrhythmias: Role of oscillatory afterpotentials. Prog. Cardiovasc. Dis., 19:459, 1977.
7. Cranefield, P.F.: Action potentials, afterpotentials and arrhythmias. Circ. Res., 41:415, 1977.
7a. Rosen, M.R., Merker, C., Gelband, H., et al.: Mechanisms of digitalis toxicity: Effects of ouabain on phase 4 of canine Purkinje fiber transmembrane potentials. Circulation, 47:681, 1973.
8. Hashimoto, K., and Moe, G.K.: Transient depolarizations induced by acetylstrophanthidin in specialized tissue of dog atrium and ventricle. Circ. Res., 32:618, 1973.
9. Ferrier, G.R., Saunders, J.H., and Mendez, C.: A cellular mechanism for the generation of ventricular arrhythmias by acetylstrophanthidin. Circ. Res., 32:600, 1973.
9a. Wit, A.L., Fenoglio, J.J., Hordof, A.J., et al.: Ultrastructure and transmembrane potentials of cardiac muscle in human anterior mitral valve leaflet. Circulation, 59:1284, 1979.
9b. Zipes, D.P., Arbel, E., Knope, R.F., et al.: Accelerated cardiac escape rhythms caused by ouabain intoxication. Am. J. Cardiol., 33:248, 1974.
9c. Zipes, D.P., Foster, P.R., Troup, P.J., et al.: Atrial induction of ventricular tachycardia: Reentry or triggered automaticity. Am. J. Cardiol., 44:1, 1979.
9d. Rosen, M.R., Fisch, C., Hoffmann, B.F., et al.: Can accelerated atrioventricular junction escape rhythms be explained by delayed afterdepolarizations? Am. J. Cardiol., 45:1272, 1980.
9e. Wellens, H.J.J., Brugada, P., Vanagt, E.J.D.M., et al.: New studies with triggered automaticity. In Cardiac Arrhythmias: A Decade of Progress. Boston, G.K. Hall, 1981, p. 601.
10. Moe, G.K.: Evidence for reentry as a mechanism of cardiac arrhythmias. Rev. Physiol. Biochem. Pharmacol., 72:55, 1975.
11. Reynolds, A.K., Chiz, J.F., and Pasquet, A.F.: Pacemaker migration and sinus node arrest with methoxyflurane and halothane. Can. Anaesth. Soc. J., 18:137, 1971.
12. Reynolds, A.K., Chiz, J.F., and Tanikella, T.K.: On the mechanism of coupling in adrenaline-induced bigeminy in sensitized hearts. Can. J. Physiol. Pharmacol., 53:1158, 1975.
13. Sasyniuk, B.I., and Dresel, P.E.: Mechanism and site of origin of bigeminal rhythm in cyclopropane-sensitized dogs. Am. J. Physiol., 220:1857, 1971.
14. Zink, J., Sasyniuk, B.I., and Dresel, P.E.: Halothane-epinephrine-induced cardiac arrhythmias and the role of heart rate. Anesthesiology, 43:548, 1975.
15. Hashimoto, K., et al.: Effects of halothane on automaticity and contractile force of isolated blood-perfused canine ventricular tissue. Anesthesiology, 42:15, 1975.
16. Atlee, J.L., and Rusy, B.F.: Halothane depression of A-V conduction studied by electrograms of the bundle of His in dogs. Anesthesiology, 36:112, 1972.
16a. Atlee, J.L., and Rusy, B.F.: Atrioventricular conduction times and atrioventricular nodal conductivity during enflurane anesthesia in dogs. Anesthesiology, 47:498, 1977.
17. Atlee, J.L., and Alexander, S.C.: Halothane effects on conductivity of the AV node and His-Purkinje system in the dog. Anesth. Analg. (Cleve.), 56:378, 1977.
18. Atlee, J.L., et al.: Supraventricular excitability in dogs during anesthesia with halothane and enflurane. Anesthesiology, 49:407, 1978.
19. Atlee, J.L., Homer, L.D., and Tobey, R.E.: Diphenylhydantoin and lidocaine modification of A-V conduction in halothane anesthetized dogs. Anesthesiology, 43:49, 1975.
20. Morrow, D.H., Logic, J.R., and Haley, J.V.: Antiarrhythmic anesthetic action 1: The effect of halothane on canine intracardiac impulse conduction during sinus rhythm. Anesth. Analg. (Cleve.), 56:187, 1977.
21. Geha, D.G., et al.: Pancuronium bromide enhances atrioventricular conduction in halothane-anesthetized dogs. Anesthesiology, 46:342, 1977.
22. Singh, B.N., and Hauswirth, O.: Comparative mechanisms of action of antiarrhythmic drugs. Am. Heart J., 87:367, 1974.
22a. Singh, B.N., and Mandel, W.J.: Antiarrhythmic drugs: Basic concepts of their actions, pharmacokinetic characteristics, and clinical characteristics. In Cardiac Arrhythmias. Mandel, W.J., (ed.), Philadelphia, J.B. Lippincott Co., 1980.
22aa. Zipes, D.P.: Management of cardiac arrhythmias: Pharmacological, electrical and surgical techniques. In Heart Disease. Braunwald, E., (ed.), Philadelphia, W.B. Saunders Co., 1984, p. 648.

22b. Singh, B.N.: The rationale basis of antiarrhythmic therapy: the clinical pharmacology of commonly used antiarrhythmic drugs. Angiology, 29:206, 1978.
22c. Singh, B.N., and Vaughan Williams, E.M.: A fourth class of antidysrhythmic action? Effect of verapamil on ouabain toxicity, on atrial and ventricular intracellular potentials and on other features of cardiac function. Cardiovasc. Res., 6:109, 1972.
22d. Bigger, J.T., Jr., and Mandel, W.J.: Effect of lidocaine on conduction in canine Purkinje fibers and at the ventricular muscle Purkinje fiber junction. J. Pharmacol. Exp. Ther., 174:487, 1970.
22e. Rosen, M.R., Merker, C., and Hoffmann, B.F.: Effects of blood perfusion on electrophysiological properties of isolated canine Purkinje fibers. Circ. Res., 30:574, 1972.
22f. Singh, B.N., and Vaughan Williams, E.M.: Local anesthetic and antiarrhythmic actions of alprenolol relative to its effects on intracellular potentials and other properties of isolated cardiac muscle. Br. J. Pharmacol., 38:749, 1970.
22g. Jewitt, D.E., and Singh, B.N.: The role of beta-adrenergic blockade in myocardial infarction. Prog. Cardiovasc. Dis., 16:421, 1974.
22h. Bacaner, M.B.: Bretylium tosylate for suppression of induced ventricular fibrillation. Am. J. Cardiol., 17:528, 1966.
22i. Bacaner, M.B.: Treatment of ventricular fibrillation and other acute arrhythmias with bretylium tosylate. Am. J. Cardiol., 21:530, 1968.
22j. Gill, E.W., and Vaughan Williams, E.M.: Local anesthetic activity of the β-receptor antagonist, pronethalol. Nature, 118:657, 1964.
22l. Vaughan Williams, E.M.: Classification of antiarrhythmic drugs. J. Pharmacol. Ther., 1:115, 1975.
22m. Freedberg, A.S., Papper, J.G., and Vaughan Williams, E.M.: The effect of altered thyroid state on atrial intracellular potentials. J. Physiol., 207:357, 1970.
22n. Singh, B.N., and Vaughan Williams, E.M.: The effect of amiodarone, a new anti-anginal drug on cardiac muscle. Br. J. Pharmacol., 39:657, 1970.
22o. Rosenbaum, M.B., Chiale, P.A., Ryba, D., et al.: Control of tachyarrhythmias associated with Wolff-Parkinson-White syndrome by amiodarone hydrochloride. Am. J. Cardiol., 34:215, 1975.
22p. Rosenbaum, M.B., Chiale, P.A., Halpern, M.S.: Clinical efficacy of amiodarone as an antiarrhythmic agent. Am. J. Cardiol., 38:934, 1976.
22q. Grayboys, T.B., Podrid, P.J., and Lown, B.: Efficacy of amiodarone for refractory supraventricular tachyarrhythmias. Am. Heart J., 106:870, 1983.
22r. Heger, J.J., Prystowsky, E.N., and Zipes, D.P.: Clinical efficacy of amiodarone in treatment of recurrent ventricular tachycardia and ventricular fibrillation. Am. Heart J., 106:887, 1983.
22s. Charlier, R.: Cardiac actions in the dog of a new antagonist of adrenergic excitation which does not produce competitive blockade of adrenoreceptors. Br. J. Pharmacol., 39:668, 1970.
23. Bigger, J.T., and Jaffe, C.C.: The effect of bretylium tosylate on the electrophysiological properties of ventricular muscle and Purkinje fibers. Am. J. Cardiol., 27:82, 1971.
24. Papp, J.G., and Vaughan Williams, E.M.: The effect on intracellular atrial potentials of bretylium in relation to its local anesthetic potency. Br. J. Pharmacol., 35:352, 1969.
25. Cranefield, P.F.: The Conduction of the Cardiac Impulse. Mount Kisco, New York, Futura, 1975.
25a. Rickensberger, R.L., Prystowsky, E.N., Heger, J.J., et al.: Effects of intravenous and chronic oral verapamil administration in patients with supraventricular tachyarrhythmias. Circulation 62:996, 1980.
25b. Sung, R.J., Elser, B., and McAllister, R.G., Jr.: Intravenous verapamil for termination of reentrant supraventricular tachycardias. Intracardiac studies correlated with plasma verapamil concentrations. Ann. Intern. Med., 93:682, 1980.
25c. Hammer, A., Peter, T., Platt, M., et al.: Effects of verapamil on supraventricular tachycardia in patients with overt and concealed Wolff-Parkinson-White syndrome. Am. Heart J., 101:600, 1981.
25d. Wellens, H.J.J., Farre, J., and Bar, F.W.: The role of the slow inward current in genesis of ventricular tachycardias in man. In The Slow Inward Current and Cardiac Arrhythmias. Zipes, D.P., et al. (eds.), The Hague, Martinus Nijhoff, 1980, p. 507.
26. Way, W.L., Katzung, B.G., and Larson, C.P., Jr.: Recurarization with quinidine. J.A.M.A., 200:163, 1967.
27. Johnson, L.W., et al.: Prophylactic digitalization for coronary artery bypass surgery. Circulation, 53:819, 1976.
27a. Tyras, D.H., Stothert, J.C., Kaiser, G.C., et al.: Supraventricular tachyarrhythmias after myocardial revascularization: A randomized trial of prophylactic digitalization. J. Thorac. Cardiovasc. Surg., 77:310, 1979.
27b. Morrison, J., and Killip, T.: Serum digitalis and arrhythmia in patients undergoing cardiopulmonary bypass. Circulation, 47:341, 1973.
27c. Atlee, J.L., Ammendrup, P., and Malkinson, C.E.: Halothane and hypocapnia: Effects on electrically stimulated atrial arrhythmias in digitalized dogs. Anesth. Analg., 60:302, 1981.
28. Basta, J.W., and Lichtiger, M.: Comparison of metocurine and pancuronium—myocardial tension-time index during endotracheal intubation. Anesthesiology, 46:366, 1977.
29. Miller, R.D., et al.: Pancuronium-induced tachycardia in relation to alveolar halothane, dose of pancuronium, and prior atropine. Anesthesiology, 42:352, 1975.
30. Stoelting, R.K.: The hemodynamic effects of pancuronium and d-tubocurarine in anesthetized patients. Anesthesiology, 36:612, 1972.
31. Edwards, R., Winnie, A.P., and Ramamurthy, S.: Acute hypocapneic hypokalemia: An iatrogenic anesthetic complication. Anesth. Analg. (Cleve.), 56:786, 1977.
32. Miller, R.D., and Roderick, L.: Diuretic-induced hypokalemia, pancuronium neuromuscular blockade and its antagonism by neostigmine. Br. J. Anaesth., 50:541, 1978.

33. Warner, H.: Therapy of common arrhythmias. Med. Clin. North Am., 58:995, 1974.
34. Sprague, D.H., and Mandel, S.D.: Paroxysmal supraventricular tachycardia during anesthesia. Anesthesiology, 46:75, 1977.
35. Marriott, H.J.L., and Bieza, C.F.: Alarming ventricular acceleration after lidocaine administration. Chest, 61:682, 1972.
36. Jeresaty, R.M., Kahn, A.H., and Landry, A.B., Jr.: Sinoatrial arrest due to lidocaine in a patient receiving quinidine. Chest, 61:683, 1972.
37. Galindo, A., Wyte, S.R., and Wetherhold, J.W.: Junctional rhythm induced by halothane anesthesia—Treatment with succinylcholine. Anesthesiology, 37:261, 1971.
38. Galindo, A., and Davis, T.B.: Succinylcholine and cardiac excitability. Anesthesiology, 23:32, 1962.
39. Dowdy, E.G., and Fabian, L.W.: Ventricular arrhythmias induced by succinylcholine in digitalized patients. Anesth. Analg. (Cleve.), 42:501, 1963.
40. Birch, A.A.B., Mitchell, G.D., and Playford, G.A.: Changes in serum potassium response to succinylcholine following trauma. J.A.M.A., 210:490, 1969.
40a. Lebowitz, P.W., Ramsey, F.M., Savarese, J.J., et al.: Combination of pancuronium and metocurine: Neuromuscular and hemodynamic advantages over pancuronium alone. Anesth. Analg., 60:12, 1981.
41. Miller, R.D., Way, W.L., and Katzung, B.G.: The potentiation of neuromuscular blocking agents by quinidine. Anesthesiology, 28:1036, 1967.
42. Harrah, M.D., Way, W.L., and Katzung, B.G.: The interaction of d-tubocurarine with antiarrhythmic drugs. Anesthesiology, 33:406, 1970.
43. Prys-Roberts, C., et al.: Studies of anaesthesia in relation to hypertension V: Adrenergic beta-receptor blockade. Br. J. Anaesth., 45:671, 1973.
43a. Mason, J.W., Winkle, R.A., Rider, A.K., et al.: The electrophysiologic effect of quinidine in the transplanted human heart. J. Clin. Invest., 59:481, 1977.
43b. Mirro, M.J., Manalan, A.S., Bailey, J.C., et al.: anticholinergic effects of disopyramide and quinidine on guinea pig myocardium: Mediation by direct muscarinic receptor blockade. Circ. Res., 47:855, 1980.
43c. Fenster, P.E., and Perrier, D.: Applications of pharmacokinetic principles to cardiovascular drugs. Mod. Conc. Cardiovasc. Dis., 51:91, 1982.
43d. Schenck-Gustaffsson, K., Jogestrand, T., Nordlander, R., et al.: Effect of quinidine on digoxin concentration in skeletal muscle and serum in patients with atrial fibrillation. Evidence for reduced binding of digoxin in muscle. N. Engl. J. Med., 305:209, 1981.
43e. Ball, W.J., Jr., Tse-Eng, D., Wallick, E.T., et al.: Effects of quinidine on the digoxin receptor in vitro. J. Clin. Invest., 68:1065, 1981.
43f. Bigger, J.T., and Hoffman, B.F.: Antiarrhythmic drugs, In The Pharmacological Basis of Therapeutics. 6th Ed. Gilman, A.G., Goodman, L.S., and Gilman, A., (eds.), New York, Macmillan Publishing Co., Inc., 1980.
44. Stern, S.: Conversion of chronic atrial fibrillation to sinus rhythm with combined propranolol and quinidine treatment. Am. Heart J., 74:170, 1967.
45. Fors, W.J., Vanderark, C.R., and Reynolds, E.W., Jr.: Evaluation of propranolol and quinidine in the treatment of quinidine-resistant arrhythmias. Am. J. Cardiol., 27:190, 1971.
46. Scarpa, W.J.: The sick sinus syndrome. Am. Heart J., 92:648, 1976.
46a. Fisch, C., Zipes, D.P., and Noble, R.J.: Digitalis toxicity: Mechanisms and recognition. Yu P., and Goodwin R. (eds.): Progress in Cardiology, 4:37, 1975.
47. Helfant, R.H., Scherlag, B.J., and Damato, A.N.: The electrophysiological properties of diphenylhydantoin sodium as compared to procainamide in the normal and digitalis-intoxicated heart. Circulation, 36:108, 1967.
48. Bigger, J.T.: Arrhythmias and anti-arrhythmic drugs. Adv. Intern. Med., 18:251, 1972.
49. Lang, T.W., et al.: The use of diphenylhydantoin for the treatment of digitalis toxicity. Arch. Intern. Med., 116:573, 1965.
50. Bigger, J.T., Jr., Schmidt, D.H., and Kutt, H.: Relationship between plasma level of diphenylhydantoin sodium and its cardiac antiarrhythmic effects. Circulation, 38:363, 1968.
50a. Leach, A.J., Brown, J.E., and Armstrong, P.W.: Cardiac depression by intravenous disopyramide in patients with left ventricular function. Am.J. Med., 68:839, 1980.
50b. Smith, W.M., and Gallagher, J.J.: "Les torsades de pointes." An unusual ventricular arrhythmia. Ann. Intern. Med., 93:578, 1980.
50c. Morady, F., Scheinman, M.M., and Desai, J.: Disopyramide. Ann. Intern. Med., 96:337, 1982.
50d. Tzivoni, D., Keren, A., Stern, S., et al.: Disopyramide-induced torsades de pointes. Arch. Intern. Med., 141:946, 1981.
50e. Katoh, T., Karagueuzian, H., Jordan, J., and Mandel, W.: The cellular electrophysiologic mechanism of the dual actions of disopyramide on rabbit sinus node function. Circulation, 66:1216, 1982.
50f. Bigger, J.T., Jr.: Management of Arrhythmias. In Heart Disease: A Textbook of Cardiovascular Management. Braunwald, E., (ed.), Philadelphia, W.B. Saunders Co., 1980, p. 717.
50g. Gillis, R.A., Clancy, M.M., and Anderson, R.J.: The deleterious effects of bretylium in cats with digitalis-induced ventricular tachycardia. Circulation, 47:976, 1973.
50h. Singh, B.N., Collett, J.T., and Chew, C.Y.C.: New perspectives in the pharmacologic therapy of cardiac arrhythmias. Prog. Cardiovasc. Dis., 22:243, 1980.
50i. Wellens, H.J.J., Tan, S.L., Bar, F.W.H., et al.: Effects of verapamil studied by programmed electrical stimulation of the heart in patients with paroxysmal reentrant supraventricular tachycardia. Br. Heart J., 39:1058, 1977.
50j. Schamroth, L.: Immediate effects of intravenous verapamil on atrial fibrillation. Cardiovasc. Res., 5:419, 1971.
50k. Waxman, H.L., Myerburg, R.J., Appel, R., et al.: Verapamil for control of ventricular rate in par-

oxysmal supraventricular tachycardia and atrial fibrillation or flutter: A double-blind randomized cross-over study. Ann. Intern. Med., 94:1, 1981.

50l. Rasmussen, K., Wang, H., and Fausa, D.: Comparative efficiency of quinidine and verapamil in the maintenance of sinus rhythm after DC conversion of atrial fibrillation. A controlled clinical trial. Acta Med. Scand., 23(Suppl.):645, 1981.

50m. Podrid, P.J., and Lown, B.: Amiodarone therapy and symptomatic sustained refractory atrial and ventricular tachyarrhythmias. Am. Heart J., 101:374, 1981.

50n. Coumel, P., and Fidelle, J.: Amiodarone in the treatment of cardiac arrhythmias in children: 135 cases. Am. Heart J., 100:1063, 1980.

50o. Marcus, F.T., Fontaine, G.H., Frank, R., et al.: Clinical pharmacology and therapeutic applications of the antiarrhythmic agent, amiodarone. Am. Heart J., 101:480, 1981.

50p. Zipes, D.P., Gaum, W.E., Foster, P.R., et al.: Aprindine for the treatment of supraventricular tachycardias with particular application to the WPW syndrome. Am. J. Cardiol., 40:586, 1977.

50q. Heger, J.J., Prystowsky, E.N., and Zipes, D.P.: Clinical choice of antiarrhythmic drugs. *In* Ventricular Tachycardia—Mechanisms and Management. Josephson, M.E. (ed.), Mt. Kisco, N.Y., Futura Publishing Co., 1982.

50r. Cocco, G., Strozzi, C., Chu, D., et al.: Torsades de pointes as a manifestation of mexiletine toxicity. Am. Heart J., 100:878, 1980.

|18|

ANTIEPILEPTIC AGENTS

ROBERT M. JULIEN

Currently there are an estimated 2 million individuals in the United States suffering from seizure disorders. Of these, approximately 25,000 per year will receive an anesthetic procedure. Since these patients are maintained on long-term medication, the anesthesiologist must be aware of the special considerations concerning seizure control as well as the pharmacology, pharmacokinetics, and drug interactions involved. In addition, certain preoperative and perioperative principles should be observed in the management of such patients.

In the preoperative consultation, the anesthesiologist should consider the following questions:

1. Is the patient currently in the optimal state of seizure control?
2. If not, can the therapy be optimized (see below) before surgery?
3. If not, should surgery be delayed until the optimal degree of control can be achieved?
4. How should seizure control be maintained through the period of perioperative fasting?
5. What anesthetic techniques will be most suited for this patient?
6. How will the patient's antiepileptic medication affect the anesthetic; what are the drug interactions involved between anesthetic agents and antiepileptic medication?

Table 18–1 lists the antiepileptic drugs currently available in the United States. Thirteen of these agents were introduced between 1946 and 1960. Only one agent, diazepam, was introduced between 1960 and 1974, although its initial primary indication was not epilepsy. With a resurgence of interest in epilepsy during the 1960s and the 1970s, three new agents have been introduced into therapy: carbamazepine, clonazepam (an anticonvulsant benzodiazepine), and valproic acid, and two additional benzodiazepines (clorazepate and lorazepam) have found uses as anticonvulsants. Concomitant with this has been the development of chemical analysis of antiepileptic drug concentrations in plasma (as well as in other body fluids, such as saliva) and the correlation between these levels and seizure control. With the routine use of these analytical techniques and with careful adjustment of drug dosage, 80% of epileptic patients can become seizure free with currently available drugs, while in the remaining 20%, seizure frequency can be greatly reduced.

The pharmacology of these drugs and their interactions with each other have been extensively reviewed in recent monographs.[1,2]

PHARMACOKINETICS OF ANTIEPILEPTIC DRUGS

Antiepileptic drug therapy was one of the first areas of medicine to benefit from

Table 18-1
Antiepileptic Drugs Available in the United States

Year Introduced	Generic Name	U.S. Trade Name	Manufacturer
1912	phenobarbital	Luminal	Winthrop
1935	mephobarbital	Mebaral	Winthrop
1938	phenytoin	Dilantin	Parke-Davis
1946	trimethadione	Tridione	Abbott
1947	mephenytoin	Mesantoin	Sandoz
1949	paramethadione	Paradione	Abbott
1951	phenacetamide	Phenurone	Abbott
1952	metharbital	Gemonil	Abbott
1953	phensuximide	Milontin	Parke-Davis
1954	primidone	Mysoline	Ayerst
1957	methsuximide	Celontin	Parke-Davis
1957	ethotoin	Peganone	Abbott
1960	ethosuximide	Zarontin	Parke-Davis
1968	diazepam	Valium	Roche
1974	carbamazepine	Tegretol	Geigy
1975	clonazepam	Clonopin	Roche
1978	valproic acid	Depakene	Abbott
1981	clorazepate	Tranxene	Abbott
	lorazepam	Ativan	Wyeth

clinical pharmacokinetics and the use of plasma drug level correlations with seizure control.[3,4] Knowledge of therapeutically effective ranges of plasma drug concentrations and drug half-lives assists in the perioperative management of the epileptic patient. Hence, the answer to the first preanesthetic question (is the patient under optimal control?) should be provided by blood level determination of the antiepileptic drug and by correlation with the medical, neurologic and pharmacologic history of the patient.

Table 18-2 summarizes the relevant pharmacokinetic data for antiepileptic drugs. The discussion which follows expands on the perioperative maintenance of the therapeutic levels of these agents when oral medications have been suspended and on the alternative medication if necessary. The discussion presumes that the patient's dosage of antiepileptic medications has been maintained relatively constant before surgery and that additional antiepileptic drugs have been neither added nor deleted in the immediate preoperative period. If such alterations in medication have occurred, plasma levels of current medications may be unstable and neurologic consultation may be needed. Woodbury[2] delineates the numerous interactions of antiepileptic drugs with each other. Here, only those interactions of most direct relevance to the anesthesiologist will be reviewed.

Phenytoin

CASE REPORT

Patient is a 68-year-old white male admitted for a cholecystectomy. The patient's history is significant for ethanol abuse (2 years post abstention) and a subdural hematoma suffered several years before admission. One year before admission, the patient experienced several grand mal (major motor) seizures requiring intravenous diazepam for control and oral phenytoin (300 mg/day) for maintenance. The patient had not taken phenytoin for several weeks prior to the present admission and no seizure activity had occurred. As preanesthetic medication, 300 mg phenytoin was administered orally at bedtime the night before surgery and again at 0700 the morning of surgery. Induction was accomplished with thiopental, 280 mg, and atracurium, 30 mg. The patient was maintained on isoflurane and nitrous oxide with controlled ventilation calculated to avoid hyperventilation. Diazepam 6 mg, IV, was administered 1 hour after induction. In the recovery room, the patient received meperidine, 75 mg IM, and morphine sulphate, 4 mg, IV. Phenytoin, 300 mg, was administered intravenously at 2000 hours and again at 0800 the morning after surgery. On the second postoperative day, oral phenytoin was restarted at 100 mg

Table 18-2
Pharmacokinetic Parameters of Antiepileptic Drugs

Drug	Daily Dose (mg/kg)	Half-life (hours)	Therapeutic Blood Level (µg/ml)
Phenytoin	3–5	22 (20–24)	10–20
Phenobarbital	1.5–3.5	96 (50–140) adults 55 (40–70) children	15–35
Carbamazepine	10–20	37 (20–50) initially 16 (5–26) chronic therapy	4–10
Primidone	10–15	10 (5–18) (primidone) 56 (PEMA) 96 (phenobarbital)	10–13 (primidone) 15–25 (phenobarbital)
Ethosuximide	20–25	36 (15–68) children 60 adults	60 (40–100)
Diazepam	0.2–0.4	36 (30–40)	0.3–0.7
Clonazepam	0.05–0.15	26 (20–40)	0.03–0.06
Valproic Acid	10–25	9 (6–12)	50–100
Acetazolamide	10	11 (10–12)	10–14
Methylphenobarbital	3–4	49 (30–60) initially 19 (12–24) chronic therapy	15–20 (phenobarbital) 1–4 (methylphenobarbital)
Trimethadione	50	16 (trimethadione) 240 (dimethadione)	35 (20–40) (trimethadione) 700 (500–1200) (dimethadione)
Clorazepate	0.5	48	1–2
Lorazepam	4–8, acute i.v.	18	0.03–0.1
Methsuximide	5–15	1–2 (methsuximide) 38 (desmethylmethsuximide)	0.04 (methsuximide) 28 (20–40) (desmethylmethsuximide)

tid. No epileptiform activity was noted during the hospitalization or over the subsequent several weeks.

Phenytoin (diphenylhydantoin, Dilantin) is useful in grand mal (generalized major motor), complex partial (temporal lobe), and focal cortical seizures. It is generally ineffective in absence (petit mal), febrile, and myoclonic seizures.

Phenytoin has a half-life of about 22 hours.[5] Thus, a once daily dosage (e.g., 300 mg at bedtime) is therapeutically as effective as a divided dosage (e.g., 100 mg three times daily). Drug which would be ordinarily taken on the day of surgery can therefore be administered as part of a preanesthetic medication the morning of surgery (e.g., 300 mg po, 0630). Oral medications can be resumed on the first postoperative day without a significant decrease in therapeutic concentrations (10 to 20 µg/ml). If oral medications cannot be resumed on postoperative days, phenytoin can be administered by slow intravenous infusion (i.e., over 15 to 30 minutes). Alcoholics and patients who require large daily doses of phenytoin are likely to be rapid metabolizers of the drug. Therefore, significantly shorter half-lives should be expected and shorter dosage intervals planned.

The often quoted therapeutic range of plasma concentrations of phenytoin is 10 to 20 µg/ml and, indeed, such a level is a good preoperative rule-of-thumb. It should be noted, however, that some patients are seizure-free at levels of 2 or 3 µg/ml, and some require levels around 25 µg/ml.[6] This explains the importance of correlating the current plasma level with the preoperative assessment of the patient and of correlating this value with those recorded during past periods of adequate control.

Intramuscular injection of phenytoin should be avoided since such injection is painful (crystals are deposited at the site of injection, causing local tissue necrosis) and absorption is erratic, producing lower than expected blood levels.[7,8]

Side effects from phenytoin are common, and several are relevant to anesthesia. Peripheral neuropathies may develop after years of use,[9] necessitating close physical examination of the extremities before peripheral nerve blocks are placed. Hepatitis and bone marrow depression are rare occurrences. Folic acid depletion may occur and may progress to megaloblastic anemia. Folate administration will resolve the anemia and allow continuation of phenytoin. More infrequent hematologic toxicities include aplastic anemia, leukopenia and agranulocytosis. (See Ref. 10 for extensive review of the hematologic toxicities of phenytoin.)

Several drug interactions involving phenytoin are important in anesthesia. Halothane can increase the serum levels of phenytoin, possibly secondary to a toxic effect of halothane on the liver with a secondary decrease in the metabolism of phenytoin.[11] Phenytoin may stimulate the hepatic metabolism of fluroxene to a hepatotoxin.[12] Thus, epileptics receiving phenytoin (and possibly phenobarbital) may constitute a high-risk group for hepatic damage after halothane- or vinyl-radical-containing anesthetics. Patients taking phenytoin chronically and subsequently given benzodiazepines may exhibit increases in phenytoin levels secondary to a depressed phenytoin metabolism. Also, the half-life of benzodiazepines decreases in phenytoin- or phenobarbital-treated patients secondary to an increase in the rate of benzodiazepine metabolism. Tricyclic antidepressants in high doses may reduce seizure thresholds; thus, if an epileptic patient is started on such drugs, the dose of anticonvulsant may have to be increased. Phenytoin-treated patients given barbiturates acutely, for example, during thiopental induction, probably exhibit increases in phenytoin levels in plasma and can be more susceptible to the barbiturates than are nonepileptics. Cimetidine inhibits phenytoin metabolism, increasing serum phenytoin levels.[13] One case of severe neutropenia in a phenytoin- and cimetidine-treated patient has been reported.[14]

Phenobarbital

CASE REPORT

Patient is a 42-year-old female with chronic pelvic pain admitted for a total abdominal hysterectomy. History is significant for 3 years of major motor seizures of unknown etiology. The EEG demonstrates a left frontal focus. She was initially treated with phenytoin, 300 mg daily. A morbiliform rash developed, and primidone was substituted. This latter drug, however, produced weakness, tight chest, headache, disturbances in vision and a loss of motor control. The patient was placed on phenobarbital, 30 mg tid. This compound was well tolerated. Preanesthetic medication consisted of phenobarbital 60 mg p.o. the night before surgery and 90 mg p.o. 1 hour prior to surgery. In the operating room, the patient received diazepam, 5 mg, nalbuphine, 20 mg, and droperidol, 1.25 mg, all IV. An epidural catheter was placed at the L3–4 interspace and 19 ml of 1.5% lidocaine with 1:200,000 epinephrine was injected. An additional 5 ml lidocaine was injected 1 hour later. The surgery proceeded uneventfully. Postoperative analgesia was maintained with epidural bupivacaine (0.25%). Phenobarbital, 30 mg tid, was reinstituted the following morning.

Phenobarbital has the longest half-life among the commonly used antiepileptic drugs, averaging 96 hours (range, 50 to 140 hours) in adults and 50 hours (range, 37 to 133) in infants (Table 18–2). Approximately 12 to 25% of the total body phenobarbital is eliminated per day.[15] Thus, the drug can be given orally the night prior to surgery or as premedication the morning of surgery. Postsurgical doses can be given either orally or parenterally (intravenously or intramuscularly) the morning of the first postoperative day. In contrast to phenytoin, phenobarbital is well absorbed following intramuscular administration.

The range of therapeutic levels of phenobarbital are not as narrow as those of phenytoin, and range from 10 to 40 µg/ml. Children require slightly higher concentrations than do adults. While levels of 10 to 15 µg/ml are often effective in children, some require levels in excess of 30 µg/ml, and such levels are often tolerated without noticeable toxicity. As a general observation, preoperative levels of 20 to 25 µg/ml are probably optimal for most patients (children and adults). (See Ref. 16 for review.)

The relationship between the administered dose (in mg/kg) and the resulting blood level of drug (in µg/ml) is well established for phenobarbital. For *initial "loading,"* each 1 mg/kg yields a plasma level of about 1 µg/ml. Thus, 20 mg/kg (1 g in a 50-kg adult) should yield a level of about 20 µg/ml and this level should persist for 12 to 24 hours. For *maintenance*, each 1 mg/kg per day in adults yields a plasma level of about 10 µg/ml. Thus, to maintain a plasma level of 20 µg/ml, an adult would require a daily dose of about 2 mg/kg. Doses in children are about 1.0 to 1.5 times the adult dose. Infants require 2 times the adult dose.

Drug interactions related to phenobarbital are many, most involving the induction of hepatic drug-metabolizing enzymes[17-19] (see Chap. 20). An additional, important interaction involves phenobarbital and valproic acid. Giving the latter compound to a patient taking phenobarbital results in an approximately 50% increase in the plasma level of phenobarbital without an increase in the phenobarbital dose. This appears to result either from a valproate-induced reduction in the renal excretion of phenobarbital or from a reduced metabolism of phenobarbital to hydroxylated metabolites.[20] The clinical manifestation of this is increasing somnolence, sometimes resulting in coma, within days or weeks after the initiation of valproate administration. One may postulate from this that valproate may intensify and prolong the sedation produced by other barbiturates such as thiopental, if especially large doses are administered.

Other Barbiturates

Methylphenobarbital (mephobarbital, Mebaral) and *metharbital* (Gemonil) are two barbiturates occasionally encountered as antiepileptic agents. Both appear to be somewhat shorter acting than phenobarbital; methylphenobarbital has a half-life in chronically treated epileptics of about 12 to 24 hours. Patients chronically treated with methylphenobarbital have plasma levels of phenobarbital (produced in the metabolism of methylphenobarbital) which exceed the plasma level of the parent drug. At a methylphenobarbital dose of 3 to 4 mg/kg/day, phenobarbital levels of about 20 µg/ml result. Plasma levels of methylphenobarbital are about $\frac{1}{7}$ to $\frac{1}{10}$ those of phenobarbital.[21]

Half-life and plasma blood level data for metharbital are not available.

Eterobarbital (dimethoxymethylphenobarbital) is a barbiturate derivative currently undergoing investigation as an antiepileptic compound. Eterobarbital is rapidly metabolized to methoxymethyl phenobarbital (which also has a short half-life) and then to phenobarbital which is probably the active antiepileptic compound.[22] The remarks made above for phenobarbital therefore apply to eterobarbital.

Primidone

Primidone (Mysoline) is closely related to the barbiturates and is used for the treatment of major motor and complex partial seizures. Primidone is metabolized in the body to two active metabolites; phenobarbital and phenylethylmalonamide (PEMA). The half-lives of primidone and its two metabolites are 10 hours (range, 5 to 18 hours) for primidone, 56 hours for PEMA, and 96 hours for phenobarbital.[23] Since phenobarbital probably contributes a prominent portion of the antiepileptic activity of primidone, it is generally assumed that enough primidone should be administered to achieve a plasma phenobarbital concentration of at least 15 µg/ml. This level of phenobarbital can usually be achieved with a total daily dose of primidone of about 10 mg/kg, a dose that will also yield a plasma primidone concentration of about 11 µg/ml (range, 10 to 13 µg/ml), a level about 70% that of phenobarbital. Thus, in patients treated with primidone, one should seek preoperative serum levels of primidone of about 10 to 13 μg/ml and of phenobarbital of 15 μg/ml or greater.[24] Preoperative administration of primidone should follow the same protocol as for other oral antiepileptic medications: i.e., any drug intended for the day of surgery should be given orally at the time of preanesthetic medication.

Since primidone is not available in parenteral form, patients unable to take oral medication on postoperative days should be switched postoperatively to phenobarbital at a dose calculated to increase the preoperative phenobarbital level by about 30 to 50% until the primidone can be reinstituted orally. Thus, if preoperative plasma assay reveals 11 μg/ml primidone and 16 μg/ml phenobarbital, a postoperative phenobarbital level of about 20 to 24 μg/ml will compensate for the reduced level of primidone. The other metabolite of primidone, PEMA, is assumed to be of little importance as an anticonvulsant in humans.

Carbamazepine

CASE REPORT

Patient is a 14-year-old, 68-kg, mentally retarded, institutionalized male admitted for removal under general anesthesia of a foreign body in his right ear. He has a history of a life-time seizure disorder, currently treated with primidone (250 mg tid) and carbamazepine (200 mg tid). The most recent laboratory determinations of blood levels were performed six months before admission. At that time the primidone level was 8 μg/ml and the carbamazepine level was 18 μg/ml. On the preanesthetic evaluation, the patient was combative and therefore a poor candidate for insertion of an intravenous catheter. Preanesthetic medication consisted of oral primidone, 250 mg, and diazepam, 5 mg. Induction was achieved with intramuscular ketamine, 7 mg/kg. About 1 minute after injection, the patient experienced a major motor seizure during which oxygenation was maintained by face mask. During the subsequent postictal period the foreign body was successfully removed and an intravenous line established. The patient experienced a second seizure as he was being placed on the transport gurney and, over the next 3 hours, had several additional seizures requiring intravenous diazepam and phenytoin. Note that aside from the primidone and diazepam premedication, the patient received no medications over the 32-hour period between admission to the hospital and the induction of anesthesia.

Carbamazepine (Tegretol) is an aminostilbene derivative structurally related to the tricyclic antidepressant imipramine.[25] It is a major antiepileptic drug for the treatment of generalized major motor seizures and/or partial seizures with complex symptomatology. It is ineffective in absence seizures. Carbamazepine is only slowly and incompletely absorbed orally and is not available in parenteral form. Following oral administration, however, half-life values of 20 to 50 hours (mean = 37 hours) have been reported in human nonepileptic volunteers and 5 to 26 hours (mean = 16 hours) in epileptics. The reduced half-life in epileptics occurs because of an autoinduction phenomenon: carbamazepine inducing its own metabolism, reducing its half-life over a period of about 3 to 5 weeks.[26] Due to this enzyme induction, carbamazepine will increase the metabolism (reducing the effectiveness and duration of action) of oral anticoagulants, antibiotics, barbiturates and other drugs metabolized by the liver. Because of the short half-life in epileptics, divided daily dosage is necessary (i.e., 2 to 4 doses per day). Therapeutic concentrations of carbamazepine in plasma range between 4 and 10 μg/ml at a mean daily dose of 14 mg/kg (range, 10 to 20 mg/kg).[27] On the day of surgery, the drug should be administered as a single oral dose before surgery. Divided daily administration should be resumed on the first postoperative day. If the patient has fasted for more than 24 hours, parenteral phenobarbital or phenytoin should be substituted until oral carbamazepine can be reinstituted. Preoperative blood and platelet counts are necessary owing to the infrequent but persistent reports of hematologic toxicities including aplastic anemia, leukopenia, agranulocytosis, and thrombocytopenia.[28,29]

Since carbamazepine is chemically related to the tricyclic antidepressants, it is theoretically possible, but not yet ascertained, that it may increase myocardial catecholamine sensitization, especially when halothane and epinephrine are used intraoperatively. Thus it might be prudent to avoid the use of halothane in carbamazepine-treated patients unless the benefits of halothane outweigh the possible risks.

Propoxyphene (Darvon) inhibits the metabolism of carbamazepine, increasing the blood levels of carbamazepine.[30] Thus, one should use analgesics other than propoxyphene in carbamazepine-treated patients.

Valproic Acid

Valproic acid (dipropylacetic acid, Depakene, Depakote) was synthesized in 1882, its antiepileptic properties discovered in 1963, its clinical efficacy verified in 1964, and its approval for use in the United States received in 1978. It is effective in a wide variety of seizure disorders, especially absence seizures, primary generalized seizures and febrile seizures.[31]

Available as a liquid-filled capsule or as a syrup under the trade name of Depakene, peak plasma levels occur within 2 hours after oral administration. A newer enteric coated tablet (Depakote) delays absorption and plasma levels peak 3 to 6 hours after oral administration. This delay in absorption does not prolong the pharmacokinetic half-life of valproic acid, but since absorption is slower, the resultant *clinical* half-life is longer. The mean elimination half-life in epileptic adults and children is approximately 9 hours (range, 6 to 12 hours),[32] increasing to 18 hours in patients with liver disease. Due to this short half-life in epileptics with normal liver function, variations in plasma levels occur and the drug must be given in divided doses.

In addition, should the patient be fasting for longer than 12 to 18 hours, one should consider substituting a parenteral antiepileptic agent such as diazepam (0.2 to 0.4 mg/kg/day, IV). Intravenous phenytoin is usually not indicated, since it is ineffective against either absence or febrile seizures and, indeed, may intensify such seizure activity.[34]

Valproic acid is metabolized in the liver and interferes with the biotransformation of other drugs.[20] Thus, one can expect prolongation of the duration of action of other drugs subject to hepatic metabolism. This would include many drugs used in anesthesia: barbiturates, benzodiazepines and narcotics. Clonazepam used concomitantly with valproic acid has been reported to produce absence status epilepticus.[35] However, this is probably a rather rare complication.[36]

The accepted range of therapeutically effective plasma levels of valproic acid is 50 to 100 µg/ml.[31] This range can usually be achieved by a total daily dose of 20 mg/kg, higher doses producing a linear increase in plasma concentrations. Doses above about 30 mg/kg/day, however, increase the incidence of serious side effects, including neutropenia, thrombocytopenia, bleeding abnormalities (inhibition of platelet aggregation), and liver dysfunction (increased SGOT, SGPT, and ammonia; centrilobular necrosis).[37] Thus patients taking valproic acid should be evaluated by a preoperative CBC, platelet count, PT/PTT, bleeding time, and liver enzyme studies. Because of this association with hepatic toxicity (23 fatalities secondary to hepatotoxicity in the United States from 1978–1981), it might be wise to avoid the use of halothane in patients receiving valproic acid.

Ethosuximide

Ethosuximide (Zarontin) is an effective and widely used drug for the treatment of absence (petit mal) seizures in children, although its popularity has been diminished by the introduction of valproic acid. Ethosuximide is generally ineffective in complex partial (temporal lobe) or grand mal seizures.

In children, an average daily dose of 20 mg/kg orally can be expected to produce a plasma level of about 60 µg/ml (range, 40 to 100 µg/ml) with a 90% reduction in seizure frequency, the mean ratio of plasma ethosuximide (μg/ml) to dose (mg/kg) was about 3.0. Dosage is adjusted after plasma determination to obtain a level of 60 to 70 μg/ml. The plasma half-life of ethosuximide ranges from 15 to 68 hours (mean, 35 hours).[38]

Perioperative considerations therefore include:

1. a preoperative plasma ethosuximide level of 60 to 70 μg/ml
2. oral administration of the daily dose on the morning of surgery
3. avoidance of hyperventilation
4. preoperative medications to avoid anxiety and hyperventilation (see below).

Specific organ sensitivities have been reported only rarely with ethosuximide. These include hematologic, dermatologic and immunologic (lupus-like) disorders.[39]

Methsuximide

Methsuximide (Celontin) is occasionally used as an alternative agent for the treatment of absence seizures in children. It is rapidly metabolized (plasma half-life, 1.4 hours) to desmethylmethsuximide which has a half-life averaging 38 hours and which exerts the major antiepileptic effect. The plasma level of desmethylmethsuximide needed for seizure control is estimated to be 20 to 40 μg/ml with a mean of 28 μg/ml.[40]

Trimethadione

Although no longer a drug of choice, trimethadione (Tridione) is still an effective drug for the control of absence seizures in children. Its use, however, is reserved for refractory cases because of its toxicity. The therapeutic effect is produced by its metabolite, dimethadione, which has a half-life of about 10 days.[41] Plasma levels of dimethadione in the range of about 500 to 1200 μg/ml (mean, 700 μg/ml) are necessary to assure control of seizures. The plasma level of the parent drug, trimethadione, will be about $\frac{1}{20}$ that of its metabolite.[42] Bone marrow depression and nephrotic syndrome[43] have limited the use of trimethadione in favor of valproic acid and ethosuximide.

Because of the extremely long half-life of the active metabolite, dimethadione, a reduced intake of trimethadione in the perioperative period should result in little or no alteration in either plasma drug concentrations or antiseizure protection.

Diazepam

Diazepam (Valium) became rapidly the drug of choice for the intravenous treatment of status epilepticus, but such use is declining in favor of lorazepam (see below). The plasma half-life of diazepam is about 30 to 35 hours, a value which increases to about 80 to 100 hours in the elderly. Plasma concentrations of about 300 to 700 ng/ml appear to be needed for initial control of status epilepticus. Such can be achieved by the intravenous administration of 0.14 to 0.35 mg/kg.[44] Orally, diazepam is mainly useful for the associated psychiatric problems of the epileptic patient. The recommended daily maintenance dose is 0.2 to 0.4 mg/kg.

Clonazepam

CASE REPORT

Patient is a 29-year-old female admitted with right temporomandibular joint syndrome for arthroplasty and joint implant. The past medical history is significant for diazepam abuse (detoxified for 2 years) and absence seizures for which she is treated with clonazepam, 0.5 mg tid. Premedication consisted of clonazepam, 0.5 mg at 0800 and 1130 and oxymorphone 1.5 mg intramuscularly on call to surgery. Following thiopental-succinylcholine induction and nasotracheal intubation, anesthesia was maintained with halothane and nitrous oxide with spontaneous ventilation in order to maintain the patient in a state of modest respiratory acidosis. Clonazepam 0.5 mg tid was resumed the day following surgery.

Clonazepam (Clonopin) is a benzodiazepine anticonvulsant useful in a variety of seizure disorders including absence, myoclonic and atonic seizures. The drug is well absorbed orally and plasma concentrations of 0.03 to 0.06 μg/ml follow oral administration of 1.5 mg clonazepam to adults. The daily maintenance dose is about 0.05 to 0.15 mg/kg. Half-lives range from 20 to 40 hours in both adults and children.[45] At present, there is no precise correlation between antiepileptic efficacy and plasma clonazepam levels. However, abrupt discontinuation of clonazepam should be avoided because of the possibility of precipitating either major motor seizures or status epilepticus.[46] A parenteral form of clonazepam has not been marketed. Intravenous diazepam can be used as a substitute in fasting patients.

Clorazepate

Clorazepate (Tranxene) is a benzodiazepine sedative and antianxiety agent approved in 1981 for use in the treatment of complex partial seizures. It is used primarily as adjunctive therapy with other anticonvulsants or in patients who do not respond to ethosuximide or valproic acid.[47,48] The half-life of clorazepate is about 2 days. At present, there are no reports correlating serum levels with antiepileptic effectiveness.

Lorazepam

Lorazepam (see Chap. 20) is yet another benzodiazepine used both as an antianxiety sedative and as an anticonvulsant. It is particularly useful in the management of status epilepticus. One mg intravenous increments (to a total dose of 4 to 8 mg) effectively control status epilepticus and abolish paroxysmal EEG discharges in approximately 90% of patients, a value significantly exceeding that obtained with diazepam.[49,50] Other advantages of lorazepam over diazepam include a prolonged duration of effectiveness such that repeated injections are not required for maintenance of seizures in responding patients.[51] Studies of plasma drug levels suggest that most patients attain good seizure control at concentrations between 30 and 100 ng/ml.[52]

Acetazolamide

Acetazolamide (Diamox) is a sulfonamide that inhibits the enzyme carbonic anhydrase and exhibits antiepileptic usefulness in humans. The rapid development of tolerance limits its long-term usefulness to about 3 to 6 months.

Since the only documented biological effect of acetazolamide is inhibition of carbonic anhydrase with a secondary accumulation of carbon dioxide, the antiepileptic effect is thought to be mediated through this action. As might be predicted, hyperventilation will decrease the antiepileptic effect and should be avoided. Its half-life in humans is about 10 to 12 hours and doses of 250 mg three times daily (about 10 mg/kg/day) produce plasma concentrations of about 10 to 14 µg/ml. Its use and indications have been reviewed by Woodbury and Kemp.[53]

PREMEDICATION FOR THE EPILEPTIC PATIENT

In addition to commonly observed side effects (sedation, ataxia, GI disturbances, skin eruptions), antiepileptic drugs may occasionally affect the bone marrow and liver. Thus preoperative laboratory studies in all patients taking antiepileptic drugs should include a recent blood count, bleeding studies, and baseline liver function studies. Patients on trimethadione should also have preoperative renal function studies.

As outlined above, the preanesthetic medications for the epileptic patient should include his/her routine antiepileptic medications for the day of surgery. Other appropriate preanesthetic medications can be used to increase antiepileptic protection if desired. Of the commonly used preanesthetic medications, the only drugs that reliably increase seizure threshold (lower brain excitability) are the sedative-hypnotic drugs such as the barbiturates and benzodiazepines. Examples of orally administered sedatives for adults include diazepam (5 to 15 mg), lorazepam (2 to 4 mg), secobarbital (50 to 100 mg) and pentobarbital (75 to 150 mg). All are administered with a sip of water 1 to 2 hours preoperatively. For children, a barbiturate suppository can produce sedation and antiepileptic protection without the discomfort of an intramuscular injection.

Major tranquilizers (phenothiazines and butyrophenones) and hydroxyzine can actually induce a modest lowering of seizure threshold (increase seizure susceptibility),[54-55] and should be avoided in epileptic patients.

Belladonna alkaloids do not appear to exert clinically significant changes in seizure threshold[56] and may be used at the discretion of the anesthesiologist. One study suggests that the concurrent use of barbiturates, scopolamine and promethazine may increase the incidence of perioperative agitation.[57]

Therapeutic doses of narcotic analgesics have traditionally been thought not to exert significant effects on brain excitability. Convulsions from opiates were observed only at toxic doses.[58] Recently, however, considerable interest and controversy have centered on narcotic-induced seizures resulting from the interactions of limbic system opiate receptors with various opiate antagonists.

In rats, morphine produces disinhibition of limbic system (hippocampal) neurons leading to electrographic seizure discharges,[59] while opioid peptides produce similar seizures which can be blocked by naloxone.[60,61] In both animals[62,63] and man,[64-66] intravenous fentanyl has been reported to produce clinical seizure activity. In addition, Murkin et al.[68] have strongly refuted the occurrence of seizures following high-dose fentanyl. Unfortunately no EEG was recorded in any of these reports and it is possible that rigidity could have been misinterpreted as "seizures." On the basis of 110 patients, Rudehill et al. concluded that the use of Innovar did not increase the incidence of epileptiform activity following injection of metrizamide. At this point in time, a conservative statement is that the low doses of narcotics prescribed for intramuscular premedication are not associated with reductions in seizure thresholds. Thus, a history of epilepsy is not presently a contraindication to the use of a narcotic for preanesthetic medication. However, anesthetic techniques utilizing large doses of narcotics in epileptics may need modification until the effects of such techniques on these patients are clarified. At present, there have been no studies of high-dose narcotic techniques in epileptics.

CHOICE OF ANESTHETIC PROCEDURE

In my opinion, if the planned surgical procedure can be performed under a regional anesthetic procedure, this is to be preferred to general anesthesia. This opinion is supported by the following considerations

1. The patient experiences only minimal alterations in the level of consciousness.

2. The patient is not likely to experience abrupt withdrawal of an anesthetic from the CNS at the completion of surgery.

3. Wide swings in seizure susceptibility are avoided.

4. The local anesthetics used for regional nerve blocks are effective anticonvulsants at the doses and blood levels often encountered in regional anesthesia. Lidocaine is the best studied of all local anesthetics in this regard and thus may be the agent of choice.[69,70]

5. The sedative drugs used intravenously for sedation of regionally anesthetized patients provide additional long-lasting antiepileptic protection. Diazepam, with a half-life of about 30 hours, is especially useful.

6. Patients are more alert postoperatively for earlier neurologic evaluation.

7. Patients can usually resume oral med-

ications at an earlier time than can patients recovering from general anesthesia.

If it is necessary to administer a general anesthetic, consideration should be given to the effects of each agent on brain excitability.

GENERAL ANESTHESIA FOR THE EPILEPTIC PATIENT

In 1912, the antiepileptic properties of a general anesthetic were exploited therapeutically when Lundy introduced phenobarbital as part of a "balanced anesthesia" to decrease the central toxicity of local anesthetics.

Berger,[71] in his eighth report on the electroencephalogram of man, demonstrated the characteristic increase in voltage with slow waves and "spindles" which accompany barbiturate-induced sleep and unresponsiveness to pain. Berger postulated a depressant action of phenobarbital on the "sleep regulating center of the brain stem in the region of the thalamus." He called phenobarbital a brainstem hypnotic and postulated that "brain sleep" occurred secondary to deafferentation. From 1912 until the 1940s, the general presumption was that the sedative, anesthetic, and antiepileptic properties of barbiturates are secondary to generalized, nonspecific CNS neuronal depression.

In 1949, Moruzzi and Magoun[72] demonstrated in cats that stimulation of the brainstem reticular formation produced both EEG and behavioral arousal. They postulated that waking is an activated state and that sleep is passive. Sleep, therefore, occurs secondary to the elimination of the waking influence of the ascending reticular activating system (ARAS) of the brainstem.

In 1953, French, Verzeano, and Magoun[73] demonstrated that barbiturates suppress the activity of the ARAS, an observation verified by Arduini and Arduini,[74] Killam and Killam,[75] and Bradley and Key.[76] From these studies developed the first postulate of the neural basis of anesthesia: neuronal depression leads to the sedative, hypnotic, anesthetic, and antiepileptic properties of general anesthesia.

Shimoji and Bickford[77,78] studied in cats the effects of thiopental, halothane, diethyl ether, and nitrous oxide on the spontaneous discharge of mesencephalic reticular formation (MRF) neurons and on their evoked responses to forepaw stimulation. All anesthetics depressed spontaneous activity of neurons and similarly depressed stimulus-evoked neuronal discharges, especially those with long (presumably polysynaptic) latencies. Shimoji and Bickford concluded that "the anesthetic state is not a simple neuronal depression, but a complex depressed state, when viewed at the level of the MRF."

Thus, until the early 1970s, there appeared to be general agreement that most general anesthetics were antiepileptic and sedative. They depressed evoked potentials in the CNS, decreased the discharge of brainstem neurons, and increased the voltage and slowed the frequency of the EEG. Such anesthetics included nitrous oxide,[79] halothane,[80-82] methohexital,[83] pentobarbital,[84] and isoflurane,[85,86] although a recent report documents an isoflurane-induced seizure in an unpremedicated adult undergoing a "gas-induction" by face mask.[87]

Julien et al.[88] and Kavan et al.[89] described more complicated effects of inhalation anesthetics on cortical and subcortical electrographic activity in cats with chronically implanted electrodes. Especially noteworthy were the electrographic alterations produced by enflurane. With this agent, EEG activity progressed from high voltage waves to epileptoid-like bursts of spikes separated by periods of burst suppressions. Unlike other inhalation anesthetics, such activity was accompanied by *increases* in the amplitude of evoked responses.[90] These studies verified and extended earlier studies.[91-94] In addition, residual effects persisted for up to 2 weeks, an observation verified in man by Ohm et al.[95] and Burchiel et al.,[96] but refuted by Heavner and Amory.[97]

Thus, it is generally accepted that while other available inhalation anesthetics and barbiturates are antiepileptic, enflurane may be epileptogenic and therefore it might be wise to avoid its use in epileptics.[98-105] However, it is important to note that despite these disquieting effects on the EEG, clinical (behavioral) seizures during enflurane anesthesia are extremely rare and recent papers have described the *antiepileptic properties* of enflurane.[80,81,106-109a] Our studies (unpublished) are in agreement with this concept of an antiepileptic property of enflurane, since the drug, like halothane and thiopental, markedly increases the threshold of electrically induced cortical afterdischarges. The three reports by Opitz and co-workers document the acceptability of enflurane anesthesia in epileptics. However, if one contemplates such use of enflurane, a few precautions are indicated: (1) proper preoperative preparation with antiepileptic medications (see above) and (2) avoidance of hyperventilation.[110] In addition, enflurane probably should not be used in epileptics taking tricyclic antidepressants;[103] inductions with etomidate probably should be avoided in such patients;[109,111] and the lowest possible concentrations of enflurane should be used.[99]

Of all anesthetic agents affecting brain excitability, ketamine is perhaps the most interesting. Ketamine, in man and in various laboratory models of epilepsy, has been reported to increase, decrease, or exert no effect on seizure activity. Reports of *pro-convulsant* effects include those of Mori et al.,[112] Kayama and Iwama,[113] Thompson,[114] Manohar et al.,[115] Bennett et al.,[116] Ferrer-Allado[117] and Black et al.[118] The editorial by Winters[119] and the review by Steen and Michenfelder[120] reinforced the pro-convulsant impression of ketamine anesthesia. Reports of the *antiepileptic* effects of ketamine include those by Corssen et al.,[121] Reder et al.,[122] and Bowyer et al.[123] Studies reporting that ketamine has *little or no effect* on seizure discharges in either epileptic or nonepileptic patients include those by Corssen et al.,[121] Celesia and Chen,[124] and Celesia et al.[125,126] Interestingly, these reports were not included in the proconvulsant argument put forth by Steen and Michenfelder in 1979.[120]

Celesia et al.[125] studied 26 epileptic patients induced with ketamine (2.0 mg/kg). The drug's effects on clinical seizures and on the EEG were compared with similar time periods during the alert and the sleep states. No seizures were precipitated or aggravated by ketamine, and the drug was less effective than natural sleep as an activator of epileptic discharges. Our data (unpublished) on the effects of ketamine on electrically induced cortical after discharges in cats indicate that after discharge thresholds are unaffected by ketamine, the drug exerting little effect on brain excitability. Thus, ketamine may neither increase nor decrease the likelihood that an epileptic patient will have either an electrographic or a clinical seizure while anesthetized.

The patient in the case report on p. 250 exhibited seizures following ketamine induction. While it is tempting to ascribe his seizures to ketamine-induced reduction in seizure threshold, one cannot overlook the fact that preoperative levels of carbamazepine were not obtained, the drug can have a half-life as short as 5 hours, and none was administered for at least 32 hours preoperatively. Seizures may therefore have resulted either from the ketamine or spontaneously due to an inadequate level of the anticonvulsant agent.

The following principles therefore should guide the use of ketamine in epileptics:

1. Therapeutic blood levels of the patient's antiepileptic medications as outlined above, with continuation of oral anticonvulsants preoperatively

2. Premedication with an antiepileptic sedative such as diazepam or lorazepam

3. Minimization of the dose of ketamine (e.g., 0.5 to 1.0 mg/kg)
4. Supplementation with intravenous barbiturates or benzodiazepines as tolerated
5. Avoidance of the concurrent use of etomidate with ketamine until this combination is further studied
6. Avoidance of hyperventilation
7. Avoidance in patients taking sympathomimetics such as tricyclic antidepressants or aminophylline, since seizures have resulted from such combinations.[127]

Seizures can occur after a general anesthetic as a consequence of the too rapid elimination of the inhalation anesthetic (resulting in loss of antiepileptic protection) or of hyperventilation. This possibility can be minimized by the administration of diazepam (5 to 15 mg, IV), of lorazepam (2 to 4 mg, IV), and by early reinstitution of the patient's normal antiepileptic medications as discussed above.

REFERENCES

1. Glasser, G.H., Penry, J.K., and Woodbury, D.M., editors: Antiepileptic Drugs; Mechanisms of Action Advances in Neurology, 27. New York, Raven Press, 1980.
2. Woodbury, D.M., Penry, J.K., and Pippenger, C.E., editors: Antiepileptic Drugs, 2nd ed. New York, Raven Press, 1982.
3. Guelen, P.J.M., and Van der Kleijn, E.: Rational antiepileptic drug therapy. North Holland, Amsterdam, Elsevier, 1978.
4. Morselli, P.L., and Franco-Morselli, R.: Clinical pharmacokinetics of antiepileptic drugs in adults. Pharmacol. Therap. 10:65, 1980.
5. Arnold, K., and Gerber, N.: The rate of decline of diphenylhydantoin in human plasma. Clin. Pharmacol. Ther., 11:121, 1970.
6. Kutt, H.: Phenytoin: Relation of plasma concentration to seizure control. In Antiepileptic Drugs, 2nd ed., New York, Raven Press. 1982, pp. 241–246.
7. Wilensky, A.J., and Lowden, J.A.: Inadequate serum levels after intramuscular administration of diphenylhydantoin. Neurology (Minneap.) 23:318, 1973.
8. Wilder, B.J., and Ramsay, R.E.: Oral and intramuscular phenytoin. Clin. Pharmacol. Ther. 19:360, 1976.
9. Lovelace, R.E., and Horwitz, S.J.: Peripheral neuropathy in long-term diphenylhydantoin therapy. Arch. Neurol., 18:69, 1968.
10. Pisciotta, A.V.: Phenytoin: Hematological toxicity. In: Antiepileptic Drugs, 2nd Ed., New York, Raven Press, 1982, pp. 257–268.
11. Karlin, J.M., and Kutt, H.: Acute diphenylhydantoin intoxication following halothane anesthesia. J. Pediatrics, 76:941, 1970.
12. Reynolds, E.S., et al.: Massive hepatic necrosis after fluroxene anesthesia—a case of drug interaction? New Engl. J. Med., 286:530, 1972.
13. Hetzel, D.J., Bochner, F., Hallpike, J.F., et al.: Cimetidine interaction with phenytoin. Br. Med. J., 282:1512, 1981.
14. Sazie, E., and Jaffe, J.P.: Severe granulocytopenia with cimetidine and phenytoin. Ann. Intern. Med., 93:151, 1980.
15. Maynert, E.W.: Phenobarbital: Absorption, Distribution and Excretion. In: Antiepileptic Drugs, 2nd ed., New York, Raven Press, 1982, pp. 309–327.
16. Booker, H.E.: Phenobarbital: relation of plasma concentration to seizure control. In Antiepileptic Drugs, 2nd ed., Edited by D.M. Woodbury, J.K. Penry and C.E. Pippenger. New York, Raven Press, 1982, pp. 341–350.
17. Hansten, P.D.: Drug Interactions, 5th ed., Philadelphia, Lea & Febiger, 1985.
18. Stockley, I.: Drug Interactions, Oxford, Blackwell, 1981.
19. Kutt, H., and Paris-Kutt, H.: Phenobarbital: Interactions with other drugs. In Antiepileptic Drugs, 2nd ed., New York, Raven Press. 1982, pp. 329–340.
20. Mattson, R.H.: Valproate: Interactions with other drugs. In Antiepileptic Drugs, 2nd ed., New York, Raven Press, 1982, pp. 579–589.
21. Eadie, M.J., Bochner, F., Hooper, W.D., et al.: Preliminary observations on the pharmacokinetics of methylphenobarbitone. Clin. Exp. Neurol., 15:131, 1978.
22. Goldberg, M.A.: Eterobarb: Absorption, Distribution, Biotransformation, and Excretion. In Antiepileptic Drugs, 2nd ed., New York, Raven Press, 1982, pp. 803–811.
23. Gallagher, B.B., Baumel, I.P., and Mattson, R.H.: Metabolic disposition of primidone and its metabolites in epileptic subjects after single and repeated administration. Neurology (Minneap.) 22:1186, 1972.
24. Fincham, R.W., and Schottelius, D.D.: Primidone: Relation of plasma concentration to seizure control. In Antiepileptic Drugs, 2nd ed., New York, Raven Press, 1982, pp. 429–440.
25. Julien, R.M., and Hollister, R.P.: Carbamazepine: Mechanisms of action. Adv. Neurol., 11:263, 1975.
26. Morselli, P.L., and Bossi, L.: Carbamazepine: Absorption, Distribution and Excretion. In Antiepileptic Drugs, 2nd ed., New York, Raven Press, 1982, pp. 465–482.
27. Cereghino, J.J.: Carbamazepine: Relation of plasma concentration to seizure control. In Antiepileptic Drugs, 2nd ed., New York, Raven Press, 1982, pp. 507–519.
28. Pisciotta, A.V.: Hematologic toxicity of carbamazepine. Adv. Neurol., 11:355, 1975.

29. Pisciotta, A.V.: Carbamazepine: Hematological toxicity. In Antiepileptic Drugs, 2nd ed., New York, Raven Press, 1982, pp. 533–541.
30. Dam, M., and Christianson, J.: Interaction of propoxyphene with carbamazepine. Lancet, 2:509, 1977.
31. Wilder, B.J., and Karas, B.J.: Valproate: Relation of plasma concentration to seizure control. In Antiepileptic Drugs, 2nd ed., New York, Raven Press, 1982, pp. 591–599.
32. Mattson, R.H., Cramer, J.A., Williamson, P.D., et al.: Valproic acid in epilepsy: Clinical and pharmacological effects. Ann. Neurol., 3:20, 1978.
33. Klotz, U., Rapp, T., and Muller, W.R.: Disposition of valproic acid in patients with liver disease. Eur. J. Clin. Pharmacol., 13:55, 1978.
34. Julien, R.M., and Fowler, G.W.: A comparative study of the efficacy of newer antiepileptic drugs on experimentally-induced febrile convulsions. Neuropharmacology, 16:719, 1977.
35. Jeavons, P.M., and Clark, J.E.: Sodium Valproate in treatment of epilepsy. Br. Med. J., 2:584, 1974.
36. Browne, T.R.: Valproic acid. Medical intelligence. N. Engl. J. Med., 302:661, 1980.
37. Jeavons, P.M.: Valproate: Toxicity. In Antiepileptic Drugs, 2nd ed., New York, Raven Press, 1982, pp. 601–610.
38. Sherwin, A.L.: Ethosuximide: Relation of plasma concentration to seizure control. In Antiepileptic Drugs, 2nd ed., New York, Raven Press, 1982, pp. 637–645.
39. Dreifuss, F.E.: Ethosuximide: Toxicity. In Antiepileptic Drugs, 2nd ed., New York, Raven Press, 1982, pp. 647–653.
40. Porter, R.J., Penry, J.K., Lacy, J.R., et al.: Plasma concentration of phensuximide, methsuximide and their metabolites in relation to clinical efficacy. Neurology (Minneap.), 29:1509, 1979.
41. Jensen, B.: Trimethadione in the serum of patients with petit mal. Dan. Med. Bull., 9:74, 1962.
42. Chamberlin, H., Waddell, W., and Butler, T.: A study of the product of demethylation of trimethadione in the control of petit mal epilepsy. Neurology (Minneap.), 15:449, 1965.
43. Wells, C.: Trimethadione: Its dosage and toxicity. Arch. Neurol. Psychiat., 77:140, 1957.
44. Schmidt, D.: Benzodiazepines: Diazepam. In Antiepileptic Drugs, 2nd ed., New York, Raven Press, 1982, pp. 711–735.
45. Dreifuss, F.E., and Sato, S.: Benzodiazepines: Clonazepam. In Antiepileptic Drugs, 2nd ed., New York, Raven Press, 1982.
46. Browne, T.R., and Penry, J.K.: Benzodiazepines in the treatment of epilepsy. Epilepsia, 15:277, 1973.
47. Troupin, A.S., Friel, P., Wilensky, A.J., et al.: Evaluation of clorazepate (Tranxene) as an anticonvulsant—a pilot study. Neurology, 29:458, 1979.
48. Troupin, A.S., Friel, P., Wilensky, A.J., et al.: Clorazepate as an anticonvulsant. In Antiepileptic Therapy: Advances in Drug Monitoring. Edited by S.I. Johannessen, P.L. Morselli, C.E. Pippenger, A., et al.: New York, Raven Press, 1980, pp. 291–298.
49. Scott, D.F., and Moffet, A.: Lorazepam: Its effect on the EEG paroxysmal activity in patients with epilepsy. Acta Neurol Scand., 64:353, 1981.
50. Leppik, I.E., Derivan, A.T., Homan, R.W., et al.: Double-blind study of lorazepam and diazepam in status epilepticus. J.A.M.A., 249:1452, 1983.
51. Homan, R.W., and Walker, J.E.: Clinical studies of lorazepam in status epilepticus. Adv. Neurol., 34:493, 1983.
52. Tasker, W.G.: Lorazepam in status epilepticus. Ann. Neurol., 6:207, 1979.
53. Woodbury, D.M., and Kemp, J.W.: Other antiepileptic drugs: Sulfonamides and derivatives: Acetazolamide. In Antiepileptic Drugs, 2nd ed., New York, Raven Press, 1982, pp. 771–789.
54. Preston, J.B.: Effects of chlorpromazine on the central nervous system of the cat: a possible neural basis for action. J. Pharmacol. Exp. Ther., 118:100, 1956.
55. Meldrum, B.S., Anlezark, G., Balzamo, E., et al.: Photically induced epilepsy in *Papio Papio* as a model for drug studies. Adv. Neurol., 10:119, 1975.
56. Weiner, N.: Atropine, scopolamine, and related antimuscarinic drugs. In Goodman and Gilman's The Pharmacological Basis of Therapeutics. 6th ed., A.G. Gilman, L.S. Goodman and A. Gilman, editors. New York, Macmillan, 1980, pp. 120–137.
57. Macris, S.G., and Levy, L.: Preanesthetic medication: untoward effects of certain drug combinations. Anesthesiology, 26:256, 1965.
58. Jaffe, J.H., and Martin, W.R.: Opioid Analgesics and Antagonists. In Goodman and Gilman's The Pharmacologic Basis of Therapeutics. 6th ed., A.G. Gilman, L.S. Goodman and A. Gilman, editors. New York, Macmillan, 1980, pp. 494–534.
59. Linseman, M.A., and Corrigall, W.A.: Effects of morphine on CA1 versus dentate hippocampal field potentials following systemic administration in freely moving rats. Neuropharmacology, 21:361, 1982.
60. Frenk, H., Urca, G., and Liebeskind, J.C.: Epileptic properties of leucine and methionine-enkephalin: Comparison with morphine and reversibility by naloxone. Brain Res., 147:327, 1978.
61. Frenk, H.: Pro- and anticonvulsant actions of morphine and the endogenous opioids: Involvement and interactions of multiple opiate and non-opiate systems. Brain Res., 287:197, 1983.
62. Tommasino, C., Maekawa, T., and Shapiro, H.M.: Fentanyl-induced seizures activate subcortical brain metabolism. Anesthesiology 60:283, 1984.
63. Sebel, P.S., Bovill, J.G., Wauquir, A., et al.: Effects of high dose fentanyl anesthesia on the electroencephalogram. Anesthesiology, 55:203, 1981.
64. Rao, T.L.K., Mummaneni, N., and El-Etr, A.A.:

Convulsions: An unusual response to intravenous fentanyl administration. Anesth. Analg., 61:1020, 1982.
65. Safwat, A.M., and Daniel, D.: Grand mal seizure after fentanyl administration. Anesthesiology, 59:78, 1983.
66. Hoen, A.O.: Another case of grand mal seizure after fentanyl administration. Anesthesiology, 60:387, 1984.
67. Rudehill, A., Gordon, E., Grepe, A., et al.: The epileptogenicity of neurolept anaesthesia in patients during and after neuroradiological examinations with metrizamide. Acta Anaesth. Scand., 27:285, 1983.
68. Murkin, J.M., Moldenhauer, C.C., Hug, C.C., et al.: Absence of seizures during induction of anesthesia with high dose fentanyl. Anesth. Analg., 63:489, 1984.
69. Julien, R.M.: Lidocaine in experimental epilepsy: Correlation of anticonvulsant effect with blood concentrations. Electroenceph. Clin. Neurophysiol., 34:639, 1973.
70. Browne, T.R.: Paraldehyde, chlormethiazole and lidocaine for treatment of status epilepticus. In Advances in Neurology. Edited by A.V. Delgado-Escueta, C.G. Wasterlain, D.M. Treiman, et al. New York, Raven Press, 1983, pp. 509–517.
71. Berger, H.: On the electroencephalogram of man. Archiv fur Psychiatrie und Nervenkrankheiten 101:452–469, 1934. Reprinted: Electroenceph. Clin. Neurophysiol., Suppl., 28:209, 1969.
72. Morruzi, G., and Magoun, H.W.: Brain stem reticular formation and activation of the EEG. Electroenceph. Clin. Neurophysiol., 1:455, 1949.
73. French, J.C., Verzeano, M., and Magnoun, H.W.: A neural basis of the anesthetic state. AMA Arch. Neurol. Psychiat., 69:519, 1953.
74. Arduini, A., and Arduini, M.G.: Effects of drugs and metabolic alterations on brain stem arousal mechanism. J. Pharmacol. Exp. Ther., 110:76, 1954.
75. Killam, E.K., and Killam, K.F.: A comparison of the effects of reserpine and chlorpromazine to those of barbiturates on central afferent systems in the cat. J. Pharmacol. Exp. Therap., 116:35, 1956.
76. Bradley, P.B., and Key, B.J.: The effects of drugs on arousal responses produced by electrical stimulation of the reticular formation of the brain. Electroenceph. Clin. Neurophysiol., 10:97, 1958.
77. Shimoji, K., and Bickford, R.G.: Differential effects of anesthetics on mesencephalic reticular neurons. I. Spontaneous firing patterns. Anesthesiology, 35:68, 1971.
78. Shimoji, K., and Bickford, R.G.: Differential effects of anesthetics on mesencephalic reticular neurons. II. Responses to repetitive somatosensory electrical stimulation. Anesthesiology, 35:76, 1971.
79. Stevens, J.E., Oshima, E., and Mori, K.: Effects of nitrous oxide on the epileptogenic property of enflurane in cats. Br. J. Anaesth., 55:145, 1983.
80. Triner, L., Vulliemoz, Y., Verosky, M., et al.: Anticonvulsant effect of halothane and enflurane. Anesthesiology, 51:S8, 1979.
81. Opitz, A., and Oberwetter, W.D.: Enflurane or halothane anesthesia for patients with cerebral convulsive disorders? Acta. Anaesth. Scand., Supp. 71:43, 1979.
82. Mecarelli, O., DeFeo, M.R., Romanini, L., et al.: EEG and clinical features in epileptic children during halothane anaesthesia. Electroenceph. Clin. Neurophysiol., 52:486, 1981.
83. Ford, E.W., Morelli, F., and Whisler, W.W.: Methohexital anesthesia in the surgical treatment of uncontrollable epilepsy. Anesth. Analg., 61:997, 1982.
84. Goldberg, M.A., and McIntyre, H.B.: Barbiturates in the treatment of status epilepticus. Advances in Neurol., 34:499, 1983.
85. Julien, R.M., and Kavan, E.M.: Electrographic studies of isoflurane. Neuropharmacology, 13:677, 1974.
86. Kavan, E.M., and Julien, R.M.: Central nervous systems' effects of isoflurane (Forane). Canad. Anaesth. Soc. J., 21:390, 1974.
87. Poulton, T.J., and Ellingson, R.J.: Seizure associated with induction of anesthesia with isoflurane. Anesthesiology, 61:471, 1984.
88. Julien, R.M., Kavan, E.M., and Elliot, H.W.: Effects of volatile anaesthetic agents on EEG activity in limbic and sensory systems. Canad. Anaesth. Soc., 19:263, 1972.
89. Kavan, E.M., Julien, R.M., and Lucero, J.J.: Electrographic alterations induced in limbic and sensory systems during induction of anaesthesia with halothane, methoxyflurane, diethyl ether and enflurane (Ethrane). Br. J. Anaesth., 44:1234, 1972.
90. Julien, R.M., and Kavan, E.M.: Electrographic studies of a new volatile anesthetic agent: Enflurane (Ethrane). J. Pharmacol. Exp. Therp., 183:393, 1972.
91. Bart, A.J., Homi, J., and Linde, H.W.: Changes in power spectra of electroencephalograms during anesthesia with fluroxene, methoxyflurane and Ethrane. Anesth. Analg., 50:53, 1971.
92. Neigh, J.L., Garman, J.K., and Harp, J.R.: The electrographic pattern during anesthesia with Ethrane. Anesthesiology, 35:482, 1971.
93. Joas, T.A., Stevens, W.C., and Eger, E.I.: Electrographic seizure activity in dogs during anaesthesia. Br. J. Anaesth., 43:739, 1971.
94. deJong, R.H., and Heavner, J.E.: Correlation of the Ethrane electroencephalogram with motor activity in cats. Anesthesiology, 35:474, 1971.
95. Ohm, W.W., Cullen, B.F., Amory, D.W., et al.: Delayed seizure activity following enflurane anesthesia. Anesthesiology, 42:367, 1975.
96. Burchiel, K.J., Stockard, J.J., Caverley, R.K., et al.: Relationship of pre- and postanesthetic EEG abnormalities on enflurane-induced seizure activity. Anesth. Analg., 56:509, 1977.
97. Heavner, J.E., and Amory, D.W.: Lidocaine and pentylenetetrol seizure thresholds in cats are not reduced after enflurane anesthesia. Anesthesiology, 54:403, 1981.
98. Niejadlik, K., and Galindo, A.: Electrocortico-

graphic seizure activity during enflurane anesthesia. Anesth. Analg., 54:722, 1975.
99. Furgang, F.A., and Sohn, J.J.: The effect of thiopentone on enflurane-induced cortical seizures. Br. J. Anaesth., 49:127, 1977.
100. Darimont, P.C., and Jenkins, L.C.: The influence of intravenous anaesthetics on enflurane-induced central nervous system seizure activity. Canad. Anaesth. Soc. J., 24:42, 1977.
101. Moorthy, S.S., Reddy, R.V., Paradise, R.R., et al.: Reduction of enflurane-induced spike activity by scopolamine. Anesth. Analg., 59:417, 1980.
102. Kruczek, M., Albin, M.S., Wolf, S., et al.: Postoperative seizure activity following enflurane anesthesia. Anesthesiology, 53:175, 1980.
103. Sprague, D.H., and Wolf, S.: Enflurane seizures in patients taking amitriptyline. Anesth. Analg., 61:67, 1982.
104. Flemming, D.C., Fitzpatrick, J., Fariello, R.G., et al.: Diagnostic activation of epileptogenic foci by enflurane. Anesthesiology, 52:431, 1980.
105. Fariello, R.G.: Epileptogenic properties of enflurane and their clinical interpretation. Electroenceph. Clin. Neurophysiol., 48:595, 1980.
106. Opitz, A., Brecht, S., and Stenzel, E.: Enfluraneanaesthesien bei epileptikern. Anaesthesist, 26:329, 1977.
107. Gallagher, T.J., Galindo, A., and Richey, E.T.: Inhibition of seizure activity during enflurane anesthesia. Anesth. Analg., 57:130, 1978.
108. Vulliemoz, Y., Verosky, M., Alpert, M., et al.: Effect of enflurane on cerebellar cGMP and on motor activity in the mouse. Br. J. Anaesth., 55:79, 1983.
109. Opitz, A., Marschall, M., Degen, R., et al.: General anesthesia in patients with epilepsy and status epilepticus. Adv. Neurol. 34: Status Epilepticus, ed. by C.G. Waserlain, P.M. Treiman, A.V. Delgado-Escueta, and R.J. Porter. New York, Raven Press, 1983.
109a.Oshina, E., Urabe, W., Shingu, K., and Mori, K.: Anticonvulsant actions of enflurane on epilepsy models in cats. Anesthesiology, 63:29, 1985.
110. Lebowitz, M.H., Blitt, C.D., and Dillon, J.B.: Enflurane-induced central nervous system excitation and its relation to carbon dioxide tension. Anesth. Analg., 51:355, 1972.
111. Gancher, S., Laxer, K.D., and Krieger, W.: Activation of Epileptogenic Activity by Etomidate. Anesthesiology, 61:616, 1984.

112. Mori, K., Kawamata, M., Mitani, H., et al.: A neurophysiologic study of ketamine anesthesia in the cat. Anesthesiology, 35:373, 1971.
113. Kayama, Y., and Iwama, K.: The EEG, evoked potentials and single-unit activity during ketamine anesthesia in cats. Anesthesiology, 36:316, 1972.
114. Thompson, G.E.: Ketamine-induced convulsions. Anesthesiology, 37:662, 1972.
115. Manohar, S., Maxwell, D., and Winters, W.D.: Development of EEG seizure activity during and after chronic ketamine administration in the rat. Neuropharmacology, 11:819, 1972.
116. Bennett, D.R., Madsen, J.A., Jordon, W.S., et al.: Ketamine anesthesia in brain-damaged epileptics. Neurology, 23:449, 1973.
117. Ferrer-Allado, T., Brechner, V.L., Dymond, A., et al.: Ketamine-induced electroconvulsive phenomena in the human limbic and thalamic regions. Anesthesiology, 38:333, 1973.
118. Black, J.A., Golder, G.T., and Fariello, R.G.: Ketamine activation of experimental corticoreticular epilepsy. Neurology, 30:315, 1980.
119. Winters, W.D.: Epilepsy or anesthesia with ketamine. Anesthesiology, 36:309, 1972.
120. Steen, P.A., and Michenfelder, J.D.: Neurotoxicity of anesthetics. Anesthesiology, 50:437, 1979.
121. Corssen, G., Little, S.C., and Tavakoli, M.: Ketamine and epilepsy. Anesth. Analg., 53:319, 1974.
122. Reder, B.S., Trapp, L.D., and Troutman, K.C.: Ketamine suppression of chemically induced convulsions in two-day-old leghorn cockerel. Anesth. Analg., 59:406, 1980.
123. Bowyer, J.F., Albertson, T.E., Winters, W.D., et al.: Ketamine induced changes in kindled amygdaloid seizures. Neuropharmacology, 22:887, 1983.
124. Celesia, G.G., and Chen, R-C.: Effects of ketamine on EEG activity in cats and monkeys. Electroenceph. Clin. Neurophysiol., 37:345, 1974.
125. Celesia, G.G., Chen, R-C., and Bamforth, B.J.: Effects of ketamine in epilepsy. Neurology, 25:169, 1975.
126. Celesia, G.G., Bamforth, B.J., and Chen, R-C.: Letters to the editor. Anesth. Analg., 55:445, 1976.
127. Hirshman, C.A., Kreiger, W., Littlejohn, G., et al.: Ketamine-aminophylline induced decrease in seizure threshold. Anesthesiology, 54:464, 1982.

19

PSYCHOTROPIC AGENTS

ESTHER C. JANOWSKY, S. CRAIG RISCH and DAVID S. JANOWSKY

Psychotropic drugs are important in the treatment of schizophrenia, mania, and severe depression and play an essential role in the practice of medicine. Psychotropic drugs, often given in combination and/or with nonpsychiatric drugs, in general profoundly affect central and peripheral neurotransmitter and ionic mechanisms. Hence, prior intake of these drugs is an important consideration in the management of the surgical patient. The drugs reviewed in this chapter include: (1) antidepressants (tricyclic antidepressants and monoamine oxidase inhibitors), (2) dopamine blocking antipsychotic drugs (phenothiazines, thioxanthenes, and butyrophenones), (3) the catecholamine-depleting antipsychotic agent, reserpine, and (4) the antimanic agent, lithium. In addition, (5) the anesthetic implications of anticholinergic agents, used to antagonize the extrapyramidal side effects of the antipsychotic drugs, will be considered. Generally, each group of drugs will be discussed under the headings of psychiatric indications, proposed psychobiologic mechanism of action, effects on various anesthetic agents and the mechanism of these effects, and clinical implications and management of these effects.

ANTIPSYCHOTIC DRUGS (TABLE 19-1)

Phenothiazines, thioxanthenes, and butyrophenones are widely used to treat psychotic symptoms in patients affected by schizophrenia, mania, and organic brain syndromes associated with psychosis. All antipsychotic drugs elevate serum prolactin and block dopaminergic receptors.[1] However, antipsychotic drugs differ from one another in their central and peripheral antiadrenergic and anticholinergic properties, and thus in their side effects. Chlorpromazine and thioridazine possess anticholinergic and antiadrenergic actions, and therefore their predominant side effects are hypotension, sedation, and anticholinergic symptoms. Obvious antidopaminergic effects, such as extrapyramidal symptoms, occur less frequently. Conversely, haloperidol, fluphenazine, trifluoperazine, and butaperazine induce few autonomic ac-

Table 19-1
Some Interactions Between Phenothiazines and Butyrophenones and Drugs Used in Anesthesia

Phenothiazine Butyrophenone	Interaction
Inhalation Drugs	↓ arterial blood pressure (halothane, enflurane)
Narcotics	↑, ↓ analgesia ↑ respiratory depression ↑ sedation
Barbiturates	↑ sleep time
Anticholinergics	↑ peripheral activity ↑ central activity
Sympathomimetics	↓ *Alpha*-adrenergic activity

tions, and their predominant side effects are antidopaminergic-extrapyramidal.[2]

Presently, the dominant neurochemical theory explains the mechanism of action of antipsychotics in terms of their dopamine blocking properties.[1] In fact, phenothiazines and butyrophenones effectively block dopamine receptors, a characteristic not found in related compounds devoid of antipsychotic properties.

Antipsychotic agents have been important in anesthetic practice since the 1950s, with the introduction in Europe of the "lytic cocktail," that is, a mixture of chlorpromazine, meperidine, and promethazine.[3] This combination never gained popularity in the United States, and later it became obsolete abroad because of hypotension, extrapyramidal signs, and prolonged somnolence.[1] However, in the last decade, a form of neuroleptanesthesia has again become popular, with the use of droperidol, which is a butyrophenone congener of haloperidol, combined with fentanyl citrate, a synthetic opioid.

Effects on Narcotic Analgesics

Generally, the antipsychotic drugs exert additive and/or synergistic effects in combination with narcotic analgesics.[10–12] The depth of meperidine, morphine, and other narcotic-induced analgesia is increased in the presence of some phenothiazine antipsychotic agents, although this effect may simply be additive rather than synergistic.[10] Among phenothiazines, promethazine appears to be antianalgesic, and others, such as perphenazine, prochlorperazine, fluphenazine, and trifluoperazine, appear to possess slight antianalgesic properties.[13] In rodents and in man, the respiratory-depressant effects of narcotic analgesics are enhanced by the presence of antipsychotic agents, probably through a synergistic interaction.[12] There is an additive sedative-hypnotic effect when meperidine is combined with promethazine.[10] A recent study of the interaction of morphine and methotrimeprazine, a congener of chlorpromazine, in ten human volunteers showed that while methotrimeprazine alone (7.5 mg IM) caused sedation, it did not alter the effects of morphine 5 mg on pain threshold or ventilatory response to carbon dioxide.[13a] Narcotic and antipsychotic drug-induced hypotension may combine to cause dramatic hypotensive episodes.[13] The mechanisms of action by which antipsychotic drugs potentiate the effects of narcotic analgesics is uncertain.

Antipsychotic compounds enhance the effects of narcotic analgesics used in anesthetic practice.[7,8] Innovar, a combination of a butyrophenone droperidol, and an opioid fentanyl, may be effective partly because of the synergism of its components' properties.[5] However, the anesthesiologist must realize that antipsychotic drugs generally decrease narcotic requirements, and that significant respiratory depression as well as hypotension can occur in patients who receive therapeutic doses of an opioid and who are concurrently treated with antipsychotic drugs.[11,12,14]

Interactions with Central Nervous System Depressants

In animal experiments, antipsychotic drugs increase barbiturate and sedative/hypnotic-induced sleep time, and deepen barbiturate coma. Thus antipsychotic drugs, such as chlorpromazine and trifluoperazine, decrease the narcosis threshold and increase respiratory depression in the presence of central nervous system (CNS) depressants.[15–19] The few clinical reports available in man confirm these animal findings.[4,20,21] The mechanism for this interaction is uncertain at present. In patients who take antipsychotic drugs and to whom a barbiturate is administered either as a premedicant for electroconvulsant treatment or as part of a general anesthetic induction, caution is necessary in view of this drug interaction. In one study of 50 patients, chlorpromazine prolonged thiopental sleep time and reduced the thiopental requirement by 60%.[20] Thus lower doses of sedative hypnotics, or barbiturates, are probably indicated when a patient has received antipsychotic medications.

Sympathomimetic Drug Interactions

Since antipsychotic drugs exert central and peripheral antiadrenergic and antidopaminergic effects, their potential interactions with various pressor agents are relevant.[2] Antipsychotic agents usually block the pressor effects of norepinephrine and related *alpha*-adrenergic stimulating drugs. However, it has been shown in dogs that pretreatment with chlorpromazine can slightly enhance the pressor response to norepinephrine, an effect which is attributed to the depression of baroreceptor reflexes.[22] Conversely, antipsychotic drugs, especially chlorpromazine and thioridazine, can intensify the effects of other drugs on *beta*-adrenergic receptors. This selective blockade of *alpha*-adrenergic receptors can lead to a *beta*-adrenergic preponderance by agents, such as epinephrine, that usually exert both *alpha*- and *beta*-adrenergic effects, thus causing vasodilation and subsequent hypotension. The combination of epinephrine and chlorpromazine predictably causes hypotension in animals.[22] If paradoxical *beta*-adrenergic activation occurs in individuals receiving antipsychotic drugs, treatment with the *beta*-adrenergic blocking agent, propranolol, is indicated.

Dopamine is currently used as a vasoactive agent in anesthesia. Phenothiazines and butyrophenones are especially active in blocking dopamine receptors. Thus, theoretically, dopamine pressor action may be attenuated in the presence of these drugs. To date, however, this hypothesis has not been clinically verified.[2,23]

Anticholinergic Drug Interactions

Antipsychotic drugs, especially chlorpromazine and thioridazine, possess inherent anticholinergic effects that can be additive with other anticholinergic drugs, such as the antiparkinsonian agents or those anticholinergics used for preanesthetic medication. Since side effects from anticholinergic agents increase with age, the risk of such side effects during or after anesthesia in patients subject to antipsychotic drug therapy is greatest in the elderly. Patients who take antipsychotic drugs, especially combined with an antiparkinsonian agent, in addition to atropine or to scopolamine, may develop peripheral anticholinergic effects, such as adynamic ileus, glaucoma, and urinary retention, as well as central anticholinergic effects, such as confusion, fever, delirium, and agitation.[24-26]

The use of noncentrally acting preanesthetic anticholinergic drugs, such as methscopolamine or glycopyrrolate, may reduce the risk of these complications.[27]

Interactions with Inhalation Anesthetics

In addition to the interactions already discussed, the halogenated anesthetics, enflurane and isoflurane, given in combination with antipsychotic agents including chlorpromazine, may cause hypotensive episodes.[28,29] Similarly, a combination of halothane and droperidol may increase the incidence of hypotension.[6] The mechanism by which antipsychotic drugs augment the effects of halogenated general anesthetics is not known. The adrenergic blocking effects, along with ganglionic blockade and myocardial depression, may be contributory.[20,28,29] Hypotension caused by a combination of inhalation anesthetics and antipsychotic agents may be treated with moderate doses of *alpha*-adrenergic vasopressors, such as norepinephrine or phenylephrine. Since this type of hypotension is often associated with hypovolemia, the replacement of fluids and/or blood is indicated.

Additional Antipsychotic Anesthetic Interactions

Several other interactions may occur when antipsychotic drugs are used in anesthesia. Promethazine and antipsychotic drugs enhance one another's side effects.[32] Furthermore, there has been at least one report of prolonged apnea following succinylcholine administration in a patient treated with promazine, possibly due to the inhibition of plasma cholinesterase activity.[33] In addition, antipsychotic drugs intensify the effects of *alpha*-adrenergic blocking agents, such as phentolamine, and this increases a patient's tendency to develop hypotension. Furthermore, phenothiazine antipsychotic drugs, particularly thioridazine, may possess some direct myocardial-depressant effects, similar to quinidine. Concurrent use of phenothiazine antipsychotic drugs and quinidine may lead to additive myocardial depression, and this combination should probably be avoided.

Several papers have discussed the cardiovascular complications occurring in young patients who take phenothiazine medication on a regular basis.[34-36] These complications include sudden death, cardiac dysrhythmias, disturbances of conduction, and electrocardiographic changes suggestive of infarction. Biopsy and autopsy specimens of cardiac tissue may show areas of focal myocardial necrosis similar to those found after the administration of catecholamines to animals. The mechanism that produces these abnormalities is not clear and the reversibility of the lesions after discontinuance of the drug is questionable. The butyrophenones do not seem to share the myocardiotoxic potential of the phenothiazines.

Chlorpromazine and the other phenothiazines also lower the convulsive seizure threshold. Thus in theory their use with enflurane and ketamine, which can cause seizures during anesthesia, presents a potential problem. No reports of this interaction have appeared.[30] Loxapine, a dibenzoxazepine, is a relatively new drug for the treatment of acute and chronic schizophrenia. It, too, may lower the convulsive threshold; 6 of 10 patients with loxapine overdosage had generalized motor seizures as one manifestation of toxicity.[30a]

On the other hand, antipsychotic agents prevent postoperative vomiting, presumably by blocking the medullary chemoreceptor trigger zone.[9] However, early studies of their use as antiemetics show that their advantages in this area are outweighed by their disadvantages, which include hypotension and delayed emergence from anesthesia.[4,20] Promethazine may decrease lower esophageal sphincter tone, thus facilitating reflux; prochlorperazine seems to enhance lower esophageal sphincter tone, thereby providing more of a barrier to reflux.[30b]

Interactions with Conduction Anesthesia

Serious hypotensive episodes have been reported when a patient taking chlorpromazine receives spinal or epidural anesthesia or celiac plexus block.[31] It was postulated that the effects of sympathetic blockade following spinal, epidural, or celiac plexus block are additive with the hypotensive effects of chlorpromazine. As with inhalation anesthetics, an infusion of phenylephrine or norepinephrine may be indicated. However, two of the three patients described had conditions associated with deranged intravascular volume (intestinal obstruction, carcinomatosis). Furthermore, no mention was made of evaluating and restoring circulating volume, an important procedure prior to any technique that causes major sympathectomy. The role of chlorpromazine under these circumstances is unclear.

Finally, one retrospective report has indicated an increased postoperative mortality rate in patients receiving long-term phenothiazine therapy.[37] In this report, 12 patients generally received ether or halothane anesthesia in combination with muscle relaxants and nitrous oxide. The 11 deaths that occurred within the first 12 postoperative days were due to several causes, including cardiac problems, respi-

Table 19–2
Some Interactions Between Reserpine and Drugs Used in Anesthesia

Reserpine	Interaction
Inhalation	↓ MAC (halothane)
Barbiturates	↑ sleep time
Sympathomimetics	↓ effect of indirect-acting agents
	↑ effect of direct-acting agents
Muscle Relaxants	↑ duration of block with d-tubocurarine (animals)

ratory arrest, and complications following adynamic ileus, a condition to which, apparently, patients receiving long-term phenothiazine therapy seem particularly susceptible.[24] Adrenocorticotropic hormone (ACTH) and "steroid hormones" have been recommended as a preventive measure during the pre- and intraoperative periods in such patients. Discontinuance of antipsychotic drugs has been recommended preoperatively and intensive monitoring has been recommended postoperatively to prevent postoperative mortality. The overall significance of the contribution of long-term phenothiazine therapy to perioperative morbidity and mortality is still undetermined. However, the autonomic imbalance created in these patients and the potential for toxic cardiomyopathy reinforce the need for careful preoperative evaluation—especially of the cardiovascular system—and the importance of intra- and postoperative monitoring.

RESERPINE (TABLE 19–2)

The rauwolfia alkaloids, including reserpine, continue to be used as effective antihypertensive agents.[2] During the 1950s, these drugs were widely used to treat mania and schizophrenia.[2,38] With the introduction of chlorpromazine as an antischizophrenic agent in the early 1950s, and with the subsequent development of related antipsychotic agents that presumably possessed fewer depressant, hypotensive, and cholinomimetic side effects, reserpine became clinically obsolete. At the height of its popularity as an antipsychotic agent, reserpine appeared to be successful in the treatment of manic and schizophrenic psychosis.[2,38]

During the past decade, psychiatrists and psychopharmacologists have become aware that the more recent antipsychotic agents (the phenothiazines, butyrophenones, and thioxanthenes) also have serious drawbacks. Predominant among these drawbacks is that it has been discovered that long-term treatment with these agents often causes irreversible choreoathetoid tongue, body, and extremity movements, labeled "tardive dyskinesias." Considerable medicolegal and professional concern has centered on this problem.[39] Since reserpine does not cause tardive dyskinesias, it is possible that it will regain popularity and will be widely used as an alternative antipsychotic drug, especially in the treatment of chronically ill psychotic patients.

Mechanism of Action

Reserpine depletes intraneuronally bound central and peripheral dopamine, norepinephrine, and serotonin, presumably by interfering with storage. Reserpine may also activate central and peripheral cholinoceptive sites. Catecholamine depletion is considered to underlie reserpine's antipsychotic and antihypertensive effects.[2,38]

Anesthetic Implications

The anesthetic management of patients receiving reserpine deserves attention in several areas. These include: (1) anesthetic considerations in patients receiving electroconvulsive therapy, (2) anesthetic precautions in the administration of reserpine to patients receiving inhalation anesthetic agents, (3) anesthetic dose reduction in patients given reserpine and receiving barbiturates, and (4) analogous precautions in the administration of vasopressors.

Electroconvulsive Therapy

In the 1950s, prolonged apnea and/or sudden death was reported in patients who had been given reserpine and who were receiving electroconvulsive therapy (ECT). In addition to apnea, patients developed profound hypotension and cardiac dysrhythmias, leading to death in some cases. Details as to the type of anesthetics used for ECT, and, indeed, whether anesthetics were used at all, are not included in these early reports. Furthermore, the amount of reserpine administered to the patients preceding ECT was large, approximately 10 mg intramuscularly. The information on this interaction is incomplete, and, until more information is available, the use of reserpine probably should contraindicate ECT. A two-week reserpine-free period is suggested for patients who are recommended for ECT.[40,41] Alternative antihypertensive drugs should be used if possible for the patient who takes reserpine for blood pressure control and who requires ECT.

Inhalation Anesthetic Agents

Until the early 1960s, reserpine was incriminated in dangerous hypotensive reactions or in vascular instability when used in conjunction with such inhalation agents as cyclopropane, ether, halothane, methoxyflurane, and trichoroethylene. The literature recommended that any patient receiving general anesthesia, especially ether and halothane, be kept reserpine-free for a period of at least 2 weeks.[42–44] However, several well-controlled studies have demonstrated that reserpine treatment of hypertensive patients increases neither hypotensive reactions nor other adverse cardiovascular effects during general anesthesia. Currently, the consensus of opinion is that attention should be paid to the potential complications of reserpine therapy, and that its parasympathetic effects should be pretreated with an anticholinergic agent, such as atropine, in order to avoid discontinuing reserpine preoperatively.[45,46]

Reserpine decreased the minimum alveolar concentration (MAC) of halothane in an animal study; the effect appeared to be dose-dependent.[47] Speculation as to the mechanism of this interaction focused on the relationship between central catecholamine levels and anesthetic requirements. Interestingly, no comments were made as to the presence or absence of cardiovascular instability in these animals pretreated with reserpine and anesthetized with halothane.

Barbiturate-Reserpine Interactions

Several animal studies have demonstrated that reserpine increases barbiturate-induced sleeping time in small rodents and that the drug may increase sleeping time and sedation in man.[17,48–51] The mechanism for this effect is unknown, although it could be due to the depletion of central catecholamines and/or the augmentation of barbiturate-induced central nervous system depression. Since reserpine increases the effectiveness of a given dose of barbiturate, a lower dose of barbiturates in the patient who is given reserpine is suggested. However, few human experiments have demonstrated this interaction.[50]

Similarly, it has also been noted in rodents that reserpine decreases the ability of phenobarbital and diazepam to raise seizure thresholds, an observation that might be significant to the seizure-prone patient who receives anesthetics such as ketamine and enflurane, which are associated with the increased incidence of convulsive episodes.[52]

Interactions Between Reserpine and Sympathomimetic Drugs

Reserpine may affect exogenously administered sympathomimetic drugs. Since reserpine releases stored catecholamines, indirect-acting pressor amines, such as metaraminol, ephedrine, amphetamine, tyramine, mephentermine, phenylpropanolamine, and methylphenidate, are less effective in animals given reserpine, and theoretically may decrease response in the patient who receives reserpine.[2,53] Conversely, probably because of the phenomenon of denervation hypersensitivity, an augmentation of the patient response to direct-acting sympathetic pressors, such as dopamine, phenylephrine, norepinephrine, and epinephrine, may occur if these agents are administered after reserpine pretreatment. Thus, in the reserpinized patient, conservative infusion of direct-acting sympathomimetic agents, rather than indirect-acting agents, is preferred for treating hypotension, should pressor agents be necessary.

Reserpine-Narcotic Analgesic Interactions

The data on reserpine-morphine interactions in animals are difficult to evaluate. Potentiation of analgesia is apparent in some species, such as rats and rabbits. In mice, depending on the test system employed, reserpine may either potentiate or antagonize morphine analgesia.[54-56] The ability of reserpine to alter the effects of narcotic analgesics has not been well studied in man. Hence the importance of a narcotic analgesic-reserpine interaction is uncertain.

Additional Reserpine-Anesthetic Interactions

In rabbits, the neuromuscular blocking effect of d-tubocurarine is antagonized by reserpine.[57] This is consistent with reserpine's cholinomimetic activity. Similarly, in rats, reserpine pretreatment increases the lethality of sublethal doses of physostigmine and of neostigmine. This effect is prevented by prior administration of anticholinergic drugs.[58] No information on the significance of these interactions in human beings is available at present.

Digitalis glycosides may cause interactions when administered in patients who have received reserpine. These interactions include cardiac dysrhythmias, bradycardia, and decreased ionotropic effect.[32,59] Reserpine may heighten the patient's responsiveness to thiazide diuretics. This interaction may require a readjustment of the dose of the diuretic.[59]

ANTICHOLINERGIC AGENTS

Anticholinergic agents are routinely used in the practice of psychiatry. These drugs, which include trihexyphenidyl and benztropine mesylate, are employed as antidotes to the frequent dystonias and parkinsonian side effects caused by the neuroleptic blockade of dopamine receptors. These agents treat related symptoms such as tremor, rigidity, shuffling gait, and drooling.[2]

Mechanism of Action

Anticholinergic agents used in psychiatry generally exert their effects through their central and peripheral antimuscarinic actions. Thus, in addition to alleviating parkinsonian symptoms, anticholinergic drugs can cause hyperpyrexia, constipation, mydriasis, adynamic ileus, urinary retention, and other signs of heightened anticholinergic activity.[2]

Anesthetic Implications

Patients who receive anticholinergic agents for the management of drug-induced parkinsonism, or who take anticholinergic drugs, such as tricyclic antidepressants, chlorpromazine, or thioridazine, are at greater risk of developing a central anticholinergic syndrome, consisting of disorientation, hallucinations, and memory loss, if centrally acting anticholinergic agents are added preoperatively.[25] Similarly, in the intraoperative and postoperative period, peripheral anticholinergic side effects are increased in patients who receive anticholinergic drugs.[24] The anticholinergic effects of various agents are additive; thus the effects of atropine or scopolamine, used preoperatively, may be augmented by the prior administration of other anticholinergics.[25] In addition, cen-

Table 19-3
Some Interactions Between Tricyclic Antidepressants and Drugs Used in Anesthesia

Tricyclic Antidepressants	Interaction
Narcotics	↑ analgesia
	↑ respiratory depression
Barbiturates	↑ sleep time
Anticholinergics	↑ central activity
	↑ peripheral activity
Sympathomimetics	↑ effect of direct-acting agents

tral and peripheral anticholinergic effects appear to be increased by methylphenidate, barbiturates, and procainamide. Anticholinergic agents and sympathomimetic drugs also may interact to enhance sympathetic effects caused by a shift in autonomic control (adrenergic-cholinergic imbalance).[24-60] Furthermore, meperidine has anticholinergic effects that may be additive to those of other anticholinergic agents.[61] To prevent a central anticholinergic syndrome, it may be appropriate either to eliminate completely or to reduce doses of atropine or scopolamine preoperatively, or to use a noncentrally acting anticholinergic drug, such as homatropine, glycopyrrolate, or methscopolamine as a preoperative medication.[27]

TRICYCLIC ANTIDEPRESSANTS (TABLE 19-3)

The tricyclic antidepressants are used to treat various psychiatric symptoms. These compounds, which include imipramine, amitriptyline, desipramine, nortriptyline, doxepin, and protriptyline, are related in structure to the phenothiazines; and indeed tricyclic antidepressants were originally developed as antipsychotic drugs, but were unsuccessful as such. Tricyclic antidepressants are used effectively in the treatment of severe depression. They may also be used in the treatment of chronic pain, phobic anxiety, and other psychosomatic disorders.

Tricyclic antidepressants block the uptake of norepinephrine and/or of serotonin or dopamine into the presynaptic nerve ending, thereby increasing central and peripheral adrenergic tone. This effect has been linked to their antidepressant activity. The majority of tricyclic antidepressants also possess moderate anticholinergic effects, which may also alleviate depression. The anticholinergic and catecholamine uptake-blocking properties of the tricyclic antidepressants seem to cause their most significant clinical interactions with anesthetic agents.[2]

Vasopressor Interactions

The tricyclic antidepressants, imipramine and desipramine, increase two- to tenfold the pressor response to injected, direct-acting sympathetic amines including norepinephrine, epinephrine, and phenylephrine. This response has resulted in hyperthermia, sweating, hypertensive crises, severe headache, rupture of cerebral blood vessels, and death. Indeed, these effects, elicited under controlled conditions, are more dramatic than the effects of a combination of direct-acting sympathetic amines and a monoamine oxidase inhibitor, a more widely feared drug-drug interaction.[62-65] Furthermore, tricyclic antidepressant-sympathetic amine interaction has occurred clinically in dental patients in Great Britain following the administration of local anesthetics to which norepinephrine was added as a vasoconstrictor.[66-68] The potentiation of the pressor action of epinephrine is not as pronounced as that of norepinephrine. However, epinephrine-induced changes in heart rate and rhythm may be dangerously potentiated by a tricyclic antidepressant.[64] Whether the same potential for hypertension and/or for disturbances in cardiac rate and rhythm exists in man with other drugs used during anesthesia that have sympathomimetic and/or anticholinergic effects, such as ketamine, pancuronium, gallamine, and fluroxene, is not known. However, pancuronium caused ventricular tachycardia and fibrillation in 40% of dogs anesthetized with halothane after 2 weeks of imipramine pretreatment.[168a] On the other hand, a study was designed to evaluate the effect of pretreatment with antidepressant drugs on the LD_{50} of intraperitoneal ketamine in rats. Although non-fatal additive toxicity was not ruled out, mortality from ketamine was not increased either by pretreatment with a tricyclic (amitriptyline) or monoamine oxidase inhibitor (tranylcypromine) antidepressant.[68a] A single case report suggests that amitriptyline may have contributed to, as well as prolonged, postoperative rebound hypertension and tachycardia associated with clonidine withdrawal.[68b] The mechanism of action by which hypertension and dysrythmias occur has been tentatively linked to the amine reuptake-blocking properties of tricyclic antidepressants.[63] This ability to block amine reuptake is shared with several other drugs, including cocaine. Alternatively, it is possible that the induction of receptor hypersensitivity by the tricyclic antidepressant affects this drug interaction.[64]

Frequently it is not possible to discontinue tricyclic antidepressant therapy before surgery either because of the patient's psychiatric condition or because of the emergent nature of the surgery. Indeed, it may not even be necessary to discontinue tricyclic antidepressant therapy if the anesthetist formulates a plan to avoid potential drug interactions, as well as a plan to treat such interactions should they occur. If direct-acting sympathetic pressor amines are necessary, e.g., for the treatment of hypotension, they should be used in reduced dosage and carefully titrated. Treatment of hypertensive crises, if they develop, consists in the administration of chlorpromazine or of an *alpha*-adrenergic blocking agent, such as phentolamine, or of the vasodilator, sodium nitroprusside. Cooling measures should be instituted if the patient is hyperpyretic.

The synthetic peptide vasoconstrictor felypressin (2-phenylalanine, 8-lysine vasopressin) does not interact adversely with tricyclic antidepressants. It has been recommended as a vasoconstrictor in a concentration of 0.03 IU/ml not to exceed a total of 8 ml, for use in conjunction with local anesthetics in patients receiving tricyclic antidepressants.[64,66] Currently, felypressin is not available in the United States.

Anticholinergic Drug Interactions

As mentioned previously, tricyclic antidepressants possess central and peripheral anticholinergic activity. Since the anticholinergic side effects of various drugs are additive, preoperative treatment with centrally active anticholinergic drugs may interact with tricyclic antidepressants and cause confusion and delirium (a central anticholinergic syndrome) during the postoperative period.[25,69] Preoperative use of noncentrally acting anticholinergic agents is suggested in the presence of tricyclic antidepressants, especially in elderly patients.[27]

Narcotic Analgesic Interactions

Although little data exist to support the contention that tricyclic antidepressants augment the analgesic and other effects of narcotic analgesics in human beings, imipramine and amitriptyline potentiate morphine analgesia in mice, and increase meperidine-induced respiratory depression.[70] These effects are theoretically important to the anesthesiologist and suggest lower doses of narcotics in patients taking tricyclic antidepressants.

Barbiturate-Sedative Hypnotic Interactions

Some animal experiments suggest that tricyclic antidepressants increase the sedative and hypnotic effects of barbiturates. Increased tricyclic antidepressant lethality occurs in the presence of a barbiturate and vice versa. Imipramine has been known to prolong hexobarbital narcosis, possibly by means of enzyme inhibition, and to prolong apnea following thiopental administration in man. Thus tricyclic antidepressants probably enhance the CNS-depressant effects of barbiturates and related sedative hypnotics.[18] Awareness of this potential interaction suggests lower doses of barbiturates in patients receiving tricyclic antidepressants.

OTHER INTERACTIONS

Tricyclic antidepressants, like the phenothiazines to which they are structurally related, lower the convulsive threshold; these compounds can induce seizure activity in nonanesthetized patients with and without a history of seizure disorder. Two cases of seizures during enflurane anesthesia in patients taking amitriptyline have been reported; seizure activity in both cases ceased when enflurane was removed from the system.[70a] In addition, several other tricyclic antidepressant-anesthetic interactions have been described. In rabbits, the tricyclic antidepressants imipramine, amitriptyline, and protriptyline have increased the local anesthetic effect of lidocaine and procaine on the cornea.[71] This is probably related to the sedating effect of the tricyclic antidepressants, although other mechanisms may be implicated.

Experimental data suggest that reversal of neuromuscular blockade with neostigmine-atropine in cats with chronic amitriptyline treatment produces significant ST-T wave changes and disturbances in myocardial conduction. The changes were not seen if the amitriptyline was discontinued at least 24 hours prior to reversal. The relevance of this information to humans is not known at present.[71a] Also in animal experiments, tricyclic antidepressants antagonize the cardiovascular effects of propranolol. The mechanism of this interaction is probably related to the anticholinergic ac-

Table 19–4
Some Interactions Between Monoamine Oxidase Inhibitors (MAOI) and Drugs Used in Anesthesia

MAOI	Interaction
Inhalation Drugs	muscle stiffness, hyperpyrexia, (halothane in animals)
Narcotics	meperidine → excitatory syndrome → ↑ narcotic effect and coma
Barbiturates	↑ sleep time
Anticholinergics	↑ central activity
Sympathomimetics	↑ ↑ effects of indirect-acting agents ↑ effects of direct-acting agents ↑ dopamine effects
Muscle Relaxants	↑ duration of block with succinylcholine (phenelzine decreases plasma cholinesterase)

tivity of antidepressants. The significance of this interaction in human beings is not known, although propranolol has successfully treated the cardiotoxicity associated with tricyclic antidepressant toxicity in man.[72,73]

New Antidepressants

Amoxapine is a new tricyclic antidepressant, the demethylated metabolite of the antipsychotic agent, loxapine.[71b] Severe cardiovascular reactions, e.g., hypotension, supraventricular tachydysrhythmias, conduction blocks, and ventricular dysrhythmias, which may occur with other tricyclic antidepressant toxicity seem less likely to occur with amoxapine. The drug is characterized by less anticholinergic activity than the other tricyclic compounds, but has dopamine blocking activity similar to that of the antipsychotic drugs and may be associated with extrapyramidal side effects.[71c,71d]

Maprotiline is a tetracyclic antidepressant which has a greater tendency than most to lower seizure thresholds. It may be prudent to avoid the use of anesthetics such as enflurane and possibly ketamine, either of which may be associated with seizure activity, in patients taking a drug known to lower the seizure threshold.[71e] It has low anticholinergic properties, similar to the less anticholinergic of the conventional tricyclic antidepressants. There is conflicting evidence as to its effect on intracardiac conduction.[71f,71g] However, in an overdose, maprotiline is quite cardiotoxic, causing ventricular dysrhythmias. In general, the same anesthetic considerations for tricyclic antidepressants would apply to maprotiline. As yet, no adverse interactions of this drug with anesthetics have been reported.

Trazodone, a nontricyclic antidepressant, is being used with increasing frequency in the United States. Its principal advantages include a negligible incidence of anticholinergic and a low incidence of cardiovascular side effects, although two cases of increased ventricular ectopy have been reported in patients who had preexisting cardiac disease (mitral valve prolapse) and who were treated with trazodone.[71b] There is also a single case report of reversible first-degree heart block associated with trazodone administration in an elderly man.[71i] Drowsiness and dizziness have been the major side effects and one case of hepatic toxicity following a therapeutic trial of the drug has been published, as have several cases of priapism.[71j,71k] There have been no reports of adverse interactions with anesthetics to date.

MONOAMINE OXIDASE INHIBITORS (TABLE 19–4)

Prior to the development and popularization of tricyclic antidepressants, a variety of monoamine oxidase inhibitors (MAOI) were developed and were found to be effective as antidepressant agents. Although they have been superseded by the tricyclic antidepressants, MAOI are still used in psychiatry. At a time when the medicolegal sanctions against ECT are increasing, MAOI are not infrequently used as a "second line" of drugs to treat depression. Indeed, some reviews suggest that these drugs may be used safely in combination with tricyclic antidepressants in the refractory-depressed patient. Currently, in the United States, the MAOI tranylcypromine and phenelzine are approved for the treatment of depression. Another, pargyline, is approved as an antihypertensive agent. However, other MAOI are used outside the United States.

Mechanism of Action

MAOI are considered effective in the treatment of depression because they inhibit monoamine oxidase. These drugs also inhibit other enzymes, particularly hepatic microsomal enzymes involved in the metabolism of many drugs. Monoamine oxidase enzymes are ubiquitous in the body, with high concentrations in liver and intestine.[74] Monoamine oxidase is a major intraneuronal enzyme necessary for the oxidative deamination of serotonin, norepinephrine, and dopamine. The norepinephrine (catecholamine) hypothesis of depression asserts that MAOI are effective because they allow the repletion of monoamine stores in the brain. This ability to inhibit the metabolism of sympathetic amines and of other monoamines underlies the majority of their interactions with anesthetics and contributes to the inherent dangers of MAOI.[2,75]

Sympathetic Amine Interactions

Monoamine oxidase inhibitors are infamous for their ability to interact with some sympathetic compounds to cause a dangerous and often lethal hypertensive crisis. The hypertensive crisis may consist of precipitous hypertension, hyperpyrexia, sweating, tachycardia, throbbing occipital headache, and intracranial bleeding. It appears to be caused by a "sympathetic storm" and is similar to the effects of an overdose of amphetamines.[74,76–84]

Since MAOI act primarily intraneuronally in the central and peripheral nervous system, indirect-acting sympathetic amines are more likely to interact with them to cause hypertensive crises, because these compounds release intraneuronal monoamines. Thus amphetamine-like psychostimulants, including amphetamine, methamphetamine, methylphenidate, and other related drugs, are likely to interact with MAOI in this context. Similarly, indirect-acting vasopressors, including tyramine, mephentermine, metaraminol, ephedrine, and phenylpropanolamine, all of which release norepinephrine and dopamine from bound intracellular neuronal stores, can interact with MAOI and cause hypertensive crises.[64,65,77–79,85,86] Acute administration of reserpine to MAOI-pretreated patients may also lead to a hypertensive crisis, since reserpine depletes intracellular catecholamines by causing their release from bound stores.[87] The same phenomenon occurs with guanethidine and, similarly, with L-DOPA, a dopamine precursor, which may interact with MAOI to cause reactions that closely resemble a hypertensive crisis.[88,89] The MAOI augment and prolong the pressor effects and enhance the action of dopamine, but not of norepinephrine, on the contractile force of the heart.[81]

Interestingly, direct-acting sympathetic amines, including norepinephrine and epinephrine, interact less with MAOI.[64,65] Although some anecdotal reports indicate that these agents cause hypertension, controlled studies show only mild hypertensive effects when direct-acting sympathetic amines and MAOI are used concurrently.[64,90] Pharmacologically, the reason for this lack of reaction may be that exogenous, direct-acting sympathetic amines do not flood the intracellular site of action of the MAOI with monoamines, and are in part degraded in an alternative route by the extracellular enzyme, catechol-o-methyl transferase (COMT). The hypertensive response has been proposed because of the "denervation hypersensitivity" caused by the MAOI. This hypertension has been noted primarily during repeated MAOI administration, usually after orthostatic hypotension has developed. Oral, but not intravenous, phenylephrine (a sympathetic amine with more direct than indirect action) has been reported to cause hypertensive crisis in combination with MAOI. This interaction is believed to occur because of the inhibition of gastrointestinal monoamine oxidase, which usually degrades orally administered phenylephrine before its systemic absorption.

Investigators suggest that hypertensive crises can be avoided by the discontinuance of monoamine oxidase inhibitors 2 to 3 weeks prior to anesthetic administration. If pressor amines must be used during anesthesia in patients who are receiving MAOI, it is suggested that low doses of direct-acting amines, such as norepinephrine, be used, rather than indirect-acting amines. If a hypertensive crisis occurs, it is best treated with *alpha*-adrenergic blocking agents, such as phentolamine and/or chlorpromazine, or with the vasodilator, sodium nitroprusside, in addition to cooling the patient to alleviate hyperpyrexia.[64,83,91] Cardiac dysrhythmias may be controlled by a *beta*-adrenergic blocking drug.[81] However, one must institute an *alpha*-blockade prior to the administration of *beta*-adrenergic blocking agents in order to prevent further hypertension from unopposed *alpha* activity.

Narcotic Analgesic Interactions

In addition to interactions with sympathetic amines, MAOI have been found to interact with the narcotic analgesic, meperidine[92–97] (see Chapter 22, second case report). In this case, a syndrome manifested by agitation, excitement, restlessness, hypertension, headache, rigidity, convulsions, and hyperpyrexia (all symptoms similar to the hypertensive crisis caused by MAOI-sympathetic amine interaction) occurs. A similar reaction has been observed between phenelzine and dextromethorphan.[98] Morphine has not been implicated clinically in this phenomenon.[99] However, a study in mice did show that pretreatment with MAOI increased the mortality not only from meperidine, but from morphine, pentazocine, and phenazocine.[100] The mechanism by which this drug interaction occurs is uncertain. However, based on animal experiments, several authors postulate that the response is caused by the elevation of serotonin levels in the brain following monoamine oxidase inhibition in the presence of meperidine.[94,100,101]

Although prevention is the best treatment of a narcotic-MAOI interaction of this type, various authors recommend the administration of prednisolone hemisuccinate, 25 mg intravenously, as well as other supportive measures as indicated, and the control of the patient blood pressure if arterial blood pressure reaches excessive levels.[92,93]

Alternatively, narcotic analgesics, especially meperidine, have been reported to interact with MAOI to cause coma, depressed respiration, and hypotension, responses apparently caused by the potentiation of primary narcotic effects. The mechanism by which this interaction occurs has been attributed to the inhibition of narcotic metabolism in the liver by an action of MAOI on enzymes, other than monoamine oxidase that increase free narcotic.[96,97] Treatment, which is primarily supportive, may include the narcotic antagonist, naloxone.[102,103]

In addition, prompt acidification of the urine, using lysine or arginine hydrochloride or sodium biphosphate intravenously, and the production of a large volume of urine have been used to hasten meperidine excretion.[84]

One-quarter to one-fifth of the usual narcotic amount should be given to the patient taking MAOI who, for whatever reason, must receive a narcotic; careful observation of the patient over the succeeding 15 to 20 minutes for any changes in vital signs or level of consciousness is important. Churchill-Davidson described a "sensitivity test," using small incremental hourly injections of morphine (or meperidine), with careful observation of the patient for signs of adverse reaction.[104] However, the unpredictability of the response to meperidine of the patient receiving MAOI therapy probably warrants the avoidance of this drug altogether, with the use of morphine in reduced doses if a narcotic is necessary.

Sedative Hypnotic and Barbiturate Interactions

MAOI have been reported to augment barbiturate and sedative hypnotic effects in animals and in man.[105] The mechanism by which this occurs is probably due to MAOI inhibition of liver microsomal enzymes necessary for barbiturate detoxification. Experimentally, a combination of an MAOI and a barbiturate increases sleep time, duration of anesthesia, and lethality in animals. Similar effects have been noted in man.[105] Thus, in a patient pretreated with MAOI, lower doses of barbiturates should be used.

Muscle Relaxant Interactions

One case of prolonged apnea following succinylcholine administration for ECT has been reported in a patient receiving the MAOI phenelzine. This response was attributed to a decrease in plasma cholinesterase. Investigation of plasma cholinesterase levels in an additional series of 22 patients taking phenelzine and other MAOI revealed depressed enzyme activity in 40% of the patients taking phenelzine and normal levels in patients receiving the other MAOI.[106]

To date, no MAOI except phenelzine has been reported to exert this effect on plasma cholinesterase. After the discontinuance of phenelzine, plasma cholinesterase levels return to normal.[106]

One animal study has investigated the

effect of d-tubocurarine on long-term MAOI therapy and found that the relaxant effect is not prolonged.[107] In the absence of clinical reports on this interaction, it is probably safe to use this nondepolarizing relaxant in patients. There are no studies available on gallamine or pancuronium in this context.

Miscellaneous MAOI-Anesthetic Interactions

Several other interactions between MAOI and agents used in anesthesia have been observed. In cats, MAOI in conjunction with halothane cause muscle stiffness.[108] In addition, pheniprazine and nialamide are reported to cause hyperpyrexia during halothane inhalation. Propranolol, given in association with an MAOI, has caused a hypertensive crisis, presumably by the blockade of *beta*-adrenergic receptors and the imbalanced activation of *alpha*-adrenergic receptors.[109] Hypotension has occurred when MAOI and thiazide diuretics are given concurrently.[110] Furthermore, MAOI have enhanced anticholinergic effects when given together with atropine.[81] Finally, one patient, receiving a large dose of droperidol in addition to a monoamine oxidase inhibitor, developed cardiovascular depression that lasted 36 hours.[111]

CASE REPORT

A 45-year-old 90-kg man required emergency repair of right wrist lacerations. He was moderately obese but was otherwise in good health. He was being treated for depression with tranylcypromine, 30 mg q.d. After premedication with diazepam, 10 mg p.o., he arrived in the operating room.

This patient presents several anesthetic problems: obesity, an emergency operation, and MAOI therapy. Detailed discussion of the patient's management as related to his obesity is omitted. Airway problems are anticipated, as well as possible intraoperative and postoperative problems with ventilation. A patient who requires an emergency operation may have a full stomach, and may also have an unknown intravascular volume status. Clinical tests of volume, such as tilting, may be misleading because of the MAOI therapy, which in itself can cause orthostatic hypotension. Because the operation is an emergency, a 2-week MAOI-free period is not possible. The anesthetic technique and agents chosen must minimize the likelihood of an adverse drug interaction between anesthetic drugs and the MAOI.

Regional techniques may be considered. A brachial plexus block through the axillary route might be selected. A local anesthetic, such as bupivacaine, could offer a long-acting block, without concomitant vasoconstrictors such as epinephrine. Blood pressure change, due to sympathectomy, is not likely with this technique, although there is the possibility of inadvertent intravascular injection and subsequent hyper- and/or hypotension that might require treatment. In the event of hypotension, a direct-acting vasopressor, such as phenylephrine, in titrated amounts is preferred to indirect-acting vasopressors, such as ephedrine or mephentermine, because phenylephrine is less likely to cause extreme hypertension. Intravenous analgesic supplementation of the block with meperidine could be hazardous. Morphine should be selected if a narcotic is necessary, using small amounts of drug and watching for adverse effects such as a decreased level of consciousness or hypotension.

Alternatively, general anesthetic techniques may be considered. Balanced techniques, involving narcotics, are probably not advisable. Inhalation techniques with agents such as halothane or enflurane could be used with appropriate precautions, involving vasopressors as noted above. A rapid induction-intubation sequence is needed because of the "full stomach." Caution is indicated in the use of narcotics in the recovery room; avoiding meperidine and using small increments of morphine is suggested. Continuous temperature monitoring is important. Equip-

Table 19-5
Some Interactions between Lithium Carbonate and Drugs Used in Anesthesia

Lithium Carbonate	Interaction
Barbiturates	↑ sleep time
Muscle Relaxants	↑ duration of block with pancuronium, succinylcholine, decamethonium

ment for direct arterial pressure monitoring should be immediately available, as should agents for the rapid control of hypertension, such as sodium nitroprusside. Awareness of the patient's drug history and of the possible adverse drug interactions is crucial for the effective management of this patient.

LITHIUM CARBONATE (TABLE 19-5)

In 1949, Cade noted the effectiveness of lithium in the treatment of mania, and the drug has been used for this indication in the United States since the early 1960s.[112] More recently, lithium has proved useful in the prevention of recurrent depression.[113] In addition, lithium therapy has been tried in over 30 other disorders, psychiatric and nonpsychiatric, ranging from alcoholism and thyrotoxicosis to Huntington's chorea.[114]

Lithium is a monovalent cation, the lightest of the alkali metals, and in the same group of elements on the Periodic Table as sodium and potassium. It generally occurs in nature as a salt (lithium carbonate, lithium chloride), rather than as a free element, and is ubiquitous. The ion has no known physiologic role.[113] Approximately 95% of ingested lithium is excreted by the kidneys, complete excretion requiring 10 to 14 days in both short- and long-term therapy.[115]

At the cellular level, lithium acts as an imperfect substitute for Na^+. It moves intracellularly during depolarization, but is extruded from the cell at a rate only 10% of that of Na^+. Lithium, therefore, accumulates within the cell and is in a position to affect processes that depend on movement of monovalent cations.[115] Many studies have dealt with the effects of lithium on brain amine metabolism. Lithium inhibits the release of norepinephrine and serotonin, increases the reuptake of norepinephrine, and possibly increases the synthesis and the turnover rate of serotonin. This agent has little effect on dopaminergic systems. Lithium inhibits activation of adenylate cyclase in the CNS of experimental animals. It is not yet certain which, if any, of these actions are important for therapy.[112,113]

The anesthetic implications of lithium therapy became a concern with the appearance of several case reports that describe probable anesthetic drug interactions with lithium.[116-118]

Lithium-Muscle Relaxant Interaction

The first problem noted was prolonged neuromuscular blockade following pancuronium bromide and succinylcholine hydrochloride in patients receiving lithium carbonate.[116,118] Hill and colleagues subsequently investigated the effect of lithium treatment on the neuromuscular blockade in dogs following the administration of succinylcholine, decamethonium, d-tubocurarine, gallamine, or pancuronium.[119] They found that lithium prolonged the blockade of succinylcholine, decamethonium, and pancuronium, but that it had no effect on the blockade produced by gallamine or d-tubocurarine. Lithium also prolonged the reversal time of pancuronium by neostigmine. There was no effect on plasma cholinesterase activity in 66 manic-depressive patients receiving chronic lithium therapy.[119] The clinical significance of the interaction between lithium and neuromuscular blocking agents has recently been questioned. A retrospective study of 766 patients who received ECT over a 5-year period found no difference in the response to succinylcholine of 17 patients taking lithium when compared with the group as a whole.[119a] Waud et al., found that pretreatment with lithium caused a slight reduction in dosage requirement for d-tubocurarine in guinea pigs. There was no effect on the response to pancuronium.[119b] They concluded that at therapeutic lithium levels there is minimal interaction of lithium with competitive neuromuscular blocking agents and only a small possibility that lithium would interact significantly with succinylcholine under clinical conditions. Atracurium has yet to be evaluated in this regard.

The effect of lithium on the neuromuscular blockade of succinylcholine and of decamethonium, as well as the prolonged reversal of pancuronium, are compatible with the findings of Vizi et al., who reported that lithium inhibited acetylcholine synthesis and release in animal preparations.[120] The effect on pancuronium blockade, if this differential effect does exist, is more difficult to explain and implies differences in the mechanism of action between pancuronium and the two other nondepolarizing drugs—d-tubocurarine and gallamine. Pancuronium may have depolarizing as well as nondepolarizing activity at the neuromuscular junction. Another possibility is that, by virtue of the steroid moiety in its structure, pancuronium may have a more profound effect on the cellular distribution of sodium and potassium than either d-tubocurarine or gallamine, particularly if pancuronium possesses mineralocorticoid activity.

Lithium-Barbiturate Interaction

Jephcott and Kerry reported a case of prolonged recovery from barbiturate anesthesia following electroconvulsive therapy in a patient taking lithium carbonate.[117] The patient's serum lithium level was 3.4 mEq/L (therapeutic range 0.9 to 1.5 mEq/L), but preanesthetic evaluation had revealed no evidence of lithium toxicity. Mannisto and Saarnivaara studied the effects of short- and long-term lithium chloride treatment on sleeping time following the administration of intravenous thiopental, methohexital, ketamine, propanidid, alphaxalone-alphadolone acetate, and diazepam in white mice.[121] They found prolonged sleep time following thiopental, methohexital, and diazepam after short-term treatment with lithium chloride, but no significant effects after prolonged treatment (21 days). However, serum lithium levels in the short-term experiments were much higher (2.3 ± 0.2 mEq/L) than in the long-term experiments (0.6 ± 0.1 mEq/L), which might account for some of the difference in results.

There have been no reports to date of interactions between lithium and either inhalation anesthetics or local anesthetics.

The therapeutic range for serum lithium concentration is narrow, with levels below 0.8 mEq/L generally ineffective and levels above 1.5 mEq/L toxic. Toxic symptoms are manifested primarily in the gastrointestinal, muscular, and central nervous systems, and range from mild, such as nausea or fine tremor of the hands, to severe, including convulsions and death. It is not uncommon for patients to become intoxicated and to develop a confusional state with blood levels in the "therapeutic" range, particularly in elderly patients, who excrete lithium more slowly than do the young.[113,122,123]

Lithium crosses the placental barrier rapidly; concentrations of the ion at the time of delivery are similar in maternal, umbilical, and neonatal serum.[124] Severe maternal and neonatal lithium toxicity developed in a patient who took lithium during the last month of pregnancy. The patient received thiazide diuretics simultaneously, and in addition was on a sodium-restricted diet. Maternal serum lithium concentration immediately after delivery was 3.4 mEq/L, whereas that of the newborn was 2.4 mEq/L.[125]

Lithium-Diuretic Interaction

Administration of diuretics or restriction of sodium is an added hazard to patients receiving lithium. Sodium loading promotes the excretion of lithium, and sodium depletion causes retention of the ion through renal mechanisms at the proximal tubule.[115] Short-term diuretic therapy can cause toxicity quickly.[126] Diuretics that deplete both sodium and potassium, such as thiazides, ethacrynic acid, and furosemide, are more hazardous in this regard than are the potassium-sparing agents, namely spironolactone and triamterene.[127] Treatment of lithium toxicity includes support of vital functions. Osmotic diuresis, alkalinization of the urine, and administration of aminophylline are important therapeutic modalities. Dialysis may be used in severe cases.[113]

Several side effects of lithium therapy may interest the anesthesiologist. Repeated lithium therapy causes a benign and reversible depression of electrocardiogram T-waves. In addition, some patients may develop a nephrogenic diabetes insipidus that is resistant to antidiuretic hormone. This syndrome resolves when lithium therapy is discontinued. A few patients may develop goiter. These patients generally remain euthyroid, and the gland shrinks when lithium treatment is discontinued.[115]

CASE REPORT

A 64-year-old 70-kg man was scheduled for cataract extraction under general anesthesia. Preoperative evaluation revealed a long history of manic-depressive psychosis that had been successfully treated with lithium carbonate, 300 mg q.i.d., for the past 2 years. The remainder of his examination was unremarkable and preoperative laboratory studies including electrolytes were normal: The patient's lithium level was 1.2 mEq/L.

In considering the anesthetic management of this patient, several points are important. First, from his preoperative evaluation, he seems to be in optimal condition for an elective operation. His lithium level is in the "therapeutic" range, and he manifests no signs of lithium toxicity. Second, the operation necessitates endotracheal anesthesia, which should be accomplished by maintaining the patient's intraocular pressure at or below preinduction levels. One could proceed with an inhalation induction using halothane and endotracheal intubation at the appropriate depth of anesthesia, thereby avoiding those muscle relaxants and barbiturates whose actions might be prolonged by lithium. If a muscle relaxant is deemed necessary, a nondepolarizing drug not known to interact with lithium (gallamine or d-tubocurarine) would be the best choice. Gallamine is preferable if used with halothane because of its vagolytic effect, unless one seeks to obtain some degree of hypotension. The effect of barbiturates in man with nontoxic serum lithium levels is not known. However, in view of the animal data, low doses of barbiturate in the presence of "therapeutic" serum lithium levels are probably safe. Thus either an inhalation technique or a balanced anesthetic technique can be used in this patient, depending on the circumstances.

In conclusion, it is clear that psychotropic drugs frequently interact with drugs used in anesthesia. Psychotropic medications are widely used in the practice both of psychiatry and of general medicine. Thus it is important for an anesthesiologist to elicit a complete preoperative drug history for all patients. A close working relationship between the psychiatrist and the anesthesiologist is important for the anesthetic management of the patient who is treated with psychotropic medications.

REFERENCES

1. Snyder, S.H.: The dopamine hypothesis of schizophrenia. Am. J. Psychiatry, 133:197, 1976.
2. Gilman, A.G., Goodman, L.S., and Gilman, A. (Eds.): The Pharmacological Basis of Therapeutics. 6th Ed. New York, Macmillan, 1980.
3. Laborit, H., Huguenard, P., and Allaume, R.: Un nouveau stabilisateur végétatif (le 4460 RP). Presse Méd., 60:206, 1952.
4. Inglis, J.M., and Barrow, M.E.H.: Premedication—a reassessment. Proc. R. Soc. Med., 58:29, 1965.
5. Holderness, M.C., Chase, P.E., and Dripps, R.D.: A narcotic analgesic and a butyrophenone with nitrous oxide for general anesthesia. Anesthesiology, 24:336, 1963.
6. Kreuscher, H.: Modifications of the classic neu-

roleptoanalgesic technique. Int. Anesthesiol. Clin., 11:71, 1973.
7. Corssen, G.: Neuroleptanalgesia and anesthesia in obstetrics. Clin. Obstet. Gynecol., 17:241, 1974.
8. Sadove, M.S., et al.: Clinical study of droperidol in the prevention of the side effects of ketamine anesthesia. Anesth. Analg., (Cleve.), 50:526, 1971.
9. Foldes, F.F.: The prevention of psychotomimetic side effects of ketamine. Proceedings of the second ketamine symposium, Mainze, 1972. In Ketamine: New Information in Research and Clinical Practice. Edited by N. Gemperle, H. Kreuscherz and D. Langrehr. Anesthesiology and Resuscitation Series, Vol. 69. Berlin and Heidelberg, and New York, Springer-Verlag, 1973.
10. Keats, A.S., Telford, J., and Kurosu, Y.: "Potentiation" of meperidine by promethazine. Anesthesiology, 22:34, 1961.
11. Jackson, C.L., and Smith, D.: Analgesic properties of mixtures of chlorpromazine with morphine and meperidine. Ann. Intern. Med., 45:640, 1956.
12. Lambertsen, C.J., Wendel, H., and Longenhagen, J.B.: The separate and combined respiratory effects of chlorpromazine and meperidine in normal men controlled at 46 mm Hg alveolar P_{CO_2}. J. Pharmacol. Exp. Ther., 131:381, 1961.
13. Dundee, J.W., Nicholl, R.M., and Moore, J.: Clinical studies of induction agents. X: The effect of phenothiazine premedication on thiopentone anaesthesia. Br. J. Anaesth., 36:106, 1964.
13a. Petts, H.V., and Pleuvry, B.J.: Interactions of morphine and methotrimeprazine in mouse and man with respect to analgesia, respiration and sedation. Br. J. Anaesth., 55:437, 1983.
14. Prasad, C.R., and Kar, K.: Effect of atropine alone and in combination with tranquilizers on morphine-induced analgesia. Curr. Sci., 35:308, 1966.
15. Morris, R.W.: Effects of phenothiazines on pentobarbital-induced sleep in mice. Arch. Int. Pharmacodyn Ther., 161:380, 1966.
16. Kissil, D., and Yelnosky, J.: A comparison of the effects of chlorpromazine and droperidol on the respiratory response to CO_2. Arch. Int. Pharmacodyn. Ther., 172:73, 1968.
17. Brodie, B.B.: Potentiating action of chlorpromazine and reserpine. Nature, 175:1133, 1955.
18. Dobkin, A.B.: Potentiation of thiopental anaesthesia by derivatives and analogues of phenothiazine. Anesthesiology, 21:292, 1960.
19. Dobkin, A.B.: Potentiation of thiopental anaesthesia with Tigan, Panectyl, Benadryl, Gravol, Marzine, Histadyl, Librium and Haloperidol. Can. Anaesth. Soc. J., 8:265, 1961.
20. Dripps, R.D., et al.: The use of chlorpromazine in anesthesia and surgery. Ann. Surg., 142:775, 1955.
21. Wallis, R.: Potentiation of hypnotics and analgesics: clinical experience with chlorpromazine. N.Y. State J. Med., 55:243, 1955.
22. Eggers, G.N., Corssen, G., and Allen, C.: Comparison of vasopressor responses in the presence of phenothiazine derivatives. Anesthesiology, 20:261, 1959.
23. Campbell, J.B.: Long-term treatment of Parkinson's disease with levodopa. Neurology, 20:18, 1970.
24. Warnes, H., Lehman, H.E., and Ban, T.A.: Adynamic ileus during psychoactive medication: a report of three fatal and five severe cases. Can. Med. Assoc. J., 96:1112, 1967.
25. El-Yousef, M.K., et al.: Reversal of antiparkinsonian drug toxicity by physostigmine: a controlled study. Am. J. Psychiatry, 130:141, 1973.
26. Grant, W.M.: Ocular complications of drugs. Glaucoma. J.A.M.A., 207:2089, 1969.
27. Janowsky, D.S., and Janowsky, E.C.: Methscopolamine as a preanesthetic medication (Letter to the Editor). Can. Anaesth. Soc. J., 23:334, 1976.
28. Gold, M.I.: Tranquilizers in the surgical patient. Surgery, 56:1027, 1964.
29. Gold, M.I.: Profound hypotension associated with preoperative use of phenothiazines. Anesth. Analg. (Cleve.), 53:844, 1974.
30. Hatch, R.C.: Ketamine catalepsy and anesthesia in dogs pretreated with antiserotonergic or antidopaminergic neuroleptics or with anticholinergic agents. Pharmacol. Res. Commun., 6:289, 1974.
30a. Peterson, C.D.: Seizures induced by acute loxapine overdose. Am. J. Psychiatry, 138:1089, 1981.
30b. Brock-Utne, J.G., Rabin, J., Welman, S., et al.: The action of commonly used antiemetics on the lower oesophageal sphincter. Br. J. Anaesth., 50:295, 1978.
31. Moore, D.C., and Bridenbaugh, L.D.: Chlorpromazine: a report of one death and eight near fatalities following its use in conjunction with spinal, epidural and celiac plexus block. Surgery, 40:543, 1956.
32. Swidler, G.: Handbook of Drug Interactions. New York, Wiley-Interscience, 1971.
33. Regan, A.G., and Aldrete, J.A.: Prolonged apnea after administration of promazine hydrochloride following succinylcholine infusion. Anesth. Analg. (Cleve.), 46:315, 1967.
34. Alexander, C.S., and Nino, A.: Cardiovascular complications in young patients taking psychotropic drugs. Am. Heart J., 78:757, 1969.
35. Fletcher, G.F., Kazamias, T.M., and Wenger, N.K.: Cardiotoxic effects of Mellaril: conduction disturbances and supraventricular arrhythmias. Am. Heart J., 78:135, 1969.
36. Editorial: Cardiovascular complications from psychotropic drugs. Br. Med. J., 1:3, 1971.
37. Matsuki, A., et al.: Excessive mortality in schizophrenic patients on chronic phenothiazine treatment. Agressologie, 13:407, 1972.
38. Alper, M.H., Flacke, W., and Krager, O.: Pharmacology of reserpine and its implications for anesthesia. Anesthesiology, 24:524, 1963.
39. Fann, W.E., Davis, J.M., and Janowsky, D.S.: The prevalence of tardive dyskinesias in mental hospital patients. Dis. Nerv. Sys., 33:182, 1972.
40. Foster, M.W., Jr., and Gayle, R.F., Jr.: Dangers

in combining reserpine with electroconvulsive therapy. J.A.M.A., 154:1520, 1955.
41. Bracha, S., and Hes, J.P.: Death occurring during combined reserpine-electroshock therapy. Am. J. Psychiatry, 133:257, 1956.
42. Coakley, C.S., Alpert, S., and Boling, J.S.: Circulatory responses during anesthesia of patients on rauwolfia therapy. J.A.M.A., 161:1143, 1956.
43. Ziegler, C.H., and Lovette, J.B.: Operative complications after therapy with reserpine and reserpine compounds. J.A.M.A., 176:916, 1961.
44. Smessaert, A.A., and Hicks, R.G.: Problems caused by rauwolfia drugs during anesthesia and surgery. New York State J. Med., 61:2399, 1961.
45. Munson, W.M., and Jenicek, J.A.: Effect of anesthetic agents on patients receiving reserpine therapy. Anesthesiology, 23:741, 1962.
46. Katz, R.L., Weintraub, H.D., and Papper, E.M.: Anesthesia, surgery and rauwolfia. Anesthesiology, 25:142, 1964.
47. Miller, R.D., Way, W.L., and Eger, E.T.: The effects of *alpha*-methyldopa, reserpine, guanethidine, and iproniazid on minimum alveolar anesthetic requirement (MAC). Anesthesiology, 29:1153, 1968.
48. Child, K.J., Sutherland, P., and Tomich, E.G.: Some effects of reserpine on barbitone anesthesia in mice. Biochem. Pharmacol., 6:252, 1961.
49. Lessin, A.W., and Parkes, M.W.: The relationship between sedation and body temperature in the mouse. Br. J. Pharmacol., 12:245, 1957.
50. Ominsky, A.J., and Wollman, H.: Hazards of general anesthesia in the reserpinized patient. Anesthesiology, 30:443, 1969.
51. Tammisto, T., et al.: The effect of reserpine, chlordiazepoxide and imipramine treatment on the potency of thiopental in man. Ann. Chir. Gynaecol., 356:323, 1967.
52. Gray, W.D., and Rauh, C.E.: The anticonvulsant action of inhibitors of carbonic anhydrase: relation to endogenous amines in the brain. J. Pharmacol. Exp. Ther., 115:127, 1967.
53. Gelder, M.G., and Vane, J.R.: Interaction of the effects of tyramine, amphetamine, and reserpine in man. Psychopharmacologia, 3:231, 1962.
54. Matilla, M.J., and Saarnivaara, L.: Potentiation with indomethacin of the morphine analgesia in mice and rabbits. Ann. Med. Exp. Biol. Fenn., 45:360, 1967.
55. Ross, J.W., and Ashford, A.: The effect of reserpine and *alpha* methyldopa on the analgesic action of morphine in the mouse. J. Pharm. Pharmacol., 19:709, 1967.
56. Tabojnikova, M., and Kovalcik, V.: On the mechanism of the inhibiting effect of reserpine on morphine. Act. Nerv. Super., 9:317, 1967.
57. Carrier, G.O., Pegram, B.L., and Carrier, O.: Antagonistic effects of reserpine on d-tubocurarine action on motor function of rabbits. Eur. J. Pharmacol., 6:125, 1969.
58. Janowsky, D.S., Pechnick, R., and Janowsky, E.C.: Lethal effects of reserpine plus physostigmine and neostigmine in mice. Clin. Exp. Pharmacol. Physiol., 3:483, 1976.
59. Therapeutic Drug Interactions. Edited by M.S. Cohen. Madison, Wisconsin, Drug Information Center, University of Wisconsin Medical Center, 1970.
60. Meyler, L., and Herxheimer, A. (Eds.): Side Effects of Drugs. Baltimore, Williams & Wilkins, 1968, Vol. VI.
61. Hartshorn, E.A.: Handbook of Drug Interactions. 3rd Ed. Hamilton, Illinois, Drug Intelligence Publications, 1976.
62. Vapaatalo, H.I., and Torofi, P.: Effect of some antidepressive drugs on the blood pressure responses to the sympathomimetic amines. Ann. Med. Exp. Biol. Fenn., 45:399, 1967.
62a. Edwards, R.P., et al.: Cardiac responses to imipramine and pancuronium during anesthesia with halothane or enflurane. Anesthesiology, 50:421, 1979.
63. Svedmyr, N.: The influence of a tricyclic antidepressive agent (protriptyline) on some of the circulatory effects of noradrenaline and adrenaline in man. Life Sci., 7:77, 1968.
64. Boakes, A.J., et al.: Interactions between sympathomimetic amines and antidepressant agents in man. Br. Med. J., 1:311, 1973.
65. Boakes, A.J.: Vasoconstrictors in Local Anaesthetics and Tricyclic Antidepressants. In Drug Interactions. Edited by D.G. Grahame-Smith. Baltimore, University Park Press, 1977.
66. Verrill, P.J.: Adverse reactions to local anaesthetics and vasoconstrictor drugs. Practitioner, 218:380, 1975.
67. Goldman, V.: Local anaesthetics containing vasoconstrictors. Br. Med. J., 1:175, 1971.
68. Jori, A.: Potentiation of noradrenaline toxicity by drug antihistaminic activity. J. Pharm. Pharmacol., 18:824, 1966.
68a. Bruce, D.L., and Capan, L.: Antidepressants do not increase the lethality of ketamine in mice. Br. J. Anaesth., 55:457, 1983.
68b. Stiff, J.L., and Harris, D.B.: Clonidine withdrawal complicated by amitriptyline therapy. Anesthesiology, 59:73, 1983.
69. Milner, G., and Hills, N.: Adynamic ileus and nortriptyline. Br. Med. J., 1:841, 1966.
70. Griffin, J.P., and D'Arcy, P.F.: A Manual of Adverse Drug Interactions. 2nd ed. Bristol, John Wright and Sons, 1979.
70a. Sprague, D.H., and Wolf, S.: Enflurane seizures in patients taking amitriptyline. Anesth. Analg., 61:67, 1982.
71. Lechat, P., Fontagne, J., and Giroud, J.P.: Influence of previously given tricyclic antidepressants on the activity of local anesthetics. Therapie, 24:393, 1969.
71a. Glisson, S.N., Fajardo, L., and El-Etr, A.A.: Amitriptyline therapy increases electrocardiographic changes during reversal of neuromuscular blockade. Anesth. Analg., 57:77, 1978.
71b. Ban, T.A., Wilson, W.H., and McEvoy, J.P.: Amoxapine: a review of literature. Int. Pharmacopsychiat., 15:166, 1980.
71c. Kulig, K., Rumack, B.H., Sullivan, J.B., et al.:

Amoxapine overdose, coma and seizures without cardiotoxic effects. J.A.M.A., *248*:1092, 1982.
71d. Steele, T.E.: Adverse reactions suggesting amoxapine-induced dopamine blockade. Am. J. Psychiatry, *139*:1500, 1982.
71e. Hoffman, B.F., and Wachsmith, R.: Maprotiline and seizures. J. Clin. Psychiatry, *43*:117, 1982.
71f. Edwards, J.G., and Goldie, A.: Mianserin, maprotiline and intracardiac conduction. Br. J. Clin. Pharmac., *15*:249S, 1983.
71g. Herrmann, H.C., Kaplan, L.M., and Bierer, B.E.: QT prolongation and Torsades de Pointes ventricular tachycardia produced by the tetracyclic antidepressant agent maprotiline. Am. J. Cardiology, *51*:904, 1983.
71h. Janowsky, D.S., Curtis, G., Zisook, S., et al.: Ventricular arrhythmias possibly aggravated by trazodone. Am. J. Psychiatry, *140*:796, 1983.
71i. Irwin, M., and Spar, J.E.: Reversible cardiac conduction abnormality associated with trazodone administration. Am. J. Psychiatry, *140*:945, 1983.
71j. Chu, A.G., Gunsolly, B.L., Summers, R.W., et al.: Trazodone and liver toxicity. Ann. Intern. Med., *99*:128, 1983.
71k. Abramowicz, M. (Ed.): The Medical Letter, *26*(658):35, March 30, 1984.
72. Marshall, L.J., and Green, V.A.: Propranolol and diazepam for imipramine poisoning. Lancet, *2*:1249, 1968.
73. Vohra, J.: Cardiovascular abnormalities following tricyclic antidepressant drug overdosage. Drugs, *7*:323, 1974.
74. Goldberg, L.I.: Monoamine oxidase inhibitors, adverse reactions and possible mechanisms. J.A.M.A., *190*:456, 1964.
75. Jenkins, L.C., and Graves, H.B.: Potential hazards of psychoactive drugs in association with anesthesia. Can. Anaesth. Soc. J., *23*:334, 1976.
76. Hunter, K.R., et al.: Monoamine oxidase inhibitors and L-dopa. Br. Med. J., *3*:388, 1970.
77. Lewis, E.: Hyperpyrexia with antidepressant drugs. Br. Med. J., *2*:1671, 1965.
78. Krisko, I., Lewis, E., and Johnson, J.: Severe hyperpyrexia due to tranylcypromine-amphetamine toxicity. Ann. Intern. Med., *70*:559, 1969.
79. Hirsh, M.S., Walter, R.M., and Hasterlik, R.J.: Subarachnoid hemorrhage following ephedrine and MAO inhibitor. J.A.M.A., *194*:1259, 1965.
80. Blackwell, B., et al.: Hypertensive interactions between monoamine oxidase inhibitors and foodstuffs. Br. J. Psychiatry, *113*:349, 1967.
81. Sjoquist, F.: Psychotropic drugs. (2) Interaction between monoamine oxidase (MAOI) inhibitors and other substances. Proc. R. Soc. Med., *58*:967, 1965.
82. Elis, J., et al.: Modification by monoamine oxidase inhibitors of the effect of some sympathomimetics on blood pressure. Br. Med. J., *2*:75, 1967.
83. Raskin, A.: Adverse reactions to phenelzine, results of a nine hospital depression study. J. Clin. Pharmacol., *12*:22, 1972.
84. Editorial: Analgesics and monoamine-oxidase inhibitor. Br. Med. J., *4*:284, 1967.
85. Horler, A.R., and Wynne, N.A.: Hypertensive crisis due to pargyline and metaraminol. Br. Med. J., *2*:460, 1965.
86. Mason, A.: Fatal reaction associated with tranylcypromine and methylamphetamine. Lancet, *1*:173, 1962.
87. Davies, T.S.: Monoamine oxidase inhibitors and rauwolfia compounds. Br. Med. J., *2*:739, 1960.
88. Hunter, K.R., Stern, G.M., and Laurence, D.R.: Use of levodopa with other drugs. Lancet, *2*:1283, 1970.
89. Teychenne, P.F., et al.: Interactions of levodopa with inhibitors of monoamine oxidase and L-aromatic amino acid decarboxylase. Clin. Pharmacol. Ther., *18*:273, 1975.
90. Horwitz, D., Goldberg, L.I., and Sjoerdsma, A.: Increased blood pressure responses to dopamine and norepinephrine produced by monoamine oxidase inhibitors in man. J. Lab. Clin. Med., *56*:747, 1960.
91. Shepherd, M.: Psychotropic drugs. (1) Interaction between centrally acting drugs in man. Proc. R. Soc. Med., *58*:964, 1965.
92. Palmer, H.: Potentiation of pethidine. Br. Med. J., *2*:944, 1960.
93. Shee, J.C.: Dangerous potentiation of pethidine by iproniazid and its treatment. Br. Med. J., *2*:507, 1960.
94. Rogers, K.J.: Role of brain monoamines in the interaction between pethidine and tranylcypromine. Eur. J. Pharmacol., *14*:86, 1971.
95. Brownlee, G., and Williams, G.W.: Potentiation of amphetamine and pethidine by monoamine oxidase inhibitors. Lancet, *1*:699, 1963.
96. Eade, N.R., and Renton, K.W.: Effect of monoamine oxidase inhibitors on the n-demethylation and hydrolysis of meperidine. Biochem. Pharmacol., *19*:2243, 1970.
97. Eade, N.R., and Renton, K.W.: The effect of phenelzine and tranylcypromine on the degradation of meperidine. J. Pharmacol. Exp. Ther., *173*:31, 1970.
98. Rivers, N., and Horner, B.: Possible lethal reaction between Nardil and dextromethorphan. Can. Med. Assoc. J., *103*:85, 1970.
99. Jounela, A.J., and Mattila, M.J.: Modification by phenelzine of morphine and pethidine analgesia in mice. Ann. Med. Exp. Biol. Fenn., *46*:66, 1968.
100. Rogers, K.J., and Thornton, J.A.: The interaction between monoamine oxidase inhibitors and narcotic analgesics in mice. Br. J. Pharmacol., *36*:470, 1969.
101. Jounela, A.J.: Effect of phenelzine on the rate of metabolism of pethidine. Ann. Med. Exp. Biol. Fenn., *46*:531, 1968.
102. Vigran, I.M.: Dangerous potentiation of meperidine hydrochloride by pargyline hydrochloride. J.A.M.A., *187*:954, 1964.
103. Cocks, D.P., and Passmore-Rowe, A.: Dangers of monoamine oxidase inhibitors. Br. Med. J., *2*:1545, 1962.
104. Churchill-Davidson, H.C.: Anaesthesia and monoamine-oxidase inhibitors. Br. Med. J., *1*:520, 1965.
105. Domino, E., Sullivan, T.S., and Luby, E.D.: Bar-

biturate intoxication in a patient treated with a MAO inhibitor. Am. J. Psychiatry, 118:941, 1962.
106. Bodley, P.O., Halwax, K., and Potts, L.: Low pseudocholinesterase levels complicating treatment with phenelzine. Br. Med. J., 3:510, 1969.
107. Cheymol, J., et al.: Influence of chronic MAOI inhibitor administration on curarization. Therapie, 21:355, 1966.
108. Summers, R.J.: Effects of monoamine oxidase inhibitors on the hypothermia produced in cats by halothane. Br. J. Pharmacol., 37:400, 1969.
109. Frieden, J.: Propranolol as an anti-arrhythmic agent. Am. Heart J., 75:283, 1967.
110. Moser, M.: Experience with isocarboxazid. J.A.M.A., 176:276, 1961.
111. Penlington, G.N.: Droperidol and monoamine oxidase inhibitors. Br. Med. J., 1:483, 1966.
112. Byck, R.: Drugs and the treatment of psychiatric disorders. In The Pharmacological Basis of Therapeutics. Edited by L.S. Goodman and A. Gilman, New York, Macmillan, 1975.
113. Davis, J.M., Janowsky, D.S., and El-Yousef, M.K.: The use of lithium in clinical psychiatry. Psychiatric Annals, 3:78, 1973.
114. Greist, J.H., et al.: The lithium librarian. Arch. Gen. Psychiatry, 34:456, 1977.
115. Peach, M.J.: Cations: calcium, magnesium, barium, lithium, and ammonium. In The Pharmacological Basis of Therapeutics. Edited by L.S. Goodman and A. Gilman. New York, Macmillan, 1975.
116. Borden, H., Clarke, M., and Katz, H.: The use of pancuronium bromide in patients receiving lithium carbonate. Can. Anaesth. Soc. J., 21:79, 1974.
117. Jephcott, G., and Kerry, R.J.: Lithium: an anesthetic risk. Br. J. Anaesth., 46:389, 1974.
118. Hill, G.E., Wong, K.C., and Hodges, M.R.: Potentiation of succinylcholine neuromuscular blockade by lithium carbonate. Anesthesiology, 44:439, 1976.
119. Hill, G.E., Wong, K.C., and Hodges, M.R.: Lithium carbonate and neuromuscular blocking agents. Anesthesiology, 46:122, 1977.
119a. Waud, B.E., Farrell, L., and Waud, D.R.: Lithium and neuromuscular transmission. Anesth. Analg., 61:399, 1982.
119b. Martin, B.A., and Kramer, P.M.: Clinical significance of the interaction between lithium and a neuromuscular blocker. Am. J. Psychiatry, 139:1326, 1982.
120. Vizi, E., et al.: The effect of lithium on acetylcholine release and synthesis. Neuropharmacology, 11:521, 1972.
121. Mannisto, P.T., and Saarnivaara, L.: Effect of lithium and rubidium on the sleeping time caused by various intravenous anaesthetics in the mouse. Br. J. Anaesth., 48:185, 1976.
122. Solomon, R., and Vickers, R.: Dysarthria resulting from lithium carbonate, a case report. J.A.M.A., 231:280, 1975.
123. Wharton, R.: Geriatric Doses (Letter to the Editor). J.A.M.A., 233:22, 1975.
124. Mackay, A.V.P., Loose, R., and Glen, A.I.M.: Labour on lithium. Br. Med. J., 1:878, 1976.
125. Wilbanks, G.D., et al.: Toxic effects of lithium carbonate in a mother and newborn infant. J.A.M.A., 213:865, 1970.
126. Macfie, A.C.: Lithium poisoning precipitated by diuretics. Br. Med. J., 1:516, 1975.
127. Ascione, F.J.: Lithium with Diuretics. Drug Ther. (Hosp.), 7:125, 1977.

20

SEDATIVES AND HYPNOTICS

N. TY SMITH

The designation "sedative-hypnotic" is probably one of the least appropriate of modern therapeutics. It does not denote a specific drug action, but rather implies a spectrum of activity from sedative through hypnotic to general anesthesia and finally to coma.[1] We shall include under this heading a large group of chemically unrelated drugs that are, after aspirin, among the most used, as well as abused. The habitual intake of these drugs to relieve insomnia or to achieve tranquility is a common preanesthetic finding. Thus the anesthesiologist should specifically inquire about the use of these agents, and should be aware of other drugs that might interact with them.

Although these agents are administered by several routes for several purposes, we shall consider mainly their long-term oral use and their short-term use as preanesthetic medication.

CASE REPORT

A 58-year-old man was admitted to the hospital for an acute myocardial infarction. In the hospital, he received digoxin, lidocaine, phenobarbital, and dicumarol. The latter agent was titrated according to the patient's prothrombin time, which, at the end of the stabilization period, was 18.4 sec, with a control of 12.1 sec. After 2 weeks, his barbiturate therapy was discontinued, but his anticoagulant therapy was maintained, without a readjustment in dosage. One week later the patient was brought to the operating room with gastric bleeding. The anesthesiologist requested a prothrombin time before he would proceed with the anesthetic. The prothrombin time was 34 seconds, with a control of 11.8 seconds. Vitamin K was administered to the patient, with a subsequent lowering of prothrombin times to the therapeutic range of dicumarol—and with the cessation of the gastric bleeding.

This case occurred long before the barbiturate/dicumarol interaction was suspected. The mechanism for the interaction responsible for this patient's problems is covered in detail in this chapter. The case report brings up several important points. It demonstrates that one drug can alter the rate of metabolism, and hence the action, of another drug. It emphasizes a less well-appreciated fact: that discontinuing an interacting drug, in this case phenobarbital, can also have an impact. Finally, it points out that the anesthesiologist should be alert for *every* drug interaction, whether or not it may directly affect the course of the anesthetic management.

In the following paragraphs I describe the basic mechanisms of the sedative-hypnotics, some of the more common agents, their mechanisms of action and uses, the more common drug interactions in which these agents participate and a commentary on the clinical importance of these interactions. The drugs include the barbiturates, ethanol, the benzodiazepines, chloral hydrate, paraldehyde, the antihistaminics, meprobamate, ethchlorvynol, glutethimide, and marijuana.

PHARMACOLOGIC MECHANISMS

The purpose of sedative therapy is to reduce anxiety or tension without interfering with the normal activities of the patient. The sedation produced can alleviate anxiety associated either with neurosis or with somatic disease. Sedatives are generally more useful in emotionally upset or neurotic persons than in psychotic patients. Drugs intended for the latter group of patients are discussed extensively in Chapter 19.

Although the sedative-hypnotic agents act at all levels in the central nervous system (CNS), the reticular-activating system is especially sensitive to their depressant effects. This action appears to be responsible for the sleep-inducing properties of these drugs.[2] The clinical effects of sedative-hypnotics are typified by the barbiturates, which are rapidly absorbed after oral administration and distributed throughout the body. Normal hypnotic doses can impair motor performance, judgment, and the performance of simple intellectual tasks.[3-6] It is unclear whether their action is at the cellular or synaptic level, and many theories have been advanced to explain their effects.[2] The barbiturates have an anticonvulsant activity, a property that may be shared by other sedative-hypnotic drugs. The sedative and anticonvulsant activities of barbiturates have been recognized as being separate, however.[7]

The CNS depression that the sedative and hypnotic agents produce accounts for a substantial number of potentially serious interactions with other CNS-depressant drugs. Alcohol is a primary culprit in this regard. Although the legendary potency of the classic "Micky Finn," a mixture of chloral hydrate and ethanol, has not been documented, the interaction of ethanol with CNS-depressant drugs can be serious.

Probably most of the interactions of sedative-hypnotics as preanesthetic medication have to do with additive central nervous system effects. Certainly most of us intuitively decrease the dosage of one preanesthetic medication when we add another. For example, we do not give as much pentobarbital in the presence of hydroxyzine as we would by itself. However, these interactions have not been well documented.

Even less clear is the effect of preanesthetic medication on anesthetic agents themselves. Preanesthetic agents certainly seem to alter anesthetic management. They facilitate the approach to the patient, and they may make the induction of anesthesia smoother. Whether these effects can be called true drug interactions is questionable. Similarly, a poorly timed or excessive dose of preanesthetic medication can prolong a patient's recovery time. How much of this phenomenon is due to interactions among the central nervous system effects of the agents and how much is due simply to the much longer action of the premedicant has not been determined.

Little information is available on the ability of the sedative-hypnotics to alter anesthetic depth when given as preanesthetic medication. A major problem is that the standard measurement of anesthetic depth (MAC) is related to pain, and most sedative-hypnotics have no analgesic action. To my knowledge, other, more appropriate types of MAC, such as MAC awake, have not been used to study the effects of the sedative-hypnotics on anesthetic depth or duration. Another type of indicator of anesthetic depth has been used to assess the impact of preanesthetic medication on the induction dose of thiopental in children. Children receiving a combination of trimeprazine, droperidol, and physeptone with atropine required only 4.2 mg/kg of thiopental to abolish the lid reflex in 90% of patients, vs. 5.2 mg/kg with trimeprazine and atropine, 5.0 mg/kg for papaveretum and hyoscine, and 10.5 mg/kg for placebo.[7a]

When given in ordinary doses as preanesthetic medication, individual sedative-hypnotics may have little impact on the potency of inhalation anesthetics. Even morphine, with its known analgesic properties, changes the MAC of halothane by only 0.05 vol %.[8] On the other hand, if 0.2 mg/kg of diazepam are given intravenously 30 minutes before a surgical incision, halothane MAC is decreased from 0.73 to 0.48, a decrease of 34%.[9] One can assume that if given in smaller doses, intramuscularly or by mouth, 2 to 3 hours before an incision, the impact of diazepam would be considerably less. That hypothesis, however, has not been examined. Perhaps many of the negative results arise from the difficulty in performing suitable human studies. In mice, small nonsedating doses of methotrimeprazine potentiate the analgesic effect of morphine, although the same investigators could not demonstrate this effect in man.[9a] This disagreement may relate to the differences in the methods used to measure pain, the lack of sensitivity of the method used in humans, the problems of achieving equipotent doses between species—only compounded in drug interaction studies—or simple species differences.

Many hypnotic drugs stimulate hepatic microsomal enzyme production, which is the basis of another common set of drug interactions of this class of agents. Microsomal enzyme induction appears between two and seven days after administration of such a drug.[10–13] After the discontinuance of the drug, enzyme induction may persist for up to one month.[14] Phenobarbital, the best known of the enzyme-inducing drugs, increases the rate of synthesis and decreases the breakdown of mouse microsomal protein and rat microsomal phospholipid.[15,16] Thus phenobarbital increases liver microsomal protein by 20 to 40%.[17–19] The physiologic significance of enhanced liver growth and the function produced by microsomal enzyme-inducing drugs is not known.[10] However, many drug interactions occur because of the unsuspected and rapid metabolism of drugs given concurrently with microsomal enzyme-inducing agents. The case report is but one example of such an interaction.

SPECIFIC AGENTS

Barbiturates

The barbiturates are often implicated in drug interactions. They are used by all segments of the population for many indications, legal and illegal. Overdosage and physical and psychologic dependence are common medical and social problems.

Absorption of barbiturates is generally good. They are effective orally, parenterally, and rectally. All of these routes of administration are used clinically.

The duration of activity of a barbiturate is related to redistribution from the brain and plasma to other body tissues, to metabolic degradation in the liver, and to renal excretion of unchanged drug.[2] Biotransformation by the liver is apparently clinically less important in determining the duration of the drug's effect. Although it has been recommended that barbiturates be given cautiously to patients with liver disease, hepatic dysfunction must be severe to decrease appreciably the rate of barbiturate metabolism to a clinically significant degree.[2,20,21]

The distribution of a barbiturate is determined by its lipid solubility, protein binding, and degree of ionization.[2] The more lipid-soluble barbiturates act rapidly and for a short time. Albumin and other plasma proteins reversibly bind a portion of the barbiturate. The type and degree of binding vary greatly with the physicochemical characteristics of the barbiturate.[2] Barbiturates bound by proteins are unavailable for drug action. Thus anything that decreases protein binding by competing for binding sites (for example, aspirin and sulfonamides) increases the pharmacologic effects of the barbiturates, and vice versa. The degree of ionization affects the distribution across membranes such as the "blood-brain barrier" and, therefore, the intracerebral concentration of barbiturates. Lower plasma pH increases brain tissue concentrations. The opposite is also true. Metabolic rather than respiratory acid-base alterations have a greater effect on barbiturate distribution and thus on central nervous system depression.[2]

Barbiturates alter the biotransformation and hence the action of a number of other drugs. The interaction is usually a biphasic enhancement followed by a reduction. If a barbiturate and another drug similarly metabolized are given for the first time together, the enzyme system is saturated and the effects of both drugs are enhanced.[20,22] The initially augmented effect takes place because barbiturates such as phenobarbital, by combining with cytochrome P-450, competitively inhibit the biotransformation of a number of drugs.

Probably the best-documented anesthetically related example of this acute inhibition phenomenon is the interaction between sedative premedications and ketamine in patients.[23] Secobarbital, diazepam, and hydroxyzine all prolong ketamine-induced sleep time in patients. These agents seem to work by inhibiting the metabolism of ketamine, as shown by an increase in the plasma half-life of the agent.

After prolonged use of a barbiturate, however, the subsequent administration of a drug similarly metabolized reduces the latter's effect because of the increase in the enzymes involved in its biotransformation.[24] (See Chap. 6 for further discussion.) The tolerance seen with the long-term use of barbiturates is due at least in part to this increased activity in the hepatic microsomal enzyme system.[24,25] One would expect an increased tolerance to most preanesthetic medications in patients taking long-term barbiturate therapy, but this has not been documented.

Central nervous system (CNS) depression by the barbiturates is well documented. A real danger of their abuse is seen with the additive effects of other CNS depressants (for example, ethanol, opiates).[26] Barbiturates, together with CNS stimulants such as amphetamines, can, conversely, result in agitation, although the clinical significance of this interaction is in doubt.[27]

INTERACTIONS WITH OTHER DRUGS

Beta-Adrenergic Blockers. If a *beta*-adrenergic blocker (e.g., propranolol or metoprolol) has flow-dependent hepatic elimination, the amount of orally administered agent that reaches the general circulation unchanged is markedly reduced by pretreatment with barbiturates.[27a-e] Although *beta*-blockers do not have a clear plasma concentration-effect relationship, there may be some reduction in *beta*-blockade due to this interaction. A 20% reduction in inhibition of exercise tachycardia has been reported under these circumstances, however.[27c] The kinetics of timolol, a *beta*-blocker with flow independent elimination, are not altered by phenobarbital.[27f]

Corticosteroids. The pharmacologic effects of corticosteroids may be decreased by barbiturates, with possible exacerbation of the disease being treated.[27g-m] In addition, enhanced steroid metabolic clearance and reduced renal allograft survival occur in patients receiving anticonvulsants, including phenobarbital.[27i]

Anticoagulants. The case report illustrates possibly the most common and certainly the best documented drug interaction. (Enzyme induction from barbiturates has also been incriminated in oral contraceptive failure.[28] Increasing the metabolism of some estrogen-like drugs renders these agents ineffective. This interaction does not directly affect the anesthesiologist—until the patient appears in the labor/delivery suite.) Enzyme induction secondary to the long-term use of barbiturates increases the metabolism of anticoagulants of the coumarin type.[28a-i] The result is a decreased coumarin effect, and the concomitant use of a barbiturate may create difficulties in the control of the coumarin dose and of the prothrombin time. Perhaps even more hazardous is the decrease in coagulability that follows cessation of the barbiturate if the rently. Kissin[31f] found that the tricyclic antidepressants were either synergistic or antagonistic to ethanol according to their ratio of sedative/stimulant activity. There is considerable risk of hypotension and interference with motor skills such as driving when these drugs are taken with ethanol. Tricyclic antidepressants also increase the susceptibility to convulsions and should be given cautiously during ethanol withdrawal.

Another disturbing interaction with ethanol involves its ability to trigger the release of biogenic amine neurotransmitters and cause a reaction similar to that seen between MAO inhibitors and tyramine—a hypertensive crisis with an occasionally lethal outcome.[31e]

Anticoagulants. The occasional use of small to moderate amounts of ethanol by patients who take oral anticoagulants can be risky. The blood levels reached after giving a standard dose of anticoagulants, such as warfarin, are higher if ethanol is simultaneously taken.[31f] The combination significantly increases the risks of hemorrhage. If ethanol intake is prolonged and heavy enough to produce liver dysfunction, anticoagulant therapy may also be affected.[32] In these patients, frequent determinations of prothrombin time are necessary, and the anesthetist should inquire about any sudden changes in ethanol consumption to determine if the anticoagulant status has been altered.

Barbiturates. The combined actions of barbiturates and ethanol have been described as antagonistic,[33] additive,[34] potentiating,[35] and synergistic.[36] The studies are difficult to compare, since they use different species, dose levels, and experimental designs.

Although the mechanism of the intensification of effect at the CNS level is not well understood, several theories have been proposed. One theory concerns the hepatic microsomal enzyme system, which not only is involved in metabolic transformations of numerous drugs, but also acts as an ethanol-oxidizing system and is responsible for adaptive increases in the rate of ethanol metabolism in alcoholics.[37] When the enzyme system is induced by phenobarbital, ethanol metabolism accelerates, and a greater tolerance to ethanol develops. When it is induced by long-term consumption of ethanol, phenobarbital is metabolized more quickly, and the patient becomes more tolerant to barbiturates. Thus phenobarbital appears to enhance the disappearance of ethanol from the blood, resulting in somewhat decreased blood ethanol concentrations.[38,39] The complete mechanism for this effect is not known, however. It may involve additional factors to a direct increase in hepatic metabolism of ethanol. When barbiturates and ethanol are ingested concurrently, competition for the enzyme system leads to the inhibition of oxidation and to the enhancement of CNS depressant effects.[40,41] However, this theory has been disputed[42,43] because the physiologic significance of the microsomal ethanol-oxidizing system itself has been questioned.

It is clear from the mechanisms just described (and probably from others as yet undiscovered) that the interrelationships between ethanol and the barbiturates are quite complex. Clinically the most important considerations are that they are both central nervous system depressants and that acute ethanol intoxication may impair barbiturate metabolism. Also, the enhanced drug metabolism with long-term ethanol intake may partially explain the tolerance to barbiturates seen in chronic alcoholics.

Although the precautions of combined ethanol-barbiturate use are well known, it bears repeating that the combination should be used cautiously with due attention to excessive central nervous system depression. In large doses the interaction of ethanol with barbiturates does present a particular danger. The lethal dose for barbiturates is nearly 50% lower in the presence of ethanol than it is alone.[45a] Blood levels of secobarbital or pentobarbital as low as 0.5 mg/dl combined with blood ethanol levels of 100 mg/dl can cause death from respiratory depression.[45a] Anesthesia should be administered with extreme care in patients who are already depressed by this combination.

Other Sedative-Hypnotic Agents. Ethanol given with any other sedative-hypnotic can result in a greater central nervous system depression than when either agent is taken alone. The agents involved include chloral hydrate,[45a-e] glutethimide,[38,45f] and phenothiazines.[45g-k] The mechanism varies slightly among agents, although in general it is the same as with barbiturates. Certainly the phenothiazines are metabolized by microsomal pathways, and their combination with ethanol is potentially hazardous and could cause hypotension, impaired coordination, and severe, potentially fatal respiratory depression.[45b,45c] The sedative side effect of antihistamines is increased to such an extent with ethanol that it is particularly dangerous to perform any hazardous task while under their combined effect.[45d] An exception to the general metabolic pattern is glutethimide. The combined use of ethanol and glutethimide *increases* blood ethanol concentration and decreases plasma glutethimide concentration.[38] Although these effects may be clinically significant, it is probably more important to remember that both drugs are CNS depressants.

Benzodiazepines. Studies on the interaction between ethanol and several benzodiazepines have demonstrated that these drug combinations can result in additive or synergistic adverse effects on driving skills and other measures of psychomotor performance.[46-49] Most of the benzodiazepines tested have produced this phenomenon, including diazepam,[50] flunitrazepam,[50a] lorazepam,[50b,c] lormetazepam,[50d] midazolam,[50d] and triazolam.[50e] Although a predominantly pharmacodynamic mechanism is likely, ethanol does alter the rate of absorption, decrease the volume of distribution, and impair the elimination of diazepam and other benzodiazepines.[50f-j] Changes in kinetics do not always predict changes in action, however. Chronic alcoholics have lower benzodiazepine levels,[48,50k] yet they manifest enhanced sedation.

Benzodiazepines of low intrinsic clearance (demoxepam and desmethyldiazepam) have a reduced clearance in dogs given ethanol acutely. Ethanol impairs the rate of disappearance from the plasma of benzodiazepines that have a high intrinsic clearance (diazepam, chlordiazepoxide) when these are given orally, but not when given intravenously.[50l] Clinically significant potentiation has been reported.[50m,n] In mice pretreated with ethanol, the main inhibitory effect is on the microsomal degradation of desmethyldiazepam.[50o] This metabolite of diazepam is more active than the parent compound, accumulates in the brain, and may be responsible for the supra-additive effect of the ethanol-diazepam combination on motor coordination.[50o] If benzodiazepines are taken with ethanol or barbiturates, however, respiratory depression can be severe. This interaction, which is not entirely understood, is the most dangerous effect associated with the benzodiazepines. Some investigators believe that the phenomenon occurs because ethanol increases membrane permeability and allows benzodiazepines to enter areas of the central nervous system that are usually somewhat resistant to their transport, such as the brainstem.[50p]

The recently discovered benzodiazepine binding site does not bind ethanol and is not altered after chronic ethanol administration.[50q] This finding implies that ethanol is acting by a different mechanism. This may explain the usual relative lack of synergism between the benzodiazepines and ethanol.

More than 100 scientific papers have appeared on the subject of the pharmacokinetic and clinical consequences of the coadministration of benzodiazepines and ethanol, and the interested reader is referred to a detailed review by Sellers and Busto.[50r]

Chloral Hydrate. Chloral hydrate is synergistic with ethanol and thus resembles most barbiturates.[50s] The combination of the two agents illustrates the potentially complex nature of drug and ethanol interactions. These interactions involve additive, synergistic, and cross-tolerance phenomena, with both direct and indirect mechanisms. Chloral hydrate is metabolized to trichloroethanol, an active metabolite with CNS depressant effects. When chloral hydrate and ethanol are taken at the same time, increased metabolism of chloral hydrate occurs, and trichloroethanol levels increase. At the same time, metabolism to trichloroacetate, an inactive metabolite, is inhibited.[50t] Trichloroethanol also inhibits aldehyde dehydrogenase activity and causes elevated acetaldehyde levels, and thereby increased toxic effects.[50u] Finally, ethanol and chloral hydrate have directly additive sedative properties.

Perhaps these mechanisms explain the fact that, in addition to the expected sedative interaction between ethanol and chloral hydrate, an occasional chloral hydrate-treated patient who ingests ethanol may develop a syndrome similar to acute ethanol intolerance and characterized by facial flushing, headache, and tachycardia.[50v]

Chlordiazepoxide. Ethanol has a supraadditive effect on prolonging the sleep time of chlordiazepoxide in mice.[50t] As with many other agents, prolongation is believed to be mediated via a metabolite of chlordiazepoxide.

Paraldehyde. Paraldehyde also interacts synergistically with ethanol. In addition, paraldehyde is the CNS depressant pharmacologically most similar to ethanol and shows the greatest degree of cross-tolerance with it.[50s]

Guanethidine. Ethanol may enhance the antihypertensive effects of guanethidine. Guanethidine interferes with storage and release of catecholamines from postganglionic sympathetic nerve fibers and thereby causes adrenergic neuron blockade.[52] The reduction of vasomotor tone and the impairment of reflex adaptation to postural changes or to muscular exercise can lead to hypotension and syncope. Alcohol exerts profound vasodilator effects primarily on cutaneous vessels, whereas blood flow through skeletal muscle is either unchanged or decreased.[53-56] In addition, ethanol may directly depress the myocardium.[57,58] As little as 60 ml of whiskey can significantly decrease stroke volume, and thereby cardiac output, in chronic alcoholics and in patients with cardiac disease of varying causes.[59]

No specific studies have been conducted concerning the guanethidine-ethanol interaction. However, the occurrence of hypotensive episodes induced by ethanol in patients treated with guanethidine has been frequent enough to warrant numerous comments and the inclusion of a warning in the manufacturer's drug package.[52,60,61] It seems that an additional stimulus is required to produce hypotension. This stimulus could include physical exercise, showers or baths, or rising quickly from a sitting or prone position.[52] Thus it is possible, although not documented, that general or spinal anesthesia could produce profound hypotension in patients who are taking guanethidine and who have ingested ethanol.

Hypoglycemia Agents. Diabetic patients treated with phenformin should avoid the ingestion of alcoholic beverages because concurrent use may cause hypoglycemic reactions or life-threatening lactic acidosis with shock. Some patients who take phenformin also experience pronounced anorexia and intolerance to ethanol.

Sulfonylureas and ethanol interact by multiple mechanisms and cause unpredictable fluctuations in serum glucose levels. Ethanol ingestion may also precipitate a disulfiram-like reaction (for example, flushing, headache, palpitations, and a feeling of breathlessness) in patients stabilized with a sulfonylurea, particularly chlorpropamide.[62]

Ethanol impairs recovery from exogenously induced hypoglycemia in both normal individuals and, more readily, in patients with abnormal carbohydrate metabolism.[63,63a,63b] Insulin-dependent diabetic patients have been known to suffer dangerous hypoglycemic episodes after excessive ethanol intake. The concurrent use of insulin and ethanol by alcoholic patients has led to at least two deaths and three cases of permanent mental impairment.[63] In each case, patients stabilized with insulin were found comatose or semiconscious from hypoglycemia caused by the consumption of excessive amounts of ethanol. The anesthesiologist should be aware of this severe reaction in patients who ingest these combined agents; this applies not only in the operating room, but also to the physician confronted with a comatose patient in the emergency room or in the intensive care unit.

Opiates. The combination of ethanol and opiate dependency is common. Ethanol and opiates interact in many ways. In the laboratory animal, ethanol dependency is associated with increased intake of morphine as well as an increased sensitivity to morphine toxicity. Acute administration of ethanol produces elevations of plasma *beta*-endorphins similar in magnitude to those seen with acute morphine administration.[63a] Opiate antagonists can precipitate ethanol withdrawal in the ethanol-dependent animal, as well as decrease toxic reactions to ethanol and to other central nervous system depressants.[63a] These data corroborate the ethanol-opiate interactions observed in narcotic addicts, including the increased morbidity seen with concurrent ethanol use in persons on methadone maintenance.[63a] The acute hazards of this combination are well documented.[63b] There appears to be a metabolic interaction, as well as a pharmacologic synergism. For example, in rats given methadone, the administration of ethanol raises the concentration of methadone in the brain by inhibiting its microsomal N-demethylation.[63c]

General Anesthetics. Clinical experience suggests that the induction of anesthesia in a long-term abuser of ethanol is prolonged, and is often seen in conjunction with marked excitement. Maintenance of anesthesia in these patients is characterized by the need for high anesthetic concentrations. These impressions are corroborated in part by Han, who showed an increase in the MAC of halothane in chronic alcoholics.[64] On the other hand, Munson could detect no motor response to a surgical incision at MAC concentrations.[65] One might expect lessened anesthetic requirements with the acutely intoxicated patient. Although this has not been documented in human beings, the interaction between ethanol and other CNS depressants is striking enough to warrant caution when anesthetizing the acute alcoholic patient.[66]

The interaction between ethanol and any of the general anesthetic agents can be delayed, so that ethanol consumed too soon after an anesthetic can be disastrous. Hugin has suggested handing a form to all patients who receive anesthetics on an outpatient basis. On the form they should acknowledge that they are not to drink ethanol or to drive a vehicle until the next day.[67]

Benzodiazepines

The benzodiazepines—chlordiazepoxide, clonazepam, clorazepate, diazepam, flurazepam, lorazepam, oxazepam, and prazepam—are used as antianxiety agents (anxiolytics), sedatives, hypnotics, anticonvulsants, and/or skeletal muscle relaxants. The drugs appear to act at the limbic, thalamic, and hypothalamic levels of the CNS. The relatively recent discovery of specific benzodiazepine receptors promises to produce an explosion both in new agents—agonists and antagonists—and in

Benzodiazepine Binding Sites. Benzodiazepines exert their main actions in the central nervous system by an enhancement of GABAergic synaptic transmission,[67a,b] following an interaction between the benzodiazepine and a specific neuronal membrane receptor.[67c,d]

The mechanism of action of the benzodiazepines can be more easily understood in terms of the relation among gamma amino butyric acid (GABA), the benzodiazepine receptors, chloride channels, and picrotoxin receptors. Gamma amino butyric acid elicits its action by opening channels in the nerve membrane, channels that are permeable to the negatively charged chloride ion, thus forcing the membrane potential to become more negative and decreasing its excitability. Additionally, open chloride channels themselves can reduce the actions of excitatory input, thereby also decreasing activity. It would appear that in the presence of therapeutic concentrations of benzodiazepines, the chloride channels open more frequently and remain open longer, thus potentiating the actions of GABA.[67e]

The interaction between benzodiazepines and GABA was strengthened further by the discovery in 1977 of specific ligand binding sites for benzodiazepines in the brain.[67f,g] These membrane binding sites bind with clinically relevant benzodiazepines with an order of affinity that closely approximates their pharmacologic potency as therapeutic agents.[67h] Moreover, the binding of these compounds is specific: neither GABA nor any other endogenous neurotransmitter displaces benzodiazepines from these sites.[67h] Association with GABA is reflected, however, as an ability of GABA to increase the interaction of the benzodiazepines with their binding sites, as well as the reciprocal ability of benzodiazepines to increase the binding of GABA to its receptor.[67i,j] Thus, one can envision a macromolecular complex located within the nerve membrane. This complex consists of the GABA receptor, benzodiazepine binding site, and chloride channel acting in concert to regulate the excitability of individual neurones.

The usefulness of this concept is expanded when one considers the action of other agents which act to regulate the excitability of the brain, either as convulsants or as anticonvulsants. Picrotoxin exerts its actions by reducing chloride permeability. This reduction is effected when picrotoxin attaches itself close to the chloride channel, thereby reducing chloride influx.[67k] Thus we can expand the model to include three separate binding sites on the complex, all closely associated with the chloride channel: the GABA receptor, the benzodiazepine binding site, and the picrotoxin binding site.

The picrotoxin binding site has attracted attention not only for its ability to bind picrotoxin and structurally related compounds, but also for the ability of several other agents, both convulsants and anticonvulsants, to bind at this site. Thus far, both valproic acid (see Chap. 18) and barbiturates with anticonvulsant actions have been demonstrated to compete with picrotoxin at this site.[67l,m] The binding of these compounds is also paralleled by physiologic responses of the tissue. Both pentobarbital[67n] and valproic acid[67o] have the ability to potentiate the actions of GABA on central nervous system neurones, while the physiologic actions of the convulsant compounds are similar to those of picrotoxin.[67p] Other pharmacologic interactions at this complex include the increase in the binding of GABA[67q] and benzodiazepines[67r] in the presence of pentobarbital.

The benzodiazepines' ability to relieve muscle spasticity is believed to involve GABA receptors in the brainstem and spinal cord.[67s]

As with the endogenous opioid systems, the fact that certain brain sites bind benzodiazepines with high affinity raises the question whether there exists an endogenous benzodiazepine-like compound or whether the binding of these agents is simply incidental. The discovery of a series of compounds that are competitive antagonists of benzodiazepines has enabled studies to proceed along these lines.[67t-v] Again as with the opioid system, some of these compounds are ostensibly pure antagonists. Several newly synthesized imidazodiazepines inhibit the binding of diazepam but produce *in vivo* none of the typical benzodiazepine effects.[88e] Of these compounds Ro 15-1788 has shown low toxicity and intense ability to block the actions of several benzodiazepines. It is a potent and specific antagonist of benzodiazepine binding *in vitro* and *in vivo*[67w] and blocks the sedative, hypnotic, muscle relaxant, and anticonvulsant actions of conventional benzodiazepines without demonstrating any intrinsic activity.[67u,v,x,y] Other benzodiazepine antagonists do possess agonist as well as antagonist activity. The main class of these compounds belongs to the carboline family. *Beta*-Carboline carboxylate esters are potent ligands for benzodiazepine recognition sites, and these compounds reverse or prevent the major central effects of benzodiazepines in animals.[67z] They also antagonize several effects of other compounds, such as barbiturates.[67aa,bb] In addition, these agents elicit behavioral and neurophysiologic effects opposite to those of the benzodiazepines.[67bb,cc] The stable *beta*-carboline derivative, methyl-*beta*-carboline-3-carboxamide (FG 7142), appears to produce signs of anxiety in man.[67dd] Methyl-*beta*-carboline-3-carboxylate is a potent convulsant in baboons,[67ee] cats,[67ff] and rodents.[67gg,hh] Methylamide-*beta*-carboline has proconvulsant (enhances the convulsant effects of other agents) actions in mice and baboons[67ii] and anxiogenic (anxiety-producing) effects in man.[67jj,kk] Ethyl-*beta*-carboline-3-carboxylate has been extracted from human urine and may be related to an endogenous ligand for the benzodiazepine receptor. It reverses the effects of the benzodiazepines *in vitro*[67ll] and *in vivo*,[67mm,nn] but also has intrinsic activity, since it lowers the seizure threshold to drugs antagonistic to GABA.[67mm,oo] For example, it has proconvulsant actions on pentylenetetrazol-induced convulsions[67pp] and in photosensitive baboons.[67qq]

The "pure" antagonist Ro 15-1788 may in fact possess some intrinsic activity. Nutt et al.[67rr] suggest that it may have a benzodiazepine-like activity in rats in high doses, while File et al.[67ss] reported that it has an anxiogenic effect at smaller doses, again in the rat.[67ss] This latter effect could arise from antagonism of an anxiolytic endogenous ligand, or by interfering with the uptake or metabolism of an anxiogenic endogenous ligand. To add to the interest, Ro 15-1788, mentioned above, interacts with the central effects of *beta*-carbolines[67bb] and reverses the effects of FG 7142,[67bb] indicating that the *beta*-carbolines interact with the benzodiazepine recognition sites as "inverse agonists."[67bb]

In a recently reported study, 3-hydroxymethyl-*beta*-carboline induced a dose-dependent increase in sleep latency in rats.[67tt] This may be partly responsible for the anxiogenic actions of this class of compounds. In addition, the agent, at a low dose that by itself did not affect sleep, blocked sleep induction by a large dose of flurazepam. These two observations indicate that the benzodiazepine receptor may play a role in both the physiologic regulation and pharmacologic induction of sleep.

The compound Ro 15-1788 has been used clinically to reverse benzodiazepine-induced coma. In 9 patients in deep benzodiazepine-induced coma (diazepam, clonazepam, or flunitrazepam), it usually almost completely reversed the coma, as shown both clinically and by changes in the EEG. Perhaps these agents will be useful in future anesthetic practice. Even with considerably smaller doses of diazepam in humans,[67uu] the duration of Ro 15-1788 was shorter than that of diazepam. Thus we may be presented with a clinical situation similar to that of opioids/opioid antagonists, where the action of naloxone is shorter than that of most of the available opioids.

Flurazepam. Flurazepam shares the actions of other benzodiazepines, but is approved by the FDA only as a hypnotic agent. It is administered orally at bedtime. The dosage must be individualized and the smallest effective dose used, especially in elderly or debilitated patients or in those with liver disease or low levels of serum albumin.

Flurazepam has become a popular nighttime hypnotic in recent years. Because it is a benzodiazepine compound, it might be expected to share the same interactions as diazepam. To date, however, no clinically significant interaction has been documented with flurazepam.[67vv-zz] As with diazepam, this agent does not seem to change the activity of any anticoagulants and thus can be used safely with them.[67yy]

Lorazepam. Lorazepam also shares the actions of other benzodiazepines and is approved by the FDA for use in the therapy of states characterized by anxiety and tension and for insomnia. It has also been used IM or IV to produce sedation or light anesthesia, as well as anterograde amnesia.

Midazolam. The rapidly acting benzodiazepine, midazolam, is discussed in Chapter 21. It should be noted that this agent demonstrates *in-vitro* anticonvulsant effects in the brains of rats or mice.[67aaa] These studies were prompted by a case of diazepam-resistant status epilepticus which responded to midazolam.

Diazepam

Diazepam is a long-acting agent and is demethylated into active metabolites. One must certainly use less of other induction agents in the company of this drug, particularly if the total dose of diazepam is 20 mg or more.

The lack of interaction with the oral anticoagulants has been mentioned previously. In addition, diazepam, given as a preanesthetic medication, prolongs ketamine-induced sleep time (see below).[23] Interestingly enough, patients premedicated with diazepam had higher plasma ketamine levels on awaking than did patients in any other group.

Cimetidine. Cimetidine seems to inhibit hepatic microsomal oxidizing capacity and thereby impair the metabolic clearance of certain benzodiazepine derivatives when the two are administered together (see Chap. 13).[67ww,xx] The coadministration of cimetidine does indeed reduce the metabolic clearance of the oxidatively biotransformed benzodiazepines chlordiazepoxide, diazepam, desmethyldiazepam, alprazolam, and triazolam.[67yy-67ddd] Cimetidine, however, has little influence on the clearance of benzodiazepines transformed by glucuronide conjugation, including lorazepam, oxazepam, and temazepam.[67eee-fff]

INTERACTIONS WITH OTHER DRUGS

Lidocaine-Induced Seizures. Diazepam participates in other interactions. One of the most notable of these is its ability to protect against lidocaine-induced seizures. There is good evidence in several species of animals that diazepam, administered intramuscularly in doses in the range of those safe for premedication, can specifically antagonize the convulsant effect of lidocaine.[68-76] Thus a larger dose and a higher plasma concentration of lidocaine are required to produce seizures. Although this antagonism has not been shown in man, an anesthetist may wish to administer diazepam before performing a regional block that may require a large amount of lidocaine. Something could be gained and little should be lost. The use of diazepam should not create a false sense of security, however. Seizures can occur. And if they do develop, they seem to be more difficult to control in that they require doses of an anticonvulsant drug that are larger than normally needed.

The *therapy* of lidocaine-induced seizures

is another matter, since controversy exists over the desirability of using diazepam as opposed to an ultrashort-acting barbiturate. Several points should be examined in considering the treatment of an individual patient. Equiprophylactic doses of pentobarbital potentiate the cardiorespiratory depressant effects of local anesthetics more than does diazepam.[69,72,73,75] This property, combined with the lesser central nervous system effects of diazepam under the same conditions, would seem to give this drug the advantage over oxybarbiturates. Certainly, diazepam can prevent local anesthetic-induced convulsions seen with increasing lidocaine cardiovascular toxicity.[77] I prefer, however, to use a thiobarbiturate such as thiopental for several reasons. First, the onset of action of the barbiturate is more rapid than that of diazepam, and allows quick titration of anticonvulsant effects. Second, since small amounts of thiopental (25 to 50 mg) can abort a lidocaine-induced seizure, the chances of producing respiratory or cardiovascular depression are minimal. Third, its duration of action is less than that of diazepam. Thus if small amounts of the barbiturate have been given and the patient has a prolonged awakening, one can probably attribute it to a postictal phenomenon, rather than to a pharmacologic effect. The short-acting benzodiazepine midazolam may, by virtue of its shorter action and possibly more specific anticonvulsant activity,[77a] solve some of the problems accompanying diazepam in the therapy of local anesthetic-induced seizures.

Since diazepam antagonizes the central nervous system toxicity of lidocaine, it was feared that it might also antagonize the antidysrhythmic action of lidocaine. However, studies in dogs have indicated that diazepam actually enhances the antidysrhythmic effect of lidocaine.[78] Perhaps a straw horse was set up in this study.

Meperidine/Normeperidine. Diazepam not only potentiates the analgesic effects of meperidine, it decreases the proconvulsant and lethal effects of normeperidine.[77b] Normeperidine is believed to be involved in the dramatic interaction between MAOI and meperidine; MAOI increase the metabolism of meperidine to normeperidine. If this is true, diazepam could be a useful adjunct in the prevention or therapy of this dangerous interaction. On the other hand, it is consistently recommended that the combination of MAOI and meperidine be avoided (see Chapters 19 and 22).

Physostigmine. Physostigmine is unique among commonly used cholinesterase inhibitors in that it has a tertiary rather than a quaternary nitrogen. Therefore, it can rapidly cross the blood-brain barrier to exert its effect in the central nervous system. There have been several case reports that suggest that physostigmine can reverse the sedative or respiratory depressant effects of diazepam or lorazepam.[79–83] Although physostigmine has reversed the effects of anticholinergic agents, such as atropine, scopolamine, the phenothiazines, or the tricyclic antidepressants, it would be surprising that it could have such an action with the benzodiazepines.

There are, of course, many problems with the case reports described. It is possible that physostigmine is acting as a nonspecific analeptic. It does cause an arousal response in the electroencephalogram of cats, presumably by acting on the reticular activating system.[84] In many of the case reports, other agents were given, some of them capable of being reversed by physostigmine. Thus it is impossible to separate out simple two-drug interactions. More importantly, none of the reports attempted to use a placebo in a double-blind fashion. This may be significant in light of an unfortunately uncompleted study.[85] When diazepam was the only agent administered during spinal anesthesia, there was no difference between a saline placebo and physostigmine in producing arousal. There was, however, a suggestion of a greater incidence of side effects in the physostigmine group. Although only 12 patients were studied, in subsequent patients *if* physostigmine had produced arousal in every patient and *if* saline had had no effect, 23 additional patients would have had to be studied before a significant difference could have been obtained. Corroborating the impressions of the incomplete study of Karen are the results of a more recent study. In this equally well-controlled study, the authors could demonstrate no effect of physostigmine on the clinical, psychomotor, or EEG effects of lorazepam.[85a]

On the other hand, preliminary evidence indicates that physostigmine does shorten the duration of somnolence induced by diazepam in rats[86] and rapidly reverses that induced in healthy volunteer subjects.[87] The latter group involved a randomized, double-blind, cross-over study. Accompanying the arousal in these latter studies were definite signs of electroencephalographic arousal. In addition, 3 recent case reports suggested that physostigmine reversed the effects of midazolam in patients postoperatively.[87a] The administration of other agonists and antagonists did once again confuse the picture, however.

Physostigmine is not a benign drug, however. During the investigations by Karen[85] and by Avant et al.,[87] 2 of the 20 patients experienced atrial dysrhythmia—one atrial flutter and one atrial fibrillation. These did convert to normal after one to two hours. In addition, the incidence of side effects was high in Pandit et al.'s study.[85a] Almost every patient suffered from nausea, vomiting, pallor, and sweating.

Sodium Valproate. This antiepileptic agent interacts with many drugs. In normal volunteers, it has been shown to displace diazepam from plasma protein binding sites and to inhibit its metabolism.[87b] In fact, during the administration of valproate, the unbound fraction of diazepam can increase twofold. Whether this translates into a clinically significant enhancement of diazepam action remains to be demonstrated.

Xanthines. On the other hand, the xanthines have a demonstrated impact on benzodiazepine effects. Theophylline antagonized diazepam-induced psychomotor impairment in healthy volunteer subjects.[87c] This interaction was apparently not mediated through pharmacokinetic mechanisms. Aminophylline (theophylline ethylenediamine) can reverse the sedative[87d,e] and psychomotor impairment[87f] effects induced by diazepam. A well-controlled study by Arvidsson et al.[87d] demonstrated that the reversal was dramatic and could be accomplished with relatively low doses of aminophylline and minimal side effects. These effects of theophylline and aminophylline on benzodiazepine depression may arise from several mechanisms. First, a direct physiologic antagonism is probably involved. The methylxanthines have a stimulant action on the central nervous system, probably mainly by blocking adenosine receptors.[87g,h] The ability of methylxanthines to antagonize various effects of benzodiazepines[87i,j] may be a result of competition for benzodiazepine receptor sites.[87] Second, diazepam enhances adenosine release and depresses acetylcholine release from the rat cerebral cortex. The latter effect can be blocked by theophylline.[87k] The potentiation of the adenosine-induced depression of neuronal activity has been proposed to account for some of the central effects of benzodiazepines.[87l] Third, a calcium-related mechanism may be involved. Peyton and Borowitz reported that chlordiazepoxide increased calcium content in synaptosomes from rat brain cortex, while theophylline decreased it.[87m] Finally, the benzodiazepine-xanthine interaction may be mediated by caffeine. Theophylline is in part metabolized to caffeine.[87n] Caffeine antagonizes not only some of the psychomotor effects of lorazepam, but at the higher doses, some of the antianxiety effects.[87o] Caffeine is itself an anxiogenic drug, that is, it can produce anxiety. In addition, there is evidence that caffeine and the benzodiazepines compete for the same site.[87p]

Ketamine. In patients receiving a continuous intravenous infusion of ketamine plus nitrous oxide 65%, the hemodynamic stimulation of ketamine was significantly less in patients who were given diazepam for preanesthetic medication as compared with controls.[87q] These same patients required a lower rate of ketamine infusion during the initial 30 minutes of anesthesia. Patients on long-term diazepam or barbiturates had high concentrations of hydroxylated metabolites, with levels higher than norketamine, while patients receiving diazepam for preanesthetic medication had low levels of hydroxylated metabolites. The biological half-life of ketamine was significantly shortened in the former group and lengthened in the latter group. Those receiving clorazepate for preanesthetic medication showed none of the effects described above.

Neuromuscular Blocking Agents. A preliminary clinical study indicated that diazepam increased the duration of action of gallamine and decreased the duration of succinylcholine activity.[88] Subsequent work, however, has not substantiated these findings,[89,90] and it appears likely that diazepam itself does not significantly affect the response to numerous neuromuscular blocking agents.

Chlordiazepoxide

Since several studies have demonstrated a lack of interaction between chlordiazepoxide and oral anticoagulants, no special precautions appear necessary when administering this agent to patients who are taking oral anticoagulants.[91-93]

Chloral Hydrate

Chloral hydrate is still a popular oral hypnotic. It is rapidly metabolized in the liver and in other tissues to trichloroethanol, which is responsible for its CNS depressant effects. Excretion of its metabolites is through the urine and the bile.

Some disagreement exists as to the ability of chloral hydrate or of trichloroethanol to induce the microsomal enzyme system.[94-95] Although one report has suggested such an induction, most studies, both laboratory and clinical, have not demonstrated this phenomenon.[12,14,94,96-102] This is not surprising, since neither agent is metabolized by the hepatic microsomal enzyme system.[94]

However, chloral hydrate can affect the action of the anticoagulants, probably by another mechanism. A major metabolite, trichloroacetic acid, can displace acidic drugs from plasma proteins, resulting in a shortened half-life but in increased blood levels. Thus, trichloroacetic acid appears to displace warfarin from plasma-protein binding. This causes a transient increase in the amount of free (active) plasma warfarin and also in its rate of metabolism. Bishydroxycoumarin is probably affected similarly, but almost all available data deal with warfarin. Results from several clinical studies indicate that chloral hydrate temporarily increases the hypoprothrombinemic effect of warfarin in some patients.[96,98,99,103] Reports to the contrary have dealt with longer-range effects, thus demonstrating that continued administration of the two drugs probably normalizes the hypoprothrombinemic effect of warfarin.[104,105] The interaction resulting from the administration of chloral hydrate to patients already receiving long-term warfarin therapy is likely to be adverse.

Paraldehyde

Paraldehyde is a hypnotic drug used in the management of convulsions, tetanus, eclampsia, and status epilepticus. It is effective orally, but is a local irritant when given parenterally. After administration, 70 to 80% is metabolized by the liver, 11 to 28% is exhaled, and 0.1 to 2.5% is excreted in the urine.

Paraldehyde is metabolized to acetaldehyde by the liver. Thus disulfiram may impair the metabolism of acetaldehyde by inhibiting acetaldehyde dehydrogenase. Consequently, paraldehyde is not advised in patients receiving disulfiram.

Antihistaminics

Concurrent administration of an antihistaminic and a barbiturate may enhance the central nervous system depression caused by either drug. There is no clinical documentation, however, that this enhanced effect occurs.[106] However, one should still be cautious when concomitantly administering agents from these two classes.

Although frequently discussed in the scientific literature, no clinically significant interactions between warfarin and the antihistamines have been reported. Therefore, no additional precautions are necessary when these drugs are given concurrently.[104] This also means that sedative antihistaminics, such as diphenhydramine, would be satisfactory for preanesthetic medication in a patient who is receiving an oral anticoagulant. An exception to the apparent benignity of most of the antihistaminics in the area of drug interactions is the H_2 blocker, cimetidine. This interesting drug is discussed in Chapter 13.

Meprobamate

Meprobamate is a tranquilizer with central nervous system depressant actions similar to those of the barbiturates. It is well absorbed from the gastrointestinal tract and, like the barbiturates, can induce hepatic microsomal enzymes.[10] It interacts with ethanol in that short-term ethanol ingestion may decrease meprobamate metabolism, whereas the long-term use of ethanol and the resultant enzyme induction hasten the metabolism of meprobamate.[10,108] The suspicion that meprobamate may interfere with coumarin-type anticoagulants has not been sufficiently documented.

Ethchlorvynol

Ethchlorvynol is an alcohol used as a nighttime sedative. It is effective orally and metabolized by the liver, although up to 10% may be excreted unchanged. This drug has been reported to increase the metabolism of coumarin-type anticoagulants in a fashion similar to the barbiturates.[109,109a,109b,109c] Reports suggest that this interaction occurs to a variable degree in most patients.[113a,113b]

Glutethimide

Glutethimide has central nervous system depressant effects similar to those of the barbiturates, although the mechanism of action of the drug is not known. The agent is used primarily as an hypnotic in the treatment of simple insomnia. Since glutethimide loses its effectiveness after 2 weeks, the anesthetist will rarely encounter a patient using it chronically.

Although data conflict,[109d] most studies support an interaction between warfarin and glutethimide.[28e,28g,109e-f] Expect an interaction in the majority of patients treated.

A recent epidemiologic study demonstrated that the combination of glutethimide and codeine taken orally as a street drug results in a far greater mortality than would be expected from the incidence of its usage.[109f] Although several mechanisms could explain this phenomenon, one cannot rule out the possibility that combinations of these agents are unusually dangerous. The capricious occurrence of these episodes may be partly related to the notorious propensity for glutethimide to produce unpredictable and unmanageable intoxication.

Δ-9-Tetrahydrocannabinol (THC) ("Marijuana")

Although one could argue that marijuana is not primarily a sedative-hypnotic agent, it does produce sedation, and a significant fraction of the American population has been exposed to this plant.[110-111] The question must arise, then, whether this drug alters the response to anesthetic agents. In mice and rats, THC markedly potentiates barbital sleeping time.[111a] Since the magnitude of this effect was greatly enhanced by enzyme inhibition, one assumes that THC itself, not a metabolite, is responsible for this observation. In independent studies, Stoelting et al.[112] and Vitez et al.[113] observed a decrease in anesthetic requirement for halothane (dogs) and for cyclopropane (rats) after the short-term administration of Δ-9-tetrahydrocannabinol (THC), an active, purified component of marijuana. Long-term administration, on the other hand, did not alter the MAC of either agent. Marijuana is often consumed together with ethanol, and the acute additive effects of this combination might decrease anesthetic requirements.[118] Enzyme induction[115,116] after long-term marijuana smoking might alter biotransformation and potential toxicity of certain agents. On the other hand, single doses of cannabis extracts do block the enzyme induction produced by phenobarbital,[118a] an observation which adds to the complexity of the situation.

The purified agent THC had interesting effects when administered *after* either oxymorphone or pentobarbital.[117] The administration of THC further increased the sedation and the respiratory depression caused by oxymorphone. Although oxymorphone alone caused no significant cardiovascular changes, the addition of THC induced hallucinations and anxiety in five of seven volunteers. The cardiovascular effects of the addition of THC were the same as with oxymorphone. Again, the experimental protocol did not imitate the clinical situation, but these studies must give us pause.

That THC must be administered within a few hours before the administration of the anesthetic or during it to affect anesthetic requirements might seem to minimize the clinical significance of these observations; presumably few patients smoke marijuana the morning of an operation.[102,103] On the other hand, some patients admitted for an emergency operation may have been exposed to street drugs, and the possibility of altered anesthetic requirement must always be kept in mind. In addition, the recent increased incidence of outpatient surgery and of inpatient surgery performed on the day of admission has increased greatly the possibility of a patient's not following instructions completely—or of not even realizing that certain actions may not be to his advantage. Perhaps more pertinent in the studies cited above is that the experimental doses of THC were 10 to 20 times those needed to produce a satisfactory "high." However, one or more of the agents contained in marijuana may ultimately become a routine preanesthetic medication, and it is at present impossible to predict the dosage that will be used. Furthermore, street drugs are notoriously variable as to the range of dosages supplied and ingested.

In summary, the anesthesiologist is probably more likely to encounter patients taking the sedative-hypnotic agents than any other type of agent, particularly if one includes ethanol in this group. It would seem that the interaction between these agents and the oral anticoagulants represents the most commonly encountered of all interactions. This impression is partly enhanced by the ease with which the interaction is detected; few agents are served by a laboratory test that defines their action so precisely as does the prothrombin time for the anticoagulant agents. Other common interactions involve those among the sedative-hypnotic agents themselves. In general, they produce additive CNS depression if given concomitantly. On the other hand, cross-tolerance is common after long-term administration of many of these agents. Awareness of the possibility of these interactions facilitates their detection and control. Because there is more awareness among physicians of these interactions than of many others, the incidence *seems* to be high. Actually, the number of serious interactions has been small, considering the enormous amount of these agents given and the theoretical potentials for interactions.

REFERENCES

1. Way, W.L., and Trevor, A.J.: Sedative-hypnotics. Anesthesiology, 34:170, 1971.
2. Harvey, S.C.: Hypnotics and sedatives. The barbiturates. In The Pharmacological Basis of Therapeutics. 6th Ed. Edited by A.G. Gilman, L.S. Goodman and A. Gilman. New York, Macmillan, 1980.
3. Kornetsky, C.O., et al.: Comparison of psychological effects of certain centrally acting drugs in man. Arch. Neurol. Psychiat., 77:318, 1957.
4. Goldstone, S., et al.: Effect of quinalbarbitone, dextroamphetamine and placebo on apparent time. Br. J. Psychol., 49:324, 1958.
5. Smith, G.M., and Beecher, H.K.: Amphetamine, secobarbital and athletic performance III: Quantitative effects on judgment. J.A.M.A., 172:623, 1960.
6. Goldstein, A.B., et al.: Effects of secobarbital and of d-amphetamine on psychomotor performance of normal subjects. J. Pharmacol. Exp. Ther., 130:55, 1960.
7. MacDonald, R.L., and Barker, J.L.: Different actions of anticonvulsant and anesthetic barbiturates revealed by use of cultured mammalian nerves. Science, 200:775, 1978.
7a. Duncan, B.B.A., Zaimi, F., Newman, G.B., et al.: Effect of premedication on the induction dose of thiopentone in children. Anaesthesia., 39:426, 1984.
8. Saidman, L.J., and Eger, E.I.: Effect of nitrous oxide and of narcotic premedication on the alveolar concentration of halothane required for anesthesia. Anesthesiology, 25:302, 1964.
9. Perisko, J.A., Buechel, D.R., and Miller, R.D.: The effect of diazepam (Valium) on minimum alveolar anesthetic requirement in man. Can. Anaesth. Soc. J., 18:536, 1971.
9a. Petts, H.V., and Pleuvry, B.J.: Interactions of morphine and methotrimeprazine in mouse and man with respect to analgesia, respiration and sedation. Br. J. Anaesth., 55:437, 1983.
10. Conney, A.H.: Pharmacological implications of microsomal enzyme induction. Pharmacol. Rev., 19:317, 1967.
11. Corn, M.: Effect of phenobarbital and glutethimide on the biological half-life of warfarin. Thromb. Diath. Haemorrh., 16:606, 1966.
12. Cucinell, S.A., et al.: The effect of chloral hydrate on bishydroxycoumarin metabolism. J.A.M.A., 197:366, 1968.
13. Robinson, D.S., and MacDonald, M.G.: The effect of phenobarbital administration on the control of coagulation achieved during warfarin therapy in man. J. Pharmacol. Exp. Ther., 153:250, 1966.
14. MacDonald, M.G., et al.: The effects of phenobarbital, chloral betaine, and glutethimide administration on warfarin plasma levels and hypoprothrombinemic response in man. Clin. Pharmacol. Ther., 10:80, 1969.
15. Shuster, L., and Jick, H.: The turnover of microsomal protein in the livers of phenobarbital-treated mice. J. Biol. Chem., 241:5361, 1966.
16. Holtzman, J.L., and Gillette, J.R.: The effect of phenobarbital on the synthesis of microsomal phospholipid in female and male rats. Biochem. Biophys. Res. Commun., 24:639, 1966.
17. Conney, A.H., et al.: Adaptive increases in drug-metabolizing enzymes induced by phenobarbital and other drugs. J. Pharmacol. Exp. Ther., 130:1, 1960.
18. Conney, A.N., and Gilman, A.G.: Puromycin inhibition of enzyme induction by 3-methylcholanthrene and phenobarbital. J. Biol. Chem., 238:3682, 1963.
19. Remmer, H., and Merker, H.J.: Drug-induced changes in the liver endoplasmic reticulum: Association with drug metabolizing enzymes. Science (N.Y.), 142:1657, 1963.
20. Brodie, B.B., Burns J.J., and Weiner, M.: Metabolism of drugs in subjects with Laennec's cirrhosis. Med. Exp., 1:290, 1959.
21. Sessions, J.T., Jr., et al.: The effect of barbiturates in patients with liver disease. J. Clin. Invest., 33:1116, 1954.
22. Rubin, A., Tephly, T.R., and Mannering, G.J.: Kinetics of drug metabolism by hepatic microsomes. Biochem. Pharmacol., 13:1007, 1964.
23. Lo, J.N., and Cumming, J.F.: Interaction between sedative premedicants and ketamine in man and in isolated perfused rat livers. Anesthesiology, 43:307, 1975.
24. Fingl, E., and Woodbury, D.M.: General principles. In The Pharmacological Basis of Therapeutics. 6th Ed. Edited by A.G. Gilman, L.S. Goodman and A. Gilman. New York, Macmillan, 1980.
25. Ascione, F.J.: Sedative and hypnotic therapy. In Evaluations of Drug Interactions. 2nd Edition. Washington, D.C., American Pharmaceutical Association, 1976.
26. Hansten, P.D.: Drug Interactions. 3rd Ed. Philadelphia, Lea & Febiger, 1975, p. 201.
27. Hansten, P.D.: Drug Interactions. 3rd Ed. Philadelphia, Lea & Febiger, 1975, p. 198.
27a. Alvan, G., Lind, M., Mellström, B., et al.: Importance of 'first pass elimination' for interindividual differences in steady-state concentrations of the adrenergic beta-receptor antagonist alphrenolol. J. Pharmacokinet. Biopharm., 5:193, 1977.
27b. Alvan, G., Piafsky, K., Lind, M., et al.: Effect of pentobarbital on the disposition of alphrenolol. Clin. Pharmacol. Ther., 22:316, 1977.
27c. Collste, P., Seideman, P., Borg, K.O., et al.: Influence of pentobarbital on effect and plasma levels of alphrenolol and 4-hydroxy-alphrenolol. Clin. Pharmacol. Ther., 25:423, 1979.
27d. Haglund, K., Seideman, P., Collste, P., et al.: Influence of pentobarbital on metoprolol plasma levels. Clin. Pharmacol. Ther., 26:326, 1979.
27e. Sotaniemi, E.A., Anttila, M., Pelkonen, R.O., et al.: Plasma clearance of propranolol and sotalol

and hepatic drug-metabolizing enzyme activity. Clin. Pharmacol. Ther., 26:153, 1979.
27f. Mäntylä, R., Männistö, P., Nykänen, S., et al.: Pharmacokinetic interactions of timolol with vasodilating drugs, food and phenobarbitone in healthy human volunteers. Eur. J. Clin. Pharmacol., 24:227, 1983.
27g. Morselli, P.L., Marc, V., Garattini, S., et al.: Metabolism of exogenous cortisol in humans. Influence of phenobarbital treatment on plasma cortisol disappearance rate. Rev. Eur. Etud. Clin. Biol., 15:195, 1970.
27h. Brooks, S.M., Werk, E.E., Ackerman, S.J., et al.: Adverse effects of phenobarbital on corticosteroid metabolism in patients with bronchial asthma. N. Engl. J. Med., 286:1125, 1972.
27i. Stjernholm, M.R., and Katz, F.H.: Effects of diphenylhydantoin, phenobarbital, and diazepam on the metabolism of methylprednisolone and its sodium succinate. J. Clin. Endocrinol. Metab., 41:887, 1975.
27j. Brooks, P.M., Buchanan, W.W., Grove, M., et al.: Effects of enzyme induction on metabolism of prednisolone: Clinical and laboratory study. Ann. Rheum. Dis., 35:339, 1976.
27k. Wassner, S.J., Malekzadeh, M.H., Pennisi, A.J., et al.: Allograft survival in patients receiving anticonvulsant medications. Clin. Nephrol., 8:293, 1977.
27l. Hancock, K.W., and Levell, M.J.: Primidone/dexamethasone interaction (letter). Lancet, 2:97, 1978.
27m. Barriere, S.L., Gambertoglio, J., Stagg, R.J., et al.: Pharmacokinetics of cefonicid in patients with varying degrees of renal function. (Abst.) Clin. Pharmacol. Ther., 31:202, 1982.
28. Janz, D., and Schmidt, D.: Anti-epileptic drugs and failure of oral contraceptives (Letter). Lancet, 1:1113, 1974.
28a. Goss, J.E., and Dickhaus, D.W.: Increased bishydroxycoumarin requirements in patients receiving phenobarbital. N. Engl. J. Med., 273:1094, 1965.
28b. Cucinell, S.A., Conney, A.H., Sansur, M.S., et al.: Drug interactions in man. I. Lowering effect of phenobarbital on plasma levels of bihydroxycoumarin (Dicumarol) and diphenylhydantoin (Dilantin). Clin. Pharmacol. Ther., 6:420, 1965.
28c. Robinson, D.S., and MacDonald, M.G.: The effect of phenobarbital administration on the control of coagulation achieved during warfarin therapy in man. J. Pharmacol. Exp. Ther., 153:250, 1966.
28d. MacDonald, M.G., and Robinson, D.S.: Clinical observations of possible barbiturate interference with anticoagulation. J.A.M.A., 204:97, 1968.
28e. MacDonald, M.G., Robinson, D.S., Sylwester, D., et al.: The effects of phenobarbital, chloral betaine, and glutethimide administration on warfarin plasma levels and hypothrombinemic responses in man. Clin. Pharmacol. Ther., 10:80, 1969.
28f. Aggeler, P.M., and O'Reilly, R.A.: Effect of hepatabarbital on the response to bishydroxycoumarin in man. J. Lab. Clin. Med., 74:229, 1969.

28g. Robinson, D.S., and Sylwester, D.: Interaction of commonly prescribed drugs and warfarin. Ann. Intern. Med., 72:853, 1970.
28h. Udall, J.A.: Clinical implications of warfarin interactions with five sedatives. Am. J. Cardiol., 35:67–71, 1975.
28i. O'Reilly, R.A., Trager, W.F., Motley, C.H., et al.: Interaction of secobarbital with warfarin pseudoracemates. Clin. Pharmacol. Ther., 28:187, 1980.
28j. Orme, M., Breckenridge, A., and Brooks, R.V.: Interactions of benzodiazepines with warfarin. Br. Med., J., 3:611, 1972.
29. Hansten, P.D.: Drug Interactions. 3rd Ed. Philadelphia, Lea & Febiger, 1975, p. 129.
29a. Data, J.L., Wilkinson, G.R., and Nies, A.S.: Interaction of quinidine with anticonvulsant drugs. N. Engl. J. Med., 294:699, 1976.
29b. Chapron, D.J., Mumford, D., and Pitegoff, G.I.: Apparent quinidine-induced digoxin toxicity after withdrawal of pentobarbital: a case of sequential drug interactions. Arch. Intern. Med., 139:363, 1979.
30. Hansten, P.D.: Drug Interactions. 3rd Ed. Philadelphia, Lea & Febiger, 1975, p. 191.
31. Hansten, P.D.: Interaction between anticonvulsant drugs: primidone, diphenylhydantoin and phenobarbital. Northwest Med. J., 1:17, 1974.
31a. Preskorn, S., and Hughes, C.: Ethanol effects on brain concentrations of amitriptyline and the relationship to psychomotor function. Psychopharmacology, 80:L217, 1983.
31b. Rubin, E., and Lieber, C.S.: Hepatic microsomal enzymes in man and rat: Induction and inhibition by ethanol. Science, 162:690, 1968.
31c. Cott, J.M., and Ogren, S.O.: Antidepressant drugs and ethanol: Behavioral and pharmacokinetic interactions in mice. J. Neural Transm., 48:223, 1980.
31d. Preskorn, S.H., Hartman, B.K., Irwin, G.H., et al.: The role of the central adrenergic system in mediating diabenzazepine (tricyclic antidepressant)-induced alteration in the mammalian blood-brain barrier in vivo. J. Pharmacol. Exp. Ther., 223:388, 1982.
31e. Tacker, M., Creavin, P.J., and McIsaac, W.M.: Alterations in tyramine metabolism by ethanol. Biochem. Pharmacol., 19:1470, 1970.
31f. Kissin, B.: Interaction of ethyl alcohol and other drugs. In Kissin B., Begleiter, H., (eds). The Biology of Alcoholism, Vol. 3, Clinical Pathology. New York, Plenum Press, 1974, 109.
32. Ascione, F.J.: Warfarin-alcohol. In Evaluations of Drug Interactions. 2nd Edition. Washington, D.C., American Pharmaceutical Association, 1976.
33. Carriere, G., et al.: Etude experimental des injections intraveineuses d'alcool au cours d'intoxications par le gardenal. C.R. Soc. Biol. (Paris), 116:188, 1934.
34. Gruber, C.M., Jr.: A theoretical consideration of additive and potentiated effects between drugs with a practical example using alcohol and barbiturates. Arch. Int. Pharmacodyn. Ther., 102:17, 1955.

35. Morselli, P.L., et al.: Further observations on the interaction between ethanol and psychotropic drugs. Arzneim. Forsch., 21:20, 1971.
36. Jetter, W.W., and McLean, R.: Poisoning by the synergistic effect of phenobarbital and ethyl alcohol. An experimental study. Arch. Pathol., 36:112, 1943.
37. Ascione, F.J.: Phenobarbital-alcohol. In Evaluations of Drug Interactions. 2nd Edition. Washington, D.C., American Pharmaceutical Association, 1976.
38. Mould, G.P., et al.: Interaction of glutethimide and phenobarbitone with ethanol in man. J. Pharm. Pharmacol., 24:894, 1972.
39. Mezey, E., and Robles, E.A.: Effects of phenobarbital administration on rates of ethanol clearance and on ethanol-oxidizing enzymes in man. Gastroenterology, 66:248, 1974.
40. Lieber, C.S., and DeCarli, L.M.: Effect of drug administration on the activity of the hepatic microsomal ethanol oxidizing system. Life Sci., 9:267, 1970.
41. Lieber, C.S., and DeCarli, L.M.: The role of the hepatic microsomal ethanol oxidizing system (MEOS) for ethanol metabolism in vivo. J. Pharmacol. Exp. Ther., 181:279, 1972.
42. Khanna, J.M., et al.: Significance in vivo of the increase in microsomal ethanol-oxidizing system after chronic administration of ethanol, phenobarbital and chlorcyclizine. Biochem. Pharmacol., 21:2215, 1972.
43. Roach, M.K., et al.: Ethanol metabolism in vivo and the role of hepatic microsomal ethanol oxidation. Quart. J. Stud. Alc., 33:751, 1972.
44. Khanna, J.M., and Kalant, H.: Effect of inhibitors and inducers of drug metabolism on ethanol metabolism in vivo. Biochem. Pharmacol., 19:2033, 1970.
45. Carter, E.A., and Isselbacher, K.J.: Hepatic microsomal ethanol oxidation. Mechanism and physiologic significance. Lab. Invest., 27:283, 1972.
45a. Bogan, J., and Smith, H.: Analytical investigation of barbiturate poisoning description of methods and survey of results. J. Forensic Sci., 7:47, 1974.
45b. Zirkle, G.A., King, P.D., McAtee, O.B., et al.: Effects of chlorpromazine and alcohol on coordination and judgment. J.A.M.A., 171:1496, 1959.
45c. Milner, G., and Landauer, A.A.: Alcohol, thioridazine and chlorpromazine effects on skills related to driving behaviour. Br. J. Psychiatry, 118:351, 1971.
45d. Lieber, C.S., and Pirola, R.C.: Clinical relevance of alcohol-drug interactions. In Recent Advances in the Biology of Alcoholism. New York, The Haworth Press, 1982, pp. 41–65.
46. Linnoila, M., and Mattila, M.J.: Drug interaction on psychomotor skills related to driving: Diazepam and alcohol. Eur. J. Clin. Pharmacol., 5:186, 1973.
47. Linnoila, M., and Häkkinen, S.: Effects of diazepam and codeine, alone and in combination with alcohol, on simulated driving. Clin. Pharmacol. Ther., 15:368, 1974.
48. Linnoila, M., Saario, I., and Maki, M.: Effect of treatment with diazepam or lithium and alcohol on psychomotor skills related to driving. Eur. J. Clin. Pharmacol., 7:337, 1974.
49. Palva, E.S., and Linnoila, M.: Effect of active metabolites of chlordiazepoxide and diazepam, alone or in combination with alcohol, on psychomotor skills related to driving. Eur. J. Clin. Pharmacol., 13:345, 1978.
50. Willumeit, H.P., Ott, H., Neubert, W., et al.: Alcohol interaction of lormetazepam, mepindolol sulphate and diazepam measured by performance on the driving simulator. Pharmacopsychiat., 17:36, 1984.
50a. Seppälä, T., Nuotto, E., and Dreyfus, J.F.: Drug-alcohol interactions on psychomotor skills: Zopiclone and flunitrazepam. Pharmacology, 27:suppl. 2, 126, 1983 and Int. Pharmacopsychiat., suppl. 2, 127, 1982.
50b. Lister, R.G., and File, S.E.: Performance impairment and increased anxiety resulting from the combination of alcohol and lorazepam. J. Clin. Psychopharmacol., 3:2:66, 1983.
50c. Seppälä, T., Aranko, K., Matilla, M.J., et al.: Effects of alcohol on buspirone and lorazepam actions. Clin. Pharmacol. Ther., 32:2:201, 1983.
50d. Subhan, Z., and Hindmarch, I.: The effects of midazolam in conjunction with alcohol on iconic memory and free-recall. Neuropsychology, 9:230, 1983.
50e. Ochs, H.R., Greenblatt, D.J., Arendt, R.M., et al.: Pharmacokinetic noninteraction of trazolam and ethanol. J. Clin. Psychopharmacol., 4:2:106, 1984.
50f. Hayes, S.L., Pablo, G., Radomski, T., et al.: Ethanol and oral diazepam absorption. N. Engl. J. Med., 296:186, 1977.
50g. MacLeod, S.M., Giles, H.G., Patzalek, G., et al.: Diazepam actions and plasma concentrations following ethanol ingestion. Eur. J. Clin. Pharmacol., 11:345, 1977.
50h. Whiting, B., Lawtence, J.R., Skellern, G.G., et al.: Effect of acute alcohol intoxication on the metabolism and plasma kinetics of chlordiazepoxide. Br. J. Clin. Pharmacol., 7:95, 1979.
50i. Desmond, P.V., Patwardhan, R.V., Schenker, S., et al.: Short-term ethanol administration impairs the elimination of chlordiazepoxide (Librium) in man. Eur. J. Clin. Pharmacol., 18:275, 1980.
50j. Sellers, E.M., Naranjo, C.A., Giles, H.G., et al.: Intravenous diazepam and oral ethanol interaction. Clin. Pharmacol. Ther., 28:638, 1980.
50k. Sellman, R., Pekkarinen, A., Kangas, L., et al.: Reduced concentrations of plasma diazepam in chronic alcohol patients following an oral administration of diazepam. Acta Pharmacol. Toxicol. 36:25, 1975.
50l. Hoyumpa, A., Desmond, P., Roberts, T., et al.: Effect of ethanol on benzodiazepin disposition in dogs. Clin. Res., 27:454A, 1979.
50m. Morland, J., Setekliev, J., Haffner, J.F.W., et al.: Combined effects of diazepam and ethanol on

mental and psychomotor functions. Acta Pharmacol. Tox., 34:5, 1974.
50n. Bo, O., Haffner, J.F.W., Langard, O., et al.: Ethanol and diazepam as causative agents in road traffic accidents. In Israelstam, S., Lambert, S., eds. Alcohol, Drugs and Traffic Safety. Toronto. Addiction Research Foundation of Ontario, 1975, pp. 439–448.
50o. Paul, C.J., and Whitehouse, L.W.: Metabolic basis for the supra-additive effect of the ethanol-diazepam combination in mice. Br. J. Pharmacol., 60:83, 1977.
50p. Digregorio, G.J.: Benzodiazepines. AFP Clin. Pharmacol., 29:2:256, 1984.
50q. Karobath, M., Rogers, J., and Bloom, F.: Benzodiazepine receptors remain unchanged after chronic ethanol administration. Neuropharmacology, 19:125, 1980.
50r. Sellers, E.M., and Busto, U.: Benzodiazepines and ethanol: Assessment of the effects and consequences of psychotropic drug interactions. J. Clin. Pharmacol., 22:249, 1982.
50s. Weller, R.A., and Preskorn, S.H.: Psychotropic drugs and alcohol: pharmacokinetic and pharmacodynamic interactions. Psychosomatics, 25:4:301, 1984.
50t. Chan, A.W.K., Greizerstein, H.B., and Strauss, W.: Alcohol-chlordiazepoxide interaction. Pharmacol. Biochem. Behav., 17:141, 1982.
50u. Creaven, P.J., and Roach, M.K.: The effect of chloral hydrate on the metabolism of ethanol in mice. J. Pharm. Pharmacol., 21:332, 1969.
50v. Sellers, E.M., Carr, G., Bernstein, J.G., et al.: Interaction of chloral hydrate and ethanol in man. II. Hemodynamics and performance. Clin. Pharmacol. Ther., 13:50, 1972.
51. Johnstone, R.E., and Reier, C.E.: Acute respiratory effects of ethanol in man. Clin. Pharmacol. Ther., 14:501, 1973.
52. Nickerson, M., and Collier, B.: Drugs inhibiting adrenergic nerves and structures innervated by them. In The Pharmacological Basis of Therapeutics. 5th Edition. Edited by L.S. Goodman and A. Gilman. New York, Macmillan, 1975.
53. Cook, E., and Grown, G.: The vasodilating effects of ethyl alcohol on the peripheral arteries. Proc. Mayo Clin., 7:449, 1932.
54. Docter, R., and Perkins, R.: The effects of ethyl alcohol on autonomic and muscular responses in humans. Quart. J. Stud. Alc., 22:374, 1960.
55. Fewings, E., et al.: The effects of ethyl alcohol on the blood vessels of the hand and forearm in man. Br. J. Pharmacol. Chemother., 27:93, 1966.
56. Gillespie, J.: Vasodilator properties of alcohol. Br. Med. J., 2:274, 1967.
57. Gimena, A., et al.: Effects of ethanol on cellular membrane potentials and contractility of isolated rat atrium. Am. J. Physiol., 203:194, 1962.
58. Regan, T., et al.: The acute metabolic and hemodynamic responses of the left ventricle to ethanol. J. Clin. Invest., 45:270, 1966.
59. Gould, L., et al.: Cardiac effects of a cocktail. J.A.M.A., 218:1799, 1971.
60. Bienvenu, O.: Essential hypertension. Med. Clin. North Am., 51:967, 1967.
61. Meyer, F.H., et al.: Review of Medical Pharmacology. Los Altos, Calif., Lange Medical Publications, 1968.
62. Arky, R.A., et al.: Irreversible hypoglycemia, A complication of alcohol and insulin. J.A.M.A., 206:575, 1968.
63. Ascione, F.J.: Tolbutamide-alcohol. In Evaluations of Drug Interactions. 2nd Edition. Washington, D.C., American Pharmaceutical Association, 1976.
63a. Ho, A.K.S., and Allen, J.P.: Alcohol and the opiate receptor: interactions with the endogenous opiates. In Advances in Alcohol and Substance abuse, Vol. 1(1), 1981, pp. 53–75.
63b. Kissin, B.: Interaction of ethyl alcohol and other drugs. In Kissin, B., and Begleiter, H., eds. The Biology of Alcoholism. Vol. 3, Clinical Pathology, New York, Plenum Press, 1974, pp. 109–161.
63c. Borowsky, S.A., and Lieber, C.S.: Interaction of methadone and ethanol metabolism. J. Pharmacol. Exp. Ther., 207:123, 1978.
64. Han, Y.H.: Why do chronic alcoholics require more anesthesia? Anesthesiology, 30:341, 1969.
65. Munson, E.A.: Unpublished data.
66. Fitzgerald, M.G., et al.: Alcohol sensitivity in diabetics receiving chlorpropamide. Diabetes, 11:40, 1962.
67. Hugin, W.: Intentional beneficial and accidental or undesirable drug interactions in anesthesia. In Drug Interactions. Edited by P.L. Morselli, S. Garattini, and S.N. Cohen. New York, Raven Press, 1974.
67a. Haefely, W., Kulcsar, A., Moehler, H., et al.: Possible involvement of GABA in the central actions of benzodiazepines; in Costa Greengard, Mechanism of action of benzodiazepines. New York, Raven Press, 1975, pp. 131–151.
67b. Hafely, W., Pieri, L., Polc, P., et al.: General pharmacology and neuropharmacology of benzodiazepine derivatives. In Hoffmeister and Stille. Handbook of Experimental Pharmacology. vol. 55, Psychotropic agents, Part 2. Berlin, Springer, 1981, pp. 13–262.
67c. Hunkeler, W., Moehler, H., Pieri, L., et al.: Selective antagonists of benzodiazepines. Nature, 290:514, 1981.
67d. Moehler, H., Battersby, M.K., and Richards, J.G.: Benzodiazepine receptor protein identified and visualized in brain tissue by a photoaffinity label. Proc. Natl. Acad. Sci. USA, 77:1666, 1980.
67e. Study, R.E., and Barker, J.L.: Diazepam and pentobarbital: Fluctuation analysis reveals different mechanisms for potentiation of γ-aminobutyric acid responses in cultured central neurons. Proc. Natl. Acad. Sci. USA, 78:180, 1981.
67f. Mohler, H., and Okada, T.: Properties of ^{3}H-diazepam binding to benzodiazepine receptors in rat cerebral cortex. Life Sciences, 20:2101, 1977.
67g. Squires, R.F., and Braestrup, C.: Benzodiazepine receptors in rat brain. Nature, 266:732, 1977.
67h. Braestrup, C., and Squires, R.F.: Pharmacological characterization of benzodiazepine receptors in the brain. Br. J. Pharmacol., 48:263, 1978.

67i. Skerritt, J.H., Willow, M., and Johnston, G.A.R.: Diazepam enhancement of low affinity GABA binding to rat brain membranes. Neurosci Lett., 29:63, 1982.
67j. Tallman, J.F., Thomas, J.W., and Gallagher, D.W.: GABAergic modulation of benzodiazepine binding site sensitivity. Nature, 274:383, 1978.
67k. Geller, H.M.: Pharmacological basis of therapeutics: anticonvulsant agents. J. Med. Soc. New Jersey, 81:4:322, 1984.
67l. Olsen, R.W., Leeb-Lundberg, F., and Napias, C.: Picrotoxin and convulsant binding sites in mammalian brain. Brain Res. Bull., 2:217, 1980.
67m. Ticku, M.K., and Davis, W.C.: Effect of valproic acid on ³H-dihydropicrotoxinin binding sites at the benzodiazepine-GABA receptor-ionophore complex. Brain Res., 223:218, 1981.
67n. Nicoll, R.A., Eccles, J.C., Oshima, T., Rubia, F.: Prolongation of hippocampal inhibitory postsynaptic potentials by barbiturates. Nature, 258:625, 1975.
67o. Baldino, F., Jr., and Geller, H.M.: Sodium valproate enhancement of GABA inhibition: Electrophysiological evidence for anticonvulsant activity. J. Pharmacol. Exp. Ther., 217:445, 1981.
67p. Geller, H.M.: Water soluble benzodiazepines with agonistic and antagonistic actions on GABA-induced inhibition in cultured hypothalamus. Neurosci. Lett., 15:313, 1979.
67q. Willow, M., and Johnston, G.A.R.: Enhancement by anesthetic and convulsant barbiturates of GABA binding to rat brain synaptosomal membranes. J. Neurosci., 1:364, 1981.
67r. Leeb-Lundberg, F., Snowman, A., and Olsen, R.W.: Barbiturate receptor sites are coupled to benzodiazepine receptors. Proc. Natl. Acad. Sci. USA, 77:7468, 1980.
67s. Digregorio, G.J.: Benzodiazepines. AFP Clinical Pharmacology, 29:2:256, 1984.
67t. Haefely, W., Bonetti, E.P., Burkard, W.P., et al.: Benzodiazepine antagonists. In Costa E. (ed.). Benzodiazepines—From Molecular Pharmacology to Clinical Practice, New York, Raven Press, 1983.
67u. Braestrup, C., and Nielsen, M.: [3H] Propyl beta-carboline-3-carboxylate as a selective radioligand for the BZ1 benzodiazepine receptor subclass. J. Neurochem., 27:333, 1981.
67v. Gee, K.W., Yamamura, S.H., Roeske, W.R., et al.: Benzodiazepine receptor heterogeneity: Possible molecular basis and functional significance. Fed. Proc., 43:2767, 1984.
67w. Möhler, H., Burkard, W.P., Keller, A.H., et al.: Benzodiazepine antagonist Ro 15-1788: binding characteristics and interaction with drug-induced changes in dopamine turnover and cerebellar cGMP levels. J. Neurochem., 37:714, 1981.
67x. Hunkeler, W., Möhler, H., Pieri, L., et al.: Selective antagonists of benzodiazepines. Nature, 290:514, 1981.
67y. Darragh, A.: Reversal of benzodiazepine-induced sedation by intravenous Ro 15-1788 (Letter). Lancet, 2:1042, 1981.
67z. Braestrup, C., and Nielsen, M.: Anxiety. The Lancet, 2:1030, 1982.
67aa. Braestrup, C., Nielsen, M., and Olsen, C.E.: Urinary and brain beta-carboline-3-carboxylates as potent inhibitors of brain benzodiazepine receptors. Proc. Natl. Acad. Sci. USA, 77:2288, 1980.
67bb. Hunkeler, W., Möhler, H., Pieri, L., et al.: Selective antagonists of benzodiazepines. Naure, 290:514, 1981.
67cc. Kemp, J.R., and Kaada, B.R.: The relation of hippocampal theta activity to arousal, attentive behavior and somato-motor movements in unrestrained cats. Brain Res., 95:323, 1975.
67dd. Mariotti, M., and Ongini, E.: Differential effects of benzodiazepines on EEG activity and hypnogenic mechanisms of the brain stem in cats. Arch. Int. Pharmacodyn., 264:203, 1983.
67ee. Schoemaker, H., Boles, R.G., Horst, W.D., et al.: Specific high-affinity binding sites of [3H] Ro 5-4864 in rat brain and kidney. J. Pharmacol. Exp. Ther., 225:61, 1983.
67ff. de Carvalho, L.P., Venault, P., Cavalheiro, E., et al.: Distinct behavioral and pharmacological effects of two benzodiazepine antagonists: Ro 15-1788 and methyl beta-carboline. In Biggio, G., and Costa E. (eds.) Benzodiazepine Recognition Site Ligands: Biochemistry and Pharmacology. New York, Raven Press, 1983.
67gg. Schoemaker, H., Bliss, M., and Yamamura, H.I.: Specific high-affinity saturable binding of [3H] Ro 5-4864 to benzodiazepine binding sites in the rat cerebral cortex. Eur. J. Pharmacol., 71:173, 1981.
67hh. Le Fur, G., Mizoule, H., Burgevin, M.C., et al.: Multiple benzodiazepine receptors: Evidence of a dissociation between anticonflict and anticonvulsant properties by PK 8165 and PK 9084 (Two quinoline derivatives). Life Science, 28:1439, 1981.
67ii. Regan, J.W., Roeske, W.R., Malick, J.B., et al.: Gamma-Aminobutyric acid enhancement of CL 218,872 affinity and evidence of benzodiazepine receptor heterogeneity. Mol. Pharmacol., 20:477, 1981.
67jj. Orrenius, S.: Alcohol and drug interactions: basic concepts. Advances in Alcohol and Substance Abuse, 1:53, 1981.
67kk. Litchfield, J.R., and Wilcoxon, F.: A simplified method of evaluating dose-effect experiments. J. Pharmacol. Exp. Ther., 96:99, 1949.
67ll. Mitchell, R., and Martin, I.: Ethyl beta-carboline-3-carboxylate antagonises the effect of diazepam on a functional GABA receptor. Eur. J. Pharmacol., 68:513, 1980.
67mm. Tenen, S.S., and Hirsch, J.D.: Beta-carboline-3-carboxylic acid ethyl ester antagonizes diazepam activity. Nature, 288:609, 1980.
67nn. Oakley, N.R., and Jones, B.J.: The proconvulsant and diazepam-reversing effects of ethyl-beta-carboline-3-carboxylate. Eur. J. Pharmacol., 68:381, 1980.
67oo. Cowen, P.J., Green, A.R., and Nutt, D.J.: Ethyl beta-carboline carboxylate lowers seizure thresh-

old and antagonises flurazepam-induced sedation in rats. Nature, 290:54, 1981.
67pp. Davies, L.R., and Huston, V.: Peripheral benzodiazepine binding sites in heart and their interaction with dipyridamole. Eur. J. Pharmacol., 73:209, 1982.
67qq. Braestrup, C., Schmiechen, R., Nielsen, M., et al.: Benzodiazepine receptor legands, receptor occupancy, pharmacological effects and GABA receptor coupling. In Pharmacology of Benzodiazepines, Usdin E., et al. (eds.), London, Macmillan Press, 1983, pp. 71–86.
67rr. Nutt, D.J., Cowen, P.J., and Little, H.J.: Unusual interaction of benzodiazepine receptor antagonists. Nature, 295:436, 1982.
67ss. File, S.E., Lister, R.G., and Nutt, D.J.: The anxiogenic action of benzodiazepine antagonists. Neuropharmacology, 21:1033, 1982.
67tt. Mendelson, W.B., Cain, M., Cook, J.M., et al.: A benzodiazepine receptor antagonist decreases sleep and reverses the hypnotic actions of flurazepam. Science, 219:141, 1983.
67uu. Darragh, A., Lambe, R., Kenny, M., et al.: RO 15-1788 antagonises the central effects of diazepam in man without altering diazepam bioavailability. Br. J. Clin. Pharmac., 14:677, 1982.
67vv. Ascione, F.J.: Amitriptyline-chlordiazepoxide. In Evaluations of Drug Interactions. 2nd Ed. Washington, D.C., American Pharmaceutical Association, 1976.
67ww. Ascione, F.J.: Diazepam-alcohol. In Evaluations of Drug Interactions. 2nd Ed. Washington, D.C., American Pharmaceutical Association, 1976.
67xx. Ascione, F.J.: Gallamine triethiode-diazepam. In Evaluations of Drug Interactions. 2nd Ed. Washington, D.C., American Pharmaceutical Association, 1976.
67yy. Ascione, F.J.: Levodopa-diazepam. In Evaluations of Drug Interaction. 2nd Ed. Washington, D.C., American Pharmaceutical Association, 1976.
67zz. Ascione, F.J.: Warfarin-chlordiazepoxide. In Evaluations of Drug Interactions. 2nd Ed. Washington, D.C., American Pharmaceutical Association, 1976.
67aaa. Kaneko, S., Kurahashi, K., Fujita, S., et al.: Potentiation of GABA by midazolam and its therapeutic effect against status epilepticus. Folia Psychiatrica et Neurologica Japonica, 37:307, 1983.
67bbb. Divol, M., Greenblatt, D.J., Abernethy, D.R., and Shader, R.I.: Cimetidine impairs clearance of antipyrine and desmethyldiazepam in the elderly. J. Am. Geriatr. Soc., 30:684, 1982.
67ccc. Klotz, U., and Reimann, I.: Influence of cimetidine on the pharmacokinetics of desmethyldiazepam and oxazepam. Eur. J. Clin. Pharmacol., 18:517, 1980.
67ddd. Abernethy, D.R., et al.: Differential effect of cimetidine on drug oxidation (antipyrine and diazepam) vs. conjugation (acetaminophen and lorazepam): Prevention of acetaminophen toxicity by cimetidine. J. Pharmacol. Exp. Ther., 224:508, 1983.
67eee. Patwardhan, R.V., et al.: Cimetidine spares the glucuronidation of lorazepam and oxazepam. Gastroenterology, 79:912, 1980.
67fff. Greenblatt, D.J., et al.: Noninteraction of temazepam and cimetidine. J. Pharm. Sci., 73:399, 1984.
68. De Jong, R.H., and Heavner, J.E.: Diazepam prevents and aborts lidocaine convulsions in monkeys. Anesthesiology, 41:226, 1974.
69. Feinstein, M.B., Lenard, W., and Mathias, J.: The antagonism of local anesthetic induced convulsions by the benzodiazepine derivative diazepam. Arch. Int. Pharmacodyn. Ther., 187:144, 1970.
70. Wale, N., and Jenkins, L.C.: Site of action of diazepam in the prevention of lidocaine induced seizure activity in cats. Can. Anaesth. Soc. J., 20:146, 1973.
71. De Jong, R.H., and Heavner, J.E.: Diazepam prevents local anesthetic seizures. Anesthesiology, 34:523, 1971.
72. Aldrete, J.A., and Daniel, W.: Evaluation of premedicants as protective agents against convulsive (LD$_{50}$) doses of local anesthetic agents in rats. Anesth. Analg. (Cleve.), 50:127, 1971.
73. Wesseling, H., Bovenhorst, G.H., and Wiers, J.W.: Effects of diazepam and pentobarbitone on convulsions induced by local anesthetics in mice. Eur. J. Pharmacol., 13:150, 1971.
74. Munson, E.S., and Wagman, I.H.: Diazepam treatment of local anesthetic-induced seizures. Anesthesiology, 37:523, 1972.
75. De Jong, R.H., and Heavner, J.E.: Local anesthetic seizure prevention: Diazepam versus pentobarbital. Anesthesiology, 36:449, 1972.
76. Munson, E.S., Gutnick, M.J., and Wagman, I.H.: Local anesthetic drug-induced seizures in rhesus monkeys. Anesth. Analg. (Cleve.), 49:986, 1970.
77. De Jong, R.H., and Heavner, J.E.: Diazepam and lidocaine-induced cardiovascular changes. Anesthesiology, 39:633, 1973.
77a. Kaneko, S., Kurahashi, K., Fujita, S., et al.: Potentiation of GABA by midazolam and its therapeutic effect against status epilepticus. Folia Psychiatrica et Neurologica Japonica, 37(3)307, 1983.
77b. Leander, J.D.: Interaction of diazepam with meperidine or normeperidine on analgesia and lethality. Pharmacol. Biochem. Behav., 16:1005, 1982.
78. Dunbar, R.W., et al.: The effect of diazepam on the antiarrhythmic response to lidocaine. Anesth. Analg. (Cleve.), 50:685, 1971.
79. Larson, G.F., Hurlbert, B.J., and Wingard, D.W.: Physostigmine reversal of diazepam-induced arousal. Anesth. Analg. (Cleve.), 56:348, 1977.
80. Bernards, W.: Case history number 74: Reversal of phenothiazine-induced coma with physostigmine. Anesth. Analg. (Cleve.), 52:938, 1973.
81. DiLiberti, J., O'Brien, M.L., and Turner, T.: The use of physostigmine as an antidote in accidental diazepam intoxication. J. Pediatr., 86:106, 1975.
82. Rosenberg, H.: Physostigmine reversal of sedative drugs (letter). J.A.M.A., 229:1168, 1974.
83. Blitt, C.D., and Petty, W.C.: Reversal of lorazepam delirium by physostigmine. Anesth. Analg. (Cleve.), 54:607, 1975.
84. Bradley, P.B., and Elkes, J.: The effect of atropine, hyoscyamine, physostigmine, and neo-

stigmine on electrical activity of the conscious cat. J. Physiol., 120:14, 1953.
85. Karen, D.: Unpublished observations.
85a. Pandit, U.A., Kothary, S.P., Satwant, K.S., et al.: Physostigmine fails to reverse clinical, psychomotor, or EEG effects of lorazepam. Anesth. Analg., 62:679, 1983.
86. Berman, M.L., and Harbison, R.D.: Induction of consciousness by physostigmine. Pharmacologist, 18:Abstract 406, 1976.
87. Avant, G.R., et al.: Physostigmine reversal of diazepam-induced hypnosis in human volunteers. In Abstracts of Scientific Papers. Park Ridge, Ill., American Society of Anesthesiologists, 1978.
87a. Caldwell, C.V., and Gross, J.B.: Physostigmine reversal of midazolam-induced sedation. Anesthesiology, 57(2)125, 1982.
87b. Dhillon, S., and Richen, A.: Valproic acid and diazepam interaction in vivo. Br. J. Clin. Pharmacol., 13:553, 1982.
87c. Henauer, S.A., Hollister, L.E., Gillespie, H.K., et al.: Theophylline antagonizes diazepam-induced psychomotor impairment. Euro. Clin. Pharmacol., 25:743, 1983.
87d. Arvidsson, S.B., Ekströ-Jodal, B., Martinell, S.A.G., et al.: Aminophylline antagonises diazepam sedation. Lancet, 1:467, 1982.
87e. Stirt, J.A.: Aminophylline is a diazepam antagonist. Anes. Analg., 60:767, 1981.
87f. Henauer, S.A., Hollister, L.E., Gillespie, H.K., et al.: Theophylline antagonizes diazepam-induced psychomotor impairment. Eur. J. Clin. Pharmacol., 25:743, 1983.
87g. Clyde, D.J.: Manual for the Clyde Mood Scale. Miami Clyde Computing Service, USA, 1963.
87h. Costa, E., and Guidotti, A.: Molecular mechanisms in the receptor action of benzodiazepines. Ann. Rev. Pharmacol. Toxicol., 19:531, 1979.
87i. Derogatis, L.R., Lipman, R.S., and Covi, L.: SCL-90: An outpatient psychiatric rating scale—preliminary report. Psychopharmacol. Bull., 9:13, 1973.
87j. Ferguson, J.L., and Couri, D.: Electron capture gas chromatography determination of benzodiazepines and metabolites. J. Analyt. Toxicol., 1:171, 1977.
87k. Hills, M., and Armitage, P.: The two-period cross-over clinical trial. Br. J. Clin. Pharmacol., 8:7, 1979.
87l. Hindmarch, I.: Psychomotor function and psychoactive drugs. Br. J. Clin. Pharmacol., 10:189, 1980.
87m. Peyton, J.C., and Borowitz, J.L.: Chlordiazepoxide and theophylline after calcium levels in subcellular fractions of rat brain cortex. Proc. Soc. Exp. Biol. Med., 161:178, 1979.
87n. Berry, C., Gelder, M.G., and Summerfield, A.: Experimental analysis of drug effects on human performance using information theory concepts. Brit. J. Psychol., 56:225, 1965.
87o. File, S.E., Bond, A.J., and Lister, R.G.: Interaction between effects of caffeine and lorazepam in performance tests and self-ratings. J. Clin. Psychopharm., 2:102, 1982.
87p. Marangos, P.J., Paul, S.M., Parma, A.M., et al.: Purinergic inhibition of diazepam binding to rat brain (in vitro). Life Sci., 24:851, 1979.
87q. Idvall, J., Aronsen, K.F., Stenberg, P., et al.: Pharmacodynamic and pharmacokinetic interactions between ketamine and diazepam. Eur. J. Clin. Pharmacol., 24:337, 1983.
88. Feldman, S.A., and Crawley, B.E.: Interaction of diazepam with the muscle-relaxant drugs. Br. Med. J., 2:336, 1970.
89. Dretchen, K., et al.: The interaction of diazepam with myoneural blocking agents. Anesthesiology, 34:463, 1971.
90. Webb, S.N., and Bradshaw, E.G.: Diazepam and neuromuscular blocking drugs (Letter). Br. Med. J., 3:640, 1971.
91. Whitfield, J.B., et al.: Changes in plasma α-glutamyl transpeptidase activity associated with alterations in drug metabolism in man. Br. Med. J., 1:316, 1973.
92. Robinson, D.S., and Sylwester, D.: Interaction of commonly prescribed drugs and warfarin. Ann. Intern. Med., 72:853, 1970.
93. Lackner, H., and Hunt, V.E.: The effect of Librium on hemostasis. Am. J. Med. Sci., 256:368, 1968.
94. Harvey, S.C.: Hypnotics and sedatives. Miscellaneous agents. In The Pharmacological Basis of Therapeutics. 6th Ed. Edited by A.G. Gilman, L.S. Goodman and A. Gilman. New York, Macmillan, 1980.
95. Ascione, F.J.: Warfarin-chloral hydrate. In Evaluations of Drug Interactions. 2nd Edition. Washington, D.C., American Pharmaceutical Association, 1976.
96. Weiner, M.: Species differences in the effect of chloral hydrate on coumarin anticoagulants. Ann. N.Y. Acad. Sci., 179:226, 1971.
97. Griner, P.F., et al.: Chloral hydrate and warfarin interaction: Clinical significance. Ann. Intern. Med., 74:540, 1971.
98. Sellers, E.M., and Koch-Weser, J.: Kinetics and clinical importance of displacement of warfarin from albumin by acidic drugs. Ann. N.Y. Acad. Sci., 179:213, 1971.
99. Sellers, E.M., and Koch-Weser, J.: Potentiation of warfarin-induced hypoprothrombinemia by chloral hydrate. N. Engl. J. Med., 283:827, 1970.
100. Van Dam, I.E., and Gribnau-Overkamp, M.J.H.: The effect of some sedatives (phenobarbital, glutethimide, chlordiazepoxide, chloral hydrate) on the rate of disappearance of ethyl biscoumacetate from the plasma. Folia Med. Neerl., 10:141, 1967.
101. Breckeneridge, A., et al.: Drug interactions with warfarin: Studies with dichloralphenazone, chloral hydrate and phenazone (Antipyrine). Clin. Sci., 40:351, 1971.
102. Breckenridge, A., and Orme, M.: Clinical implications of enzyme induction. Ann. N.Y. Acad. Sci., 179:421, 1971.
103. Boston Collaborative Drug Surveillance Program: Interaction between chloral hydrate and warfarin. N. Engl. J. Med., 286:53, 1972.
104. Ascione, F.J.: Gallamine triethiode-diazepam. In

Evaluations of Drug Interactions. 2nd Ed. Washington, D.C., American Pharmaceutical Association, 1976.
105. Udall, J.A.: Chloral hydrate and warfarin therapy (Letter). Ann. Intern. Med., 75:141, 1971.
105a. Drug Interaction Facts. The Mediphor Editorial Group, Facts and Comparisons Division. St. Louis, C.V. Mosby Co., 1984, p. 32.
106. Ascione, F.J.: Chlorcyclizine-phenobarbital. In Evaluations of Drug Interactions. 2nd Edition. Washington, D.C., American Pharmaceutical Association, 1976.
107. Ascione, F.J.: Warfarin-diphenylhydramine. In Evaluations of Drug Interactions. 2nd Edition. Washington, D.C., American Pharmaceutical Association, 1976.
108. Hunninghake, D.B., and Azarnoff, D.L.: Drug interactions with warfarin. Arch. Intern. Med., 121:349, 1968.
109. Ascione, F.J.: Anticoagulant therapy. In Evaluations of Drug Interactions. 2nd Edition. Washington, D.C., American Pharmaceutical Association, 1976.
109a. Martin, Y.C.: The effect of ethchlorvynol on the drug-metabolizing enzymes of rats and dogs. Biochem. Pharmcol., 16:2041, 1967.
109b. Cullen, S.I., and Catalano, P.M.: Griseofulvin-warfarin antagonism. J.A.M.A., 199:582, 1967.
109c. Johansson, S.A.: Apparent resistance to oral anticoagulant therapy and influence of hypnotics on some coagulation factors. Acta. Med. Scand., 184:297, 1968.
109d. Corn, M.: Effect on phenobarbital and glutethimide on biological half-life of warfarin. Thromb. Diath. Haemorrh., 16:606, 1966.
109e. Taylor, P.J.: Hemorrhage while on anticoagulant therapy precipitated by drug interaction. Ariz. Med., 24:697, 1967.
109f. Feuer, E., and French, J.: Descriptive epidemiology of mortality in New Jersey due to combinations of codeine and glutethimide. Am. J. Epidemiol., 119:2:202, 1984.
109g. Sofie, R.D., and Barry, III, H.: The effects of SKF 525-A on the analgesic and barbiturate-potentiating activity of Δ-9-tetrahydrocannabinol in mice and rats. Pharmacology, 27:223, 1983.
110. Hollister, L.E., Richard, R.K., and Gillespie, H.K.: Comparison of tetrahydrocannabinol and synhexyl in man. Clin. Pharmacol. Ther., 9:783, 1968.
111. Brill, N.Q.: The marihuana problems. Ann. Intern. Med., 73:449, 1970.
111a. Sanz, P., Villar, P., and Repetto, M.: Effect of cannabis on enzyme induction by phenobarbital. Arch. Toxicol., Suppl. 6, 115, 1983.
112. Stoelting, R.K., et al.: Effects of delta-9-tetrahydrocannabinol on halothane MAC in dogs. Anesthesiology, 38:521, 1973.
113. Vitez, T.S., et al.: Effects of delta-9-tetrahydrocannabinol on cyclopropane MAC in the rat. Anesthesiology, 38:525, 1973.
114. Beaconsfield, P., Ginsburg, J., and Rainsbury, R.: Marihuana smoking. Cardiovascular effects in man and possible mechanisms. N. Engl. J. Med., 287:209, 1972.
115. Berman, M.L.: "Pot" and anesthetics—how do they mix. J.A.M.A., 220:914, 1972.
116. Lemberger, L., Axelrod, J., and Kopin, I.: Metabolism and disposition of delta-9-tetrahydrocannabinol in man. Pharmacol. Rev., 23:371, 1971.
117. Johnstone, R.E., et al.: Combination of Δ-9-Tetrahydrocannabinol with oxymorphone or pentobarbital: Effects on ventilatory control and cardiovascular dynamics. Anesthesiology, 42:674, 1975.

|21|

INTRAVENOUS ANESTHETIC AGENTS

J.G. REVES and IGOR KISSIN

No intravenous anesthetic induction agent is a total anesthetic. Total anesthesia requires several intravenous adjuvant drugs to accomplish the necessary degree of analgesia, hypnosis, amnesia, muscle paralysis, and attenuation of noxious reflexes. Hence, the potential for drug interactions is greatly increased with the use of these agents. Furthermore, patients who require intravenous induction may be also exposed to other pharmacologic agents which may provoke additional interactions. This chapter reviews the commonly used intravenous anesthetics, along with their interactions with each other and with other commonly used drugs.

THIOPENTAL

General Characteristics

Since its introduction in 1934, thiopental has become the most widely used agent for induction of anesthesia, owing to its rapid and usually predictable effect, lack of vascular irritation, and general safety. Despite its well-known potential for cardiovascular depression when administered rapidly in large doses, thiopental can produce minimal hemodynamic effects in normal patients or those with heart disease, provided it is administered slowly or by continuous infusion. The tachycardia that often accompanies the use of thiopental, however, may constitute a serious problem in patients with ischemic heart disease. The drug is biotransformed by the liver and has a relatively low hepatic extraction. Prompt awakening from thiopental is due to its rapid redistribution. Its distribution half-life is 2.5 minutes, while its elimination half-life varies from 5 to 12 hours. Thiopental's protein binding has been reported to vary from 72 to 86%. It appears to be inversely related to the dose of the drug; i.e., the larger the dose, the more restricted the protein binding. Thiopental remains the drug of choice for induction of anesthesia in healthy patients.

Interactions

Some of the potential perioperative interactions between thiopental and other drugs are pharmacokinetic in nature because the administration of one drug affects the elimination or distribution of the other, thus altering the concentration of that drug at the receptor site. For example, since the concentration of thiopental in the cerebral spinal fluid (CSF) is directly proportional to the concentration of the unbound thiopental in plasma,[1] a decrease in the protein binding of thiopental will increase its effect. Accordingly, the effect of thiopental is potentiated by the injection of contrast media. In 1956, McAfee and Willson[2] observed that the duration and depth of thiopental anesthesia after aortography were greater than usually seen in surgical patients receiving a similar dose of thiopental. Lasser et al.[3] found that, in rat experiments, several iodinated organic compounds used as contrast media prolong the duration of pentobarbital anesthesia. The authors suggested that the tendency of iodipamide to potentiate pentobarbital anesthesia is due to its ability to compete with barbiturates for the same binding sites on plasma proteins. Csogor and Kerek[4] demonstrated that sulfonamides can potentiate the effect of thiopental by a similar mechanism. They found that sulfafurasol decreased the hypnotic dose of thiopental in surgical patients. It has been reported also that chloramphenicol can prolong the action of thiopental and other barbiturates via an inhibition of hepatic mixed-function oxidases. This experimental finding, however, does not play a major role with usual clinical induction doses, since the effect is terminated by distribution.[5]

Thiopental can decrease the minimum alveolar concentration (MAC) of halothane in dogs. Eger et al.[6] found that an induction dose of thiopental (150 to 200 mg) reduced MAC by 5 to 20% for 2 to 4 hours. Rusy et al.[7] also reported that thiopental, 225 mg, decreased cyclopropane requirement for at least 45 minutes. Manani et al.[8] demonstrated that thiopental in large doses reduced the intensity of succinylcholine-induced fasciculations. The authors suggest that this phenomenon was due to a pharmacodynamic interaction between succinylcholine and thiopental consequent to thiopental's postsynaptic depressant effect at the neuromuscular junction. It is interesting to note, however, that thiopental did not affect the incidence and duration of succinylcholine-induced myalgia.

Data regarding the possible interaction between lithium and barbiturates have demonstrated that lithium significantly increased the duration of pentobarbital anesthesia in mice.[9] However, this interaction has not been studied in man.

METHOHEXITAL

General Characteristics

Methohexital is an ultrashort-acting methylbarbiturate. It is approximately three times as potent as thiopental and has similar actions and uses. Early claims of a less pronounced cardiovascular depression of methohexital versus thiopental have not been confirmed. Its most important advantage is the quicker recovery of consciousness. Methohexital is inactivated in the body more rapidly than thiopental and has an elimination half-life of 1 to 2 hours, as opposed to 6 hours for thiopental. The recovery of consciousness after a single dose of methohexital is due to the redistribution of the drug from the central nervous system into the muscle compartment mass. This process occurs more rapidly with methohexital than with thiopental. The protein binding of methohexital is identical to that of thiopental. Abnormal muscle movement and laryngospasm occur more frequently with methohexital than with thiopental.

Interactions

Since the induction of anesthesia with methohexital is followed by an appreciable incidence of excitatory effects (spontaneous involuntary muscle movement, rigidity, tremor), Dundee investigated the effect of a number of drugs that might affect the frequency and severity of the excitatory phenomena.[10] He observed that the incidence of excitatory effects was reduced by either premedication with meperidine or the administration of fentanyl immediately before the induction of anesthesia. According to this study, meperidine decreased the incidence of excitatory effects from 17 to 7%, while promethazine, hyoscine, and their combinations showed an opposite effect and increased the incidence of excitatory responses during anesthesia with methohexital. For example, when promethazine was given, methohexital 1.6 mg/kg^{-1} caused excitatory effects in 70% of the patients, as compared to 17% without.

KETAMINE

General Characteristics

Ketamine was developed in the United States and introduced into practice in 1970. It is a phencyclidine derivative whose anesthetic actions differ so markedly from barbiturates and other central nervous system depressants that Corssen and Domino defined its effects as "dissociative anesthesia."[11] Although ketamine produces rapid hypnosis and profound analgesia, respiratory and cardiovascular function are not depressed as much as with most other induction agents. Disturbing psychotomimetic activity (described as vivid dreams, hallucinations, or emergence phenomena), as well as undesirable increases in myocardial oxygen consumption and intracranial pressure, have limited its use.

Interactions

Stimulation of the cardiovascular system by ketamine is not always desirable, and a number of pharmacologic antagonists have been employed to block ketamine-induced tachycardia and systemic hypertension. Nishimura used adrenergic blocking drugs to attenuate the cardiovascular effects of ketamine[12] and found that the combination of propranolol (*beta*-blockade) and phenoxybenzamine (*alpha*-blockade) was superior to either drug alone as well as to trimethaphan or chlorpromazine in attenuating the increases in heart rate and blood pressure.[12] Droperidol (200 µg/kg IV) also blocks the hemodynamic response to ketamine apparently by a central sympathetic and peripheral *alpha*-adrenergic blockade.[13] The calcium-channel blocker and vasodilator, verapamil, successfully attenuates ketamine-induced hypertension, although it increases its tachycardic response.[13]

Perhaps the most useful approach to the prevention of ketamine-induced hypertension and tachycardia consists in the prior administration of benzodiazepines. Diazepam, flunitrazepam, or midazolam attenuates the hemodynamic effects of ketamine.[15-21] For example, in a study involving 16 patients with valvular heart disease, ketamine (2 mg/kg) did not produce significant hemodynamic changes when preceded by diazepam (0.4 mg/kg).[18] Indeed, heart rate, mean arterial blood pressure, and rate-pressure product were unchanged, although cardiac index was significantly reduced.[18] The combination of diazepam and ketamine rivals the recently introduced technique of high-dose fentanyl with regard to hemodynamic stability. When diazepam and ketamine were used concomitantly in cardiac surgery, hemodynamics remained stable. No patient experienced hallucinations, although 2% complained of dreams and 1% recalled events occurring in the operating room.[17] The combination of the new short-acting benzodiazepine, midazolam, with ketamine is attractive, since both possess relatively similar pharmacokinetic profiles.[15]

Many studies have examined the interaction between ketamine and other anesthetic drugs. In general, other agents, such as benzodiazepines, prevent the hemodynamic changes that occur during induction with ketamine. The administration of pentobarbital, 4 mg/kg, meperidine, 0.8 mg/kg, and scopolamine, 0.01 mg/kg, prior to ketamine, 2 mg/kg IV, attenuates the hypertension and tachycardia and maintains the ejection fraction in children with congenital heart disease.[22] Ketamine, 2 mg/kg, given to healthy patients anesthetized with halothane produced a 10 to 28% reduction in blood pressure, but no change in heart rate.[23-24] Cardiac index, stroke index, and blood pressure decreased when ketamine was administered to patients already anesthetized with halothane or enflurane. The hemodynamic depression produced by ketamine is more pronounced in the presence of halothane than enflurane.[24] A plausible explanation for this is that the inhalation drug blocks the ketamine-induced sympathetic hyperactivity, which normally antagonizes ketamine's direct myocardial depressant effects.

Ketamine produces a uniformly high incidence of illusions, but no hallucinations.[25] Illusion is defined as "the misinterpretation of a real, external sensory experience," while hallucination is defined as "a false sensory perception in the absence of an external sensory experience." The incidence of illusions and other emergence phenomena may be markedly reduced by the concomitant use of benzodiazepines or some other sedative hypnotic drugs, as illustrated in the following case report.[26-27]

CASE REPORT

A 30-year-old 60-kg woman sustained severe third-degree burns of the trunk and back. Care for this patient required frequent dressing changes, as well as painful debridements and grafting. On her first debridement procedure, the patient was anesthetized with intravenous ketamine, 120 mg, followed at 20- to 30-minute intervals by incremental doses of 20 mg during the hour-long procedure. Upon emergence from anesthesia in the recovery room, she appeared frightened and experienced vivid dreams related to her accident and other terrifying experiences. When seen on postoperative rounds, she requested some remedy for such unpleasant postanesthetic sequelae. For her next debridement and grafting operation, she received 15 mg of diazepam followed by 60 mg of ketamine and nitrous oxide plus oxygen 50:50 with one subsequent 30-mg injection of ketamine for the hour-long procedure. Emergence after this operation was completely normal, without dreams or illusions. On postoperative rounds, she thanked the anesthesiologist for such a pleasant experience.

Other Interactions

Ketamine and diazepam are pharmacokinetically interactive.[21,28] Both drugs are oxidized in the liver, and a competitive antagonism occurs when the two drugs are given concurrently. In man, this results in a prolongation of the elimination half-life of ketamine and its metabolites.[21] This pharmacokinetic response is also observed after premedication with hydroxyzine and secobarbital.[28] This phenomenon causes a prolongation of ketamine sleeptime. The half-life of ketamine is also extended by halothane anesthesia.[29]

A potential for interaction between ketamine and lithium exists.[30] Lithium is widely used to treat patients with affective disorders. Chronic lithium treatment of rats significantly prolongs the duration of ketamine anesthesia. This interaction apparently is mediated by dopamine, serotonin, or both in the central nervous system. The obvious clinical corollary is the avoidance of ketamine in lithium-treated patients. There is no information about the interaction in man, and one wonders if lithium may exacerbate emergence phenomena.

Ketamine reduces the MAC of halothane in a dose-related fashion. It is possible that this combination may prolong the anesthetic state. Some interactions between halothane and ketamine are listed in Table 21–1.[31] Ketamine may interact similarly with other inhalation anesthetics.

TABLE 21–1
Summary of Interaction Between Ketamine and Halothane

1.	Ketamine reduces the MAC of halothane.[29]
2.	Halothane prolongs the pharmacologic effects of ketamine.[75]
3.	Halothane decreases plasma clearance, redistribution, and metabolism of ketamine.[75]
4.	Ketamine causes hypotension when given during halothane anesthesia.[24,76]
5.	Ketamine and halothane both enhance the dysrhythmogenicity of epinephrine.[77]
6.	Ketamine and halothane both enhance a nondepolarizing neuromuscular blockade.[76]

DIAZEPAM

General Characteristics

Diazepam is probably the most widely used 1,4 benzodiazepine in the world. Synthesized by Leo H. Steinbach in 1959, it was introduced in the United States in 1963. The probable mechanism of action of diazepam and other benzodiazepines in the central nervous system is potentiation of the inhibitory effect of gamma-aminobutyric acid (GABA) on neuronal transmission[32] (see Chap. 20). All benzodiazepines show hypnotic, anticonvulsant, muscle relaxant, amnesic, and anxiolytic properties.

Pharmacokinetic Interactions

Of clinical importance is the administration of diazepam in combination with cimetidine, a histamine (H_2) blocker which is also a hepatic enzyme inhibitor. Cimetidine inhibits the plasma clearance of diazepam and prolongs the hypnotic effect.[33] Patients taking cimetidine have a significantly impaired plasma clearance of diazepam and a decreased volume of distribution.[33] These differences in kinetics were associated with marked changes in the effects of diazepam: cimetidine-treated patients manifest more pronounced sedation when compared with controls. The presumed mechanism resides in the binding of cimetidine to cytochrome P-450 oxidase, which is responsible for the clearance of diazepam and many other drugs as well.[34-35] However, Klotz examined the interaction between cimetidine and the steady-state kinetics of diazepam and observed a significant effect on the kinetics, but no effect on the dynamics of the drug.[36]

Another potentially important pharmacokinetically mediated interaction, particularly for patients who are undergoing cardiopulmonary bypass and who have received diazepam, is the increase in the free concentration of diazepam after the administration of heparin.[37] There is a three-fold increase in the free concentration of diazepam after the intravenous administration of 1,000 units of heparin. It is not clear whether this increase explains the transient hypotension that occurs after the administration of heparin.[38] Since diazepam is a vasodilator, however, an increase in its free concentration may induce a decrease in blood pressure. The mechanism of action may depend on a heparin-induced release of free fatty acids, which may displace diazepam from its binding sites (presumably on albumin).[37]

Cardiopulmonary Interactions

CASE REPORT

A 52-year-old male was scheduled for elective coronary artery bypass grafting. He had a history of stable angina for which he took only nitroglycerin as needed. Cardiac catheterization showed good ventricular function with an angiographic ejection fraction of 0.50. He received a preanesthetic medication consisting of morphine (10 mg IM) and scopolamine (0.3 mg IM). His resting heart rate on entrance into the operating room was 75, and blood pressure was 120/70. After insertion of pulmonary and radial arterial catheters, anesthesia was induced with diazepam, 0.13 mg/kg intravenously. Four minutes later, an infusion of fentanyl (0.4 mg/min) was begun and metocurine (0.4 mg/kg IV) was given. After the patient had received 25 µg/kg of fentanyl, the mean arterial pressure decreased from 100 to 60 mm Hg. The hypotension was treated with phenylephrine and the fentanyl infusion resumed.

Although diazepam may be safely combined with other anesthetic drugs, there is some potential for hemodynamic depression, a phenomenon particularly well documented with the opiates.[39] The effect of the combination of diazepam and morphine in patients with ischemic heart disease (IHD)[40-41] and valvular heart disease[42] has been reported. The administration of diazepam, 0.25 to 0.35 mg/kg, over 10 minutes, to patients who have IHD and are anesthetized with morphine, 3 mg/kg, did not change the heart rate, mean aortic pressure, pulmonary arterial pressure, pulmonary vascular resistance, or systemic vascular resistance and produced modest decreases in mean arterial blood pressure (84 to 73 mm Hg) and cardiac index (2.91 to 2.36 L/min/m²).

Diazepam and fentanyl interact to produce significant hemodynamic changes. Diazepam (10 mg) administered to patients who have mitral valvular disease and who are anesthetized with fentanyl (up to 50 µg/kg) produced mild, but statistically significant, hemodynamic depression of cardiac output (21%), mean arterial blood pressure (10%), and stroke volume (17%), while heart rate was unchanged.[43] The induction of anesthesia with a combination of diazepam and 50% nitrous oxide in oxygen produced hemodynamic changes similar to those consequent to induction with diazepam alone, except that adding N_2O caused a greater decrease in the mean arterial pressure and left ventricular stroke work index. These variables are unchanged by diazepam alone, but decrease with N_2O alone (Fig. 21–1).[44-45] There is one reported case of profound hypotension induced by the administration of diazepam and N_2O.[46] This, however, appears to be an exception rather than common type of response.[46]

Diazepam (0.5 mg/kg IV)[44-45] per se, produces minimal hemodynamic effects in patients with ischemic or valvular heart disease. Similarly, fentanyl, in doses up to 100 µg/kg, produces little or no hemodynamic change.[43,47-49] Given together, however, the two drugs, even in lower doses,[50] significantly reduce systemic vascular resistance and BP (Fig. 21–2). This interaction appears to be "synergistic," since the combination of small doses of each drug produces greater hemodynamic effects than much larger doses of the single drug. The mechanism of this interaction is probably related to diminished release of epinephrine occurring when diazepam is given to patients receiving fentanyl.[50] Singly, each drug can cause a dose-related decrease in myocardial contractility, in concentrations much higher than clinically obtainable.[51] The combination of fentanyl and diazepam induces an additive negative inotropic effect (Fig. 21–3). It appears that, whatever the underlying mechanism, the net result is a synergistic vasodilation that causes an unpredicted, greater decrease in systemic vascular resistance and mean arterial pressure.

There is preliminary evidence that diazepam and fentanyl also manifest respiratory depressant interactions. Small doses of diazepam (0.1 mg/kg IV) and fentanyl (2 µg/kg IV) depress the slope of minute-ventilation/end-tidal CO_2 (V_E/ET CO_2) curves in healthy volunteers.[52] The combination of drugs produces greater depression in V_E/ET CO_2 (53% of control) than diazepam (76% of control) and fentanyl (66% of control). This interaction, however, is purely additive, since the respiratory depression is equal to the sum of the effects of both agents given separately. This means that the dose of each drug should be reduced. It is not known how this combination would interact in elderly patients or in those with lung disease, but caution in prescribing the combination in these patients seems warranted.

Effect of Diazepam on MAC of Halothane and on Muscle Relaxants

Diazepam, 0.2 mg/kg, given intravenously, decreases the minimum alveolar concentration (MAC) of halothane in man by approximately 34%.[53] Doubling the dose of diazepam did not alter this effect. One possible mechanism is the effect of diazepam on gamma-aminobutyric acid (GABA) in the CNS.[32] Since the diazepam was administered after an induction with halothane, the precise relevance for diazepam used as a preanesthetic medication or as an induction agent is unknown, although the former use may be quite valid, using a moderate dose of diazepam.

Any postulated effect of benzodiazepines on muscle relaxants is thought to be related to the potentiation of GABA.[32] It has been established, however, that the administration of diazepam does not significantly affect the neuromuscular blockade from succinylcholine or from nondepolarizing muscle relaxants such as pancuronium and curare.[54-55]

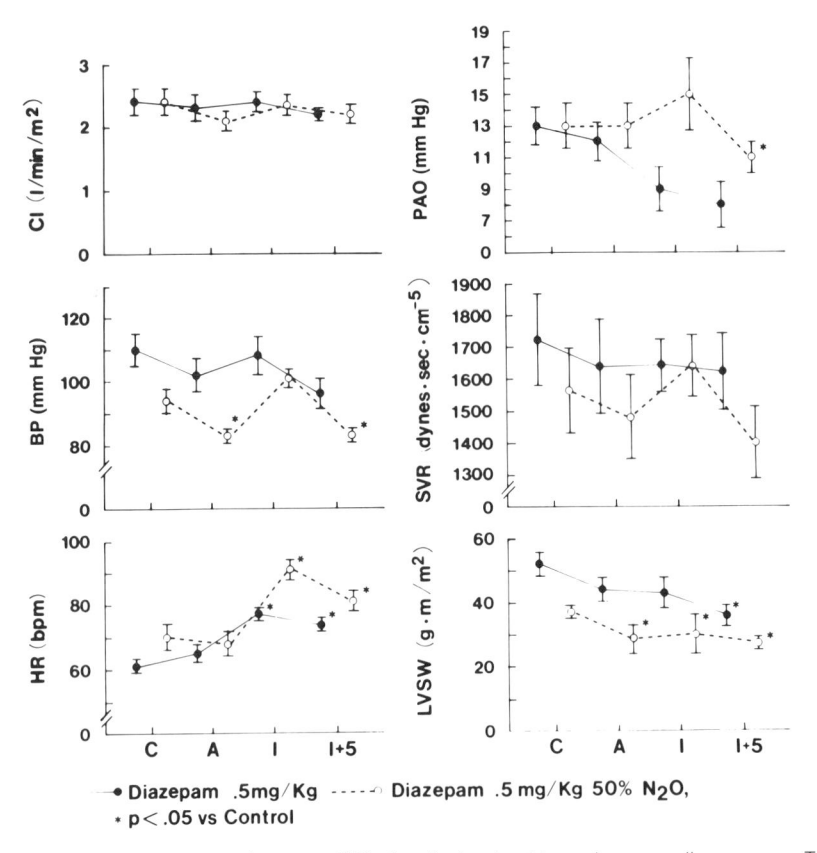

Fig. 21–1. Hemodynamic response (mean ± SD) of patients about to undergo cardiac surgery. Ten patients were anesthetized with diazepam and oxygen, and 10 patients were anesthetized with diazepam and N$_2$O:O$_2$ (50:50). Note that addition of N$_2$O reduced blood pressure significantly and tended to elevate PAO and lower SVR. C = control, A = anesthesia induction, I = intubation, I+5 = intubation plus 5 minutes, PAO = pulmonary artery occluded pressure, LVSW = left ventricular stroke work, CI = cardiac index, HR = heart rate. (Reproduced with permission from Reves, J.G., and Kissin, I.: Pharmacology of anesthetic drugs: intravenous anesthetics. In Cardiac Anesthesia. Vol. 2. Edited by J.A. Kaplan. New York, Grune & Stratton, 1983.)

MIDAZOLAM

General Characteristics

Midazolam is a water-soluble benzodiazepine that was synthesized in 1975. It is unique among the benzodiazepines because of its water solubility, rapid onset, short duration of action, and relatively rapid plasma clearance.[56] Midazolam is biotransformed in the liver to four known metabolites,[57] some of which are active, although less active and shorter acting than the parent compound.

Interactions

Because midazolam is still a relatively new drug, little is known about its interactions with other drugs. Premedication with morphine and scopolamine decreases time required to induce anesthesia.[56] The combination of N$_2$O (50%) with midazolam (0.2 mg/kg) does not produce cardiovascular depression.[45] The safety of the combination of N$_2$O and midazolam contrasts to the well-known additive depression of N$_2$O and narcotics.[47,58] Patients tolerate midazolam plus halothane[59] although dP/dt max does decrease.[60] Midazolam, 0.15 mg/kg, and ketamine, 1.5 mg/kg, have proved to be a safe and useful combination for a rapid-sequence induction for emergency surgery.[15] This method appeared to be superior to thiopental alone, since it

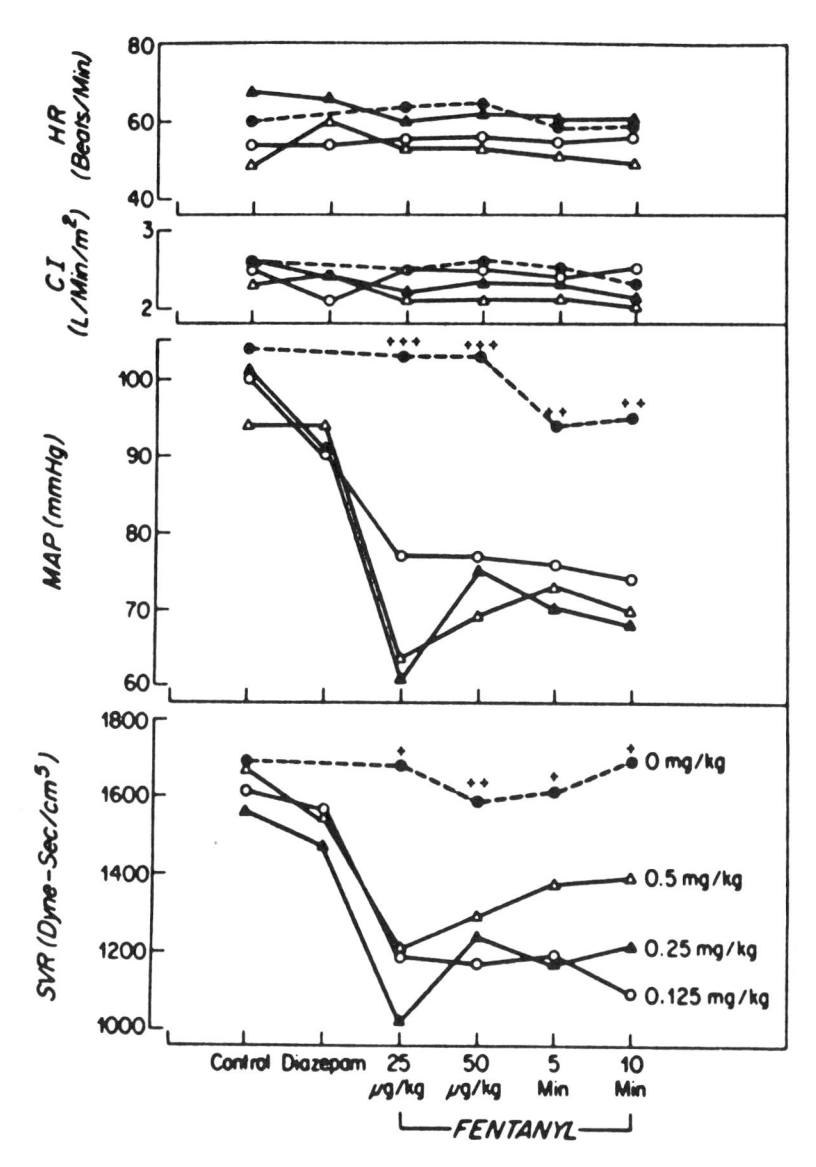

Fig. 21–2. Hemodynamic data for four groups of patients: group 1, control, no diazepam; group 2, 0.125 mg/kg^{-1} diazepam; group 3, 0.25 mg/kg^{-1} diazepam; and group 4, 0.5 mg/kg^{-1} diazepam. Significant intergroup difference designated by + ($p < 0.05$), + + ($p < 0.01$), or + + + ($p < 0.001$). Note that there is a significant reduction in SVR and MAP when fentanyl and diazepam are combined. The diazepam effect is not dose related. HR = heart rate, MAP = mean arterial pressure, CI = cardiac index, and SVR = systemic vascular resistance. (Reprinted with permission from the International Anesthesia Research Society from Diazepam and fentanyl interaction–hemodynamic and hormonal effects in coronary artery surgery, by R.C. Tomicheck, et al., Anesth. Analg., 62:881, 1983.)

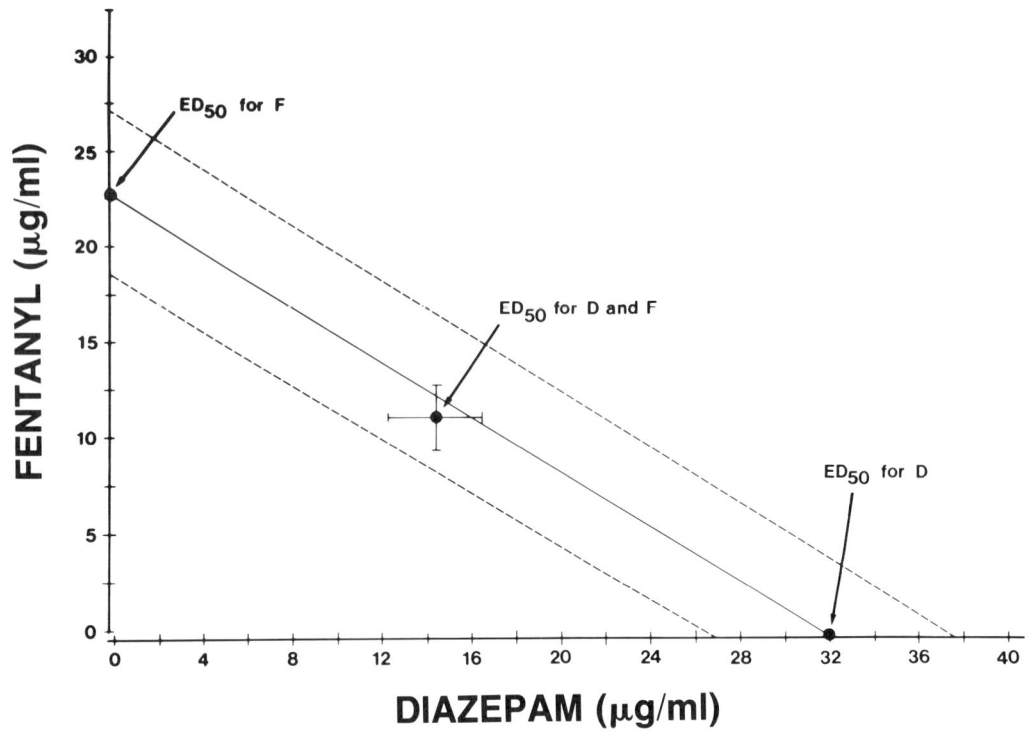

Fig. 21-3. Isobologram for the interaction between the negative inotropic effects of fentanyl and diazepam at ED_{50} level (50% decrease from control in dP/dt_{max}). ED_{50} values for fentanyl and diazepam alone are plotted on the ordinate and abscissa, respectively. ED_{50} for an equipotent combination of fentanyl and diazepam is plotted in the dose field. The ED_{50} additive line was generated by connecting the ED_{50} for fentanyl with the ED_{50} for diazepam (solid line). All ED_{50} points are plotted with SD. The dotted lines connect the end points of 67% confidence limits for fentanyl and diazepam. Note that the combined drug value falls along the additive line, indicating that the combination of fentanyl and diazepam has an additive negative inotropic effect at ED_{50}. Had the point been above and to the right of the additive line, the interaction would have been infraadditive, and had it been to the left and under the additive line, the interaction would have been supraadditive. (Reprinted with permission from the International Anesthesia Research Society from Additive negative inotropic effect of a combination of diazepam and fentanyl, by J.G. Reves, et al., Anesth. Analg., 63:97, 1984.)

caused less cardiovascular depression, more amnesia, and less postoperative somnolence. Midazolam can be safely combined with etomidate, fentanyl, and $N_2O:O_2(2:1)$.[61] After induction with midazolam, endotracheal intubation produces tachycardia and hypertension. The administration of fentanyl, 5 to 7.5 μg/kg, before endotracheal intubation blocks this sympathetic response.

It appears that midazolam, like diazepam, has little effect on succinylcholine and pancuronium neuromuscular blockade.[62-63] After the administration of midazolam, the doses of pancuronium and succinylcholine are not different from those required after thiopental. Therefore, the muscle-relaxant properties of midazolam do not seem to have clinically important effects on neuromuscular blocking drugs administered during anesthesia.

When given 35 to 45 minutes before the incision, midazolam, 0.6 mg/kg, decreases the MAC of halothane[64] by approximately 30%. Since midazolam has a relatively short half-life, the effect of MAC might have been greater had the administration and incision times been closer together. The fact that the dose used, 0.6 mg/kg, is about three times that required for induction may partly compensate for this relatively long interval, however. Apnea[65] and respiratory depression induced by midazolam are more likely to occur in patients given opiates for preanesthetic medication. The use of the opiates fentanyl[66] and alfentanil[67] reduces the induction dose of midazolam and the interindividual variation in response to a given dose of midazolam. The use of opiates tends to prolong the recovery from midazolam, however.[68]

ETOMIDATE

General Characteristics

Etomidate, a carboxylated imidazol derivative, has a rapid onset (one circulation time) and brief duration of action. In comparative studies with other anesthetic drugs, etomidate is usually characterized as the drug that affects cardiovascular variables the least. However, in dogs[69] etomidate produced a dose-dependent depression of myocardial contractility. The presence of valvular heart disease may influence the hemodynamic responses to etomidate, and its cardiodepressant potential may be realized more frequently than in healthy patients. Etomidate is hydrolyzed primarily in the liver, although some breakdown takes place in the blood as well. Pharmacokinetic investigations revealed that etomidate is rapidly distributed, with a distribution half-life of approximately 3 minutes, and an elimination half-life of about 4 hours. Etomidate's binding to serum albumin is approximately 80%. The administration of etomidate was accompanied by a significant incidence of venous sequelae, which probably is higher than with most other drugs. Myoclonic movements after administration of etomidate are also rather high (approximately 40 to 50%). They are not associated with an epileptiform pattern on EEG. None of these complications is sufficiently severe, however, to prohibit the use of etomidate.

Interactions

The cardiovascular effects of etomidate are not significantly altered by the simultaneous administration of many other anesthetic drugs, although the drug has not been systematically studied with all agents. The administration of 66% N_2O and oxygen has little effect on the hemodynamic changes observed after induction with etomidate.[70] Nor does the presence of basal neuroleptanesthesia produce any effect.[71] Etomidate, 0.3 mg/kg, reduced the dP/dt 18% in patients anesthetized with neurolept drugs, but there was no change in either heart rate or blood pressure. Systemic vascular resistance and left ventricular dP/dt decreased when etomidate, 0.3 mg/kg, was given to normal patients anesthetized with halothane 0.3% in 66% nitrous oxide.[72]

A number of investigations, including Dundee's,[73] evaluated the effects of various preanesthetic medications on the spontaneous involuntary muscle movements, tremor, and hypertonus often noted after induction with etomidate. He showed that, compared with unpremedicated patients, diazepam reduced the incidence of excitatory effects. Dundee also observed that meperidine caused an even greater reduction of this involuntary muscle movement. Premedication with meperidine decreased the incidence of excitatory effects from 80% without meperidine to 30% with meperidine. Other studies indicate that fentanyl can also reduce the incidence of myoclonic movements. Unfortunately, the pain on intravenous administration of etomidate can be decreased but not eliminated by pretreatment with fentanyl.[74]

Summary

From the foregoing discussion, it is evident that a variety of drug interactions involving intravenous anesthetics may occur. Some of these interactions involve pharmacokinetics, but have no major pharmacodynamic effect. Some of the dynamic actions are potentially hazardous, while others may be beneficial. The anesthesiologist should make use of this knowledge in choosing the particular combinations of drugs, as well as the doses of these drugs.

REFERENCES

1. Brodie, B.B., Kurz, H., and Schanker, L.: The importance of dissociation constant and lipid-solubility in influencing the passage of drugs into the cerebrospinal fluid. J. Pharmacol. Exp. Ther. 130:20, 1960.
2. McAfee, J.G., and Willson, J.K.V.: A review of the complications of translumbar aortography. Am. J. Roentgenol. 75:956, 1956.
3. Lasser, E.C., Elizondo-Martel, G., and Granke, R.C.: Potentiation of pentobarbital anesthesia by competitive protein binding. Anesthesiology. 24:665, 1963.
4. Csogor, S.I., and Kerek, S.F.: Enhancement of thiopentone anaesthesia by sulphafurazole. Br. J. Anaesth. 42:988, 1970.
5. Reiche, R., and Frey, H.H.: Interactions between chloramphenicol and intravenous anesthetics. Anaesthesist. 30:504, 1981.
6. Eger, E.I., II, Saidman, L.J., and Brandstater, B.: Minimum alveolar anesthetic concentration: A standard of anesthetic potency. Anesthesiology. 26:756, 1965.
7. Rusy, B.F., Witherspoon, C.D., Montaner, C.G., et al.: Effect of reserpine on cardiac function during thiopental-cyclopropane anesthesia in the dog. Anesthesiology. 26:14, 1965.
8. Manani, G., Valenti, S., Segatto, A., et al.: The influence of thiopentone and alfathesin on succinylcholine-induced fasciculations and myalgias. Can. Anaesth. Soc. J. 28:253, 1981.
9. Diamond, B.I., Havdala, H.S., and Borison, R.L.: Potential of lithium as anaesthetic premedicant. Lancet 2:1229, 1977.
10. Dundee, J.W.: The present status of barbiturates. In Intravenous Anaesthetic Agents. London, Edward Arnold Ltd., 1979, p. 6.
11. Corssen, G., and Domino, E.F.: Dissociative anesthesia: further pharmacologic studies and first clinical experience with the phencyclidine derivative CI-581. Anesth. Analg. 45:29, 1966.
12. Nishimura, K., Kitamura, Y., Hamai, R., et al.: Pharmacological studies of ketamine hydrochloride in the cardiovascular system. Osaka City Med. J. 19:17, 1973.
13. Balfors, E., Haggmark, S., Nyhman, H., et al.: Droperidol inhibits the effects of intravenous ketamine on central hemodynamics and myocardial oxygen consumption in patients with generalized atherosclerotic disease. Anesth. Analg. 62:193, 1983.
14. Johnstone, M.: The cardiovascular effects of ketamine in man. Anaesthesia 31:873, 1976.
15. White, P.F.: Comparative evaluation of intravenous agents for rapid sequence induction—thiopental, ketamine and midazolam. Anesthesiology. 57:279, 1982.
16. Jackson, A.P.F., Dhadphale, P.R., Callaghan, M.L., et al.: Haemodynamic studies during induction of anaesthesia for open-heart surgery using diazepam and ketamine. Br. J. Anaesth. 50:375, 1978.
17. Hatano, S., Keane, D.M., Boggs, R.E., et al.: Diazepam-ketamine anaesthesia for open heart surgery a "micro-mini" drip administration technique. Can. Anaesth. Soc. J. 23:648, 1976.
18. Dhadphale, P.R., Jackson, A.P.F., and Alseri, S.: Comparison of anesthesia with diazepam and ketamine vs morphine in patients undergoing heart-valve replacement. Anesthesiology. 51:200, 1979.
19. Kumar, S.M., Kothary, S.P., and Zsigmond, E.K.: Plasma free norepinephrine and epinephrine concentrations following diazepam-ketamine induction in patients undergoing cardiac surgery. Acta. Anaesth. Scand. 22:593, 1978.
20. Freuchen, I., Ostergaard, J., Kohl, J.B., et al.: Reduction of psychotomimetic side effects of ketalar (ketamine) by rohypnol (flunitrazepam). Acta Anaesth. Scand. 20:97, 1976.
21. Idvall, J., Aronsen, K.F., Stenberg, P., et al.: Pharmacodynamic and pharmacokinetic interactions between ketamine and diazepam. Eur. J. Clin. Pharmacol. 24:337, 1983.
22. Bini, M., Reves, J.G., Berry, D., et al.: Ejection fraction during ketamine anesthesia in congenital heart diseased patients. Anesth. Analg. 63:186, 1984.
23. Stanley, T.H.: Blood-pressure and pulse-rate responses to ketamine during general anesthesia. Anesthesiology. 39:648, 1973.
24. Bidwai, A.V., Stanley, T.H., Graves, C.L., et al.: The effects of ketamine on cardiovascular dynamics during halothane and enflurane anesthesia. Anesth. Analg. 54:588, 1975.
25. Garfield, J.M., Garfield, F.B., Stone, J.G., et al.: A comparison of psychologic responses to ketamine and thiopental-nitrous oxide-halothane anesthesia. Anesthesiology. 36:329, 1972.
26. Kothary, S.P., and Zsigmond, E.K.: A double-blind study of the effective antihallucinatory doses of diazepam prior to ketamine anesthesia. Clin. Pharmacol. Ther. 21:108, 1977.
27. Liang, H.S., and Liang, H.G.: Minimizing emergence phenomena: Subdissociative dosage of ketamine in balanced surgical anesthesia. Anesth. Analg. 54:312, 1975.
28. Lo, J.N., and Cumming, J.F.: Interaction between sedative premedicants and ketamine in man and in isolated perfused rat livers. Anesthesiology. 43:307, 1975.
29. White, P.F., Johnston, R.R., and Pudwill, C.R.: Interaction of ketamine and halothane in rats. Anesthesiology. 42:179, 1975.
30. Rubin, E.H., and Wooten, G.F.: Lithium-ketamine interaction: An animal study of potential clinical and theoretical interest. J. Clin. Psychopharmacol. 2:211, 1982.
31. Miller, R.D., and Booij, L.D.H.J.: Intravenous agents. In Drug Interactions in Anesthesia. Edited

by Smith, N.T., Miller, R.D., Corbascio, A.N., Philadelphia, Lea & Febiger, 1981, pp. 211–220.
32. Richter, J.J.: Current theories about the mechanisms of benzodiazepines and neuroleptic drugs. Anesthesiology. 54:66, 1981.
33. Klotz, U., and Reimann, I.: Delayed clearance of diazepam due to cimetidine. N. Engl. J. Med. 302:1012, 1980.
34. Ruffalo, R.L., Thompson, J.F., and Segal, J.L.: Diazepam-cimetidine drug interaction: A clinically significant effect. South. Med. J. 74:1075, 1981.
35. Feely, J.: Interaction of cimetidine with other drugs. South. Med. J. 76:753, 1983.
36. Klotz, U., and Reimann, I.: Elevation of steady-state diazepam levels by cimetidine. Clin. Pharmacol. Ther. 30:513, 1981.
37. Routledge, P.A., Kitchell, B.B.: Bjornsson, T.D., et al.: Diazepam and N-desmethyldiazepam redistribution after heparin. Clin. Pharmacol. Ther. 27:528, 1980.
38. Konchigeri, H.N.: Hemodynamic effects of heparin in patients undergoing cardiac surgery. Anesth. Analg. 63:235, 1984.
39. Stanley, T.H.: Pharmacology of intravenous narcotic anesthetics. Anesthesia. Volume 1. Edited by Miller, R.D. New York, Churchill Livingstone, 1981, pp. 425–449.
40. Melsom, M., Andreassen, P., Melsom, H., et al.: Diazepam in acute myocardial infarction. Clinical effects and effects on catecholamines, free fatty acids, and cortisol. Br. Heart J. 38:804, 1976.
41. Hoar, P.F., Nelson, N.T., Mangano, D.T., et al.: Adrenergic response to morphine-diazepam anesthesia for myocardial revascularization. Anesth. Analg. 60:406, 1981.
42. Stanley, T.H., Bennett, G.M., Loeser, E.A., et al.: Cardiovascular effects of diazepam and droperidol during morphine anesthesia. Anesthesiology. 44:255, 1976.
43. Stanley, T.H., and Webster, L.R.: Anesthetic requirements and cardiovascular effects of fentanyl-oxygen and fentanyl-diazepam-oxygen anesthesia in man. Anesth. Analg. 57:411, 1978.
44. Samuelson, P.N., Lell, W.A., Kouchoukos, N.T., et al.: Hemodynamics during diazepam induction of anesthesia for coronary artery bypass grafting. South. Med. J. 73:332, 1980.
45. Samuelson, P.N., Reves, J.G., Kouchoukos, N.T., et al.: Hemodynamic responses to anesthetic induction with midazolam or diazepam in patients with ischemic heart disease. Anesth. Analg. 60:802, 1981.
46. Falk, R.B., Jr., Denlinger, J.K., Nahrwold, M.L., et al.: Acute vasodilation following induction of anesthesia with intravenous diazepam and nitrous oxide. Anesthesiology. 49:149, 1978.
47. Lunn, J.K., Stanley, T.H., Eisele, J., et al.: High dose fentanyl anesthesia for coronary artery surgery: plasma fentanyl concentrations and influence of nitrous oxide on cardiovascular responses. Anesth. Analg. 58:390, 1979.
48. Waller, J.L., Hug, C.C. Jr., Nagle, D.M., et al.: Hemodynamic changes during fentanyl-oxygen anesthesia for aortocoronary bypass operation. Anesthesiology. 55:212, 1981.
49. Sebel, P.S., Bovill, J.G., Boekhorst, R.A.A., et al.: Cardiovascular effects of high-dose fentanyl anaesthesia. Acta Anaesthesiol. Scand., 26:308, 1982.
50. Tomicheck, R.C., Rosow, C.E., Philbin, D.M., et al.: Diazepam-fentanyl interaction-hemodynamic and hormonal effects in coronary artery surgery. Anesth. Analg. 62:881, 1983.
51. Reves, J.G., Kissin, I., Fournier, S.E., et al.: Additive negative inotropic effect of a combination of diazepam and fentanyl. Anesth. Analg. 63:97, 1984.
52. Bailey, P.L., Andriano, K.P., Pace, N.L., et al.: Small doses of fentanyl potentiate and prolong diazepam induced respiratory depression. Anesth. Analg. 63:175, 1984.
53. Perisho, J.A., Buechel, D.R., and Miller, R.D.: The effect of diazepam (Valium) on minimum alveolar anaesthetic requirement (MAC) in man. Can. Anaesth. Soc. J. 18:536, 1971.
54. Asbury, A.J., Henderson, P.D., Brown, B.H., et al.: Effect of diazepam on pancuronium-induced neuromuscular blockade maintained by a feedback system. Br. J. Anaesth. 53:859, 1981.
55. Bradshaw, E.G., and Maddison, S.: Effect of diazepam at the neuromuscular junction. A clinical study. Br. J. Anaesth. 51:955, 1979.
56. Reves, J.G., Samuelson, P.N., and Vinik, H.R.: Midazolam, New Pharmacologic Vistas in Anesthesia, Contemporary Anesthesia Practice. Edited by Brown, B.R. Jr. Philadelphia, F.A. Davis Co., 1983, pp. 147–162.
57. Woo, G.K., Kolis, S.J., and Schwartz, M.A.: In vitro metabolism of an imidazobenzodiazepine. Pharmacologist 19:164, 1977.
58. Lappas, D.G., Buckley, M.J., Laver, M.B., et al.: Left ventricular performance and pulmonary circulation following addition of nitrous oxide to morphine during coronary-artery surgery. Anesthesiology. 43:61, 1975.
59. Melvin, M.A., Johnson, B.H., Quasha, A.L., et al.: Induction of anesthesia with midazolam decreases halothane MAC in man. Anesthesiology 53:S10, 1980.
60. Hilfiker, O., and Kettler, D.: Die wirkung von midazolam auf die allgemeine hamodynamik und die hirndurchblutung beim tier und beim menschen. Arzneim Forsch Drug Res. 31:2236, 1981.
61. Massaut, J, d'Hollander, A., Barvais, L., et al.: Haemodynamic effects of midazolam in the anaesthetized patient with coronary artery disease. Acta Anaesthesiol. Scand. 27:299, 1983.
62. Cronnelly, R., Morris, R.B., and Miller, R.D.: Comparison of thiopental and midazolam on the neuromuscular responses to succinylcholine or pancuronium in humans. Anesth. Analg. 62:75, 1983.
63. Reves, J.G., Vinik, R., Hirschfield, A.M., et al.: Midazolam compared with thiopentone as a hypnotic component in balanced anaesthesia: A randomized, double-blind study. Can. Anaesth. Soc. J. 26:42, 1979.

64. Melvin, M.A., Johnson, B.H., Quasha, A.L., et al.: Induction of anesthesia with midazolam decreases halothane MAC in humans. Anesthesiology 57:238, 1982.
65. Kanto, J., Sjovall, S., and Vuori, A.: Effect of different kinds of premedication on the induction properties of midazolam. Br. J. Anaesth. 54:507, 1982.
66. Fragen, R.J., and Caldwell, N.J.: Awakening characteristics following anesthesia induction with midazolam for short surgical procedures. Arzneim Forsch. Drug Res. 31:2261, 1981.
67. De Castro, P.J., Andrieu, S., Dubois, A., et al.: Etude du midazolam comme inducteur, correcteur et potentialisateur d'une anesthesie analgesique a base d'alfentanil. Arzneim Forsch. Drug Res. 31:2251, 1981.
68. deJong, R.H., and Bonin, J.D.: Benzodiazepines protect mice from local anesthetic convulsions and deaths. Anesth. Analg. 60:385, 1981.
69. Kissin, I., Motomura, S., Aultman, D.F., et al.: Inotropic and anesthetic potencies of etomidate and thiopental in dogs. Anesth. Analg. 62:961, 1983.
70. Firestone, S., Kleinman, C.S., Jaffe, C.C., et al.: Human research and noninvasive measurement of ventricular performance: An echocardiographic evaluation of etomidate and thiopental. Anesthesiology. 51:S22, 1979.
71. Hempelmann, G., Piepenbrock, S., Hempelmann, W., et al.: Influence of althesine and etomidate on blood gases (continuous PO_2-monitoring) and hemodynamics in man. Acta Anaesth. Belg. 25:402, 1974.
72. Patschke, D., Bruckner, J.B., Eberlein, H.J., et al.: Effects of althesin, etomidate and fentanyl on haemodynamics and myocardial oxygen consumption in man. Can. Anaesth. Soc. J. 24:57, 1977.
73. Dundee, J.W.: Etomidate, Intravenous Anaesthetic Agents. London, Edward Arnold Ltd., 1979, p. 52.
74. Stanley, T.H.: Pharmacology of intravenous nonnarcotic anesthetics. In Anesthesia. Volume 1. Edited by Miller, R.D. New York, Churchill Livingstone, 1981, p. 471.
75. White, P.F., Marietta, M.P., Pudwill, C.R., et al.: Effects of halothane anesthesia on the biodisposition of ketamine in rats. J. Pharmacol. Exp. Ther. 196:545, 1976.
76. Johnston, R.R., Miller, R.D., and Way, W.L.: The interaction of ketamine with d-tubocurarine, pancuronium and succinylcholine in man. Anesth. Analg. 53:496, 1974.
77. Koehntop, D.E., Liao, J.C., and Van Bergen, F.H.: Effects of pharmacologic alterations of adrenergic mechanisms by cocaine, tropolone, aminophylline, and ketamine on epinephrine-induced arrhythmias during halothane-nitrous oxide anesthesia. Anesthesiology. 46:83, 1977.
78. Reves, J.G., and Kissin, I.: Pharmacology of anesthetic drugs: intravenous anesthetics. In Cardiac Anesthesia: Vol. 2. Edited by Kaplan, J.A. New York, Grune & Stratton, Inc., 1983, pp. 3–29.

22

NARCOTICS AND NARCOTIC ANTAGONISTS

CARL C. HUG, JR. and DAVID E. LONGNECKER

Narcotic analgesics are widely used in the practice of medicine, in anesthesia in particular and in nonmedical circumstances (so-called "street use"), where their abuse is frequent. There are two fundamental pharmacologic actions of narcotics that account for their widespread use: analgesia and euphoria. Perhaps the most striking examples of the use of opiates as analgesics are the high-dose narcotic techniques frequently employed in anesthesia for cardiovascular surgery. On the other end of the spectrum, the illicit user of narcotics consumes these drugs for their euphoric effect rather than for their analgesic properties. The most frequent medical applications for narcotics are in cases where both analgesia and euphoria are desirable. The alleviation of acute or chronic pain by narcotics results from both properties of these compounds and accounts for their prevalent use in medical practice.

Because opiates are used so commonly, the potential for significant interactions with other drugs is considerable. Although many interactions with opiates may occur, some of the most important involve their analogues, the narcotic antagonists. Narcotic antagonists antagonize both the acute and chronic effects of narcotic analgesics. In persons who suffer from narcotic addiction, the antagonists are used to prevent the euphoria that the abuser craves and to antagonize toxic side effects. In the physically dependent addict, a narcotic antagonist precipitates an acute abstinence syndrome. In anesthetic practice, the antagonists are used postoperatively to treat respiratory depression that remains from the intraoperative administration of narcotic analgesics.

The classification of narcotic drugs as (pure) agonists or partial agonists (agonist-antagonists) refers to their effects when binding to the opiate receptor sites (see below). Narcotic analogues which lack any intrinsic effect when binding to the opiate receptors are called (pure) antagonists (examples are naloxone and naltrexone). This chapter reviews briefly: (1) the pharmacology of the narcotic agonists and illustrates some drug-drug interactions that may occur with narcotic agents; (2) the pharmacology and interactions of narcotic agonist-antagonist analgesics; and (3) the pharmacology of narcotic antagonists and their interactions with narcotic and other drugs.

NARCOTIC AGONISTS

Pharmacology

CNS. Narcotic agonists and antagonists are used and abused mainly because of their CNS effects. The major therapeutic use of opiates is the alleviation of pain, an indication for which they are uniquely effective. Although there is some evidence that narcotics may act peripherally, it is generally believed that the principal site of action of opiates is in the CNS. They possess not only intrinsic analgesic properties, but also the ability to modify the perception of pain.

In the absence of pain, opiates can induce a state of euphoria and apathy or more frequently dysphoria. If the dose of the narcotic is increased, progressive drowsiness, inability to concentrate, mental clouding, and, finally, loss of consciousness occur. All narcotics administered in large enough doses can induce convulsions.[1] This has seldom, if ever, been observed in man except for a few anecdotal reports (without EEG documentation) of "seizures" following bolus injections of fentanyl, and even these reports have been called into question.[2,3]

Cardiovascular System. The widespread and growing use of narcotic anesthetic techniques in patients with impaired myocardial performance attests to the mildness of their effects on the human cardiovascular system.[4,5] In general, arterial blood pressure, heart rate, heart rhythm, and cardiac output are not altered by opiates if the recipient is recumbent. In the standing position, however, hypotension is likely to follow the administration of opiates. Such hypotension is due primarily to the peripheral vascular effects of opiates on the capacitance vessels, with pooling of blood in dependent veins and a consequent decrease in venous return, cardiac output, and arterial blood pressure.

Another important hypotensive mechanism of certain opiates is related to their tendency toward endogenous histamine release. Flacke et al.[6] studied the release of histamine in patients receiving equipotent doses of meperidine, morphine, fentanyl, or sufentanil (a new, more potent fentanyl analogue). Fentanyl and sufentanil administration did not result in significant histamine liberation. However, in 10% of morphine-treated and 42% of meperidine-treated patients, the authors observed a significant increase in plasma histamine levels. Pretreatment with histamine receptor (H-1 and H-2) blocking drugs can prevent the possible hazards of histamine release secondary to narcotic administration.

Respiratory System. Because of its potentially lethal consequences, respiratory depression is perhaps one of the most important components of the pharmacology of narcotics. Marked slowing of respiratory rate or even complete apnea may occur with large doses of opiates. Respiratory depression results from direct effects of the drugs on the respiratory control centers in the central nervous system. Ventilatory depression is rapid in onset and has been shown to persist for several hours when sensitive tests, such as the carbon dioxide challenge test, are used to evaluate respiratory function. Death from narcotic overdose is almost invariably due to respiratory depression.

Miscellaneous Effects. Nausea and vomiting are common side effects of narcotic administration and result from the stimulation of the chemoreceptor trigger zone in the medulla oblongata. Large (anesthetic) doses of narcotics depress the vomiting center so that nausea and vomiting tend to occur when the concentrations of narcotics in the body are low. Bowel peristalsis is reduced, whereas sphincter tone is increased, leading to paralytic ileus in some patients. Narcotics may produce spasm of the sphincter of Oddi, with resultant biliary colic. Enhanced bladder sphincter tone occasionally produces urinary retention.

Chest wall rigidity is frequently observed during the induction of anesthesia with fentanyl, sufentanil, or alfentanil.[7,8] It may also occur when morphine and other narcotic analgesics are combined with nitrous oxide.[8] Occasionally, rigidity is observed in the postoperative period.[8] It may cause ventilatory problems in patients who have not received sufficient muscle relaxation. As reported by Scamman,[10] part of the fentanyl-induced increase in resistance to ventilation may be due to glottic closure rather than to rigidity of chest wall or abdominal muscles. Recent work by Ben-

Drug Interactions with Narcotics

Unfortunately, there are few clinical studies of drug interactions between the narcotics and other drugs. Although numerous single-case reports exist, the absence of both systematic investigation and controlled studies is striking. Much of what is known about drug interactions with narcotics has been derived from animal studies, and even these results are inconsistent and often confusing. In part, the lack of clinical studies and the conflicting laboratory data reflect the difficulties in the reliable documentation of the effects of these drugs. The degree of analgesia is difficult to quantitate in human beings, and inconsistent data may result from placebo effects, suggestion, tolerance, and measurement errors. The subjective properties of these compounds are also difficult to quantitate in humans, and almost impossible in animals. Perhaps the one property of opiates that can be assessed quantitatively is the respiratory depressant effect. It must be remembered, however, that respiratory depression is usually regarded as a side effect rather than the desired therapeutic effect. Although it is tempting to do so, one must not conclude that interactions in the respiratory system can be extrapolated either quantitatively or qualitatively to any other system. No doubt one could increase respiratory depression if d-tubocurarine were administered along with morphine, but it is difficult to imagine that increased analgesia or euphoria could result from this combination.

Thus the literature on the subject is not illuminating. One finds reports that show both potentiation and inhibition of narcotic potency for each of the following drugs: dopamine, reserpine, phenoxybenzamine, MAO inhibitors, L-dopa, dexamethasone, and chlorpromazine. In light of these problems, the following discussion focuses only on those interactions that appear to be well documented in either human beings or animals, or on those interactions founded in clinical experience despite the lack of firm laboratory confirmation.

CASE REPORT

A 27-year-old man with a suspected fracture of the right femur was brought to the emergency room following an automobile accident. There was a strong smell of alcohol in his expired breath. He was incoherent, frequently somnolent, and occasionally combative. There was no evidence of head trauma, and witnesses indicated that he never lost consciousness. The emergency room physician administered morphine sulfate, 15 mg IM (intramuscularly), and sent the patient for roentgenograms of the right lower extremity. Twenty minutes later the physician was urgently called to the radiology department. The technician reported that the patient had become increasingly somnolent to the point of unresponsiveness and had vomited. Examination revealed small pupils, vomitus in the pharynx, and a respiratory rate of six breaths per minute. There were coarse moist rhonchi in both upper lung fields. He was only slightly responsive to deep pain. After consultation with a colleague, a presumptive diagnosis of narcotic overdose and polydrug abuse, involving at least alcohol, was made and appropriate treatment for narcotic overdose and associated aspiration of gastric contents was instituted. Following recovery, the patient recalled that he had been at a party and had ingested approximately 500 ml of vodka and several "downers" (thought to be barbiturates) before the accident.

CNS Depressants. This case illustrates an important principle of narcotic interactions: in general, the CNS-depressant properties of narcotics add to the CNS-depressant effects of other drugs. Under ordinary circumstances, the prescription of morphine, 15 mg, would have been appropriate for this patient. However, in the presence of two other CNS-depressants (alcohol and barbiturates), this amount of narcotic was sufficient to induce a profound loss of consciousness and consequent regurgitation and possible pulmonary aspiration of gastric contents. Morphine potentiates acute alcohol intoxication in mice.[11] In humans, the incidence of mortality of former addicts in methadone maintenance programs is greater among alcohol abusers than among nonabusers.

Narcotics enhance the effects of other CNS depressants as well, including general anesthetics. In both man and animals, the anesthetic requirements for several of the inhalation anesthetics are reduced by narcotics.[12,12a]

In general, narcotics act in consort with other CNS depressants to alter states of consciousness, although the exact type of interaction (simple additivity or true synergism) is generally not known.

Although the interactions between the opiates and other CNS depressants on the level of consciousness seem well established, the effect of the CNS depressants on analgesia produced by the narcotics is less clear. For example, barbiturates (including thiopental, pentobarbital, and phenobarbital) are reported to antagonize the analgesic properties of narcotics in humans as well as animals.[13,14] Results obtained in mice suggest that the overall effect of diazepam is to antagonize morphine analgesia, although some enhancement of analgesia may occur briefly (less than 30 minutes) after both drugs are administered.[15] Of special importance to anesthesiologists are reports of the cardiovascular effects of the combined administration of fentanyl and diazepam. Regardless of the order of administration, severe arterial hypotension was observed with this drug combination in patients scheduled for valve replacement or coronary bypass surgery.[5,16] The decrease in mean arterial blood pressure was predominantly due to peripheral arterial vasodilation, although some additional negative inotropic effects could not be excluded. Additive negative inotropic effects of diazepam and fentanyl *in vitro* (Langendorff preparation of the rat heart) have been reported by Reves et al.[17]

Other Drugs. Many drugs have altered the analgesic properties of narcotics in animals, and a recent publication summarizes many of these interactions.[18] However, the mechanism of these interactions is poorly understood at best, and the clinical significance of most of them remains unknown. In general, it appears that drugs that deplete central nervous system stores of biogenic amines antagonize the analgesic actions of narcotics, while sympathomimetic agents appear to enhance narcotic analgesia in both humans and other animals. On the other hand, adrenergic blocking drugs (either *alpha* or *beta*) do not alter morphine analgesia. The cholinergic nervous system appears to be a positive modulator of narcotic analgesia. In animals, drugs that increase cholinergic activity, such as physostigmine, enhance morphine analgesia, whereas atropine antagonizes opiate analgesia.[19]

Occasionally narcotics are administered in combination with other drugs to produce sedation for cardiac catheterization or radiologic procedures. Although this is done with the intention of achieving a greater degree of sedation without increasing toxicity, this rarely occurs. Careful studies in humans of the respiratory depressant properties of meperidine and chlorpromazine, alone or in combination, revealed that potentiation of respiratory depression occurred with this drug combination, indicating that increased toxicity always accompanied increased sedation.[20] On the other hand, droperidol did not increase the ventilatory depressant effects of fentanyl in volunteers.[20a,20b] One possible confounding factor in studies of narcotic-induced ventilatory depression is the fact that natural sleep alone synergistically increases the ventilatory depression produced by morphine (and presumably other narcotics as well).[20c]

Cimetidine, widely used preoperatively to reduce gastric acid production, was reported to increase the terminal elimination half-life time of fentanyl by more than 100% in the dog.[21] In patients, fentanyl was found to alter the distribution volume and clearance of etomidate: etomidate plasma levels were increased and its elimination half-life time prolonged substantially in the presence of fentanyl.[22]

Muscle relaxants often are combined with narcotic analgesics in anesthesia. Because the narcotics tend to produce vagally mediated bradycardia, one would logically choose a relaxant like pancuronium with an anticholinergic action to prevent or to reverse the bradycardia. Apparently, however, pancuronium not only prevents narcotic-induced bradycardia, but also increases heart rate and perhaps enhances sympathetic responses to noxious surgical stimulation.[23,24] The latter responses may be undesirable in patients with certain types of cardiac disease.

CASE REPORT

A 43-year-old woman was scheduled for excision of a ganglion of the wrist. She had a long history of depression and anxiety for which she was taking phenelzine, 45 mg daily. She was anxious about the forthcoming operation and refused regional anesthesia. All medications were stopped 24 hours preoperatively. She received meperidine, 75 mg IM, with atropine, 0.4 mg IM, 60 minutes prior to the procedure. Shortly after these medications, she developed agitation, diaphoresis, stupor, and hypotension, followed by coma and marked cyanosis with slow respirations.

MAOI. This case demonstrates an uncommon but severe drug interaction involving narcotics and monoamine oxidase inhibitors (also known as MAOI) (pargyline, furazolidone, isocarboxazid, phenelzine, nialamide, and tranylcypromine).[25] These potent compounds are notorious for their toxicity and for their propensity to interact with other drugs, especially narcotics. Interaction with narcotics may produce hypertension or hypotension, tachycardia, coma, convulsions, diaphoresis, respiratory depression, and hyperpyrexia. Meperidine has been implicated most frequently but all narcotics should be considered to be potential sources for this severe interaction. The MAOI should be discontinued at least 2 weeks before any elective surgical procedure. When emergency circumstances demand narcotic treatment in patients who are receiving these drugs, therapy should be initiated cautiously with morphine. Meperidine should not be used. Although this is an infrequent reaction, it has caused deaths; it is essential therefore that this interaction be avoided.

NARCOTIC AGONIST-ANTAGONIST ANALGESICS (Table 22–1)

Drugs in this class combine the properties of morphine ("pure" agonist) and

TABLE 22–1
Narcotic Antagonist Analgesics

Currently available in USA	More prominent effect
Nalorphine (Nalline)	antagonism
Levallorphan (Lorfan)	antagonism
Pentazocine (Talwin)	analgesia (agonism)
Butorphanol (Stadol)	analgesia (agonism)
Nalbuphine (Nubain)	analgesia (agonism)
In clinical trials in USA	
Buprenorphine	analgesia (agonism)
Dezocine (Dalgan)	analgesia (agonism)

naloxone ("pure" antagonist). In the presence of a large dose or overdose of a narcotic agonist like morphine or fentanyl, an agonist-antagonist antagonizes analgesia, somnolence, and ventilatory depression. In the absence of a narcotic agonist, the agonist-antagonist will produce analgesia, ventilatory depression, and other effects, some of which resemble and others that differ from those typically produced by morphine-type agonists. Differences in the spectra of pharmacologic actions of pure agonists and mixed agonist-antagonists, (e.g., nalorphine) (Table 22–2) and the complex nature of their interactions suggest the existence of several subtypes of opioid receptors (Table 22–3).

Opioid Receptors

There is overwhelming evidence for the existence of highly specific opioid receptors in the nervous system and certain types of smooth muscle (Table 22–4). Since it is not possible to explain on the basis of a single receptor the actions and interactions among the large number of drugs included in the class of narcotic analgesics or opioids, Martin postulated the existence of subtypes of opioid receptors.[26] Initially he proposed two subtypes, one for morphine-like drugs and the other for nalorphine-like analgesics. According to his hypothesis, morphine binds to a μ receptor in a concentration-dependent manner so that the intensity of its effects is proportional to its concentration at the receptor site (dose-response relationship). Naloxone can compete with morphine for the same μ receptors and prevent or reverse the actions of

TABLE 22–2
Effects of Morphine and Nalorphine and the Ability of Naloxone to Prevent or to Reverse Them

Effects	Produced by Morphine	Produced by Nalorphine	Antagonized by Naloxone[a]
CNS			
Analgesia	++	(++)	++
Ventilatory Depression	++	(++)	++
Antitussive	++	?	++
Bradycardia	+	+	++
Miosis	++	++	++
Nausea	++	+	b
Sedation-Sleep	++	+/0	++
Amnesia	0	0	—
Coma (Anesthesia)	+	0	++
Rigidity	+	?	++
Euphoria	++	0	++
Dysphoria (in absence of pain)	+	++	++
Psychosis	0	+	?
Psychic dependence	++	0	c
Physical dependence	++	+	d
Abuse potential	++	0	++
Tolerance	++	+	e
Death-ventilatory depression	++	+/0	++
Peripheral			
Smooth muscle spasm (GI, GU) Colic, constipation	++	+	++
Vasomotor stimulation	0	?	?
Hypotension	++	+	+
Histamine release	++	?	0
Newborn depression & apnea	++	?	++

++ Strong, optimal efficacy
(++) Equivalent to morphine in lower doses; ceiling effect is evident as dose is increased
+ Mild
0 None
? Unknown

a. Larger doses of naloxone are required to antagonize nalorphine than to antagonize morphine.
b. Naloxone often produces nausea as it antagonizes narcotic effects.
c. Naloxone blocks euphoric response but does not "cure" psychic dependence.
d. Naloxone precipitates an acute abstinence syndrome that is different for nalorphine or compared with morphine.
e. Tolerance is rapidly lost with the discontinuation of morphine administration. The effect of naloxone on loss of tolerance is not known.

morphine; the degree of antagonism depends on the relative concentrations of morphine and naloxone, and in sufficiently high concentrations (doses) naloxone can completely antagonize the actions of morphine by occupying all of the μ receptors (Fig. 22–1). When naloxone occupies all the opioid receptors, no drug action is observed, since naloxone binds to but does not activate the receptors (lacks efficacy).

Naloxone per se produces no observable effect in normal subjects given doses even larger than those usually required to antagonize large doses of pure agonists.[27,28] Extremely large doses of naloxone may produce behavioral effects and CNS stimulation in animals.[29] Under certain conditions it is possible to demonstrate naloxone's antagonism of actions thought to be mediated by enkephalins and endorphins.[30]

Nalorphine, the prototype agonist-an-

TABLE 22–3
Hypothetical Interactions of Narcotic Analgesics and Antagonists with Different Types of Opioid Receptors

	Receptor Type		
	Mu	Kappa	Sigma (PCP)
Experimental measure			
Analgesia	Yes	Yes	No
Ventilation	Depression	Depression	Stimulation
Pupil size	Miosis	Miosis	Mydriasis
Behavior	Euphoria/Indifference	?	Dysphoria/Psychosis
Suppression of morphine-type abstinence syndrome	Yes	No	No
In vitro inhibition of smooth muscle contraction	Yes		
Prototypical agonists	Morphine	Dynorphin	Phencyclidine
	Fentanyl	Cyclazocine	Cyclazocine
	Beta Endorphins	Nalorphine	Nalorphine ?
Sensitivity to naloxone antagonism	High	Moderate	Low
Analgesic Classes			
Agonists (e.g., Morphine)	Ag	Ag (weak)	0
Partial agonists and Agonist-Antagonists			
Buprenorphine	Pag	0	0
Dezocine	Pag	0	0
Butorphanol	0/Pag	Pag	Pag?
Nalbuphine	Ant/Pag	Pag	Pag?
Nalorphine	Ant/Pag	Pag	Pag?
Pentozocine	Ant/Pag	Pag	Pag?
Antagonist			
Naloxone	Ant	Ant	0
Naltrexone	Ant	Ant	0

Ag—Agonist Pag—Partial agonist Ant—Antagonist 0—No interaction

TABLE 22–4
Evidence for the Existence of Opioid Receptors

1. Extremely potent analgesics (etorphine, carfentanil)
2. Structure—activity relationships
   —morphine potent analgesic
   —3-methoxymorphine (codeine) weak analgesic
   —N-allylnormorphine (nalorphine) analgesic-antagonist
3. Stereospecificity (d- vs l-morphinans)
   —levorphanol potent analgesic
   —dextrorphanol inactive as analgesic
4. Specific antagonists
   —antagonism at doses of naloxone producing no effect in the absence of an agonist
   —competitive interactions of agonists and antagonists
5. Dose—concentration—response relationships

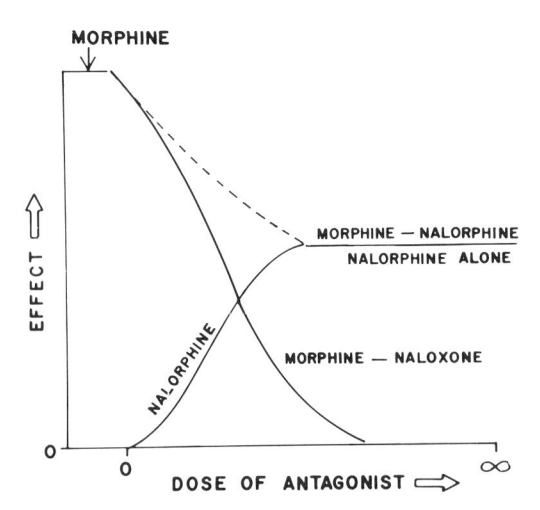

Fig. 22-1. Theoretical comparison of the effects of adding progressively larger doses of naloxone or nalorphine to an existing effect of morphine. Naloxone is able to reverse the effect of morphine completely. In contrast, high doses of nalorphine reduce the effect of morphine (dashed line) to the level of the ceiling effect of nalorphine given alone.

tagonist analgesic, can also compete with morphine for μ receptors in a concentration-dependent fashion. Nalorphine has a limited efficacy compared with morphine at these receptors and is often referred to as a partial agonist. The intensity of μ receptor-mediated actions varies, depending on the numbers of μ receptors occupied by each drug (Fig. 22-2). Small doses of morphine and nalorphine produce essentially additive effects.[31]

The effects of a large dose of morphine are attenuated by nalorphine (Figs. 22-1 and 2) and, when all the μ receptors are occupied by nalorphine, the effects observed will be those of maximum doses of nalorphine alone.[31,32] Namely, the depth of analgesia and ventilatory depression will be much less than that expected with large doses of morphine alone. In other words, there is a relatively low ceiling on the nalorphine dose-response relationship.[33] Incidentally, the effects of nalorphine (a partial agonist) at the μ receptor are antagonized by naloxone (a pure antagonist).

In addition to its morphine-like actions, nalorphine produces other effects (e.g., dysphoria, hallucinations, physical dependence characterized by signs and symptoms different from those induced by morphine dependence) that are not seen with morphine (Table 22-2). Hence, there is a need to postulate a second type of opioid receptor. As the number of agonist-antagonist analgesics synthetized by pharmaceutical chemists increased and the variety of testing procedures expanded, pharmacologic and biochemical differences among the mixed agonist-antagonists became apparent and the complexities of the interactions among pure agonists, agonist-antagonists, and pure antagonists increased. One consequence has been the need to propose the existence of additional subtypes of opioid receptors.[32,34] Another has been confusion about the designation of the receptor subtypes, especially since it is not yet possible to fit all the observations into neat single categories even for compounds reputed to be specific for a particular receptor subtype. Fortunately, these circumstances have not impeded the study and clinical application of the agonist-antagonist analgesics.

Interactions of Agonist-Antagonists

A. With Naloxone. Naloxone antagonizes the μ and κ receptor-mediated actions of the agonist-antagonist analgesics (Table 22-3). Thus, naloxone will prevent or reverse analgesia, ventilatory depression, and other effects of the agonist-antagonists except for their phencyclidine-like actions. In subjects taking these drugs chronically, naloxone will precipitate an acute abstinence syndrome which is quite different in its characteristics from that seen in morphine-dependent subjects.[35]

Buprenorphine is an exception to the above generalizations. It appears that buprenorphine dissociates slowly from opioid receptors once it is bound. Although the prior administration of naloxone can prevent or reduce buprenorphine's actions, naloxone is not an effective antagonist when given after buprenorphine.[34,36,37] It is interesting to note that buprenorphine has unique pharmacologic

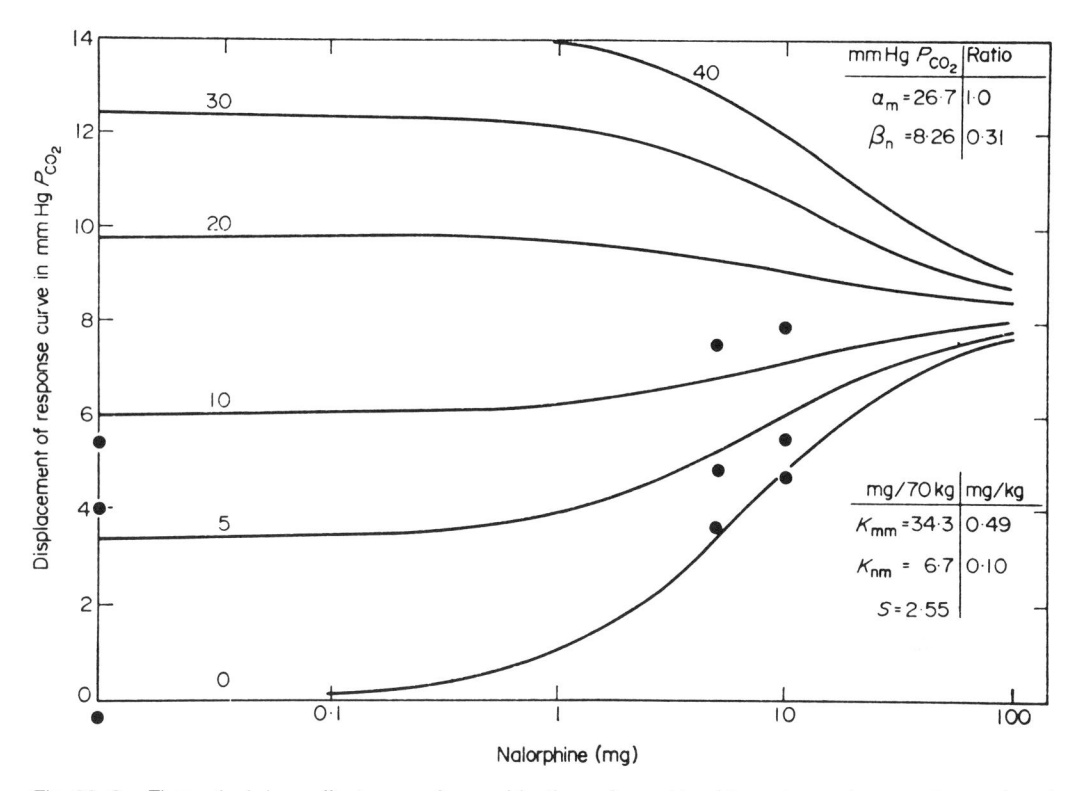

Fig. 22–2. Theoretical dose-effect curves for combinations of morphine (dose shown above each curve) and nalorphine. The data points represent the average displacement of the P_{CO_2} vs. minute ventilation response line (i.e., ventilatory depression) as observed by Bellville and Fleischli (1968). (Reprinted from Martin, W.R., Gorodetzky, C.W., and Thompson, W.O.: Receptor dualism: some kinetic implications. In Agonist and Antagonist Actions of Narcotic Analgesic Drugs. Edited by H.W. Kosterlitz, H.O.J. Collier, and J.E. Villarreal. Baltimore, University Park Press, 1973, pp. 30–44.)

features among the analgesics. Buprenorphine has much greater potency but less efficacy (lower ceiling) than morphine, is able to antagonize morphine, and does not produce dysphoria. Thus, it has been classified as a partial agonist at μ receptors. It is effective orally and sublingually, has a long duration of action, and its chronic administration is followed by a delayed and mild abstinence syndrome. It has been suggested that buprenorphine should have therapeutic applications (1) as an analgesic with low abuse potential and (2) as a drug for treatment of narcotic addiction.[38] At the moment it is gaining popularity in Europe as an analgesic administered sublingually for acute postoperative and chronic pain.

B. With Pure Agonists. Three important points should be recognized in regard to the agonist-antagonist analgesics.

1. It is customary to state the analgesic potency relative to that of morphine and the antagonistic potency relative to that of naloxone or nalorphine (Table 22–5). The analgesic and antagonistic potencies are not directly related. Thus, butorphanol is approximately five times more potent than morphine as an analgesic and an extremely weak antagonist. On the other hand, nalbuphine is equal to morphine and nalorphine in analgesic potency and is one-fourth as potent as nalorphine as an antagonist. Hence, even though butorphanol is a more potent analgesic than nalbuphine, it is almost inactive as an antagonist. This has important implications in the clinical uses and interactions of these drugs (see below).

2. Side effects of the agonist-antagonists

TABLE 22-5
Relative Potencies of Agonists and Antagonists in Relation to Morphine as an Analgesic and to Nalorphine as an Antagonist.

Drug	Analgesic Potency	Antagonistic Potency
Morphine	1	0
Naloxone (Narcan)	0	5–10
Nalorphine (Nalline)	1	1
Nalbuphine (Nubain)	1	0.25
Dezocine (Dalgan)	1	?
Butorphanol (Stadol)	3–5	0 (humans); 0–0.25 (animals)
Buprenorphine (Temgesic)	25	10
Pentazocine (Talwin)	0.25–0.33	0.02

(Data from Jasinki, D.R.: Human pharmacology of narcotic antagonists. Br. J. Clin. Pharmacol., 7:2875, 1979)

include those mediated by opioid receptors (e.g., ventilatory depression) and others apparently not involving opioid receptors (e.g., hemodynamic changes). Little information is available concerning drug interactions on the nonopioid side effects which may be important in certain patients.

3. Because of quantitative variability between subjects and even in the same subject under different conditions, it is impossible to predict the responses that will occur when a pure antagonist is combined with an agonist-antagonist.[40] Thus, it is usually best to avoid mixing members of the subclasses of narcotic analgesics together in the same patient. One possible exception to this general rule is noted below and involves the careful titration of the dose of an antagonist against unwanted degrees of ventilatory depression due to residual amounts of an agonist used in very high doses for narcotic anesthesia.

However, there are likely to be occasions when an analgesic or anesthetic plan has to be altered unexpectedly, and the physician has to choose among reasonable alternatives. For example, it may be desirable to discontinue halothane administration during general anesthesia consisting of halothane supplemented by an agonist-antagonist analgesic. What are the anesthesiologist's reasonable alternatives?

Based on pharmacologic information more than actual clinical experiences (few reports), the following guidelines seem reasonable at this time. Of course, new information may suggest modifications.

Butorphanol is a weak antagonist and it should not interfere with the use of a pure agonist to achieve analgesia or anesthesia. In fact, Moldenhauer et al. administered morphine successfully for postoperative analgesia in a group of 6 adult patients given extraordinarily large doses of butorphanol (up to 0.3 mg/kg) before the induction of anesthesia for aortocoronary artery bypass grafting.[41] The interval between the intravenous injection of butorphanol and morphine varied from 6 to 10 hours. In fact, the antagonistic ability of butorphanol has not been evident in man although weak antagonism of pure agonists has been demonstrated in animals.[37]

The administration of butorphanol after a pure agonist would appear to offer little benefit in reducing unwanted degrees of ventilatory depression due to residual high levels of the agonist. Presumably moderate degrees of analgesia could be sustained at the ceiling level of butorphanol as the pure agonist was eliminated.

Nalbuphine and pentazocine are relatively potent antagonists and should be used cautiously in the presence of a pure agonist. Each of these drugs has been shown to precipitate acute abstinence in morphine-dependent patients and also to reduce the analgesic and ventilatory depressant effects of morphine.[37,39,42,43] Nalbuphine has been used in the postoperative period following moderate and high doses of narcotic analgesics administered during anesthesia.[44–46] With nalbuphine it has been possible to antagonize unwanted degrees of ventilatory depression from residual narcotic agonists, to provide analgesia, and to avoid clinically significant hemodynamic stimulation and other manifestations of stress. The results of these preliminary studies in only 96 patients are summarized in Table 22–6. Although these results are encouraging, a much larger number of patients must be studied under a variety of clinical circumstances in order to demonstrate the efficacy and safety of this use of nalbuphine.

Pentazocine (1 mg/kg) has also been used to antagonize the ventilatory depression due to residual fentanyl administered intraoperatively.[47] Compared with nalorphine (5 mg) and naloxone (0.4 mg), pentazocine had a slower onset and was a weaker antagonist. There appeared to be little difference in the analgesic requirements and the incidence of side effects among the three groups of patients receiving an antagonist and the control group.

A note of caution should be sounded. The interactions of nalbuphine and pentazocine with pure agonists (e.g., morphine, fentanyl) are probably competitive in nature. As such, the degree of antagonism will depend on the relative concentrations of the pure agonist and agonist-antagonist. The degree of antagonism may be variable in degree and variable over time as the agonist and agonist-antagonist are removed at different rates (pharmacokinetics) from the sites of competition. Thus, there may be risks of recurrent ventilatory depression after a small dose of agonist-antagonist in the presence of a large quantity of the agonist, and as noted above, large doses of the agonist-antagonist may precipitate an acute abstinence syndrome in the patient physically dependent on a pure agonist. The rates of development of physical dependence during narcotic anesthesia have not been reported, but it is conceivable that this process commences with the first exposure to a narcotic analgesic. It is clear that the development of tolerance begins acutely during exposure to anesthetic doses of fentanyl.[48]

Narcotic Antagonist Analgesics in the Induction and Maintenance of Anesthesia

As with *analgesic doses* of any "pure" agonist, the narcotic antagonist analgesics can be used for premedication, supplementation of general and regional anesthetic drugs, and postoperative analgesia.[37] For these purposes their principal advantage over the pure agonists (limited postoperative ventilatory depression) has to be weighed against their potential disadvantages (limited analgesic efficacy and side effects, especially dysphoria in the postoperative period) and compared with those seen after analgesic doses of the morphine-like drugs. In a double-blind comparison, Fahmy found analgesic doses of nalbuphine and morphine to be equally effective as supplements to nitrous oxide-thiopental anesthesia, and nalbuphine was associated with lesser incidences of postoperative vomiting and ventilatory depression.[49] Rosow and Keegan found butorphanol to be as effective as morphine in suppressing the sympathetic responses to tracheal intubation.[50]

It is clear that none of the agonist-antagonists or partial agonists is likely to be suitable as a "narcotic anesthetic." That is, the ceiling effect on analgesia and ventilatory depression extends to their other actions in the central nervous system. Butorphanol, nalbuphine, and pentazocine are much less efficacious than the pure agonists in reducing the concentrations of inhaled anesthetics required to prevent movement to a noxious stimulus in animals (MAC).[51–53] In patients scheduled to undergo coronary artery surgery, neither butorphanol nor nalbuphine reliably induced unconsciousness, even after doses equivalent to 1.5 to 3 mg/kg doses of morphine, and these large doses also failed to obtund the autonomic and hemodynamic responses to noxious surgical stimulation after the induction of general anesthesia with potent inhaled anesthetics.[41,54]

TABLE 22-6
Use of Nalbuphine After Narcotic Anesthesia to Antagonize Excessive Ventilatory Depression While Preserving Analgesia

	\multicolumn{3}{c}{Investigators}		
	Magruder, et al.[44]	Latasch, et al.[45]	Moldenhauer, et al.[46]
Patients			
Number	15	60	21
Type of surgery	Non-cardiac	Non-cardiac	Cardiac
Age (years)	34–72	45 ± 15 SD	48–77
Anesthesia			
Narcotic analgesic	Oxymorphone, Hydromorphone	Fentanyl	Fentanyl
Total dose	6–15 mg 8–16 mg	23 ± 6 µg/kg	95–157 µg/kg
Duration of anesthesia (hours)	2.5–3	1.3 ± 0.6	>4
Other anesthetic drugs	diazepam, thiopental, lidocaine, nitrous oxide, succinylcholine, metocurine, neostigmine-glycopyrollate	hexobarbital, droperidol, nitrous oxide, succinylcholine, pancuronium	pancuronium ± diazepam ± enflurane
Premedication	cimetidine	Innovar, atropine	morphine, diazepam scopolamine
Postoperative Nalbuphine			
Nalbuphine dose	0.1 mg/kg	20 mg	45–66 µg/kg*
Satisfactory ventilation	15/15 patients	presumably 60/60	20/21 patients
Satisfactory analgesia —duration	15/15 patients 7 hours (mean)	48–59/60** 3–5 hours duration	20/21 patients —?
Hemodynamic stimulation	moderate (20% ↑ HR & BP), transient	not reported	4/21 (25% MAP) no dysrhythmias
Nausea-retching	not reported	5/60	2/21
Other side effects	not reported	12-shivering	3-renarcotization 2-restlessness

*An initial dose of 15 µg/kg was given and followed by increments of 15 to 30 µg/kg until the $PaCO_2$ was less than 48 mm Hg or until a maximum dose of 150 µg/kg had been administered (one patient).
**Patients received additional doses of nalbuphine as requested for pain relief and complete pain relief increased from 79.7% of the patients 15 minutes after the first intravenous dose to 98.3% at 2 hours (number of doses unspecified).

Some caution is indicated in generalizing from the limited observations that have been made to date. First, studies on the reduction of MAC do not necessarily reflect all of the potentially useful effects of narcotic analgesics. Second, the dose-response relationships need to be examined more closely since the overall shape of the dose-response curves published to date at least suggest that large doses of the agonist-antagonists are mainly antagonists. The ventilatory response to CO_2 not only reached a ceiling of depression, but also appeared to return toward normal as the dose of nalbuphine or dezocine was increased.[55,56] Finally, it should be noted that large doses of nalbuphine completely antagonized the MAC reduction produced by fentanyl in dogs, whereas the MAC reduction might have been expected to level off at the maximum MAC reduction produced by nalbuphine alone as illustrated in Figure 22–1.[57] Thus, more study is needed to define the actions and interactions of the agonist-antagonists more fully in the setting of general anesthesia.

The interactions of agonist-antagonist analgesics with skeletal muscle relaxants are unknown. As with the pure agonist analgesics, the concerns of anesthesiologists center on (1) the production of muscular rigidity by the analgesic and the need for a relaxant to relieve it; (2) the impairment of ventilation by the combination of an analgesic and relaxant, especially in the postoperative period; (3) cholinergic, sympathetic, and hemodynamic interactions of relaxants and the antagonist-analgesics; (4) the difficulty of determining anesthetic depth when using an agonist-antagonist analgesic to supplement nitrous oxide-relaxant anesthesia.

NARCOTIC ANTAGONISTS

CASE REPORT

A 73-year-old, 55-kg woman was scheduled for open reduction and internal fixation of a fractured hip. She had a long history of hypertension, angina, and occasional congestive heart failure. Physical examination revealed an elderly patient with bilateral ankle edema, dyspnea when supine, moderate jugular venous distension, and bilateral rates and rhonchi in the lung bases. The presumptive diagnosis was mild congestive heart failure, in addition to the hip fracture. The anesthesiologist selected a nitrous oxide-oxygen-narcotic anesthetic technique. She was anesthetized for 90 minutes, during which time she received 30 mg of morphine intravenously (IV) in addition to the 6 mg administered preoperatively. The narcotic was antagonized with naloxone, 0.3 mg intravenously, and she was taken to the recovery room in satisfactory condition. She was alert and comfortable during the first hour in the recovery room. Ninety minutes later the recovery room nurse reported that the patient had become cyanotic, lethargic, and the respiratory rate was only six breaths per minute. The presumptive diagnosis was recurrent narcotism. Naloxone, 0.3 mg, was administered again and promptly reversed both the mental clouding and the respiratory depression.

This case illustrates the principal drug interaction involving the narcotics: the antagonism of the opiates by narcotic antagonists. The following section reviews the principal features of narcotic antagonists and summarizes their interactions with the opiates. Other drugs that may interact with the antagonists are also discussed.

Pharmacology

History. The narcotic-antagonist properties of N-allylnorcodeine were first observed in 1914, and N-allylnormorphine (nalorphine) was synthesized and its narcotic antagonist properties were demonstrated in animals in 1940. Nevertheless, it was not until 1952 that nalorphine was introduced into clinical medicine. Naloxone was synthesized in 1966 and, because of the unique pharmacologic properties of this compound, it has become a popular drug for the antagonism of respiratory depression associated with narcotics.

Structure. Most opiates contain a methylated nitrogen atom, and nearly all narcotic antagonists are synthesized by replacing the methyl group with a longer side chain, usually an allyl group (Fig. 22–3). Although other substitutions are possible, the major narcotic antagonists currently available are N-allyl substitutions of an opiate. Nalorphine is the N-allyl derivative of morphine, levallorphan is the N-allyl

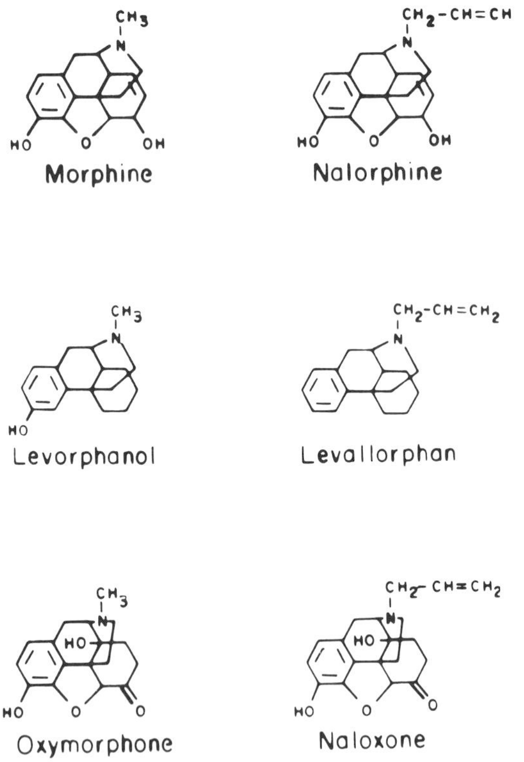

Fig. 22-3. Comparisons of the chemical structures of agonist (left) and antagonists (right). In each case, the methyl group on the nitrogen of the agonist has been replaced by an allyl group to produce an antagonist.

substitution of levorphanol, and naloxone is the N-allyl congener of oxymorphone.

Classification. Whereas there are other compounds with mixed agonist-antagonist properties, the potent antagonists are basically three: nalorphine, levallorphan, and naloxone. Narcotic antagonists may be classified into two major groups based on their agonist potential: partial agonists and pure antagonists. Both nalorphine and levallorphan are partial agonists; that is, when these drugs are administered to a patient who has not received any narcotic, there will be evidence of mild to moderate agonist activity, including respiratory depression.[58] In essence, the therapeutic rationale for these drugs is the substitution of a weak agonist for a potent one. The problems associated with this form of therapy are obvious. If, for example, a comatose patient is incorrectly diagnosed as suffering from narcotic overdose, when in fact the cause was a hypnotic or sedative agent, the administration of a partial agonist will aggravate the problem rather than correct it. Naloxone is the only pure antagonist currently available. No evidence of narcotic activity is associated with the administration of even large doses of this drug to volunteer subjects.[58] (Naltrexone, another pure antagonist, is not yet approved for human use).

Mechanism of Action. The action of narcotic antagonists can be explained in terms of the agonist-antagonist-receptor theory of drug interactions; that is, that narcotic antagonists bind to opiate receptors in the central nervous system and either displace or prevent the narcotics from binding to these receptors.

Recently, specific opiate receptors have been identified and characterized within the central nervous system.[59] These receptors are more abundant in the amygdala, hypothalamus, and thalamus of primates, and a similar distribution pattern appears to exist in man also. Opiate receptors can be isolated from other areas of the gray matter, but there is no evidence of receptor activity in white matter. Structure-activity relationships are prominent, since nonopiates do not bind to the receptor and only levorotatory forms of the narcotics exhibit agonist properties. The binding of both agonists and antagonists depends on the sodium concentration in the area of the receptor. *In vitro,* the binding of narcotic agonists is reduced by increasing sodium concentration in brain homogenates, whereas the opiate antagonists are more tightly bound to the receptor when the sodium concentration is increased. This "sodium effect" may be clinically important, since it may explain the greater potency of antagonists as compared with that of agonists (that is, small doses of naloxone antagonize large doses of narcotics). At normal body sodium concentrations, the antagonists are 10 to 100 times more tightly bound to the receptor than are the agonists and, therefore, a one-to-one antagonist/agonist ratio is not necessary to displace the narcotic from the receptor site.

Actions of Antagonists. In general, antagonists counteract nearly all the properties of the opiates. In the central nervous system, the drowsiness, apathy, lethargy, euphoria, and loss of consciousness associated with narcotics are reversed. In the cardiovascular system, the orthostatic hypotension and peripheral vasodilation induced by narcotics are abolished. By far the most important application of the opiate antagonists in anesthesia is the reversal of the respiratory depression associated with these potent analgesics. The antagonists promptly reverse the respiratory depression produced by even large doses of narcotics. In patients subjected to morphine-nitrous oxide anesthesia for approximately 2½ hours, naloxone, 5 µg/kg IV, provided rapid reversal of a total morphine dose that averaged 1.5 mg/kg.[60] These results indicate the potency of naloxone as a narcotic antagonist. Others have reported similar results and have successfully employed smaller doses of naloxone (approximately 2 µg/kg) when correspondingly smaller amounts of narcotic were used to supplement nitrous oxide anesthesia.[61,62] All investigators noted the brief duration of action of naloxone when morphine or, in many cases even fentanyl, was the agonist.

Duration of Action of Naloxone. The short duration of action of naloxone is extremely important to the clinician. It has been confirmed by clinical studies in human beings and by laboratory studies. The kinetics of both morphine and naloxone have been determined in animals.[63] After intravenous administration of naloxone, the brain concentrations of the drug exceed the plasma concentrations by a factor of 3 to 4. In contrast to naloxone, the initial brain concentration of morphine is only one-tenth that detected in the plasma. However, the brain concentration of naloxone declines much more rapidly than that of morphine, suggesting that the rapid loss of naloxone from the CNS could explain its short duration of action. The plasma half-life of naloxone was estimated to be 64 minutes in human beings, a value consistent with the clinical data, indicating that supplemental naloxone is required to ensure adequate antagonism of morphine (or large doses of fentanyl). Various protocols for supplementing intravenous naloxone have been described, but intramuscular supplements are consistently effective and the dosage schedule is much simpler than either a constant intravenous infusion or intermittent intravenous injections of the drug.[60,61] In general, up to twice the successful intravenous dose may be given intramuscularly to antagonize narcotic induced respiratory depression, but one should be aware that these relatively large doses of naloxone are not without hazards.

Side Effects of Antagonism by Naloxone. The antagonism of narcotics by naloxone is associated with four major problems: nausea and vomiting, CNS excitation, cardiovascular stimulation, and reversal of analgesia.

Nausea and vomiting appear to be closely related to the speed of injection and to the total dose of naloxone. When the drug was injected rapidly into patients who received narcotics, we observed nausea and vomiting following 60% of the injections.[60] Others have reported no greater incidence of nausea and vomiting in postoperative patients who received smaller doses of naloxone than in patients who do not receive the drug.[62] More recently, it is our impression that administering the drug slowly over 2 to 3 minutes reduces the incidence of nausea and vomiting in postoperative patients. Fortunately, arousal occurs either before or simultaneously with the vomiting, so that the patient's protective reflexes are present and aspiration has not been a problem. However, the potential does exist.

CNS stimulation is manifested by rapid and sometimes dramatic arousal which may be associated with pain, delirium, and marked anxiety in the postoperative patient.

Cardiovascular stimulation following intravenous naloxone has been reported in both humans and animals.[64–66] The prevailing response is generalized sympathetic activation manifested by hypertension and tachycardia. Interestingly, cardiovascular stimulation was noted when naloxone was administered to animals maintained at a stable depth of general anesthesia by a combination of a narcotic and potent inhalation anesthetic, and in the absence of noxious stimulation.[66,66a] Ventricular irritability associated with naloxone reversal of morphine anesthesia has been reported. These patients, however, were in the early postcardiotomy period and were also receiving other cardiovascular drugs.[67] Severe cardiovascular reactions to naloxone appear to be rare, although severe hypertension with rupture of a cerebral aneurysm has been reported, and the number of case reports of acute pulmonary edema following naloxone reversal of fentanyl anesthesia is still increasing.[65,68,69] Andree has also reported 2 cases of fatal cardiac arrest in healthy young women following naloxone reversal of narcotic anesthesia.[70] The postoperative administration of naloxone should not be considered as a risk-free procedure, and the alternatives of administering mixed agonist-antagonist agents (nalorphine or nalbuphine, for example) or of maintaining controlled ventilation postoperatively still represent valuable alternatives in the care of postoperative respiratory depression.

Although it is inevitable that some loss of analgesia will accompany the administration of naloxone to postoperative patients, this problem can be minimized by careful titration of the dose of antagonist.[61,62] After intravenous naloxone, there is prompt arousal, and some patients may complain briefly of pain. Within 2 to 3 minutes this effect is greatly reduced (again, consistent with the pharmacokinetics of the antagonist). It would be unwise to conclude that respiratory depression could be reversed without some loss of analgesia; nevertheless, clinical trials and experience suggest that the problem of loss of analgesia is not so severe as to constitute a contraindication to their proper use.[62]

Opiate Antagonist Interactions with Nonnarcotics. Although there are isolated reports of the effectiveness of naloxone in partially reversing alcohol, barbiturate, diazepam, or propoxyphene intoxications or in reversing clonidine overdosage, the efficacy of this drug in treating nonnarcotic overdoses must be questioned until convincing data are available. The role of naloxone or naltrexone (a new, long-acting pure antagonist) in antagonizing the anesthetic effects of inhalational agents, ketamine, or pentobarbital is not well established. Both antagonistic[71–75] effects as well as failure[76–80] to reverse anesthetic effects of these various anesthetic agents have been reported. At present, it appears likely that naloxone is a potent antagonist of narcotics only. Although the drug may have general analeptic properties in other circumstances, these effects have not been well documented in humans. Naloxone therefore should not be considered an appropriate treatment of CNS depression produced by nonnarcotics until more convincing data become available.

The interaction of opiate antagonists with nonnarcotic drugs has received little attention. In animals, the following drugs have been reported to potentiate narcotic antagonists: cortisone, ACTH (adrenocorticotropic hormone), L-dopa, and propranolol, whereas atropine and physostigmine appear to inhibit narcotic antagonists.[18] The clinical significance of these observations is unknown at this time.

The role and value of naloxone in treatment of hemorrhagic or septic shock remain controversial. Whereas most investigators uniformly reported increased arterial blood pressure values following administration of large doses of naloxone, its effect on improvement of tissue perfusion at the present time is not well established.[81,82] However, survival studies in dogs submitted to hemorrhagic or septic shock demonstrated an improved survival up to 72 hours in naloxone-treated animals compared with those receiving placebo.[83,84]

SUMMARY

Narcotics and narcotic antagonists are potent drugs that interact with one another as well as with other drugs. Narcotic antagonists can reverse nearly all the depressant properties of opiates, but they are usually employed therapeutically to abolish the respiratory depression associated with morphine and related compounds. Naloxone is the only pure narcotic antagonist and is the most specific drug for opiate antagonism. However, naloxone has a brief duration of action and narcotic depression may recur unless the drug is repeated intravenously, given as a continuous infusion, or administered intramuscularly. Further, cardiovascular and CNS stimulation may accompany narcotic reversal in postoperative patients, although these effects are generally infrequent if the antagonist is administered judiciously. The unwanted side effects of the pure antagonist, naloxone, have led some to use mixed agonist-antagonists for the reversal of narcotic "anesthesia" postoperatively, but naloxone remains the drug of choice for the treatment of accidental narcotic overdose.

The most important interactions of narcotics with other drugs involve additive or synergistic effects with other CNS depressants and the rare but dramatic interactions with MAOI. Narcotic antagonists are either potentiated or inhibited by several drugs in laboratory animals, but the clinical importance of these effects is undetermined at present.

REFERENCES

1. De Castro, J., de Water, A.V., Wouters, L., et al.: Comparative study of cardiovascular, neurological and metabolic side effects of eight narcotics in dogs. Acta Anaesthesiol. Belg., 3:51, 1979.
2. Rao, T.L.K., Mummaneni, N., El-Etr, A.A.: Convulsions: an unusual response to intravenous fentanyl administration. Anesth. Analg., 61:1020, 1982.
3. Murkin, J.M., Moldenhauer, C.C., and Hug, C.C., Jr., et al.: Absence of seizures during induction of anesthesia with high-dose fentanyl. Anesth. Analg., 63:489, 1984.
4. Lowenstein, E., et al.: Cardiovascular responses to large doses of intravenous morphine in man. N. Engl. J. Med., 281:1389, 1969.
5. Stanley, T.H., and Webster, L.R.: Anesthetic requirements and cardiovascular effects of fentanyl-oxygen and fentanyl-diazepam-oxygen anesthesia in man. Anesth. Analg., 57:411, 1978.
6. Flacke, J.W., van Etten, A., Flacke, W.E.: Greatest histamine release from meperidine among four narcotics: double-blind study in man. Anesthesiology, 59:A51, 1983.
7. Nauta, J., de Lange, S., Koopman, D., et al.: Anesthetic induction with alfentanil: a new short acting narcotic analgesic. Anesth. Analg., 61:267, 1982.
8. Goldberg, M., Ishak, S., Garcia, C., et al.: Postoperative rigidity following sufentanil administration. Anesthesiology, 63:199, 1985.
9. Freund, F.G., Martin, W.E., Wong, K.C., et al.: Abdominal muscle rigidity induced by morphine and nitrous oxide. Anesthesiology, 38:358, 1973.
10. Scamman, F.L.: Fentanyl-O_2-N_2O rigidity and pulmonary compliance. Anesth. Analg., 62:332, 1983.
11. Eerola, R., et al.: Acute alcohol poisoning and morphine. Ann. Med. Exp. Biol. Fenn., 33:253, 1955.
12. Eger, E.I., II: Anesthetic Uptake and Action. Baltimore, Williams & Wilkins, 1974.
12a. Murphy, M.R., and Hug, C.C., Jr.: The anesthetic potency of fentanyl in terms of its reduction of enflurane MAC. Anesthesiology, 57:485, 1982.
13. Dundee, J.W.: Alterations in response to somatic pain associated with anesthesia. II. The effects of thiopentone and pentobarbitone. Br. J. Anaesth., 32:407, 1960.
14. Neal, M.J.: The hyperalgesic action of barbiturates in mice. Br. J. Pharmacol., 24:170, 1965.
15. Fennessy, M.R., and Sawynok, J.: The effect of benzodiazepines on the analgesic effect of morphine and sodium salicylate. Arch. Int. Pharmacodyn. Ther., 204:77, 1973.
16. Tomicheck, R.C., Rosow, C.E., Schneider, R.C., et al.: Cardiovascular effects of diazepam-fentanyl anesthesia in patients with coronary artery disease. Anesth. Analg., 61:217, 1982.
17. Reves, J.G., Kissin, I., and Fournier, S.E.: Additive negative inotropic effect of a combination of diazepam and fentanyl. Anesthesiology, 59:A326, 1983.
18. Takemori, A.E.: Pharmacologic factors which alter the action of narcotic analgesics and antagonists. In: Interactions of Drugs of Abuse. Edited by E.S. Vessell and M.C. Braude. Ann. N.Y. Acad. Sci., 281:262, 1976.
19. Takemori, A.E., Tulunay, F.C., and Yano, I.: Differential effects on morphine analgesia and naloxone antagonism by biogenic amine modifiers. Life Sci., 17:21, 1975.
20. Lambertsen, C.J., Wendel, H., and Longenhagen, J.B.: The separate and combined respiratory effects of chlorpromazine and meperidine in normal men controlled at 46 mmHg alveolar PCO_2. J. Pharmacol. Exp. Ther., 131:381, 1961.
20a. Kallos, T., and Smith, T.C.: The respiratory effects of Innovar given for premedication. Br. J. Anaesth., 41:303, 1969.
20b. Harper, M.H., Hickey, R.F., Cromwell, T.H., et al.: The magnitude and duration of respiratory depression produced by fentanyl and fentanyl plus droperidol in man. J. Pharmacol. Exp. Ther., 199:464, 1976.

20c. Forrest, W.H., Jr., and Bellville, J.W.: The effect of sleep plus morphine on the respiratory response to carbon dioxide. Anesthesiology, 25:137, 1964.
21. Borel, J.D., Bentley, J.B., Nenad, R.E., et al.: Cimetidine alteration of fentanyl pharmacokinetics in dogs. Abstracts, 56th Annual Meeting, International Anesthesia Research Society, San Francisco, California, March 14–18, 1982, pp. 149–150.
22. Schüttler, J., Wilms, M., Stoeckel, H., et al.: Pharmacokinetic interaction of etomidate and fentanyl. Anesthesiology. 59:A247, 1983.
23. Salmenpera, M., Peltola, K., Takkunen, O., et al.: Cardiovascular effects of pancuronium and vecuronium during high-dose fentanyl anesthesia. Anesth. Analg., 62:1059, 1983.
24. Khoury, G.F., Estafanous, F.G., Zurick, A.M., et al.: Sufentanil/pancuronium versus sufentanil/metocurine anesthesia for coronary artery surgery. Anesthesiology, 57:A47, 1982.
25. Goldberg, L.I.: Monoamine oxidase inhibitors. Adverse reactions and possible mechanisms. J.A.M.A., 190:456, 1964.
26. Martin, W.R.: Opioid antagonists. Pharmacol. Rev., 19:463, 1967.
27. Jasinski, D.R., Martin, W.R., and Haertzen, C.A.: The human pharmacology and abuse potential of N-allylnoroxymorphone (Naloxone). J. Pharmacol. Exp. Ther., 157:420, 1967.
28. Estilo, A.E., and Cottrell, J.E.: Hemodynamic and catecholamine changes after administration of naloxone. Anesth. Analg., 61:349, 1981.
29. Sawynok, J., Pinsky, C., and LaBella, F.S.: Minireview on the specificity of naloxone as an opiate antagonist. Life Sci., 25:1621, 1979.
30. Stoelting, R.K.: Opiate receptors and endorphins: Their role in anesthesiology. Anesth. Analg., 59:874, 1980.
31. Belleville, J.W., and Fleischli, G.: The interaction of morphine and nalorphine on respiration. Clin. Pharmacol. Ther., 9:152, 1968.
32. Martin, W.R.: Pharmacology of opioids. Pharmacol. Rev., 35:283, 1984.
33. Keats, A.S., and Telford, J.: Studies of analgesic drugs. X. Respiratory effects of narcotic antagonists. J. Pharmacol. Exp. Ther., 151:126, 1966.
34. Martin, W.R.: History and development of mixed opioid agonists, partial agonists and antagonists. Br. J. Clin. Pharmacol., 7:273s, 1979.
35. Jasinski, D.R., Martin, W.R., and Hoeldtke, R.D.: Effects of short- and long-term administration of pentazocine in man. Clin. Pharmacol. Ther., 11:385, 1970.
36. Rance, M.J.: Animal and molecular pharmacology of mixed agonist-antagonist analgesic drugs. Br. J. Clin. Pharmacol., 7:281s, 1979.
37. Houde, R.W.: Analgesic effectiveness of the narcotic agonist-antagonists. Br. J. Clin. Pharmacol., 7:297s, 1979.
38. Jasinski, D.R., Pevnick, J.S., and Griffith, J.D.: Human pharmacology and abuse potential of the analgesic buprenorphine: A potential agent for treating narcotic addiction. Arch. Gen. Psychiatry, 35:501, 1979.
39. Jasinski, D.R.: Human pharmacology of narcotic antagonists. Br. J. Clin. Pharmacol., 7:287s, 1979.
40. Telford, J., and Keats, A.S.: Narcotic-narcotic antagonist mixtures. Anesthesiology, 22:465–484, 1961.
41. Moldenhauer, C.C., Hug, C.C., Jr., and Nagel, D.M.: High-dose butorphanol (Stadol) in anesthesia for aortocoronary bypass surgery (ABS). Abstracts, 3rd Annual Meeting, Society of Cardiovascular Anesthesiologists, San Francisco, California, May 10–13, 1981, pp. 59–60.
42. Jasinski, D.R., and Mansky, P.A.: Evaluation of nalbuphine for abuse potential. Clin. Pharmacol. Ther., 13:78, 1972.
43. Blumberg, H., Dayton, H.B., and Wolf, P.S.: Analgesic properties of the narcotic antagonist EN-2234A. Pharmacologist, 10:201, 1968.
44. Magruder, M.R., Delaney, R.D., and DiFazio, C.A.: Reversal of narcotic-induced respiratory depression with nalbuphine hydrochloride. Anesthesiology Review, 9:34, 1982.
45. Latasch, L., Probst, S., and Dudziak, R.: Reversal by nalbuphine of respiratory depression caused by fentanyl. Anesth. Analg., 63:814–816, 1984.
46. Moldenhauer, C.C., Roach, G.W., Finlayson, D.C., et al.: Nalbuphine antagonism of ventilatory depression following high-dose fentanyl anesthesia. Anesthesiology, 62:647, 1985.
47. Kaukinen, L., Kaukinen, S., Eerola, R., et al.: The antagonistic effect of pentazocine on fentanyl induced respiratory depression compared with nalorphine and naloxone. Ann. Clin. Res., 13:396–401, 1981.
48. Askitopoulou, H., Whitwam, J.G., Al-Khudhairi, D., et al.: Acute tolerance to fentanyl during anesthesia in dogs. Anesthesiology, 63:255, 1985.
49. Fahmy, N.R.: Nalbuphine in 'balanced' anesthesia: Its analgesic efficacy and hemodynamic effects. Anesthesiology, 53:s66, 1980.
50. Rosow, C.E., and Keegan, C.R.: Butorphanol vs morphine: Dose-related suppression of the response to intubation. Anesth. Analg., 63(2):270, 1984.
51. Murphy, M.R., and Hug, C.C., Jr.: The enflurane sparing effects of morphine, butorphanol and nalbuphine. Anesthesiology 57:489, 1982.
52. DiFazio, C.A., Moscicki, J.C., and Magruder, M.R.: Anesthetic potency of nalbuphine and interaction with morphine in rats. Anesth. Analg., 60:629, 1981.
53. Hoffman, J.C., and DiFazio, C.A.: The anesthesia-sparing effect of pentazocine, meperidine, and morphine. Arch. Int. Pharmacodyn., 188:261, 1970.
54. Lake, C.L., Duckworth, E.N., DiFazio, C.A., et al.: Cardiovascular effects of nalbuphine in patients with coronary or valvular heart disease. Anesthesiology, 57:498, 1981.
55. Romagnoli, A., and Keats, A.S.: Ceiling effect for respiratory depression by nalbuphine. Clin. Pharmacol. Ther., 27:475, 1980.
56. Romagnoli, A., and Keats, A.S.: Ceiling respiratory depression by dezocine. Clin. Pharmacol. Ther., 35:367, 1984.
57. Murphy, M.R., and Hug, C.C., Jr.: Efficacy of fentanyl in reducing isoflurane MAC; antagonism by naloxone. Anesthesiology, 59:A338, 1983.
58. Foldes, F.F., and Torda, T.A.G.: Comparative studies with narcotics and narcotic antagonists in man. Acta Anaesthesiol. Scand., 9:121, 1965.
59. Snyder, S.H.: Opiate receptors and internal opiates. Sci. Am., 236:44, 1977.
60. Longnecker, D.E., Grazis, P.A., and Eggers, G.W.N., Jr.: Naloxone for antagonism of mor-

phine induced respiratory depression. Anesth. Analg., 52:447, 1973.
61. Heisterkamp, D.V., and Cohen, P.J.: The use of naloxone to antagonize large doses of opiates administered during nitrous oxide anesthesia. Anesth. Analg., 53:12, 1974.
62. Kripke, B.J., et al.: Naloxone antagonism after narcotic-supplemented anesthesia. Anesth. Analg., 55:800, 1976.
63. Ngai, S.H., et al.: Pharmacokinetics of naloxone in rats and in man. Basis for its potency and short duration of action. Anesthesiology, 44:398, 1976.
64. Tanaka, G.Y.: Hypertensive reaction to naloxone. J.A.M.A., 228:25, 1974.
65. Flacke, J.W., Flacke, W.E., and Williams, G.D.: Acute pulmonary edema following naloxone reversal of high-dose morphine anesthesia. Anesthesiology, 47:376, 1977.
66. Patschke, D., et al.: Antagonism of morphine with naloxone in dogs: Cardiovascular effects with special reference to the coronary circulation. Br. J. Anaesth., 49:525, 1977.
66a.Flacke, J.W., Flacke, W.E., Bloor, B.C., et al.: Effects of fentanyl, naloxone, and clonidine on hemodynamics and plasma catecholamine levels in dogs. Anesth. Analg., 62:305, 1983.
67. Michaelis, L.L., et al.: Ventricular irritability associated with the use of naloxone hydrochloride. Ann. Thorac. Surg., 18:608, 1974.
68. Taff, R.H.: Pulmonary edema following naloxone administration in a patient without heart disease. Anesthesiology, 59:576, 1983.
69. Prough, D.S.: Acute pulmonary edema in healthy teenagers following conservative doses of intravenous naloxone. Anesthesiology, 60:485, 1984.
70. Andree, R.A.: Sudden death following naloxone administration. Anesth. Analg., 59:782, 1980.
71. Finck, A.D., Ngai, S.H., and Berkowitz, B.A.: Antagonism of general anesthesia by naloxone in the rat. Anesthesiology, 46:241, 1977.
72. Arndt, J.O., and Freye, E.: Perfusion of naloxone through the fourth cerebral ventricle reverses the circulatory and hypnotic effects of halothane. Anesthesiology, 51:58, 1979.
73. Gilbert, P.E., and Martin, W.R.: Antagonism of the effects of pentobarbital in the chronic spinal dog by naltrexone. Life Sci., 20:1401, 1977.
74. Finck, A.D., and Ngai, S.H.: Opiate receptor mediation of ketamine analgesia. Anesthesiology, 56:91, 1982.
75. Yang, J.C., Crawford, Clark, W., and Ngai, S.H.: Antagonism of nitrous oxide analgesia by naloxone in man. Anesthesiology, 52:414, 1980.
76. Smith, R.A., Wilson, M., and Miller, K.W.: Naloxone has no effect on nitrous oxide anesthesia. Anesthesiology, 49:6, 1978.
77. Duncalf, D., Nagashima, H., and Duncalf, R.M.: Naloxone fails to antagonize thiopental anesthesia. Anesth. Analg., 57:558, 1978.
78. Pace, N.L., and Wong, K.C.: Failure of naloxone and naltrexone to antagonize halothane anesthesia in the dog. Anesth. Analg., 58:36, 1979.
79. Bennett, P.B.: Naloxone fails to antagonize the righting response in rats anesthetized with halothane. Anesthesiology, 49:9, 1978.
80. Harper, M.H., Winter, P., Johnson, B.H., et al.: Naloxone does not antagonize general anesthesia in the rat. Anesthesiology, 49:3, 1978.
81. Chen, R.Y.Z., Muraszko, K.M., Carlin, R.D., et al.: Improvement of cerebral and myocardial blood flows by naloxone during hemorrhagic hypotension in dogs. Anesthesiology, 59:A119, 1983.
82. Coates, D.P., Seyde, W.C., Epstein, R.M., et al.: The influence of naloxone on regional hemodynamics in hemorrhaged rats. Circ. Shock (in press).
83. Vargish, T., Reynolds, D.G., Gurll, N.J., et al.: Naloxone reversal of hypovolemic shock in dogs. Circ. Shock, 7:31, 1980.
84. Reynolds, D.G., Gurll, N.J., Vargish, T., et al.: Blockade of opiate receptors with naloxone improves survival and cardiac performance in canine endotoxic shock. Circ. Shock, 7:39, 1980.

23

INHALATION ANESTHETIC AGENTS

JOHN L. NEIGH

Today multiple drug exposure prior to inhalation anesthesia is almost the rule. Not only are anesthesiologists presented with patients who receive numerous medications, but also inhalation anesthesia is often induced and maintained by a variety of agents that produce unconsciousness, analgesia, abolition of noxious reflexes, and muscle relaxation. The following case report represents a common example of a patient who undergoes anesthesia and operation and who has received multiple drug therapy.

CASE REPORT

A 54-year-old man was admitted to a hospital with a 4-day history of abdominal pain and intermittent light stools. He had noted chills and icteric sclerae on the day before admission. The patient's past medical history included 13-year treatment of hypertension; several hospitalizations for substernal pain without electrocardiographic or enzyme evidence of acute myocardial infarction; syncope and seizures; alcoholic intake of up to a gallon of wine daily; and 40-year smoking history. His current medications were *alpha*-methyldopa, 250 mg q.i.d.; hydralazine, 50 mg q.i.d.; propranolol, 40 mg q.i.d.; dyazide capsules, one daily; phenytoin (diphenylhydantoin), 100 mg t.i.d.; and phenobarbital, 15 mg q.i.d.

On admission to the hospital, icteric sclerae, cardiomegaly with a grade 3 holosystolic murmur, and right upper quadrant tenderness were noted. The patient's blood pressure was 130/90, pulse was 72, respiratory rate was 18, and oral temperature was 101.2° F. Laboratory values were hemoglobin 13.1 g/100 ml, hematocrit 41%, white blood cell count 15,400 with a shift to the left, serum sodium 141 mEq/L, serum potassium 4.2 mEq/L, serum chloride 105 mEq/L, serum bicarbonate 23 mEq/L, blood urea nitrogen 16 mg/100 ml, creatinine 1.1 mg/100 ml, and total bilirubin 9 mg/100 ml. The chest roentgenogram was normal except for cardiomegaly, the ECG (electrocardiogram) indicated left ventricular hypertrophy with a strain pattern, and a percutaneous transhepatic cholangiogram demonstrated a common duct stone. He was scheduled for cholecystectomy and for common duct exploration the following day.

This chapter discusses the interaction of inhalation anesthetics with prior drug therapy as well as the interaction of agents administered during anesthesia. It demonstrates that under optimal conditions the patient may usually continue to benefit from previous drug therapy up to the time of anesthesia and operation.

INFLUENCE OF PRIOR DRUG THERAPY

Antihypertensive Drugs

Antihypertensive drugs can be classified by their mechanism of action. A common list categorizes these agents.[1] Diuretics include the benzothiazines, and loop and distal tubule diuretics. They produce a natriuresis that decreases blood volume, extracellular fluid volume, and cardiac output via a loss of sodium chloride and, to a lesser extent, potassium. Adrenergic inhibitors function centrally or peripherally. The centrally acting agents include *alpha*-methyldopa, clonidine, and guanabenz. *Alpha*-

methyldopa enters the norepinephrine biosynthetic pathway with the formation of *alpha*-methylnorepinephrine which acts as an *alpha* 2-adrenoreceptor agonist in the central nervous system, inhibiting the outflow of sympathetic impulses. Clonidine stimulates presynaptic *alpha* 2-adrenergic receptors in the medulla thereby liberating norepinephrine, downregulating sympathetic tone, and diminishing the release of norepinephrine from peripheral adrenergic nerves. Guanabenz is a centrally acting *alpha*-adrenergic antihypertensive drug that reduces central sympathetic outflow through stimulation of central *alpha* 2-adrenergic receptors. Antihypertensives with peripheral sympathomimetic action include reserpine, guanethidine, prazosin, and the *beta*-adrenergic blocking drugs. Reserpine and guanethidine deplete norepinephrine stores. Proposed mechanisms for the hypotensive action of *beta*-blockers include a decreased heart rate and cardiac output by action on cardiac *beta*-adrenoreceptors, a central *beta*-adrenoreceptor antagonism, and an inhibition of renin secretion. The *beta*-adrenergic blocker labetalol also has significant peripheral *alpha*-adrenoreceptor activity. Hydralazine and minoxidil are direct arteriolar dilators; they are commonly used with other agents that control tachycardia and sodium retention. Other mechanisms of antihypertensive therapy include inhibition of the renin-angiotensin system by captopril and calcium-channel blockade with nifedipine, verapamil, or diltiazem.[1-3]

Our concept of the interaction between antihypertensive agents and inhalation anesthetics has changed dramatically over the last 25 years. Originally it was feared that antihypertensive agents, by altering sympathetic tone, as well as fluid and electrolyte balance, would lead to drastic changes in cardiovascular function, especially hypotension, particularly with agents such as cyclopropane that depend upon sympathetic nervous system stimulation for cardiovascular support, or with halothane, enflurane, or isoflurane, which cause myocardial depression or vasodilation.[4,5] Reports of hypotension, bradycardia, and unresponsiveness to vasopressor therapy during anesthesia in patients receiving norepinephrine-depleting antihypertensive drugs, especially reserpine, led to the practice of discontinuing reserpine and other antihypertensive agents 10 days to 2 weeks before anesthesia.

Subsequently, the impression that intraoperative hypotension could be due to other causes, such as hemorrhage or reflex response to surgical manipulations, the awareness that hypertensive patients are prone to greater oscillations in blood pressure, and the unavoidable emergency surgery and anesthesia in patients who were taking reserpine, led to the conclusion that it was not necessary to discontinue antihypertensive medication before surgery.[6] The anesthetic course of patients whose blood pressure is controlled by reserpine up to the time of surgery compares well with patients in whom reserpine has been discontinued, indicating persistence of compensatory reflexes, and confirming the safety of this form of antihypertensive therapy.[2,3,7-10]

Current practice is based on clinical experience and data gathered in two well-known studies that present some conflicting findings, and that have troublesome shortcomings.[11-13] The first study was directed toward the evaluation of a single selected anesthetic technique, halothane 1%, and nitrous oxide and oxygen, in normotensive, untreated hypertensive patients or treated hypertensive patients.[11] Patients with adequately controlled arterial pressure exhibited circulatory changes analogous to those that occur in normotensive patients who receive halothane.[11] The major alteration in cardiovascular function in the untreated patient was decreased peripheral vascular resistance with hypotension, dysrhythmias, or evidence of myocardial ischemia. Hypotension was most pronounced during the induction of anesthesia; endotracheal intubation was frequently marked by hypertension, tachycardia, and dysrhythmias.[11,14] Responses to endotracheal intubation may be controlled by *beta*-blockade.[15] The second study involved the prospective evaluation of a large number of hypertensive patients undergoing anesthesia and surgical procedures.[12] Although patients with higher preoperative blood pressure had larger absolute intraoperative blood pressure decreases, the lowest mean intraoperative systolic pressure in well-controlled hypertensive patients did not differ from that in patients with poorly treated or untreated mild to moderate hypertension. Intraoperatively the need for adrenergic agents or fluid challenges did not differ in these groups. Predictors of perioperative hypertension included the type of operation and a history of diastolic blood pressure of 110 mm Hg or higher. The data identify two factors of perioperative cardiac complications—the cardiac risk index score and development of severe decreases in intraoperative blood pressure.[12,16] These data suggest that elective surgery in the absence of ideal antihypertensive therapy need not subject patients to added clinical risk, provided diastolic pressure is stable and not higher than 110 mm Hg.

It therefore seems clear that preoperative control of blood pressure is almost obligatory, because of the potential for wide variation in arterial pressure in untreated hypertensive patients, and that elective anesthesia and surgery should be postponed if the diastolic pressure exceeds 110 mm Hg. Antihypertensive medications should be continued up to and including the morning of surgery. Discontinuance of chronic antihypertensive therapy is especially hazardous with clonidine and *beta*-adrenergic blocker therapy, since rebound hypertension and loss of protection from sympathetic stimuli during anesthesia and surgery may occur.[17-19]

Drugs that deplete central nervous system catecholamines decrease anesthetic requirements. In the dog, treatment with either *alpha*-methyldopa or reserpine reduces the minimal alveolar concentration (MAC) for halothane, whereas guanethidine, which depletes only peripheral catecholamine stores, does not alter MAC.[20]

The anesthetic management of the hypertensive patient receiving antihypertensive therapy is multifaceted. No anesthetic technique is superior to any other, but careful titration of anesthetic drugs is indicated. Invasive monitoring will allow the anesthetist to respond rapidly to alterations in blood pressure. Many drugs should be available to control blood pressure. Management of hypotension includes reduction in anesthetic concentration, change in position, modification of positive airway pressure, appropriate fluid therapy, atropine, and vasopressors. Direct-acting vasopressors, such as methoxamine and phenylephrine, are preferable to indirect-acting ones. Since direct-acting pressors may induce excessive responses owing to receptor oversensitivity in the treated patient, the dose of pressor drug should be carefully titrated. The increased systemic vascular resistance that occurs when blood pressure is increased by these agents may be dangerous if myocardial contractility is depressed by an inhalation agent or myocardial disease. The treatment of hypertension and tachycardia should include direct-acting vasodilators, *alpha*-receptor antagonists, and intravenous nitrates.

In summary, the evidence indicates the safety and the desirability of continuing antihypertensive medications up to the time of anesthesia. The value of controlling arterial pressure seems clearly established, and remains the most important consideration in the anesthetic management of the hypertensive patient.

Beta-Adrenergic Antagonists

Beta-adrenergic receptors are divided into two classes: *beta* 1-receptors, whose stimulation causes increased cardiac inotropy, chronotropy, and excitability, increased plasma renin activity and aqueous humor production; and *beta* 2-receptors, whose stimulation results in bronchodilation, vasodilation, uterine relaxation, skeletal muscle tremor, increased insulin secretion, glycogenolysis, and gluconeogenesis.[21,22] Blockade of *beta* 1-receptors reduces the strength of myocardial contraction, rate of shortening and tension development, heart rate, and blood pressure. The total oxygen demand on the heart is decreased, and this decreases myocardial oxygen consumption and exercise tolerance. Atrioventricular (AV) node refractory time and AV conduction are prolonged. Antagonism of *beta* 2-receptors inhibits *beta* 2 effects.[21,22] *Beta*-antagonists are either nonselective with mixed *beta* 1- and *beta* 2-antagonism or cardioselective with relatively more *beta* 1-antagonism. Of the *beta*-adrenergic blockers available in the United States, propranolol, nadolol, timolol, and pindolol are nonselective, with propranolol and pindolol having a membrane stabilizing, or quinidine-like, action. Pindolol also possesses intrinsic sympathomimetic activity. Metoprolol and atenolol are cardioselective in low doses.[23] *Beta*-adrenergic blockers are used in the treatment of coronary artery disease and angina, hypertension, dysrhythmias, migraine headache, glaucoma, some forms of tremor, and hypertrophic obstructive cardiomyopathy.[22,23]

Previous clinical reports of serious myocardial depression following cardiopulmonary bypass in patients on long-term propranolol therapy, as well as concern over inhalation anesthetic-propranolol interaction, led to the recommendation that oral propranolol therapy be discontinued 2 weeks before anesthesia.[24] Currently, patients are maintained on *beta*-adrenergic blocker therapy up to the time of surgery to maintain the benefits of the therapy to the patient and to avoid an increased incidence of angina, hypertension, or infarction that may follow abrupt withdrawal of these drugs, as well as because of our greater understanding of the effects of *beta*-adrenergic blockade during anesthesia.[25,26]

Although considerable data are available on the interaction of *beta*-adrenergic blockers and inhalation anesthetics, most of the studies involve propranolol. The interaction has been studied by means of the intravenous or long-term oral administration of *beta*-blockers in dogs, although intravenous administration may differ in its effects from long-term oral administration. Intravenous propranolol, 0.2 mg/kg, reduces cardiac output 47%, and decreases stroke volume, myocardial contractility, and systolic blood pressure in dogs receiving cyclopropane.[27] Similar results are obtained with diethyl ether anesthesia.[28] Dogs anesthetized with trichloroethylene show a 25% reduction in cardiac output following oral propranolol therapy.[29] An additive myocardial-depressant action, in which cardiac output is reduced by 15%, can be shown in dogs receiving methoxyflurane and intravenous *beta*-blockers.[30]

In the dog, halothane 1% and intravenous propranolol, 0.2 mg/kg, produce a decrease in heart rate with no change in cardiac output. This was part of the cyclopropane study noted above and illustrates the major cardiovascular depression produced by propranolol in combination with a sympathomimetic inhalation anesthetic such as cyclopropane. After propranolol both anesthetics behaved hemodynamically similarly.[27] Propranolol, 0.25 mg/kg, administered intravenously, and halothane 0.7% decrease cardiac output, reflecting increased afterload and increased peripheral vascular resistance and blood pressure.[31] Halothane and prolonged high-dose propranolol in dogs slightly decrease cardiac output and stroke volume without changing heart rate or systemic vascular resistance.[32,33] The added depression produced by propranolol is equivalent to an additional 0.5% halothane concentration. The intravenous administration of propranolol to dogs anesthetized with enflurane, which does not stimulate sympathetic function, causes deterioration in cardiovascular function, with large decreases in mean arterial pressure, cardiac output, and myocardial contractility.[34,35] In contrast, isoflurane plus intravenous propranolol produce either mild depression—comparable to that seen with halothane plus propranolol—or no depression in dogs anesthetized with 1 MAC or 2 MAC halothane and given propranolol, 0.1 and 0.2 mg/kg.[36,37]

Studies in man indicate a lack of cardiovascular depression when inhalation anesthetics and *beta*-adrenergic blockers are combined. Intravenous propranolol administered to healthy patients given atropine produces minimal effects.[38] Results obtained from a larger series of patients undergoing coronary artery bypass graft surgery show no difference in arterial pressure, heart rate, or incidence of hypotension, irrespective of whether propranolol had been discontinued 24, 48, or over 48 hours before the induction of nitrous-oxide, enflurane, and oxygen anesthesia.[25] In another large group of patients who were not undergoing cardiac surgery, a similar schedule of propranolol administration associated with nitrous oxide-relaxant or nitrous oxide-halothane anesthesia did not change the incidence of hypotension or of bradycardia in any group, irrespective of the anesthetic used.[26] In a group of cardiac patients given propranolol up to 6 hours before surgery and anesthetized with nitrous oxide-halothane, there was a decrease in heart rate, but no difference in cardiac output, mean arterial pressure, stroke volume, or systemic vascular resistance when compared with cardiac patients not receiving propranolol.[39] The cardiovascular stability afforded by halothane is also demonstrated in hypertensive patients who receive *beta*-adrenergic blockers and other antihypertensive drugs up to the morning of surgery. Following intravenous atropine, patients with *beta*-adrenergic blockade showed higher mean arterial pressure and cardiac output and lower systemic vascular resistance than did a group of hypertensive patients receiving only conventional antihypertensive medication.[15] Fewer dysrhythmias and less ECG evidence of myocardial ischemia are observed in patients with *beta*-adrenergic blockade following endotracheal intubation.[14]

The addition of the stress imposed by hemorrhage has been evaluated in dogs by the acute reduction of 20 to 25% of their blood volume. *Beta*-blocked dogs anesthetized with halothane both with and without experimentally induced myocardial infarction tolerate hemorrhage well, as do dogs receiving isoflurane.[36,40,41] The imposition of both hemorrhage and *beta*-blockade on trichloroethylene, methoxyflurane, and particularly enflurane anesthesia, however, is poorly tolerated.[29,30,35]

These studies in man and animals suggest that myocardial depression produced by inhalation anesthetics in the patient treated with *beta*-adrenergic blockers is additive[32,42] and that greater depression will occur with interactions involving inhalation anesthetic agents that produce sympathomimetic stimulation. Isoflurane, nitrous oxide-narcotic, or halothane may be the anesthetic agents of choice, especially in the presence of additional stress of hemorrhage or depression of left ventricular function. Intravenous doses of propranolol of 0.25 mg to 0.5 mg are recommended. High doses of cardioselective *beta*-adrenergic blockers are similar to nonselective drugs in their actions. Animal studies with oxyprenolol, which possesses intrinsic sympathomimetic activity, show that some of the depressant effects of the inhalation agent may be antagonized.[43] The use of timolol topically for glaucoma treatment may result in hypotension, bradycardia, and bronchospasm.[44]

Hypotension associated with propranolol during anesthesia is treated by decreasing the inspired anesthetic concentration, by increasing fluid administration, or by administering atropine or vasopressors. Intravenous calcium may improve myocardial performance. Since the *beta*-adrenergic block is competitive in nature, isoproterenol may overcome it. Increased doses of isoproterenol may be required, however, and dysrhythmias and tachycardia may precede inotropic effects. Glucagon and digitalis also retain their inotropic activity and *beta*-adrenergic blockade.

Calcium-Channel Blocking Drugs

The calcium-channel blocking drugs interfere with the influx of calcium through slowly activated ion channels and thereby inhibit conduction, myocardial contraction, and the contracture of vascular smooth muscle. The agents available in the United States are verapamil, nifedipine, and diltiazem. They have differing chemical structures and mechanisms of action. Verapamil is a derivative of papaverine and a racemic mixture of *d* and *l* optical isomers. The *l* isomer inhibits calcium influx by prolonging the inactivation phase of the slow calcium channels; the *d* isomer exerts a quinidine-like effect on the fast inward flux of sodium.[45,46] Nifedipine blocks the calcium channels on the cell surface but does not effect calcium-channel kinetics.[45,46] Diltiazem blocks the slow current, lowering the plateau phase of the action potential and depressing cardiac contractility. High concentrations inhibit the fast (sodium) channels.[45,46] Verapamil and diltiazem produce decreased SA node discharge and increased AV node conduction time and refractory period. Nifedipine produces major coronary and systemic arteriolar vasodilatation. Verapamil and diltiazem produce more cardiac depression than does nifedipine, possibly because of a greater reduction in afterload and less negative chronotropic and dromotropic action produced by nifedipine. The main clinical use of verapamil is in the management of supraventricular tachycardias, but it is also used in the management of angina because of its mild coronary artery and systemic arteriolar dilating properties. Nifedipine is used in the treatment of the hypertensive patient affected by coronary artery disease, in which it is frequently combined with *beta*-adrenergic blockers to control heart rate.[45,46]

Numerous investigations demonstrate the interaction between calcium-channel blockers and inhalation anesthetics. In animals, intravenous verapamil, with controlled and equipotent anesthetic concentrations, decreases myocardial contractility and arterial pressure, has varying effects on cardiac output, decreases systemic vascular resistance, and increases atrioventricular conduction time.[47-50] Increasing the doses of verapamil decreases arterial pressure, cardiac index, and left ventricular dP/dt during enflurane or isoflurane anesthesia, with the greatest depression being produced by enflurane. The only significant change during halothane anesthesia is prolongation of the PR interval. Systemic vascular resistance is unchanged.[49] Data on nifedipine show that reduction in systemic vascular resistance is the major change caused by this drug during anesthesia with a potent inhaled agent.[50,51]

Several studies involving calcium-channel blockers and inhalation anesthesia have been performed in humans. One study examined intravenous verapamil administered during halothane anesthesia for treatment of dysrhythmias and indicated a reduction in blood pressure and prolongation of the PR interval.[52] Other studies involving nitrous oxide-narcotic anesthesia in patients with good ventricular function, showed that intravenous verapamil caused a decrease in arterial pressure and systemic vascular resistance, no change in heart rate, and an increase or no change in cardiac output.[53,54] Another investigation demonstrated a small additional decrease in arterial pressure secondary to decreased systemic resistance when verapamil was given intravenously to patients who had normal left ventricular function, were anesthetized with halothane, were receiving chronic therapy with *beta*-adrenergic blockers, and were to undergo coronary artery surgery.[55]

These reported interactions between general anesthetics and calcium-channel blockers lead to several clinical considerations. Although no data exist on the effects of chronic preoperative therapy and inhalation anesthetics, there is no theoretical indication that calcium-channel blockers should be discontinued before anesthesia. Rather they should be continued because of the therapeutic benefit they afford. The effects of these drugs seem additive with inhalation anesthetics with respect to their effects on myocardial contractility, systemic vascular resistance, and PR conduction time. Reduced concentrations of the inhalation agent should be considered, and particular caution with enflurane is necessary. Plasma levels of verapamil are directly related to the development of myocardial depression. Fortunately, conduction abnormalities and the antidysrhythmic effect are evident at lower plasma levels. Therefore, low-dose IV administration during anesthesia may avoid major myocardial depression. Patients with poor ventricular function, conduction defects, hypovolemia, and preexisting *beta*-adrenergic blockade are at greatest risk with the combination of anesthesia and calcium-channel blockers. Verapamil has also been shown to exacerbate the effects of hyperkalemia during halothane anesthesia.[56] Calcium-channel blockers will not attenuate tachycardia and hypertension secondary to the sympathetic stimulation elicited by intubation.[1]

The therapy of cardiovascular depression produced by anesthesia plus calcium-channel blockers includes the use of muscarinic blocking agents. Intravenous calcium will increase cardiac output through an increase in contractility. *Alpha*-adrenergic agonists may be preferable to calcium therapy for treatment of decreased peripheral resistance, while combined *alpha*- and *beta*-adrenergic agonists may be indicated in patients with poor left ventricular function.

Levodopa

*Levo*dopa is the immediate precursor of dopamine. Unlike dopamine, it can penetrate the blood-brain barrier. Thus the rate-limiting step in catecholamine synthesis is bypassed, and *levo*dopa is rapidly converted to dopamine by dopa decarboxylase. Dopamine inhibits dopamine neurons in the basal ganglia that control extrapyramidal function. *Levo*dopa is also converted to dopamine in peripheral tissues. A decarboxylase inhibitor, such as carbidopa or benserazide, that blocks the peripheral conversion of *levo*dopa to dopamine may often be administered simultaneously; these inhibitors have no central effect. Increased amounts of dopamine are responsible for the cardiovascular side effects of *levo*dopa therapy.[57–59] Postural hypotension is due to several mechanisms, such as dopaminergic effect on the peripheral vasculature, the replacement of norepinephrine by dopamine, and a possible central action of *levo*dopa itself. Dysrythmias and hypertension also occur, although less frequently than hypotension, and a decrease in intravascular volume is seen. *Levo*dopa should be administered up to the time of anesthesia for several reasons, including its effectiveness in controlling the symptoms of Parkinson's disease, the short duration of its action, and the danger that its sudden withdrawal may precipitate chest wall rigidity and excessive salivation.[60]

The interaction between *levo*dopa and inhalation anesthetics is minor and is probably caused by rapidly diminishing peripheral dopamine concentrations. Hypotension is a potential problem owing to the hypotensive effects of dopamine combined with the vasodilation and the cardiac depression produced by inhalation anesthetic agents. Dysrhythmias may occur with anesthetics that sensitize the heart to catecholamines, although dopamine is approximately one-seventy-fifth as dysrhythmogenic as norepinephrine.[61] Since butyrophenones block the dopaminergic activity of dopamine, the droperidol used in neuroleptanesthesia can produce muscle rigidity.[62] Small doses of *levo*dopa decrease halothane MAC in dogs. This is probably due to the fact that a small increase in blood dopamine level facilitates neuromuscular blockade. When large doses of *levo*dopa are used, halothane MAC increases in the early phases of anesthesia and decreases after 3 hours. This biphasic response may be due to increased CNS norepinephrine levels, owing to its displacement by dopamine from nerve terminals in the CNS.[63]

Tricyclic Antidepressants

Tricyclic antidepressants block the mechanism of reuptake of catecholamines from the synaptic cleft to intracellular storage areas, alter the mechanism of catecholamine storage, and possess an anticholinergic effect. The most important side effects of these agents are cardiac, and an atropine-like action, myocardial depression, and dysrhythmias are seen with high therapeutic doses or with overdosage. Therapeutic doses of tricyclic antidepressants usually produce no cardiovascular side effects.[64] Tricyclic antidepressants need not be discontinued before anesthesia. However, the cardiac depressant and dysrhythmogenic potential associated with tricyclic antidepressant therapy should be considered when selecting inhalation anesthetic agents. Interaction with inhalation anesthetics is uncommon, although a delayed awakening of the patient and a decrease in MAC have been reported.[65,66] Interactions between these antidepressant and antihypertensive agents may cause problems with preoperative blood pressure control, and an exacerbated pressor response may follow the administration of vasopressors.[67,68] Ventricular dysrhythmias are common in dogs that are pretreated with a tricyclic antidepressant, anesthetized with halothane, and receiving pancuronium. The use of this combination in patients should be avoided.[69]

MAOI

At present, monoamine oxidase inhibitors (MAOI) are rarely administered as psychotherapeutic or antihypertensive agents, although increased usage does occur in elderly patients who do not respond to tricyclic antidepressants. Inhibitors of monoamine oxidase interfere with the oxidative deamination of norepinephrine, dopamine, and serotonin. There are several important drug interactions involving MAOI. Severe hypertension may follow the administration of indirect acting sympathomimetic amines.[70,71] The combination of MAOI and meperidine can be accompanied either by potentiation of the narcotic response, consisting of hypotension, respiratory depression, and coma; or by an excitatory response marked by tachycardia, hypertension, hyperthermia, and convulsions.[70,72] Other narcotics may produce similar actions and should be used carefully, although a dog study and case reports suggest the safety of fentanyl.[73,74] Delayed awakening in patients may follow barbiturate administration, perhaps owing to partial interference with barbiturate metabolism by the MAOI on liver microsomal enzymes; other sedatives may show prolonged effects. Interactions with inhalation anesthetics are not clearly defined; it has been suggested that general anesthetics be avoided in patients receiving MAOI for several reasons. Certain anesthetics and techniques may stimulate the sympathetic nervous system. Delayed awakening in patients receiving MAOI following inhalation anesthetics may occur. Halothane MAC is not increased in the dog by pretreatment with iproniazid, whereas iproniazid increases MAC in the rat.[20] Current opinion recommends that MAOI be discontinued 2 weeks before inhalation anesthesia since most of these inhibiting drugs are irreversible inhibitors of MAO. Nitrous-oxide-fentanyl anesthesia may be safe in emergency situations.[74] Hypotensive responses should be treated with small amounts of direct-acting vasopressors, whereas hypertension may be managed by adrenolytic or ganglionic blocking drugs or by direct-acting vasodilators. *Beta*-adrenergic blockade for the treatment of dysrhythmias is dangerous.

Phenothiazines

Phenothiazines and their congeners and derivatives are especially effective in the treatment of schizophrenia. These drugs are usually administered in progressive doses until a therapeutic benefit or extrapyramidal side effects occur. The cardiovascular effects and sedation induced by phenothiazines may have important consequences when inhalation anesthetics are administered.

The interaction has two important clinical aspects. Although phenothiazines are poor hypnotics, they have been used as premedicants, often in combination with narcotics. Hypotension and, less commonly, tachycardia may occur, thereby decreasing the desirability of phenothiazines for preanesthetic medication.[75-77] The administration of small doses of these agents before inhalation anesthesia does not cause major cardiovascular changes. In large doses, chlorpromazine, 400 mg or more daily, may increase hypotension during and may delay awakening after inhalation anesthesia.[78] The mechanism of the hypotension produced by phenothiazines is unclear. However, weak *alpha*-adrenergic blockade, peripheral vasodilation, and central nervous system effects have been implicated. Current opinion suggests that if phenothiazine therapy is essential to the patient's emotional stability, the drug should be administered until the induction of anesthesia. If a modification of dosage is required, phenothiazine levels may be effectively altered within 48 hours. Maintenance of adequate blood volume and appreciation of the additional cardiovascular depression produced by certain inhalation anesthetics and by other adjunct drugs is important for the successful management of these patients. The effectiveness of vasopressor agents may be compromised by increased vascular resistance, and epinephrine, an *alpha*- and *beta*-receptor stimulator, is more effective in the treatment of hypotension than are pure *alpha*-adrenergic stimulants.[79]

High-dose administration of butyrophenones may cause similar problems. Experience gained with the intravenous administration of smaller doses of droperidol in neuroleptanesthesia indicates that a brief decrease in blood pressure may occur secondary to peripheral vasodilation and to weak *alpha*-adrenergic blockade.[80,81] There is little alteration in cardiovascular function following the addition of nitrous oxide, except in patients who are hypovolemic or who have significant myocardial pathologic condition, in which cases arterial pressure may decrease.[80,81]

Aminophylline

Aminophylline is used in the pre- and intraoperative anesthetic management of patients with asthma and chronic obstructive pulmonary disease. High concentrations of the potent inhalation agents are often administered to asthmatic patients to block bronchospasm secondary to endotracheal intubation under light anesthesia. Deep anesthesia, however, may also sensitize the myocardium to catecholamines and to aminophylline.[82] The cardiovascular effects of aminophylline include an increased heart rate and a decreased systemic vascular resistance; these changes may be magnified by the potent anesthetic agents.[83] There are case reports of ventricular dysrhythmias following preoperative aminophylline in patients anesthetized with halothane.[83,84]

Animal studies with intravenous aminophylline infusions suggest that ventricular dysrhythmias are rare if the therapeutic range of aminophylline is not exceeded, and that the dysrhythmias usually resolve spontaneously.[85] In the presence of toxic aminophylline levels, there is a greater tendency for halothane to be associated with ventricular dysrhythmias than is enflurane or isoflurane.[86,87]

Ethanol

The induction of anesthesia in alcoholics is often prolonged and can be characterized by excitement and an increased anesthetic requirement. These impressions are corroborated by studies showing that continuous ethanol ingestion for 10 to 20 days increases the required anesthetizing concentration (ED_{50}, or median effective dose) of isoflurane in rats.[88] Chronic ethanol ingestion increases the minimal alveolar concentration of halothane in man.[89] Tolerance to drug-induced central nervous system depression in the chronic alcoholic may not apply to the cardiovascular system, so that serious cardiovascular depression may be associated with anesthetic concentrations required for unconsciousness.[90,91] Acute ethanol intoxication reduces the ED_{50} for isoflurane in the rat.[88] One should expect lessened anesthetic requirements for the acutely intoxicated patient, and data indicate that alcohol reduces the anesthetic requirements of halothane proportionally more than it reduces the concentration necessary to produce respiratory or cardiac failure.[90,91]

INFLUENCE OF DRUGS ADMINISTERED BY THE ANESTHETIST

Preanesthetic Medication

Barbiturates, benzodiazepines, butyrophenones, and other sedatives used for premedication minimally depress the circulation and respiration, although preanesthetic administration of phenothiazine may cause hypotension.[77,81] These agents rarely produce a clinically significant greater depression after the induction of inhalation anesthesia, although evaluations of MAC indicate that these agents do reduce the amount of inhalation anesthetic required.[92] The time for awakening after anesthesia is not prolonged. Narcotic analgesics used singly or in combination with other sedatives may increase cardiovascular or respiratory depression during inhalation anesthesia, reduce anesthetic requirements, and increase sleep time.[93,94]

Intravenous Induction Agents

The administration of thiopental decreases myocardial contractility and arterial pressure and increases heart rate, with little change in systemic vascular resistance.[95] This agent decreases systemic vascular resistance in patients with uncontrolled hypertension.[14] The cardiorespiratory-depressant effects of thiopental are so brief that they usually do not alter a patient's response to inhalation anesthesia, although in the hypovolemic patient or the patient with cardiac disease, greater cardiovascular depression may occur with the combination.

Induction with intravenous diazepam produces variable and small changes in heart rate, arterial pressure, and systemic vascular resistance, with unaltered cardiac index both in normal patients and in those with myocardial disease.[96-98] Larger induction doses may decrease blood pressure and stroke volume more significantly. Respiratory depression is common following induction with intravenous doses large enough to produce induction of anesthesia.[96,97] The addition of narcotics following diazepam for induction decreases blood pressure and systemic vascular resistance.[99] The long plasma clearance of diazepam causes the circulatory and respiratory effects to extend into anesthesia and may also produce interactions with inhalation anesthetics. Studies of anesthetic interaction involving the addition of nitrous oxide following intravenous diazepam show either no cardiovascular changes or a decrease in arterial pressure and left ventricular stroke work.[100,101] Induction with diazepam reduces anesthetic requirements.[92]

The interaction between ketamine and inhalation anesthetics is becoming an important clinical consideration with the increasing use of ketamine in a rapid-sequence induction in cases where an increase in blood pressure, heart rate, and cardiac output may be desirable in critically ill patients.[102,103]

Hypertension predominates with the subsequent administration of nitrous oxide.[102] Studies of ketamine administration to patients receiving halothane or enflurane indicate blockade of the cardiovascular stimulating properties of ketamine; a decrease in cardiac output and blood pressure is observed, with greater depression occurring in patients receiving halothane.[104–106] Ketamine reduces the minimal alveolar concentration of halothane, and a similar action with other inhalation agents would be expected.[107]

Narcotic Anesthesia

Anesthesia may be induced slowly with high-dose morphine, meperidine, fentanyl, a combination of fentanyl and droperidol, or by the new agents, alfentanil and sufentanil. Intravenous narcotics used in this fashion rarely produce major circulatory alteration, although bradycardia and hypotension due to arteriolar and venular dilation may occur, particularly with morphine.[108,109] Fentanyl-droperidol combinations may decrease arterial pressure and systemic vascular resistance.[80,81,110,111] Nitrous oxide is often used with narcotic anesthesia. Nitrous oxide has minimal cardiovascular effects by itself, although it can directly produce myocardial depression that is balanced by sympathetic stimulation through increased sympathetic outflow from the brain and inhibition of norepinephrine breakdown in the lung.[112–115]

The addition of various concentrations of nitrous oxide to morphine anesthesia can produce a variety of effects, depending on the circumstances: a decrease in heart rate and cardiac output and an increase in systemic vascular resistance, with no change in blood pressure in healthy volunteers;[116] a decrease in arterial pressure and cardiac output and an increase in systemic vascular resistance in patients with valvular or coronary artery disease;[117] a dose-related decrease in cardiac output and arterial pressure with concentrations of nitrous oxide ranging from 10 to 50% in patients with valvular disease;[118] a decrease in arterial pressure and cardiac output without change in systemic vascular resistance in patients with coronary artery disease;[119] and a decrease in arterial pressure, heart rate, and cardiac output without changes in systemic vascular resistance in a diverse group of patients undergoing orthopedic or abdominal surgery.[120]

The interaction of nitrous oxide and fentanyl shows an increase in arterial pressure and systemic vascular resistance with coronary artery disease;[121] a decrease in arterial pressure, heart rate, and cardiac output without change in systemic vascular resistance in patients for orthopedic or abdominal surgery;[120] and a decrease in arterial pressure, heart rate, and cardiac output with no change in systemic vascular resistance in patients with valvular heart disease.[111] Similar results in this patient group occurred with the addition of nitrous oxide to fentanyl (10 µg/kg) − droperidol (100 µg/kg).[111]

The most frequent pattern of cardiovascular alteration in these studies is a decrease in cardiac output and blood pressure with an increase in systemic vascular resistance.[109] Nitrous oxide will also increase pulmonary vascular resistance in patients with valvular disease and pulmonary hypertension.[122,123] The use of nitrous oxide during narcotic induction will increase the incidence of truncal rigidity.[124] The addition of low-dose halothane to morphine anesthesia reduces arterial pressure and cardiac output in patients with coronary artery disease.[125] Bennett and Stanley[126] evaluated the addition of intravenous narcotic to anesthesia produced by halogenated agents. They based their investigation on the presumption that the narcotic will permit a reduction in the concentration of the potent inhalation agent and reduce cardiovascular depression. These authors demonstrated a decrease in cardiac output and arterial pressure and no change in systemic vascular resistance following intravenous fentanyl, 200 μg, during enflurane anesthesia, but no change following fentanyl, 50 to 100 μg.[126]

Nitrous Oxide

The most common interaction between inhalation anesthetics occurs when nitrous oxide is given with other, more potent volatile agents. The results of this interaction can affect several organ systems.

The use of nitrous oxide reduces the minimum alveolar concentration of any volatile anesthetic. This interaction is additive. Assuming a MAC of nitrous oxide of 100% (actually 115%), the addition of 70% nitrous oxide would reduce the MAC of the other agent by 70%. If the halothane-oxygen MAC is 0.74%, the addition of 70% nitrous oxide would reduce MAC to 0.29%.[93] If the fluroxene-oxygen MAC is 3.4%, the addition of 70% nitrous oxide would reduce MAC to 0.8%.[127] If the methoxyflurane-oxygen MAC is 0.16%, the addition of 70% nitrous oxide would reduce MAC to 0.07%.[128] With enflurane-oxygen, MAC is 1.68%, and the addition of 70% nitrous oxide would reduce MAC to 0.7%.[129] With isoflurane-oxygen, MAC is 1.28%, and the addition of 70% nitrous oxide would reduce MAC to 0.56%.[130] Again, all of this is based on the optimistic assumption that the MAC of nitrous oxide is 100%.

Nitrous oxide increases the speed of induction when used simultaneously with another inhaled agent. This increase is due in part to the rapid equilibration of alveolar with inspired concentration of nitrous oxide. Owing to its rapid onset, nitrous oxide anesthesia helps decrease the perceived irritative properties of the other agent and thereby allows the patient to inhale this agent more readily. The rapid initial uptake of nitrous oxide increases the rate of uptake of the other anesthetic. The uptake of this other agent is higher when administered with nitrous oxide than when administered either with oxygen or with air (second-gas effect).[131] Both a concentrating effect of the second gas due to the high nitrous oxide uptake and an increase in ventilation replenishing the lung with the same initial concentration of the delivered anesthetic mixture increase the concentration of the other anesthetic.[132] Whereas the second-gas effect is of some importance, rapid induction is usually accomplished by increasing either ventilation or the inspired concentration of the volatile agent. The abrupt discontinuance of nitrous oxide accelerates the elimination of halothane by diluting its alveolar concentration, thereby increasing the expired volume (reversed second-gas effect).[133] Dilution of alveolar oxygen and carbon dioxide will also occur.[134]

The addition of nitrous oxide decreases the respiratory effects of volatile anesthetics. At equipotent anesthetic doses, the use of nitrous oxide may result in less respiratory depression than would occur with the use of the volatile agent alone. An increase in respiratory rate is responsible for the maintenance of minute ventilation. At MAC for halothane plus nitrous oxide, 70%, resting ventilation is greater and carbon dioxide retention is less than at MAC for halothane-oxygen.[135] During equi-MAC isoflurane-nitrous oxide and isoflurane-oxygen anesthesia, the respiratory rate and minute ventilation are higher with nitrous oxide, although arterial carbon dioxide tension is similar.[136] The addition of nitrous oxide, 70%, to halothane, 0.8% or 1.5%, decreases tidal volume, and increases respiratory frequency with only minor increases in carbon dioxide tension.[135] The responsiveness of respiration to inhaled carbon dioxide is not altered by the addition of nitrous oxide to halothane, 0.8 or 1.5%, in volunteers.[135] This mild respiratory stimulation of nitrous oxide can also reduce the respiratory depression following thiopental, provided that no narcotic has been administered before thiopental.[137] The use of nitrous oxide with volatile anesthetics, coupled with the respiratory stimulation consequent to surgical incision, decreases respiratory depression.[138]

Important advantages are derived from administering nitrous oxide with a potent inhaled agent. This combination minimizes the cardiovascular depression produced by the potent inhalation anesthetic. At equi-MAC levels, the cardiovascular depression with nitrous oxide plus the potent agent is less than that occurring with the potent agent with oxygen alone. Halothane, 0.3%, in nitrous oxide depresses arterial pressure and cardiac output less than does halothane, 0.8%, in oxygen in volunteers with spontaneous ventilation.[135] During controlled ventilation at 1.2 and 2.4 MAC equivalents, halothane-nitrous oxide depresses cardiac output, mean arterial pressure, and ventricular work less than does halothane-oxygen.[139] At equi-MAC levels in volunteers, enflurane-nitrous oxide depresses the cardiovascular system less than enflurane-oxygen; evidence of cardiovascular support is most pronounced in comparisons at 1.5 MAC levels than at 1 MAC.[140] Comparative studies of nitrous oxide-isoflurane and isoflurane-oxygen at equi-anesthetic concentrations show that there is less hypotension with nitrous oxide, due to higher systemic vascular resistance. Heart rate, stroke volume, and cardiac output are similarly affected by both combinations.[136]

Inconsistent changes are noted following the addition of nitrous oxide to an existing level of a potent inhalation anesthetic. Cardiovascular stimulation by nitrous oxide is seen during its addition to diethyl ether; systemic vascular resistance and arterial pressure increase, cardiac output does not change.[141] Both *alpha*- and *beta*-adrenergic simulating effects are seen with the addition of nitrous oxide to fluroxene, with *alpha*-adrenergic effects dominating at 5%, and mixed *alpha* and *beta* effects at 9%.[142] The addition of nitrous oxide to halothane, 0.8%, during spontaneous ventilation in volunteers increases cardiac output, heart rate, stroke volume, and mean arterial pressure, with no alteration in vascular resistance. Conversely, the addition of nitrous oxide to halothane, 1.5%, in these volunteers resulted in cardiovascular depression.[135] In another study, the addition of nitrous oxide for 15 minutes to light halothane (0.8 to 1.2%) during controlled ventilation in volunteers increased arterial pressure and peripheral resistance without changing cardiac output, whereas the addition of nitrous oxide to higher halothane concentrations (1.5 to 2.0%) produced a greater increase.[143] In patients with acquired valvular heart disease, the addition of nitrous oxide to halothane, 0.55%, does not change arterial pressure, heart rate, stroke volume, cardiac index, or vascular resistance.[144] Nitrous oxide added to halothane, 0.5%, in patients with coronary artery disease results in depression of cardiac performance.[145] In volunteers, the addition of nitrous oxide to steady-state enflurane-oxygen anesthesia does not alter cardiovascular function.[140] This combination decreases arterial pressure and cardiac output and increases vascular resistance in patients who are undergoing operations in which several adjunct anesthetic drugs are also administered. The combination decreases systemic vascular resistance, heart rate, cardiac output, and arterial pressure in *beta*-blocked patients who have coronary artery disease.[146,147]

Data concerning the interaction between nitrous oxide and narcotics or potent inhalation agents vary for a number of reasons: differences between volunteers and patients who may receive adjunct drug therapy as well as premedication and have altered left ventricular function; the presence or absence of surgical stimulation; alteration in ventilation and oxygenation; attempts at equipotent levels of anesthesia; variation in the sequence of administration of the two anesthetics; and duration of anesthetic administration at the time of study. Alteration in arterial oxygen tension has been implicated when shifting from high oxygen concentration as carrier gas to oxygen, 30%, during the addition of nitrous oxide. However, studies with ether, fluroxene, halothane, and enflurane that have used nitrogen to reduce oxygen tension demonstrated that there is no change when oxygen concentration is decreased.

The addition of nitrous oxide to volatile anesthetics or to narcotic anesthesia induces a combination of *alpha-* and *beta*-adrenergic stimulation, as well as myocardial depression. Sympathetic stimulation is not equally effective with every agent; for example, the degree of stimulation depends upon the agent's inherent ability to stimulate the sympathetic nervous system. It also varies with depth of anesthesia: *alpha* effects predominate with light anesthesia, *alpha* and *beta* effects are seen at deeper levels of anesthesia, and ultimate cardiovascular depression occurs with deep anesthesia. Finally, sympathetic activation is altered by the patient's ability to respond with compensatory reflexes. With volatile anesthetics, sympathetic activation associated with nitrous oxide prevails, as evidenced by pupillary dilation and increased plasma norepinephrine.[143] In the rat this effect is demonstrated by the fact that nitrous oxide increases discharge from preganglionic cervical sympathetic nerves and splanchnic nerves, even in the face of halothane depression of pre- and postganglionic sympathetic activity.[148,149] Nitrous oxide and narcotics may depress the circulation because narcotics block the sympathomimetic effects of nitrous oxide and produce their own parasympathetic effects.

In summary, the interaction between nitrous oxide and volatile anesthetics and narcotics can account for varied cardiovascular responses. Normally one would expect less cardiovascular depression when nitrous oxide is *combined* with volatile anesthetics. If nitrous oxide is added to a volatile agent, cardiovascular depression may result. Obviously, nitrous oxide should not be considered to be a benign carrier gas without important effects of its own or devoid of significant interactions with other agents.

Neuromuscular Blocking Drugs

The interaction between inhalation anesthetics and neuromuscular blocking agents is of major importance. Inhalation anesthetics produce muscle relaxation as well as potentiate or add to the action of neuromuscular blocking drugs through several mechanisms. Depression of spinal cord reflexes achieved with high concentrations of some inhalation anesthetics produces relaxation sufficient to permit abdominal operations without the use of neuromuscular blocking drugs. Diethyl ether and enflurane induce desensitization of the postjunctional membrane to depolarization. An action distal to the postjunctional membrane is demonstrated by several phenomena: fading of contraction of innervated muscle caused by high tetanic rates of stimulation, lengthening of the neuromuscular refractory period, and reduction in twitch height.[149–156] An increase in muscle blood flow seen with isoflurane may cause a large percentage of the dose of a neuromuscular blocking agent to be distributed to the end plate.[157] This may explain why potentiation has not always been observed in isolated nerve-muscle preparation and may be responsible for the potentiation of succinylcholine blockade, a phenomenon that is observed with isoflurane only and observed *in vivo* only.[158]

The potentiation or additive effects of neuromuscular blocking drugs by inhalation anesthetics has a dual aspect. First, at equipotent depths of various anesthetics, the dose of neuromuscular blocking drug needed to produce identical degrees of depression of neuromuscular function depends upon the inhalation anesthetic.[153,158-160] Potentiation is greatest with enflurane and isoflurane, less for halothane, and minimal for nitrous oxide. The potencies of *d*-tubocurarine and pancuronium are influenced to a larger degree by the choice of anesthetic than are the potencies of vecuronium and atracurium. For example, enflurane or isoflurane may augment a *d*-tubocurarine or pancuronium block by more than 100% when compared with an equipotent halothane anesthetic.[158] A vecuronium or atracurium block is augmented only 20 to 30% by isoflurane or enflurane as compared with equal depth halothane anesthesia.[161-163] Second, the greater the depth of inhalation anesthesia, the less neuromuscular blocking drug is needed to achieve the desired degree of blockade.[159] Again the influence of anesthetic depth is greater with *d*-tubocurarine or pancuronium than with vecuronium or atracurium. An increase in isoflurane depth from 1.2 to 2.2 MAC decreases the ED_{50} of pancuronium 70%, yet only decreases that of vecuronium 33%.[159,163] At equal MAC levels, the amount of succinylcholine required for an equal amount of neuromuscular block is similar during halothane and enflurane anesthesia while up to 50% more succinylcholine may be required during halothane than during isoflurane anesthesia.[158,164]

The data on interactions between inhalation agent and neuromuscular blocking agents have primarily involved the evaluation of the intensity of neuromuscular block. Although the effects of the interaction of neuromuscular blocking drugs and anesthetic concentration on the duration of block has not been determined, a profound neuromuscular block induced by an overdose of relaxant in conjunction with a potentiating inhalation anesthetic agent inevitably prolongs recovery time.

Sympathomimetic Amines

Inhalation anesthetics sensitize the myocardium to endogenous and exogenous sympathomimetic amines and produce dysrhythmias. This sensitization is due to at least three factors: alterations of phase-four depolarization of the heart, an increase in the automaticity of cardiac muscle, and the production of hypertension.[165,166] The tendency of anesthetics to produce ventricular dysrhythmias has been evaluated in numerous studies in dogs at various levels of anesthetic depth or respiratory depression, and with various epinephrine doses. In this model, the order of decreasing sensitivity among common anesthetics is trichloroethylene, cyclopropane, halothane, and various halogenated ethers.[165] The extrapolation of these results to man is controversial, but such a ranking of sensitivity among anesthetics is useful in clinical practice, and studies in man indicate the basic accuracy of this approach.

Epinephrine and norepinephrine are the drugs most likely to cause dysrhythmias. The peripheral acting agents, methoxamine and phenylephrine, as well as ephedrine, mephentermine, and dopamine, are not considered to be as dysrhythmogenic as the first two drugs.

The catecholamine-inhalation agent interaction is important because sympathomimetic amines, particularly epinephrine, produce local hemostasis when injected submucosally or subcutaneously. The greatest risk involves cyclopropane and epinephrine combinations. In one clinical series, 30% of the patients developed ventricular dysrhythmias on administration of epinephrine 1:60,000, 6 ml every 5 minutes to a total dose of 30 ml (0.5 mg).[167] Whereas trichloroethylene is sensitizing in the dog, a clinical evaluation indicates that 1:60,000 to 1:200,000 epinephrine with a total dose in a 10-minute period or 30 ml per hour may be used safely in man.[168]

The two previously mentioned anesthetics are now seldom used, but the safety of epinephrine with halothane and with the newer halogenated ethers is a topic of major concern. Studies in dogs indicate that 10 μg/kg or less of epinephrine will eventually produce ventricular extrasystoles.[165]

With halothane the amount of epinephrine needed to produce this degree of ventricular irritability is 5 μg/kg, with methoxyflurane it is 15 μg/kg, with fluroxene it is over 40 μg/kg, with enflurane it is between 10 to 17 μg/kg, and with isoflurane it is greater than 20 μg/kg.[169–171] Earlier data concerning enflurane-epinephrine combinations in the dog indicated a 45% incidence of ventricular fibrillation with 10 μg/kg but more recent studies suggest that a dose of 17 μg/kg is more likely to be dysrhythmogenic.[170,172] Clinical studies indicate a greater myocardial sensitization to epinephrine with halothane than with either enflurane or isoflurane.[173–176] Patients receiving neither preanesthetic medication nor barbiturate induction were given epinephrine submucosally at equipotent anesthetic concentrations. Three or more premature ventricular contractions were observed at the following mean concentrations of epinephrine: 2.1 μg/kg in conjunction with halothane, 3.7 μg/kg with halothane when the epinephrine was mixed with lidocaine, 6.8 μg/kg with isoflurane, and 10.9 μg/kg with enflurane.[174]

Other clinical studies show the safety of using epinephrine (1:100,000 to 1:200,000 no more than 10 ml per 10 minutes or 30 ml in an hour) during halothane or halogenated ether anesthesia, although the tolerance seems higher with the latter.[173] Ten ml of 1:200,000 epinephrine represents less than 1 μg/kg in an adult.

There are still unresolved problems. One study suggests a lower incidence of dysrhythmias when lidocaine is mixed with epinephrine, whereas most other studies do not evaluate this mixture.[174] Adequate ventilation is considered to be important in avoiding dysrhythmias, although one study suggests that increasing PA_{CO_2} will not increase the incidence of dysrhythmias with halothane, isoflurane, or fluroxene.[171] The importance of anesthetic depth or of elevated arterial pressure preceding the onset of dysrhythmias in the production of ventricular irritability is not well defined.

Sympathomimetic amines are administered during anesthesia for the treatment of hypotension. The intravenous use of epinephrine or norepinephrine can be hazardous; these drugs are used only during resuscitative efforts following major cardiovascular depression occurring with sensitizing and nonsensitizing anesthetics or following cardiopulmonary bypass. In spite of their frequent intravenous administration, other amines have not been adequately evaluated as to their interaction with inhalation anesthetics. These agents, although occasionally given for surgical vasoconstriction, are usually administered intravenously. Dysrhythmias are caused by metaraminol and, to a lesser extent, by ephedrine injected intravenously in dogs during equipotent halothane or isoflurane anesthesia; the amount of amines needed is greater with isoflurane anesthesia. Phenylephrine also produces ventricular dysrhythmias, but at relatively higher doses than either ephedrine or metaraminol.[177] These effects are dose-dependent and suggest caution in the intravenous use of sympathomimetic amines during halothane anesthesia, although the peripherally acting (*alpha*-adrenergic) pressor agents seem to be better tolerated.

Metabolism

The development of delayed organ toxicity following inhalation anesthesia can possibly be related to the metabolism of the inhalation agent (see Chap. 6). The enzymatic metabolism of volatile agents is an oxidative process of ether cleavage or dehalogenation involving cytochrome P-450.[178–180] The metabolism of halothane may also involve a reductive mechanism under certain circumstances.[181] Inhalation anesthetics are capable of enzyme induction, and this has been demonstrated by various techniques, including increased levels of cytochrome P-450 in animals and man.[182–188]

Although inhalation anesthetics are weak inducing agents, the more soluble anesthetics remain in tissues for a length of time sufficient to produce enzyme induction; chronic exposure may be a greater stimulus to induction than is a high anesthetic concentration.[189] Anesthetic enzyme induction may increase the metabolism of the same agent on subsequent administration, or other anesthetics, and of drugs administered in the postoperative period.

Prior drug therapy also induces hepatic microsomal enzymes.[182] Important enzyme inducers include barbiturates, ethanol, chlorpromazine, meprobamate, chlordiazepoxide, diphenylhydantoin, diphenhydramine, various steroids, and isoniazid. Enzymatic induction secondary to prior drug therapy will also cause increased metabolism of inhalation anesthetics.[190,191]

Toxicity of these metabolites involves the kidney and liver. High levels of serum inorganic fluoride are directly correlated with nephrotoxicity associated with methoxyflurane and, to a lesser extent, enflurane metabolism.[192–194] While the most important factor in the level of the metabolite is the total amount of anesthetic administered (dose × time), increased metabolism may occur because of genetic factors or enzyme induction, increased sensitivity of kidneys to the effects of fluoride, and concurrent treatment with drugs known to be nephrotoxic.[195,196]

The implications of harmful metabolic products in the etiology of halothane-induced hepatotoxicity is controversial. Current investigations use an animal model in which enzyme induction, hypoxia, and reductive metabolism and covalent binding of potentially toxic reactive intermediates to microsomal lipids and proteins are essential elements in the production of centrolobular hepatic necrosis.[197] Evidence suggests that the reductive metabolites may be less significant in the etiology of halothane-induced hepatotoxicity than is hypoxia.[198] The use of fasting animals exacerbates liver toxicity with halothane,[199] under certain experimental conditions. Centrolobular hepatic necrosis is also associated with enflurane or isoflurane under certain experimental conditions, although reductive intermediate metabolites are not produced during the metabolism of these agents.[200] These data suggest that the following factors may be pertinent in patients in regard to hepatotoxicity: drug-related enzyme induction, poor nutritional status, halothane anesthesia, reduced hepatic oxygenation related to an anesthetic-produced decrease in splanchnic blood flow, and a reduced arterial concentration of oxygen during abdominal surgery.[201–203]

A positive correlation in the development of halothane hepatitis has been multiple exposure to halothane.[204] A hypersensitivity or immunologic response to the reactive intermediates has also been suggested. No experimental animal model exists for the production of an immunologic mechanism associated with halothane metabolism, and the recently described halothane-related antibody may be the *result* of the hepatic injury, not the cause.[205,206]

Summary

This chapter defines interactions involving inhalation anesthetics and drugs administered pre- and intraoperatively. The interactions are described in enough detail to provide the anesthesiologist with important information on perioperative management. Except in the case of monoamine oxidase inhibitors, a patient should continue to receive the benefits of previously instituted, long-term drug therapy up to the time of anesthesia. The maintenance of a stable cardiovascular system and the control of central nervous system disorders allow the patient to withstand the stress of anesthesia and surgery more safely. The use of multiple agents to achieve satisfactory anesthesia carries with it the concerns of interaction among inhalation agents themselves as well as between these agents and narcotic analgesics, sedatives, neuromuscular blocking drugs, and sympathomimetic amines. These interactions are so important that they must be considered in the administration of every anesthetic.

REFERENCES

1. Prys-Roberts, C.: Anesthesia and hypertension. Br. J. Anaesth., 56:711, 1984.
2. Prys-Roberts, C.: Chronic antihypertensive therapy; in cardiac anesthesia, Vol. 2. Cardiovascular Pharmacology (ed. J.A. Kaplan), New York, Grune & Stratton, 1983, p. 345–362.
3. Foex, P., and Prys-Roberts, C.: Anesthesia and the hypertensive patient. Br. J. Anaesth., 46:575, 1974.
4. Price, H.L., et al.: Sympathoadrenal responses to general anesthesia in man and their relation of hemodynamics. Anesthesiology, 20:563, 1959.
5. Eger, E., II, Smith, N.T., Cullen, D.J., et al.: A comparison of the cardiovascular effect of halothane, fluroxene, ether and cyclopropane in man. Anesthesiology, 34:25, 1971.
6. Munson, W.M., and Jenicek, J.A.: Effects of anesthetic agents on patients receiving reserpine therapy. Anesthesiology, 23:741, 1962.
7. Alper, M.H., Flacke, W., and Krayer, O.: Pharmacology of reserpine and its implications for anesthesia. Anesthesiology, 24:524, 1963.
8. Katz, R.L., Weintraub, H.D., and Papper, E.M.: Anesthesia, surgery, and rauwolfia. Anesthesiology, 25:142, 1964.
9. Hickler, R.B., and Vandam, L.D.: Hypertension. Anesthesiology, 33:214, 1970.
10. Ominsky, A.J., and Wollman, H.: Hazards of general anesthesia in the reserpinized patient. Anesthesiology, 30:443, 1969.
11. Prys-Roberts, C., Meloche, R., and Foex, P.: Studies of anesthesia in relation to hypertension I: Cardiovascular responses of treated and untreated patients. Br. J. Anaesth., 43:122, 1971.
12. Goldman, L., and Caldera, D.L.: Risks of general anesthesia and elective operation in the hypertensive patient. Anesthesiology, 50:285, 1979.
13. Prys-Roberts, C.: Hypertension and anesthesia-fifty years on. Anesthesiology, 50:281, 1979.
14. Prys-Roberts, C., et al.: Studies of anaesthesia in relation to hypertension II: Hemodynamic consequences of induction and endotracheal intubation. Br. J. Anaesth., 43:531, 1971.
15. Prys-Roberts, C., et al.: Studies of anaesthesia in relation to hypertension V: Adrenergic beta-receptor blockade. Br. J. Anaesth., 45:671, 1973.
16. Goldman, L., Caldera, D.L., Nussbaum, S.R., et al.: Multifactorial index of cardiac risk in noncardiac surgical procedures. N. Engl. J. Med., 297:845, 1977.
17. Bruce, D.L., Croley, T.F., and Lee, J.S.: Preoperative clonidine withdrawal syndrome. Anesthesiology, 51:90, 1979.
18. Alderman, E.L., Coltart, D.J., Wettach, G.E., et al.: Coronary artery syndromes after sudden propranolol withdrawal. Ann. Intern. Med., 81:625, 1974.
19. Miller, R.R., Olsen, H.G., Amsterdam, E.A., et al.: Propanolol-withdrawal rebound phenomenon. N. Engl. J. Med., 293:416, 1975.
20. Miller, R.D., Way, W.L., and Eger, E., II: The effects of alpha-methyldopa, reserpine, guanethidine and iproniazid on minimum alveolar anesthetic requirement (MAC). Anesthesiology, 29:1153, 1968.
21. Lands, A.M., Arnold, A., McAuliff, J.P., et al.: Differentiation of receptor system activated by sympathomimetic amines. Nature, 214:597, 1967.
22. Shand, D.G.: Propranolol. N. Engl. J. Med., 293:280, 1975.
23. Frishman, W.H.: Beta-adrenoceptor antagonists, new drugs and new indications. N. Engl. J. Med., 305:500, 1981.
24. Viljoen, J.F., Estafanous, G., and Kellner, G.A.: Propranolol and cardiac surgery. J. Thoracic. Cardiovasc. Surg., 64:826, 1972.
25. Kaplan, J.A., et al.: Propranolol and cardiac surgery: A problem for the anesthesiologist? Anesth. Analg., 54:571, 1975.
26. Kaplan, J.A., and Dunbar, R.W.: Propranolol and surgical anesthesia. Anesth. Analg., 55:1, 1976.
27. Craythorne, N.W.B., and Huffington, P.E.: Effects of propranolol on the cardiovascular response to cyclopropane and halothane. Anesthesiology, 27:580, 1966.
28. Jorfeldt, L., et al.: Cardiovascular pharmacodynamics of propranolol during either anesthesia in man. Acta Anaesthesiol. Scand., 11:159, 1967.
29. Foex, P., et al.: Is beta-adrenergic blockade compatible with trichloroethylene anesthesia? Br. J. Anaesth., 46:798, 1974.
30. Saner, C.A., et al.: Methoxyflurane and practol: a dangerous combination? Br. J. Anaesth., 47:1025, 1975.
31. Merin, R.G., and Tonnesen, A.S.: The effect of beta-adrenergic blockade on myocardial hemodynamics and metabolism during light halothane anesthesia. Can. Anaesth. Soc. J., 16:336, 1969.
32. Roberts, J.G., et al.: Haemodynamic interactions of high-dose propranolol pretreatment and anaesthesia in the dog I: Halothane dose response studies. Br. J. Anaesth., 48:315, 1976.
33. Roberts, J.G., et al.: Haemodynamic interactions of high-dose propranolol pretreatment and anesthesia in the dog II: The effects of acute arterial hypoxaemia at increasing depths of halothane anesthesia. Br. J. Anaesth., 48:403, 1976.
34. Millar, R.A., et al.: Further studies of sympathetic actions of anesthetics in intact and spinal animals. Br. J. Anaesth., 42:366, 1970.
35. Horan, B.F., et al.: Hemodynamic responses to enflurane anaesthesia and hypovolemia in the dog, and their modification by propranolol. Br. J. Anaesth., 49:1189, 1977.
36. Horan, B.F., et al.: Haemodynamic responses to isoflurane anaesthesia and hypovolemia in the

dog and their modification by propranolol. Br. J. Anaesth., *49*:1179, 1977.
37. Philbin, D.M., and Lowenstein, E.: Lack of beta-adrenergic activity of isoflurane in the dog: a comparison of circulatory effects of halothane and isoflurane after propranolol administration. Br. J. Anaesth., *48*:1165, 1976.
38. Johnstone, M.: Propranolol (Inderal) during halothane anaesthesia. Br. J. Anaesth., *38*:516, 1966.
39. Kopriva, C.J., Brown, A.C.D., and Papas, G.: Hemodynamics during general anesthesia in patients receiving propranolol. Anesthesiology, *48*:28, 1978.
40. Roberts, J.G., et al.: Haemodynamic interactions of high-dose propranolol pretreatment and anaesthesia in the dog III: The effects of haemorrhage during halothane and trichloroethylene anaesthesia. Br. J. Anaesth., *48*:411, 1976.
41. Prys-Roberts, C., et al.: Interaction of anesthesia, beta-receptor blockade, and blood loss in dogs with induced myocardial infarction. Anesthesiology, *45*:326, 1976.
42. Slogoff, S., Keats, A.S., Hibbs, C.W., et al.: Failure of general anesthesia to potentiate propranolol activity. Anesthesiology, *47*:504, 1977.
43. Foex, P., Roberts, J.G., Saner, C.A., et al.: Oxyprenolol and the circulation during anesthesia in the dog: influence of intrinsic sympathomimetic activity. Br. J. Anaesth., *53*:463, 1981.
44. Samuels, S.I., and Maze, M.: Beta-receptor blockade following the use of eye drops. Anesthesiology, *52*:369, 1980.
45. Henry, P.D.: Comparative pharmacology of calcium antagonists: nifedipine, verapamil and diltiazem. Am. J. Cardiol., *46*:1047, 1980.
46. Reves, J.G., Kissen, I., Lell, W.A., et al.: Calcium entry blockers: Uses and implications for anesthesiologists. Anesthesiology, *57*:504, 1983.
47. Kapur, P.A., and Flacke, W.F.: Epinephrine-induced arrhythmias and cardiovascular function after verapamil during halothane anesthesia in the dog. Anesthesiology, *55*:219, 1981.
48. Kates, R.A., Kaplan, J.A., Guyton, R.A., et al.: Hemodynamic interactions of verapamil and isoflurane. Anesthesiology, *59*:132, 1983.
49. Kapur, P.A., Bloor, B.C., Flacke, W.E., et al.: Comparison of cardiovascular responses to verapamil during enflurane, isoflurane or halothane anesthesia in the dog. Anesthesiology, *61*:156, 1984.
50. Kates, R.A., Zaggy, A.P., Norfleet, E.A., et al.: Comparative cardiovascular effects of verapamil, nifedipine, and diltiazem during halothane anesthesia in swine. Anesthesiology, *61*:10, 1984.
51. Tosone, S.R., Reves, J.G., Kison, et al.: Nifedipine and halothane: addictive hemodynamics with depression in dogs. Anesth. Analg., *61*:218, 1982.
52. Brichard, G., and Zimmerman, P.E.: Verapamil in cardiac dysrhythmias during anaesthesia. Br. J. Anaesth., *42*:1005, 1970.
53. Zimpler, M., Fitzal, S., and Tonczar, L.: Verapamil as a hypotensive agent during neuroleptanesthesia. Br. J. Anaesth., *53*:885, 1981.
54. Reves, J.G., Samuelson, P.N., Lell, W.A., et al.: Myocardial damage in coronary bypass surgical patients anaesthetized with two anaesthetic techniques: A random comparison of halothane and enflurane. Can. Anaesth. Soc. J., *27*:238, 1980.
55. Schulte-Sasse, U., Hess, W., Markschies-Hornug, A., et al.: Combined effects of halothane anesthetic and verapamil on systemic hemodynamics and left ventricular myocardial contractility in patients with ischemic heart disease. Anesth. Analg., *63*:791, 1984.
56. Nugent, M., Tinker, J.H., and Moyer, T.P.: Verapamil worsens rate of development and hemodynamic effects of acute hyperkalemia in halothane-anesthetized dogs: effects of calcium therapy. Anesthesiology, *60*:435, 1984.
57. Goldberg, L.I.: Dopamine-clinical uses of an endogenous catecholamine. N. Engl. J. Med., *291*:707, 1974.
58. Goldberg, L.I.: Levodopa and anesthesia. Anesthesiology, *34*:1, 1971.
59. Liu, P.L., Kronis, L.J., and Ngai, S.H.: The effect of levodopa on the norepinephrine stores in the rat heart. Anesthesiology, *34*:4, 1971.
60. Ngai, S.H.: Parkinsonism, levodopa, and anesthesia. Anesthesiology, *37*:344, 1972.
61. Katz, R.L., Lord, C.O., and Eakins, K.E.: Anesthetic-dopamine cardiac arrhythmias and their prevention by beta-adrenergic blockade. J. Pharmacol. Exp. Ther., *158*:40, 1967.
62. Wiklund, R.A., and Ngai, S.H.: Rigidity and pulmonary edema after Innovar in a patient on levodopa therapy: report of a case. Anesthesiology, *35*:545, 1971.
63. Johnston, R.R., White, P.F., Way, W.L., et al.: The effect of levodopa on halothane anesthetic requirement. Anesth. Analg., *54*:178, 1975.
64. Williams, R.B., and Sherter, C.: Cardiac complications of tricyclic antidepressant therapy. Ann. Intern. Med., *74*:395, 1971.
65. Jenkins, L.C., and Graves, H.B.: Potential hazards of psychoactive drugs in association with anesthesia. Can. Anaesth. Soc. J., *12*:121, 1965.
66. Edwards, R. and Miller, R.D.: Personal Communication.
67. Raisfeld, I.H.: Cardiovascular complications of antidepressant therapy-interactions at the adrenergic neuron. Am. Heart J., *88*:129, 1972.
68. Boakes, A.J., Laurence, D.R., Teoh, P., et al.: Interactions between sympathomimetic amines and antidepressant agents in man. Br. Med. J., *1*:311, 1973.
69. Edwards, R.P., Miller, R.D., Roizers, M.F., et al.: Cardiac responses to imipramine and pancuronium during anesthesia with halothane or enflurane. Anesthesiology, *50*:421, 1979.
70. Campbell, G.D.: Dangers of monoamine oxidase inhibitors. Br. Med. J., *1*:750, 1963.
71. Hirsh, M.S., Walter, R.M., and Hasterlik, R.J.: Subarachnoid hemorrhage following ephedrine and MAO inhibitors. J.A.M.A., *194*:1259, 1965.
72. Janowsky, E.C., Risch, C., and Janowsky, D.S.: Effect of anesthesia on patients taking psycho-

tropic drugs. J. Clin. Psychopharmacol., *1*:14, 1981.
73. Braverman, B., Ivankovich, A.D., and McCarthy, R.: The effects of fentanyl and vasopressor on anesthetized dogs receiving MAO inhibitors. Anesth. Analg., *63*:2192, 1984.
74. Michaels, I., Serrins, M., Nicke-ha, Q.S., et al.: Anesthesia for cardiac surgery in patients receiving monoamine oxidase inhibitors. Anesth. Analg., *63*:1041, 1984.
75. Eckenhoff, J.E., Helrich, M., and Rolph, W.D.: The effects of promethazine upon respiration and circulation in man. Anesthesiology, *18*:703, 1957.
76. Dobkin, A.B., Gilbert, R.C.G., and Melville, K.I.: Chlorpromazine. A review and investigation as a premedicant in anesthesia. Anesthesiology, *17*:135, 1956.
77. Dundee, J.W., et al.: Studies of drugs given before anesthesia. VI: The phenothiazine derivatives. Br. J. Anaesth., *37*:332, 1965.
78. Gold, M.I.: Profound hypotension associated with preoperative use of phenothiazines. Anesth. Analg., *53*:844, 1974.
79. Eggers, G.W.N., Jr., Grossen, G., and Allen, C.R.: Comparison of vasopressor responses in the presence of phenothiazine derivatives. Anesthesiology, *20*:261, 1959.
80. Graves, C.L., Downes, N.H., and Browne, A.B.: Cardiovascular effects of minimal analgesic quantities of Innovar, fentanyl, and droperidol in man. Anesth. Analg., *54*:15, 1975.
81. Prys-Roberts, C., and Kelman, G.R.: The influence of drugs used in neuroleptanesthesia on cardiovascular and ventilatory function. Br. J. Anaesth., *39*:134, 1967.
82. Kingston, H.G.G., and Hirshman, C.A.: Perioperative management of the patient with asthma. Anesth. Analg., *63*:844, 1984.
83. Stirt, J.A., and Sullivan, S.F.: Aminophylline. Anesth. Analg., *60*:587, 1981.
84. Roizen, M.F., and Stevens, W.C.: Multiform ventricular tachycardia due to the interaction of aminophylline and halothane. Anesth. Analg., *57*:738, 1978.
85. Stirt, J.A., Berger, J.M., Richer, S.M., et al.: Arrhythmogenic effects of aminophylline during halothane anesthesia in experimental animals. Anesth. Analg., *59*:410, 1980.
86. Stirt, J.A., Berger, J.M., Roe, S.D., et al.: Safety of enflurane following administration of aminophylline in experimental animals. Anesth. Analg., *60*:871, 1981.
87. Stirt, J.A., Berger, J.M., and Sullivan, S.F.: Lack of arrhythmogenicity of isoflurane following administration of aminophylline in dogs. Anesth. Analg., *62*:568, 1983.
88. Johnstone, R.E., Kulp, R.A., and Smith, T.C.: Effects on isoflurane requirement in mice. Anesth. Analg., *54*:277, 1975.
89. Han, Y.H.: Why do chronic alcoholics require more anesthesia? Anesthesiology, *30*:341, 1969.
90. Wolfson, B., and Freed, B.: Influence of alcohol on anesthetic requirements and acute toxicity. Anesth. Analg., *59*:826, 1980.
91. Bruce, D.L.: Alcoholism and anesthesia. Anesth. Analg., *62*:84, 1983.
92. Perisho, J.A., Buechel, D.R., and Miller, R.D.: The effect of diazepam (Valium) on minimum alveolar anesthetic requirements in man. Can. Anaesth. Soc. J., *18*:536, 1971.
93. Saidman, I.I., and Eger, E.I., II: Effect of nitrous oxide and of narcotic premedication on the alveolar concentration of halothane required for anesthesia. Anesthesiology, *25*:302, 1964.
94. Munson, E.S., Saidman, L.J., and Eger, E.I., II: Effect of nitrous oxide and morphine on the minimum anesthetic concentration of fluroxene. Anesthesiology, *26*:134, 1965.
95. Filner, B.E., and Kasliner, J.S.: Alterations of normal left ventricular performance by general anesthesia. Anesthesiology, *45*:610, 1976.
96. Rao, S., et al.: Cardiopulmonary effects of diazepam. Clin. Pharmacol. Ther., *14*:182, 1973.
97. Dalen, J.E., et al.: The hemodynamics and respiratory effects of diazepam. Anesthesiology, *30*:259, 1969.
98. Cote, P., Gueret, T., and Bourassa, M.G.: Systemic and coronary hemodynamic effects of diazepam in patients with normal and diseased coronary arteries. Circulation, *50*:1210, 1974.
99. Tomicheck, R.C., Roscow, C.E., Schneider, R.C., et al.: Cardiovascular effects of diazepam-fentanyl anesthesia in patients with coronary artery disease. Anesth. Analg., *61*:217, 1982.
100. McCammon, R.L., Hilgenberg, J.C., and Stoelting, R.F.: Hemodynamic effects of diazepam and diazepam-nitrous oxide in patients with coronary artery disease. Anesth. Analg., *59*:438, 1980.
101. Samuelson, P.N., Rever, J.G., Kouchoukos, N.T., et al.: Hemodynamic responses to anesthetic induction with midazolam or diazepam in patients with ischemic heart disease. Anesth. Analg., *60*:802, 1981.
102. Tweed, W.A., Minuk, M., and Mymin, D.: Circulatory responses to ketamine anesthesia. Anesthesiology, *37*:613, 1972.
103. White, P.F., Way, W.L., and Trevor, A.J.: Ketamine—its pharmacology and therapeutic uses. Anesthesiology, *56*:119, 1982.
104. Johnston, R.R., Miller, R.D., and Way, W.L.: The interaction of ketamine with d-tubocurarine, pancuronium, and succinylcholine in man. Anesth. Analg., *53*:496, 1974.
105. Stanley, T.H.: Blood pressure and pulse rate responses to ketamine during general anesthesia. Anesthesiology, *39*:648, 1973.
106. Bidwai, A.V., et al.: The effects of ketamine on cardiovascular dynamics during halothane and enflurane anesthesia. Anesth. Analg., *54*:588, 1975.
107. White, P.F., Johnston, R.R., and Pudwill, C.R.: Interaction of ketamine and halothane in rats. Anesthesiology, *42*:179, 1975.
108. Lowenstein, E., et al.: Cardiovascular responses to large doses of intravenous morphine in man. N. Engl. J. Med., *281*:1389, 1969.
109. Bovill, J.G., Sebel, P.S., and Stanley, T.H.: Opioid analgesics in anesthesia: with special ref-

erences to their use in cardiovascular anesthesia. Anesthesiology, 61:731, 1984.
110. Tarhan, S., et al.: Hemodynamic and blood gas effects of Innovar in patients with acquired heart disease. Anesthesiology, 34:250, 1971.
111. Stoelting, R.D., et al.: Hemodynamic and ventilatory responses to fentanyl, fentanyl-droperidol, and nitrous oxide in patients with acquired valvular disease. Anesthesiology, 42:319, 1975.
112. Craythorne, N.W.B., and Darby, T.D.: The cardiovascular effects of nitrous oxide in the dog. Br. J. Anaesth., 37:560, 1965.
113. Goldberg, A.H., Sohn, Y.Z., and Phear, W.P.Z.: Direct myocardial effects of nitrous oxide. Anesthesiology, 43:61, 1975.
114. Eisele, J.H., and Smith, N.T.: Cardiovascular effects of forty percent nitrous oxide in man. Anesth. Analg., 51:956, 1972.
115. Eisele, J.H., Reitan, J.A., Massumi, R.A., et al.: Myocardial performance and N20 analgesia in coronary artery disease. Anesthesiology, 44:16, 1976.
116. Wong, K.C., et al.: The cardiovascular effects of morphine sulfate with oxygen and with nitrous oxide in man. Anesthesiology, 38:542, 1973.
117. Stoelting, R.K., and Gibbs, P.S.: Hemodynamic effects of morphine and morphine-nitrous oxide in valvular heart disease and coronary artery disease. Anesthesiology, 38:45, 1973.
118. McDermott, R.W., and Stanley, T.H.: The cardiovascular effects of low concentrations of nitrous oxide during morphine anesthesia. Anesthesiology, 44:89, 1974.
119. Lappas, D.G., Buckley, M.J., Laver, M.B., et al.: Left ventricular performance and pulmonary circulation following addition of nitrous oxide to morphine during coronary artery surgery. Anesthesiology, 43:61, 1975.
120. Bennett, G.M., and Stanley, T.H.: Human cardiovascular responses to endotracheal intubation during morphine-N20 and fentanyl-N20 anesthesia. Anesthesiology, 52:520, 1980.
121. Lunn, J.K., Stanley, T.H., Eisele, J., et al.: High dose fentanyl anesthesia for coronary artery surgery: plasma fentanyl concentrations and the influence of nitrous oxide on cardiovascular responses. Anesth. Analg., 58:390, 1979.
122. Hilgenberg, J.C., McCammon, R.L., and Stoelting, R.K.: Pulmonary and systemic vascular responses to nitrous oxide in patients with mitral stenosis and pulmonary hypertension. Anesth. Analg., 59:323, 1980.
123. Schulte-Sasse, U., Hess, W., and Tarnow, J.: Pulmonary vascular responses to nitrous oxide in patients with normal and high pulmonary vascular resistance. Anesthesiology, 57:9, 1982.
124. Freund, F.G., Martin, W.E., Wong, K.C., et al.: Abdominal-muscle rigidity induced by morphine and nitrous oxide. Anesthesiology, 38:358, 1973.
125. Stoelting, R.K., et al.: Circulatory effects of halothane added to morphine anesthesia in patients with coronary artery disease. Anesth. Analg., 53:449, 1974.
126. Bennett, G.M., and Stanley, T.H.: Cardiovascular effects of fentanyl during enflurane anesthesia in man. Anesth. Analg., 58:179, 1979.
127. Munson, E.S., Saidman, L.J., and Eger, E.I., II: Effect of nitrous oxide and morphine on the minimum anesthetic concentration of fluroxene. Anesthesiology, 26:134, 1965.
128. Stoelting, R.K.: The effect of nitrous oxide on the MAC of methoxyflurane needed for anesthesia. Anesthesiology, 34:353, 1971.
129. Torri, G., Dania, G., and Fabiani, M.: Effect of nitrous oxide on the anesthetic requirement of enflurane. Br. J. Anaesth., 46:468, 1974.
130. Stevens, W.C., et al.: Minimal alveolar concentrations (MAC) of isoflurane with and without nitrous oxide in patients of various ages. Anesthesiology, 42:197, 1975.
131. Epstein, R.M., et al.: Influence of the concentration effect on the uptake of anesthetic mixtures: The second gas effect. Anesthesiology, 25:364, 1964.
132. Stoelting, R.K., and Eger, E.I., II: An additional explanation for the second gas effect. Anesthesiology, 30:273, 1969.
133. Masuda, T., and Ikeda, K.: Elimination of nitrous oxide accelerates elimination of halothane: reversed second gas effect. Anesthesiology, 60:567, 1984.
134. Fink, B.R.: Diffusion anoxia. Anesthesiology, 16:511, 1955.
135. Hornbein, T.F., et al.: Nitrous oxide effects on the circulatory and ventilatory responses to halothane. Anesthesiology, 31:250, 1969.
136. Dolan, W.M., et al.: The cardiovascular and respiratory effects of isoflurane-nitrous oxide anaesthesia. Can. Anaesth. Soc. J., 21:557, 1974.
137. Eckenhoff, J.E., and Helrich, M.: The effect of narcotics, thiopental and nitrous oxide upon respiration and respiratory response to hypercapnia. Anesthesiology, 19:240, 1958.
138. Eger, E.I., II, et al.: Surgical stimulation antagonizes the respiratory depression produced by Forane. Anesthesiology, 36:544, 1972.
139. Bahlman, S.H., et al.: The cardiovascular effects of nitrous oxide-halothane anesthesia in man. Anesthesiology, 35:274, 1971.
140. Smith, N.T., et al.: Impact of nitrous oxide on the circulation during enflurane anesthesia in man. Anesthesiology, 48:345, 1978.
141. Smith, N.T., et al.: The cardiovascular responses to the addition of nitrous oxide to diethyl ether in man. Can. Anaesth. Soc. J., 19:42, 1972.
142. Smith, N.T., et al.: The cardiovascular responses to the addition of nitrous oxide to fluroxene in man. Br. J. Anaesth., 44:142, 1972.
143. Smith, N.T., et al.: The cardiovascular and sympathomimetic responses to the addition of nitrous oxide to halothane in man. Anesthesiology, 32:410, 1970.
144. Stoelting, R.K., Reis, R.R., and Longnecker, D.E.: Hemodynamic responses to nitrous oxide-halothane and halothane in patients with vascular heart disease. Anesthesiology, 37:430, 1972.
145. Moffit, E.A., Sethna, D.H., Gary, R.J., et al.: Nitrous oxide added to halothane reduces cor-

onary flow and myocardial oxygen consumption in patients with coronary artery disease. Can. Anaesth. Soc. J., 30:5, 1983.
146. Bennett, G.M., et al.: Cardiovascular responses to nitrous oxide during enflurane and oxygen anesthesia. Anesthesiology, 46:227, 1977.
147. Moffitt, E.A., Scovil, J.E., Barker, R.A., et al.: The effects of nitrous oxide on myocardial metabolism and hemodynamics during fentanyl or enflurane anesthesia in patients with coronary artery disease. Anesth. Analg., 63:1071, 1984.
148. Millar, R.A., Warden, J.C., and Cooperman, L.H.: Central sympathetic discharge and mean arterial pressure during halothane anesthesia. Br. J. Anaesth., 41:918, 1969.
149. Fukunaga, A.F., and Epstein, R.M.: Sympathetic excitation during nitrous oxide-halothane anesthesia in the rat. Anesthesiology, 39:23, 1973.
150. Ngai, S.H., Hanks, E.C., and Farhie, S.E.: Effects of anesthetics on neuromuscular transmission and somatic reflexes. Anesthesiology, 26:162, 1965.
151. Gissen, A.I., Karis, H.H., and Nastuk, W.L.: The effect of halothane on neuromuscular transmission. J.A.M.A., 197:770, 1966.
152. Karis, J.H., Gissen, A.J., and Nastuk, W.L.: Mode of action of diethyl ether in bocking neuromuscular transmission. Anesthesiology, 27:42, 1966.
153. Miller, R.D., et al.: Comparative neuromuscular effects of Forane and halothane alone and in combination with d-tubocurarine in man. Anesthesiology, 35:38, 1971.
154. Epstein, R.A., and Jackson, S.H.: The effect of depth of anesthesia on the neuromuscular refractory period of anesthetized man. Anesthesiology, 32:494, 1970.
155. Katz, R.L.: Neuromuscular effects of diethyl ether and its interaction with succinylcholine and d-tubocurarine. Anesthesiology, 27:52, 1966.
156. Lebowitz, M.H., Bliff, C.D., and Walts, L.F.: Depression of twitch response to stimulation of the ulnar nerve during Ethrane anesthesia in man. Anesthesiology, 33:52, 1970.
157. Vitez, T.S., et al.: Comparison in vitro of isoflurane and halothane potentiation of d-tubocurarine and succinylcholine neuromuscular blockades. Anesthesiology, 41:53, 1974.
158. Miller, R.D., et al.: Comparative neuromuscular effects of pancuronium, gallamine, and succinylcholine during Forane and halothane anesthesia in man. Anesthesiology, 35:509, 1971.
159. Miller, R.D., Way, W.L., and Dolan, W.M.: The dependence of pancuronium- and d-tubocurarine-induced neuromuscular blockades on alveolar concentrations of halothane and Forane. Anesthesiology, 37:573, 1972.
160. Katz, R.L., and Gissen, A.J.: Neuromuscular and electromyographic effects of halothane and its interaction with d-tubocurarine in man. Anesthesiology, 28:564, 1967.
161. Foldes, F.F., Bencini, A., and Newton, D.: Influence of halothane and enflurane on the neuromuscular effects on ORG NC45 in man. Br. J. Anaesth., 52(Suppl 1):645, 1980.
162. Rupp, S.M., Fahey, M.R., and Miller, R.D.: Neuromuscular and cardiovascular effects of atracurium during nitrous oxide-fentanyl and nitrous oxide-isoflurane anesthesia. Br. J. Anaesth., 55(Suppl 1):675, 1983.
163. Rupp, S.M., Miller, R.D., and Gencarelli, P.J.: Vecuronium-induced neuromuscular blockage during enflurane, halothane and isoflurane in human. Anesthesiology, 60:102, 1984.
164. Fogdall, R.P., and Miller, R.D.: Neuromuscular effects of enflurane, alone and in combination with d-tubocurarine, pancuronium, and succinylcholine in man. Anesthesiology, 42:173, 1975.
165. Katz, R.L., and Gail, G.J.: Surgical infiltration of pressor drugs and their interaction with volatile anesthetics. Br. J. Anaesth., 38:712, 1966.
166. Katz, R.L., and Epstein, R.A.: The interaction of anesthetic agents and adrenergic drugs to produce cardiac arrhythmias. Anesthesiology, 29:763, 1968.
167. Matteo, R.S., Katz, R.L., and Papper, E.M.: The injection of epinephrine during general anesthesia with halogenated hydrocarbons and cyclopropane in man. 3. Cyclopropane. Anesthesiology, 24:327, 1963.
168. Matteo, R.S., Katz, R.L., and Papper, E.M.: The injection of epinephrine during general anesthesia with halogenated hydrocarbons and cyclopropane in man. 1. Trichloroethylene. Anesthesiology, 23:360, 1962.
169. Bamforth, B.J., et al.: Effect of epinephrine on the dog heart during methoxyflurane anesthesia. Anesthesiology, 22:169, 1961.
170. Munson, E.S., and Tucker, W.K.: Doses of epinephrine causing arrhythmias during enflurane, methoxyflurane and halothane anesthesia in dogs. Can. Anaesth. Soc. J., 22:495, 1975.
171. Joas, T.A., and Stevens, W.C.: Comparison of the arrhythmic doses of epinephrine during Forane, halothane and fluroxene anesthesia in dogs. Anesthesiology, 35:48, 1971.
172. McDowell, S.A., Holl, K.D., and Stephen, C.R.: Difluoro-methyl 1, 1, 2-trifluoro-2-chloroethylether; experiments on dogs with a new inhalational anesthetic agent. Br. J. Anaesth., 40:511, 1968.
173. Katz, R.L., Matteo, R.S., and Papper, E.M.: The injection of epinephrine during general anesthesia with halogenated hydrocarbons and cyclopropane in man. 2. Halothane. Anesthesiology, 23:597, 1962.
174. Johnston, R.R., Eger, E.I., II, and Wilson, C.: A comparative interaction of epinephrine with enflurane, isoflurane and halothane in man. Anesth. Analg., 55:709, 1976.
175. Konchigeri, H.N., Shaker, M.H., and Winnie, A.P.: Effect of epinephrine during enflurane anesthesia. Anesth. Analg., 53:894, 1974.
176. Lippman, M., and Reisner, L.S.: Epinephrine injection with enflurane anesthesia: Incidence of cardiac arrhythmias. Anesth. Analg., 53:886, 1974.
177. Tucker, W.K., Rackstein, A.D., and Munson,

E.S.: Comparison of arrhythmic doses of adrenalin, metaraminol, ephedrine and phenylephrine during isoflurane and halothane anesthesia. Br. J. Anaesth., 46:392, 1974.
178. VanDyke, R.A.: Metabolism of volatile anesthetics III: Induction of microsomal dechlorinating and ether-cleaving enzymes. J. Pharmacol. Exp. Ther., 154:365, 1966.
179. Brown, B.R.: The diphasic action of halothane on the oxidative metabolism of drugs by the liver: an in-vitro study in the rat. Anesthesiology, 35:241, 1971.
180. Sharp, J.H., Trudell, J.R., and Cohen, E.N.: Volatile metabolites and decomposition products of halothane in man. Anesthesiology, 50:2, 1979.
181. Ahr, H.J., King, L.J., Nastainczyk, W., et al.: The mechanism of reductive dehalogenation of halothane by liver cytochrome P-450. Biochemical Pharmacology, 31:383, 1982.
182. Brown, B.R., Jr.: Hepatic microsomal enzyme induction. Anesthesiology, 39:178, 1973.
183. Linde, H.W., and Berman, M.L.: Non-specific stimulation of drug-metabolizing enzymes by inhalation anesthetic agents. Anesth. Analg., 50:656, 1971.
184. Berman, M.L., and Bochantin, B.S.: Non-specific stimulation of drug metabolism in rats by methoxyflurane. Anesthesiology, 32:500, 1970.
185. Hitt, B.A., et al.: Species, strain, sex and individual differences in enflurane metabolism. Br. J. Anaesth., 47:1157, 1975.
186. Berman, M.L., et al.: Enzyme induction by enflurane in man. Anesthesiology, 44:496, 1976.
187. Brown, B.R., Jr., and Sagalyn, A.M.: Hepatic microsomal enzyme induction by inhalation anesthetics: Mechanism in the rat. Anesthesiology, 40:152, 1974.
188. Duvaldstein, P., Mazze, R.I., Nivoche, Y., et al.: Enzyme induction following surgery with halothane and neuroleptanesthesia. Anesth. Analg., 60:319, 1981.
189. Wood, M., and Wood, A.J.J.: Contrasting effects of halothane, isoflurane and enflurane on in vivo drug metabolism in the rat. Anesth. Analg., 63:709, 1984.
190. Greenstein, L.R., Hiff, B.A., and Mazze, R.I.: Metabolism in vitro of enflurane, isoflurane and methoxyflurane. Anesthesiology, 42:420, 1975.
191. Mazze, R.I., Woodruff, R.E., and Heerdt, M.E.: Isoniazid-induced enflurane defluorination in human beings. Anesthesiology, 57:5, 1982.
192. Cousins, M.J., and Mazze, R.I.: Methoxyflurane nephrotoxicity: a study of dose-response in man. J.A.M.A., 225:1611, 1973.
193. Cousins, M.J., Greenstein, L.R., Hiff, B., et al.: Metabolism and renal effects of enflurane in man. Anesthesiology, 44:44, 1976.
194. Barr, G.A., Mazze, R.I., Cousins, M.J., et al.: An animal model for combined methoxyflurane and gentamicin nephrotoxicity. Br. J. Anaesth., 45:306, 1973.
195. Mazze, R.I., Calverley, R.K., and Smith, N.T.: Inorganic fluoride nephrotoxicity: prolonged enflurane and halothane anesthesia in volunteers. Anesthesiology, 46:265, 1977.
196. Kuzucu, E.Y.: Methoxyflurane, tetracycline and renal failure. J.A.M.A., 211:1162, 1970.
197. McLain, G.E., Sipeo, I.G., and Brown, B.R.: An animal model of halothane hepatotoxicity: roles of enzyme induction and hypoxia. Anesthesiology, 51:321, 1979.
198. Shingu, K., Eger, E.I., II, and Johnson, B.H.: Hypoxia per se can produce hepatic damage without death in rats. Anesth. Analg., 61:820, 1982.
199. VanDyke, R.A.: Hepatic centrilobular necrosis in fasting rats after exposure to halothane, enflurane or isoflurane. Anesth. Analg., 61:812, 1982.
200. Shingu, K., Eger, E.I., II, Bryute, H.J., et al.: Hepatic injury induced by anesthetic agents in rats. Anesth. Analg., 62:140, 1983.
201. Epstein, R.M., Deutsch, S., Cooperman, L.H., et al.: Splanchnic circulation during halothane anesthesia and hypercapnia in normal man. Anesthesiology, 27:654, 1966.
202. Hughes, R.L., Campbell, D., and Fitch, W.: Effects of enflurane and halothane on liver blood flow and oxygen consumption in the greyhound. Br. J. Anaesth., 52:1079, 1980.
203. Harper, M.H., Collins, P., Johnson, B.H., et al.: Postanesthetic hepatic injury in rats: influence of alterations in hepatic blood flow, surgery, and anesthesia time. Anesth. Analg., 61:79, 1982.
204. Inman, W.H.W., and Mushin, W.W.: Jaundice after repeated exposure to halothane: a further analysis of reports of the Committee on Safety in Medicine. Br. Med. J., 2:1455, 1978.
205. Dienstag, J.L.: Halothane hepatitis-allergy or idiosyncracy. N. Engl. J. Med., 303:102, 1980.
206. Neuberger, J., Gimson, A.E.S., Davis, M., et al.: Specific serologic markers in diagnosis of fulminant hepatic failure associated with halothane anesthesia. Br. J. Anaesth., 55:15, 1983.

|24|

NEUROMUSCULAR BLOCKING AGENTS

RONALD D. MILLER and N. TY SMITH

Numerous drug interactions have been reported to involve muscle relaxants or their antagonists.[1-4] Several problems confuse the interpretation of these interactions, however. It is important to establish which interactions are clinically relevant and which are exclusively of pharmacologic or academic interest. The difficulty of extrapolating animal data to man is nowhere more evident than in this context. The difference is not only quantitative, but is also qualitative, since interactions in man may depend on entirely different mechanisms (for example, decreased renal excretion, hypercapnia, increased anesthetic depth).

Ideally, all drug interactions should be detected clinically and should be confirmed by controlled clinical or animal studies. This discussion therefore concerns only those interactions that have been documented either clinically or in animal species known to respond similarly to man. Those drugs discussed include: (1) azathioprine, (2) furosemide, (3) antibiotics, (4) steroids, (5) inhalation anesthetics, (6) local anesthetics, (7) antidysrhythmics, (8) ketamine, (9) lithium, (10) magnesium sulfate, (11) other muscle relaxants, (12) acetylcholinesterase inhibitors, (13) pseudocholinesterase inhibitors, (14) hypotensive agents, and (15) agents used in the treatment of renal failure. Many interactions are illustrated by case reports drawn either from our experience or from the literature. Only those drugs known to interact with muscle relaxants and likely to have clinical relevance are included. The following case report describes a patient who experienced a prolonged *d*-tubocurarine neuromuscular blockade. In addition to renal failure, the patient received seven drugs that could have prolonged the block. Each drug is discussed after the case report.

CASE REPORT

A 38-year-old, 64-kg man with end-stage renal disease secondary to chronic glomerulonephritis was admitted to the University of California Hospitals for kidney transplantation. The patient had been previously treated by hemodialysis. Prior to operation, his arterial blood pressure was 170/100 mm Hg, hemoglobin 6.8 g/L, serum creatinine 6.0 mg/dL, and serum potassium 5.3 mEq/L. He was taking daily oral doses of azathioprine, 300 mg; prednisone, 120 mg; Lugol's solution, ten drops; and *alpha*-methyldopa, 250 mg.

The patient received no preanesthetic medications. Anesthesia was induced with halothane and nitrous oxide, 60%. His trachea was intubated without the use of other drugs. Neuromuscular function was monitored to allow recording of twitch height. Although the patient was anesthetized, the operation was delayed because of multiple traumatic attempts to insert a Foley catheter into the bladder. Since the trauma might have caused septicemia, gentamicin, 120 mg, was given intravenously. In spite of not having been given a relaxant previously, the patient's twitch height started to decrease immediately (Fig. 24–1). Twenty minutes later, a small dose of *d*-tubocurarine, 6 mg, completely abolished the twitch (Fig. 24–1). It was two hours before any further twitch began to appear. The patient started to recover from the neuromuscular block three hours after *d*-tubocurarine administration. Immediately before

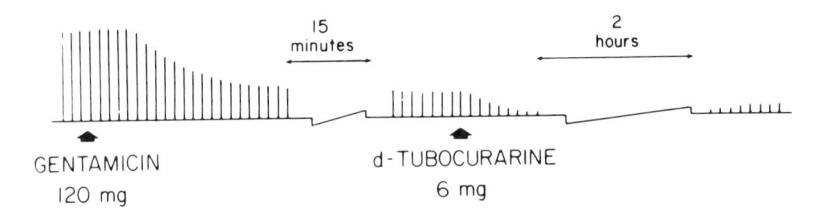

Fig. 24–1. The effect on twitch height of gentamicin, 120 mg, given intravenously to a 64-kg patient who had received no previous muscle relaxants. Six milligrams of d-tubocurarine completely abolished the twitch, which resumed only after 2 hours.

the vasculature to the kidney was opened, furosemide, 80 mg, in divided doses, and mannitol, 12.5 g, were given intravenously; neuromuscular block was augmented and prolonged (Fig. 24–2). At the end of the operation, the patient's subcutaneous tissue was irrigated with a neomycin/bacitracin solution. Despite the administration of neostigmine, 5 mg, and of atropine, 1.0 mg, intravenously, the patient was weak and dyspneic in the recovery room. After 3 hours of controlled ventilation, his neuromuscular function returned, as evidenced by a vital capacity of 3.8 L and by a sustained response to a tetanic stimulus of 50 Hz, as well as by the absence of post-tetanic facilitation.

Many drugs and/or physiologic changes could have accounted for the prolonged neuromuscular blockade, including azathioprine, furosemide, mannitol, bacitracin, neomycin, gentamicin, prednisone, renal failure, and halothane. Each is discussed separately. The particular importance of monitoring neuromuscular function is also illustrated by this case. If it had not been recognized that gentamicin had caused a partial block, perhaps more than 6 mg of d-tubocurarine might have been given, which would have caused an even greater overdose.

AZATHIOPRINE

Azathioprine, a derivative of mercaptopurine, is an immunosuppressant used in patients who undergo kidney transplantation. It antagonizes a nondepolarizing and augments a depolarizing neuromus-

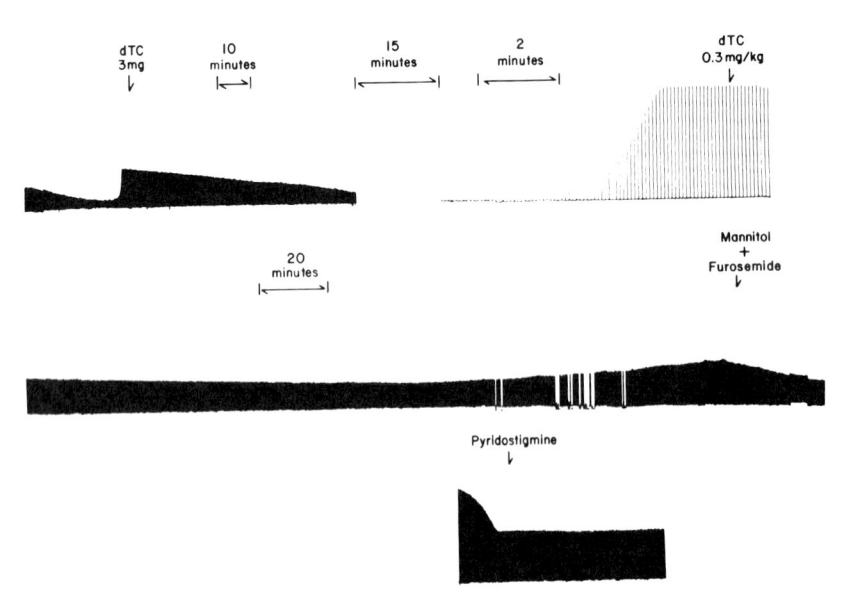

Fig. 24–2. (The panel reads from right to left) A decrease in twitch tension following intravenous administration of mannitol, 12.5 g, and furosemide, 80 mg.

cular blockade.[5] This effect is probably due to the inhibition of phosphodiesterase at the motor nerve terminal. The role of cyclic nucleotides in neuromuscular transmission has been recently emphasized by Standaert et al.[6] However, we doubt whether this interaction is important clinically. Antagonism of an existing nondepolarizing neuromuscular blockade was observed when 300 mg of azathioprine were given intravenously. Azathioprine is usually given in this dose orally a few hours before anesthesia, however. In this latter situation, azathioprine is not likely to influence significantly the neuromuscular blockade from muscle relaxants.

DIURETICS

One might predict that diuretics will hasten the elimination of nondepolarizing muscle relaxants and will thereby shorten the duration of neuromuscular blockade. Diuretics, however, do not hasten the elimination of d-tubocurarine, and some may even augment and prolong its block. Elimination of muscle relaxants is not accelerated because most diuretics act at renal sites different from those that regulate the excretion of relaxants.[7] Muscle relaxants have a low molecular weight and are filtered by renal glomeruli. They are ionized, are not reabsorbed by the tubular epithelium, and hence are promptly eliminated by the kidney. Diuretics primarily affect tubular function and have little influence on glomerular filtration, which is mainly responsible for the excretion of neuromuscular blocking agents.

Although mannitol appears to have little or no effect on neuromuscular blocking agents, furosemide may augment a nondepolarizing neuromuscular blockade by a direct effect at the neuromuscular junction, possibly by displacing the relaxant from nonactive to active sites. Proof for the latter hypothesis is weak and is based on observations in one patient in whom furosemide increased the plasma concentration of d-tubocurarine even though no d-tubocurarine had been administered during the previous hour.[8] A more likely explanation is that furosemide may exert a direct depressant effect on the neuromuscular junction, probably by reducing the influx of calcium into the motor nerve terminal that is necessary for the release of acetylcholine. This reduced influx may be the result of protein kinase inhibition.[9] Clinical concentrations of furosemide apparently do not affect twitch height, but do augment a nondepolarizing blockade.[10] The ability of neostigmine to antagonize a combined nondepolarizing-furosemide block has not been established.

ANTIBIOTICS

There are more than 120 clinical reports concerning the enhancement of neuromuscular blockade by antibiotics.[11] Although most antibiotics produce a neuromuscular blockade similar to that of d-tubocurarine, their blocking actions are antagonized unpredictably by neostigmine and by pyridostigmine (Table 24–1). Calcium does not usually produce a persistent antagonism. The neuromuscular blockade from antibiotics appears to be antagonized predictably and persistently by 4-aminopyridine.[11a] To date, this drug is not available for routine clinical use in the United States.

The search for a mechanism of antibiotic-induced neuromuscular blockade probably is confused by the possibilities inherent in the variety of antibiotics that can cause blockade. One popular theory is that streptomycin, neomycin, and kanamycin chelate calcium and produce a neuromuscular blockade by reducing serum calcium concentrations. However, determinations of ionized rather than total calcium levels have discredited this hypothesis.[11]

Attempts to clarify the mechanisms for antibiotic neuromuscular actions have frustrated us. Polymyxin B is an example. The most recent information suggests that

Table 24-1
Interaction of Antibiotics, Muscle Relaxants, Neostigmine, and Calcium

	Neuromuscular Block from Antibiotic Alone Antagonized by		Increase in Neuromuscular Block of		Neuromuscular Block from Antibiotic and d-Tubocurarine Antagonized by	
	Neostigmine	Calcium	d-Tubocurarine	Succinylcholine	Neostigmine	Calcium
Neomycin	sometimes	sometimes	yes	yes	usually	usually
Streptomycin	sometimes	sometimes	yes	yes	usually	usually
Gentamicin	sometimes	yes x	yes	*	sometimes	yes x
Kanamycin	sometimes	sometimes	yes	yes	sometimes	sometimes
Paromomycin	yes x	yes x	yes	*	yes x	yes x
Viomycin	yes x	yes x	yes	*	yes x	yes x
Polymyxin A	no	no	yes	*	no	no
Polymyxin B	no†	no	yes	yes	no†	no
Colistin	no	sometimes	yes	yes	no	sometimes
Tetracycline	no	*	yes	no	partially	partially
Lincomycin	partially	partially	yes	*	partially	partially
Clindamycin	partially	partially	yes	*	partially	partially

* Not studied
† Block augmented by neostigmine
x In spite of this, difficulty with antagonizing the block from these antibiotics is still likely to occur

polymyxin B exerts its primary neuromuscular effect by depressing the postjunctional membrane's response to acetylcholine.[12] If this were true we should be able at least partially to antagonize the block by increasing the acetylcholine concentration at the neuromuscular junction by means of neostigmine administration. The opposite occurs, however; neostigmine augments rather than antagonizes a polymyxin B block.[13] This is one example of inconsistency in the literature concerning antibiotic-induced neuromuscular blockade.

Of prime importance is the management of a combined muscle relaxant-antibiotic neuromuscular blockade. We arbitrarily administer neostigmine up to 5 mg/70 kg. Calcium is not given unless hypocalcemia is clearly established. Calcium is an inconsistent antagonist and may antagonize the antibacterial effect.[13a] The following case report, taken from an article by Fogdall and Miller, illustrates why more than 5 mg/70 kg of neostigmine or the equivalent of other drugs should not be administered to antagonize a muscle relaxant-antibiotic neuromuscular block.[14]

CASE REPORT

A 76-year-old man was admitted to a hospital in 1972 for open reduction and internal fixation of a right femoral neck fracture. With the exception of congenital ocular palsies and hip fracture, physical examination disclosed no abnormality. Anesthesia was induced and maintained with nitrous oxide, 60%, in oxygen, and with an end-tidal halothane concentration of 0.75%. The patient's trachea was intubated without additional drug. Neuromuscular function was evaluated by supramaximal stimulation of the ulnar nerve at the wrist, and the force of adduction of the thumb was measured by a force-displacement transducer. Thirty-five minutes after the induction of anesthesia, pancuronium bromide, 24 mg/m² (4.8 mg), was administered intravenously, resulting in 100% depression of twitch height. Fifty minutes later, when the twitch was still absent, the surgical wound was irrigated with one liter of 0.9% sodium chloride containing polymyxin B, 250,000 units, and bacitracin, 50,000 units.

Because 100% neuromuscular block still existed 103 minutes after the administration of pancuronium, and because the end of the surgical procedure was anticipated, antagonism of the neuromuscular blockade was attempted by a bolus intravenous injection of pyridostigmine, 14.5 mg, and atropine, 0.6 mg. This dose of pyridostigmine is equivalent to about 2.8 mg of neostigmine. Since 26 minutes later the twitch had returned to only 10% of the control height, 10 mg more of pyridostigmine were given.

Approximately 4 hours after the administration of pancuronium (and 2 hours after initial pyridostigmine administration), twitch had returned to only 80% of the control height, and the response to a tetanic stimulus of 50 Hz for 5 seconds was unsustained, with a spontaneous tidal volume of 0.35 L. Total doses of medications given were pyridostigmine, 24.5 mg, neostigmine, 1.0 mg, edrophonium, 10 mg, and calcium chloride, 1,200 mg.

Neuromuscular function was monitored continuously in the recovery room for the next 2 hours, during which time an additional 200 mg of calcium chloride was administered without benefit. The patient responded to vocal commands with a slight nod of the head but was able neither to lift his head off the bed nor to grip a pencil. Because the patient's spontaneous tidal volume was only 0.20 L, his ventilation was controlled. Six hours after administration of pancuronium, the response to tetanus still unsustained, monitoring of neuromuscular block with the force-displacement transducer was discontinued. Thirteen hours after the administration of pancuronium, the patient's vital capacity had increased to 0.60 L, but the maximum inspiratory force was less than 20 cm H₂O. Controlled ventilation was continued.

Twenty-one hours after the administration of pancuronium, the patient was able to lift his head off the pillow for at least 20 seconds, and his bilateral grip strength was equal to that of the observer. His maximum inspiratory force was greater than 40 cm H₂O, his vital capacity was 1.0 L, and his chest roentgenogram was normal. Sustained response to a tetanic stimulus of 30 Hz for 5 seconds was elicited. When the patient started breathing spontaneously without an endotracheal tube, his arterial P_{O_2}, P_{CO_2}, and pH were 122 mm Hg, 41 mm Hg, and 7.40, respectively, with oxygen administered at a flow rate of 5 L/min through a nasal cannula. The patient recovered without further complications.

This case report illustrates the problem of repeated pharmacologic attempts to antagonize an antibiotic-relaxant neuromuscular blockade. Unknown to the anesthesiologists, including the senior author, neostigmine actually *augments* a polymyxin B block.[13] Thus the patient would have recovered from the neuromuscular blockade much sooner if no attempts to antagonize the block had been made. Unfortunately, it is impossible for the anesthesiologist to assess the percentage contributed to the blockade by the antibiotic, as opposed to the effect of the nondepolarizing relaxant; only the latter can be consistently antagonized by either neostigmine or pyridostigmine. For these reasons, as indicated previously, our attempts to antagonize the neuromuscular block are limited to the administration of neostigmine, 5 mg/70 kg, or of pyridostigmine, 15 mg/kg. If this fails, controlled ventilation is indicated until the neuromuscular blockade terminates spontaneously.

RENAL FAILURE

In patients who are without kidney function, the neuromuscular block from those relaxants (gallamine and decamethonium) that depend entirely on the kidney for excretion will be prolonged unless small doses are used. Churchill-Davidson et al. reported prolonged paresis following gallamine administration in seven such patients.[15] Three of these patients required hemodialysis to eliminate the gallamine. The researchers concluded that gallamine should not be given to patients with impaired renal function, and the same conclusion probably applies to decamethonium. White et al. disagree with Churchill-Davidson and suggest that gallamine "in appropriate doses" is a satisfactory relaxant in patients who are without renal function.[16] They adduce as evidence the absence of prolonged paralysis, or "recurarization," in 17 patients who received gallamine (1 to 2 mg/kg). Although White et al. attempted to explain their results by suggesting that gallamine is metabolically degraded, there is a simpler and more likely explanation. They probably did not administer doses large enough to saturate the inactive depots. This can be quantified by determining the volume of distribution of gallamine by a pharmacokinetic analysis. If the inactive depots are saturated, urinary excretion becomes the only route by which gallamine can be removed from plasma. Since the volume of the inactive depots is small, it does not take a large amount of a highly ionized drug such as gallamine to saturate them. Therefore, as emphasized by White et al., gallamine should be used sparingly in patients with renal failure.[16] We believe that whereas White et al. may be correct on pure pharmacologic grounds, the approach of Churchill-Davidson et al. is more practical.[15,16] Only relaxants that do not entirely depend on renal excretion for their elimination should be used in patients with renal failure.

Recent studies indicate that d-tubocurarine may be preferable to pancuronium in patients with renal failure. In man, 40% of an injected dose of d-tubocurarine is eliminated in the urine.[17] Since the remaining 60% is eliminated from the body by unidentified nonrenal routes, d-tubocurarine disappears from plasma (and from neuromuscular junction) even if renal function is absent (Fig. 24–3).[17] In contrast, the elimination of pancuronium from plasma is impaired by renal failure (Fig. 24–3).[18] From the curves in Figure 24–3 it has been calculated that 80% of an injected dose of pancuronium is eliminated in the urine, although this has not been confirmed by actual measurements.

By using a pharmacokinetic computer simulation model for excretion of d-tubocurarine, Gibaldi and associates predicted that the absence of renal function should prolong the duration of action of d-tubocurarine only when large single or multiple doses are injected.[19] For example, the researchers predict that the neuromuscular blockade of d-tubocurarine, in a dose of 18 mg/m^2 (0.4 mg/kg), will last about two hours. This agrees with the data reported by Churchill-Davidson and associates.[15] Thus, if single doses smaller than 18 mg/m^2 (0.4 mg/kg) are administered, significant prolonged paralysis should not occur.

This discussion of renal failure does not deal with drug interaction as such, al-

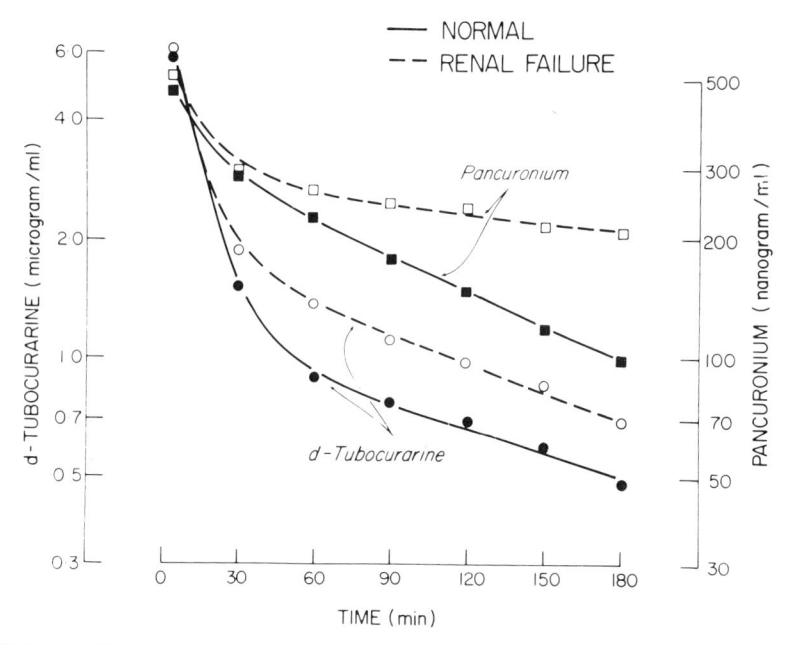

Fig. 24–3. Rates at which plasma concentrations of d-tubocurarine and pancuronium decrease in patients with normal renal function and with renal failure. Note that the decay rates (the slopes of the long lines) are about the same in patients with normal renal function. However, the decay rate is much slower in patients with renal failure receiving pancuronium than in those receiving d-tubocurarine. The data for pancuronium were obtained from McLeod et al.[90] and those for d-tubocurarine from Miller et al.[17] (From Miller, R.D.: Reversal of neuromuscular blockage. Regional Refresher Courses in Anesthesiology, 5:134, 1977.)

though any drug that depresses glomerular filtration may delay the excretion of d-tubocurarine or of pancuronium and thereby prolong the neuromuscular blockade. For example, halothane decreases glomerular filtration by approximately 40 to 50%.[18] It is not known, however, whether halothane delays the excretion of these relaxants, because the problem has not been investigated.

PREDNISONE

Animals that have undergone adrenalectomy and hypophysectomy manifest a decreased amplitude of action potentials generated from the neuromuscular junction; this can be reversed by the administration of cortisone or of ACTH (adrenocorticotropic hormone). ACTH also can improve neuromuscular function in patients with myasthenia gravis. Meyers described the anesthetic management of a patient who received long-term cortisone therapy.[19] After the induction of anesthesia, the administration of pancuronium resulted in a prolonged neuromuscular blockade that was partially antagonized by hydrocortisone. The patient was suspected of having inadequate replacement of adrenocortical hormones.

The mechanism of corticosteroid action on the neuromuscular junction is unknown. Steroids probably have little effect at the neuromuscular junction unless the patient is depleted of these compounds. In this case, it is conceivable that low prednisone levels could have contributed to the prolonged block described by Meyers.[19] Further studies are required to clarify the role of corticosteroids and neuromuscular transmission.

INHALATION ANESTHETICS

In the patient in the case report concerning kidney transplantation, halothane

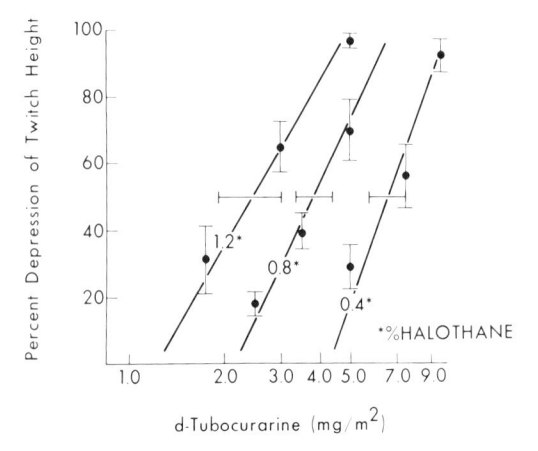

Fig. 24-4. The effects of 3 alveolar concentrations of halothane on mean depression of twitch height by d-tubocurarine. Each solid dot represents mean depression of twitch height (± 1 SE) for three patients. From these data, lines of linear regression were determined. (From Miller, R.D., et al.: The dependence of pancuronium and d-tubocurarine induced neuromuscular blockades on alveolar concentrations of halothane and Forane. Anesthesiology, 37:573, 1972.)

could have augmented the nondepolarizing block intraoperatively, but not in the recovery room, when most of the halothane should have been eliminated from the neuromuscular junction. Inhalation anesthetics augment the neuromuscular block from nondepolarizing relaxants in a dose-dependent fashion (Fig. 24-4) that, surprisingly, does not depend on the duration of anesthesia.[20,21] Of the anesthetic agents studied, inhalation anesthetics augment the muscle relaxants in decreasing order: isoflurane and enflurane, halothane, fluroxene and cyclopropane, and nitrous oxide-barbiturate-narcotic anesthesia.[22–23]

There are several theories as to the mechanisms by which inhalation anesthetics produce relaxation and augment the neuromuscular blockade from muscle relaxants. The non-neuromuscular mechanisms are:

1. Central nervous system depression.
2. Increased muscle blood flow (isoflurane).
3. Decreased glomerular filtration.
4. Decreased liver blood flow.
5. Hypothermia (poikilothermic).

Neuromuscular mechanisms are as follows:

1. Some inhalation anesthetics increase blood flow in the muscle, a phenomenom that delivers a greater fraction of the injected relaxant to the neuromuscular junction.[24] If it exists, this mechanism is probably significant only with isoflurane, which increases the amount of blood in muscle more than do other inhalation anesthetic agents.
2. Inhalation anesthetics induce relaxation at a site proximal to the neuromuscular junction, which site obviously is the central nervous system.[25]
3. Inhalation anesthetics decrease the sensitivity of the postjunctional membrane to depolarization.[29,30]
4. Inhalation anesthetics possibly act at a site distal to the cholinergic receptor and postjunctional membrane, such as at the muscle membrane.[27,28,31]

Inhalation anesthetics do not interfere with the release of acetylcholine from the motor nerve terminal, and these agents have no demonstrable effect on the cholinergic receptor.[26–28]

Although most inhalation agents such as halothane do not decrease twitch tension, conceptually they reduce the margin of safety of neuromuscular transmission. Waud indicates that halothane acts at a site distal to the cholinergic receptor, perhaps by interfering with calcium conductance or by release from depolarization, which may interfere with muscle contraction.[28,29,31] In his excellent review, Ngai points out that inhalation anesthetics are capable of producing relaxation with minimal neuromuscular blockade by acting on the central nervous system.[31] Thus these agents can induce adequate muscle relaxation without causing neuromuscular blockade.

CASE REPORT

(Conclusion of kidney transplant case report)
Of all the possibilities, decreased renal function, antibiotics, and furosemide appear to be likely causes of the prolonged d-tubocurarine neuromuscular blockade. Azathioprine and prednisone had been given several hours before the administration of muscle relaxants and their concentration in the patient's blood was presumably low. Furthermore, azathioprine antagonizes rather than augments a nondepolarizing blockade. Halothane administration had been stopped, yet the block persisted in the recovery room. Mannitol has been shown not to affect neuromuscular transmission.

LOCAL ANESTHETICS

In large doses, most local anesthetics block neuromuscular transmission; in smaller doses they enhance the neuromuscular block from both nondepolarizing and depolarizing muscle relaxants.[32,33] Telivuo and Katz found an additional decrease in twitch height and in tidal volume from lidocaine, mepivacaine, prilocaine, and bupivacaine in patients partially paralyzed with nortoxiferine.[32] Thus local anesthetics given as antidysrhythmic agents intra- or postoperatively may augment a residual neuromuscular block.

In low doses, local anesthetics depress post-tetanic potentiation, which is thought to be a neural, prejunctional effect.[34] In higher doses, local anesthetics block acetylcholine-induced muscle contractions, thereby suggesting a stabilizing effect on the postjunctional membrane.[35,36] Local anesthetics also have a direct effect on the muscle membrane by decreasing the strength of contraction of a denervated muscle or one that has received curare in response to a single shock.[37] Procaine has been shown to displace calcium from the sarcolemma and thus to inhibit caffeine-induced contraction of skeletal muscle.[38] These mechanisms of action probably apply to all the local anesthetics. In essence, local anesthetics have actions on the presynaptic, postjunctional, and muscle membranes.

Although situations may exist in which local anesthetics and muscle relaxants are given intraoperatively, probably most common is the administration of 50 to 100 mg/70 kg of lidocaine intravenously for the treatment of ventricular irritability. Whether that amount of lidocaine augments a partial neuromuscular blockade is an important question. The following case is an example of such a situation.

CASE REPORT

A 48-year-old woman was anesthetized with fluroxene and with nitrous oxide for the insertion of a cardiac pacemaker. Unknown to us at that time, her dibucaine number was 23%. Three minutes after the administration of d-tubocurarine, 3 mg, succinylcholine, 70 mg, was administered intravenously. There was a 100% neuromuscular blockade, as evidenced by the complete abolition of any response to peripheral nerve stimulation. About 40 minutes later, the twitch recurred and the patient resumed breathing spontaneously; a Phase II (desensitization) block was present, as evidenced by a fade in response to tetanic stimulus of 50 Hz and post-tetanic facilitation. Ten minutes later twitch height had fully returned and tidal volume was estimated to be 0.4 L: however, premature ventricular contractions (6 to 8/min) appeared, for which lidocaine, 50 mg, was given intravenously. The patient immediately stopped breathing and the twitch disappeared. Approximately 45 minutes later, tidal volume was 0.45 L and the response to a tetanic stimulus (50 Hz) was sustained. The patient recovered with no further difficulty.

This case demonstrates that lidocaine given as a 50- to 100-mg bolus, or possibly by intravenous infusion, may augment a Phase II block caused by succinylcholine or a nondepolarizing block caused by either d-tubocurarine or pancuronium. The interaction between lidocaine and muscle relaxants may be particularly important in the recovery room. If a patient has a slight undetected residual neuromuscular block that does not affect tidal volume, and subsequently receives lidocaine for ventricular irritability, a profound block may occur.

ANTIDYSRHYTHMIC DRUGS (EXCLUDING LOCAL ANESTHETICS)

Several drugs used for the treatment of dysrhythmias also augment the block caused by muscle relaxants, particularly by d-tubocurarine.[39] For example, patients have become "recurarized" after receiving quinidine in the recovery room. These cases may represent unrecognized residual effects of curare that are augmented by the administration of quinidine. Furthermore, when quinidine is administered to facilitate cardioversion in patients anesthetized with thiopental and succinylcholine, a prolonged neuromuscular blockade is likely to follow.[40] Quinidine potentiates the neuromuscular block caused by both nondepolarizing and depolarizing muscle relaxants;[41] edrophonium is ineffective in antagonizing a nondepolarizing blockade after quinidine. In these clinical doses, quinidine appears to act at the prejunctional membrane since it does not affect acetylcholine-evoked twitch. However, large, nonclinical doses of quinidine given intra-arterially produce a depolarizing neuromuscular blockade that is augmented by edrophonium.[42]

KETAMINE

Ketamine induces inadequate muscle relaxation, although it enhances the magnitude and duration of the neuromuscular block brought about by d-tubocurarine concomitantly administered.[43] Succinylcholine neuromuscular blockade appears not to be affected. *In vivo* (cat) and *in vitro* (frog) microelectrode studies have demonstrated that ketamine reduces the postjunctional membrane sensitivity to acetylcholine.[44]

MAGNESIUM SULFATE

Microelectrode studies performed in the frog nerve-muscle preparation suggest that magnesium has both pre- and postsynaptic activity.[45] Thus magnesium (1) decreases the amplitude of the end-plate potential, (2) decreases the depolarizing action of acetylcholine applied directly and the excitability of the muscle fiber itself, and (3) decreases the amount of acetylcholine release from the motor nerve terminal through nerve impulse.

Magnesium sulfate is used for the treatment of preeclamptic and eclamptic toxemia of pregnancy; these patients may also receive muscle relaxants during anesthesia for cesarean section. The neuromuscular blocking properties of both d-tubocurarine and succinylcholine are enhanced by magnesium, probably in an additive manner.[46,47] An increased neuromuscular block from d-tubocurarine is easily explained, since magnesium reduces the output of acetylcholine from the motor nerve terminal and reduces the sensitivity of the postjunctional membrane. These factors should antagonize the block from succinylcholine, although the opposite occurs. However, succinylcholine appears to be less affected by magnesium than does d-tubocurarine.[47]

LITHIUM CARBONATE

Lithium carbonate is used with increasing frequency in psychiatric disorders. If a patient is receiving lithium, will the neuromuscular depression from muscle relaxants be prolonged? Only one case report in the literature suggests that the block from nondepolarizing muscle relaxants may be prolonged.[48] The interaction between lithium and succinylcholine has been well documented by Hill et al.; the following case report is abstracted from their article.[49]

CASE REPORT

A 38-year-old woman was anesthetized for an emergency cesarean section. She had previously received lithium carbonate by mouth daily, which resulted in a blood level of 1.2 mEq/L. Anesthesia was induced with pancuronium, 0.5 mg, thiopental 350 mg, and succinylcholine, 150 mg, intravenously, followed by a succinylcholine drip (310 mg total in 120 minutes). A 5-lb 6-oz infant was delivered with no difficulty (Apgar scores were five and nine).

Postoperatively, the patient remained apneic for four hours. Stimulation of the ulnar nerve indicated probable Phase II block. After four hours of mechanical ventilation, she could raise her head; tidal volume was 0.45 L, and forced vital capacity was 0.9 L; her handgrip was strong. The patient's trachea was then extubated without further respiratory problem. Her dibucaine number was 73.

In order to explore further the interaction

between succinylcholine and lithium, Hill et al. performed studies in their laboratory.[49] They found that both the time it took to reach peak effect (onset) and the duration of succinylcholine neuromuscular blockade were prolonged by the concomitant administration of clinical doses of lithium. Hence this seems to be a well-established fact. However, the delayed onset of succinylcholine deserves additional comment. If a rapid induction of anesthesia is attempted in a patient pretreated with lithium, the tendency of the anesthetist will be to give repeated doses of succinylcholine because relaxation does not occur as promptly as expected. This practice will be avoided when the retardant effect of lithium is fully recognized.

The ultimate mechanism of action of lithium on the neuromuscular junction remains unknown.

INTERACTION BETWEEN NONDEPOLARIZING MUSCLE RELAXANTS AND SUCCINYLCHOLINE

Nondepolarizing (*d*-tubocurarine, pancuronium, and gallamine) and depolarizing (succinylcholine and decamethonium) muscle relaxants show antagonistic or additive properties depending on the method of testing.[50,51] Both types of relaxants are administered concomitantly in three clinical situations.

Succinylcholine is commonly given to facilitate intubation of the trachea and is usually followed by a longer-acting nondepolarizing relaxant such as *d*-tubocurarine or pancuronium. Presumably the block caused by a nondepolarizing relaxant will not be affected if the longer-acting drug is given after the block from succinylcholine has dissipated. Katz, however, reported that prior administration of succinylcholine nearly doubled the depression of twitch height induced by the same dose of pancuronium.[51] The duration of the block was similarly increased. Although succinylcholine and *d*-tubocurarine are supposedly antagonistic, Katz et al. have speculated that the end-plate may remain desensitized by the initial dose of succinylcholine.[51] If true, this may account for the unexpected increase in duration of nondepolarizing block induced by previous succinylcholine administration.

The second possible association is the injection of *d*-tubocurarine or pancuronium for prolonged relaxation, followed by the shorter-acting succinylcholine to facilitate closure of the peritoneum. The amount of succinylcholine required for adequate relaxation directly depends on the amount of residual *d*-tubocurarine or pancuronium blockade present. For example, if succinylcholine is added to a 65% neuromuscular block due to *d*-tubocurarine, the onset from succinylcholine will be delayed 150% and its duration will be decreased from 9 to approximately 7 minutes.[52] Although the onset of succinylcholine block will be delayed, its duration will be increased to 17 minutes (100% increase) when added to a preexisting partial pancuronium block. The mechanism by which pancuronium prolongs a succinylcholine neuromuscular blockade has not been established. Pancuronium inhibits plasma cholinesterase, although this inhibition is not clinically significant.[52] Despite the questionable pharmacologic reasoning, concomitant administration of an antagonist and agonist in appropriate doses appears to be effective.[53] Whether this is the best approach to the problem is disputed. Many anesthetists prefer either to give an additional dose of a nondepolarizer that can be easily antagonized at the end of the operation or to increase the anesthetic dose or concentration, since relaxation and augmentation of the effect of muscle relaxants depend on anesthetic dose.[20] We prefer the latter approach. (See Chap. 1.)

A small dose of a nondepolarizing agent is commonly given before administering succinylcholine to prevent adverse effects. Succinylcholine administration may increase intraocular and intragastric pressure, and may cause muscle pains and possibly hyperkalemia.[54-57] These adverse effects can be either attenuated or prevented by prior administration of a subparalyzing dose of *d*-tubocurarine or gallamine. Despite its advantages, this technique has been questioned for two reasons: (1) more succinylcholine is required for adequate relaxation, and (2) prolonged apnea may occur from a desensitization block. The latter effect has not been documented.[53] The former is well established, but it causes little difficulty clinically.[58,59] In an excellent study, Dery has provided further evidence of the safety of this approach.[60] We have only mentioned *d*-tubocurarine and gallamine, although theoretically pancuronium should be just as useful. However, the effectiveness of pancuronium in preventing the increase in intraocular and intragastric pressure has not been determined. In any case, the administration of *d*-tubocurarine, 3 mg/70 kg, or of gallamine, 20 mg/70 kg, prior to succinylcholine seems to be acceptable.

INTERACTION OF ATRACURIUM OR VECURONIUM WITH OTHER DRUGS

The main information on interactions of vecuronium or atracurium with other drugs comprises anesthetics, antibiotics, and succinylcholine.

Inhaled Anesthetic Agents

Anesthetics enhance a nondepolarizing neuromuscular blockade in the following order: nitrous oxide-narcotics <halothane <isoflurane and enflurane.[60a] The potencies of atracurium and vecuronium appear to be influenced less by the choice and concentration of anesthetic than are the potencies of *d*-tubocurarine and pancuronium. Enflurane and isoflurane augment a *d*-tubocurarine and pancuronium neuromuscular blockade about twice as much as does an equipotent concentration of halothane (Fig. 24-4).*[22,23,60b] For example, the ED_{50}s of *d*-tubocurarine and pancuronium are 1.70 and 0.27 mg/m², respectively, during isoflurane anesthesia and 5.60 and 0.49 mg/m², respectively, during halothane anesthesia.[22,60b] In contrast, the augmentation of a vecuronium- or atracurium-induced neuromuscular blockade by enflurane and isoflurane is only 20 to 30% greater than the augmentation produced by halothane or nitrous oxide-narcotic anesthesia (Fig. 24-4).[60c-60f]

Changes in the end-tidal concentration of inhaled anesthetics also have a lesser influence on neuromuscular blockades produced by vecuronium or atracurium than those produced by other nondepolarizing neuromuscular blockers. Increasing the anesthetic concentration from 1.2 MAC to 2.2 MAC decreases the ED_{50} of vecuronium by 51, 33, and 18% during enflurane, isoflurane, and halothane anesthesia, respectively.[60e] Yet the ED_{50}s of *d*-tubocurarine and pancuronium decreased 62 and 57%, respectively, for similar increases in halothane concentration, and 30 and 70%, respectively, for similar increases in the isoflurane concentration.[20]

Injected Anesthetic Agents. Ketamine, fentanyl, gammahydroxybutrate, and etomidate have all been shown to potentiate the neuromuscular block produced by vecuronium on the isolated rat phrenic nerve/hemidiaphragm preparation, and also in the anesthetized rat and cat.[60g] Of the four anesthetics tested, only ketamine significantly prolonged the recovery time from block due to vecuronium.

Inhaled and Injected Agents. The potentiating effect of the inhaled agents on neuromuscular block appears to take place in the presence of other drugs. Halothane (0.5%) and enflurane (1.0%) both enhance the neuromuscular block produced by an intravenous infusion of vecuronium in pa-

---

*The reasons for vecuronium or atracurium's being less influenced by the specific anesthetic and its dose or concentration are unknown.

tients anesthetized with N_2O/O_2 and fentanyl. The infusion rate of vecuronium could be decreased by 25 to 30% in the presence of halothane with balanced anesthesia or in the presence of enflurane with balanced anesthesia to achieve the same depth of block as under balanced anesthesia alone.[60h]

Succinylcholine. Prior administration of succinylcholine probably enhances the neuromuscular blockades from vecuronium or atracurium.[60i–60k] However, as with pancuronium[51,60l] and *d*-tubocurarine,[50,60m] there is a lack of agreement among investigators. Stirt et al.[60j] observed that prior administration of succinylcholine, 1.0 mg/kg, increased the intensity of the atracurium neuromuscular blockade from 52 to 84% but did not increase its duration. d'Hollander et al.[60n] reported that succinylcholine augmented both the magnitude and duration of a vecuronium-induced neuromuscular blockade. This augmentation occurred if vecuronium was given within 30 minutes of succinylcholine administration. Krieg et al.[60aa] found that vecuronium given after full recovery from succinylcholine, 1 mg/kg, caused a 19% greater depression of twitch tension than did vecuronium given without a prior dose of succinylcholine. Yet Fisher and Miller[60o] observed that prior administration of succinylcholine did not alter a vecuronium-induced neuromuscular blockade. Clearly, the response to vecuronium, and probably atracurium, varies when given after succinylcholine.

Although potentiation of nondepolarizing neuromuscular block by succinylcholine is controversial, the finding of Krieg and co-workers[60k] is interesting, since vecuronium is most likely able to inhibit butyrylcholinesterase at clinically used doses;[60p] butyrylcholinesterase is the enzyme responsible for the inactivation of succinylcholine. Although the reverse sequence (vecuronium followed by succinylcholine) has not been investigated, this would also probably result in potentiation, since vecuronium would inhibit butyrylcholinesterase and thus decrease the breakdown rate of succinylcholine by the enzyme.

Antibiotics

The same workers also investigated the effects of antibiotics on vecuronium neuromuscular block *in vitro* and *in vivo*.[60k] In the anesthetized rat or cat, an intravenous bolus injection of clindamycin (10 mg/kg), gentamicin (1 mg/kg), or neomycin (3 mg/kg) increased the 50% twitch depression produced by an intravenous infusion of vecuronium. However, the prior administration of any one of the antibiotics did not affect the depth or time course of the twitch depression produced by a bolus dose of vecuronium. In the rat or cat the tibialis anticus muscle was used to monitor neuromuscular transmission. Only neomycin was investigated *in vitro* on the isolated rat diaphragm by the same workers.[60k] At subblocking concentrations (160 μg/ml), neomycin significantly potentiated both vecuronium and pancuronium.[60k] In a similar but separate study using the isolated rat phrenic nerve-hemidiaphragm preparation, sisomicin, tobramycin, netimicin, and gentamicin were shown to potentiate the neuromuscular blocking activity of vecuronium and pancuronium.[60q]

Reversibility

There have been no reports of difficulty in antagonizing either a vecuronium- or atracurium-induced neuromuscular blockade with anticholinesterase drugs. Basta et al.[60r] determined that the doses of neostigmine required to antagonize neuromuscular blockade produced by atracurium or metocurine were similar. Also, the times from administration of neostigmine to recovery of 98% control twitch height were comparable: 8.2 minutes for atracurium and 7.6 minutes for metocurine. Conversely, Fahey et al.[60s] found that less neostigmine was required to antagonize a neuromuscular blockade induced by vecuronium than one induced by pancuronium. However, this conclusion was based on data obtained from administration of intermittent injections of neostigmine. Possibly because a neuromuscular blockade by vecuronium would terminate spontaneously more rapidly than one by pancuronium, less neostigmine would be required with vecuronium. To compensate for the possibility that this pharmacokinetic characteristic would decrease the neostigmine requirement, Gencarelli and Miller[60t] continuously infused either pancuronium or vecuronium and observed no difference in the neostigmine dose required for antagonism. They concluded that vecuronium and pancuronium effectively and equally (independent of their pharmacokinetics) are antagonized by neostigmine. Baird et al.[60u] found that edrophonium, 0.5 to 1.0 mg/kg IV, rapidly (i.e., 1 to 2 min) restored a vecuronium depressed twitch to 80% (i.e., 20% depression of twitch tension still remaining) of the control height but that an additional period of 6 to 8 minutes was required for complete restoration of neuromuscular function, as judged by the train-of-four response.

These studies indicate that both vecuronium- and atracurium-induced neuromuscular blockades are antagonized readily by edrophonium or neostigmine. Because the new neuromuscular blocking drugs produce a blockade of relatively short duration, an antagonist may not be necessary. For example, Katz et al.[60v] found it necessary to antagonize only 5 of 25 neuromuscular blockades from atracurium. Undoubtedly, administration of an antagonist is not always necessary. However, we believe spontaneous recovery should not be relied upon for termination of neuromuscular blockade unless a sustained response to a tetanic stimulus of 100 Hz for 5 seconds or a completely normal train-of-four unquestionably exists.

Antagonism of vecuronium-induced neuromuscular block by anticholinesterases has been clearly demonstrated in both animal and clinical studies. In the rhesus monkey, neuromuscular block produced by vecuronium was reversed by 35 μg/kg of neostigmine and 0.5 mg (total dose) of atropine in a significantly faster time than spontaneous recovery.[60w] In another study using anesthetized cats, a dose of 70 μg/kg of neostigmine reduced the recovery time (time from 25 to 75% recovery) from 90% twitch depression from 2.1 ± 0.3 to 0.98 ± 0.2 min.[60x] Clinically, neostigmine[60y,60z] and pyridostigmine[60aa] adequately reverse the neuromuscular block produced by vecuronium more rapidly than control recovery, and Fahey and co-workers[60y] found significantly less neostigmine was required to reverse vecuronium than pancuronium. 4-Aminopyridine and 3,4-diaminopyridine are agents that increase evoked transmitter release via an action on the nerve terminal, an effect occurring at the neuromuscular junction,[60bb,60cc] in addition to other synapses;[60dd] no anticholinesterase activity at doses that potentiate transmitter release has been reported with either drug. 3,4-Diaminopyridine (1 mg/kg) reversed vecuronium in the anesthetized rhesus monkey,[60w] and 4-aminopyridine reversed the neuromuscular block produced by an infusion of vecuronium in the anesthetized rat.[60ee] Only 4-aminopyridine has been used clinically as a reversal agent, and its use of such has been confined to Europe.[60ff] There is little clinical information available concerning reversal of vecuronium by 4-aminopyridine.

INTERACTION OF NEOSTIGMINE WITH SUCCINYLCHOLINE

The importance of the interaction between neostigmine and succinylcholine revolves around two questions: (1) Is it rational to administer succinylcholine when a nondepolarizing block has been antagonized by neostigmine? (2) Should neostigmine be used to antagonize a Phase II (desensitization) block?

The answer to the first question is that,

although this practice may be reasonable, one should realize that the neuromuscular block from succinylcholine will be prolonged.[61] This is because, in addition to inhibiting acetylcholinesterase at the endplate, neostigmine also inhibits plasma cholinesterase. As a result, the breakdown of succinylcholine, when administered after neostigmine, will be delayed. The senior author's experience indicates that when succinylcholine (0.75 to 1.5 mg/kg) is administered within 20 minutes after the administration of 2 to 3 mg/70 kg of neostigmine, the ensuing neuromuscular block may last as long as 60 to 90 minutes. This observation has been confirmed experimentally by Nastuk et al., who observed a reduction in the concentration of depolarizing drug required to produce paralysis in the presence of acetylcholinesterase inhibitors.[62] It is not known how much time should elapse after the administration of neostigmine before one can expect a normal response to succinylcholine. Neostigmine has a duration of action of 50 to 90 minutes, which is probably the necessary interval for the return of a normal response to succinylcholine.[63]

With regard to the second question, a well-defined Phase II block by succinylcholine can be antagonized with neostigmine. Our opinion differs from that of Katz and Churchill-Davidson, who suggest that neostigmine should probably be avoided altogether in patients who manifest a prolonged response to succinylcholine.[64] This difference of opinion is based on reports that neostigmine may either antagonize or enhance a Phase II (desensitizing) block from succinylcholine.[61,65,66] How can we predict successful antagonism of a desensitizing neuromuscular block? Gissen et al. attribute importance to the presence of succinylcholine in plasma.[67] In the absence of circulating succinylcholine, anticholinesterase drugs will antagonize a desensitizing block induced by succinylcholine. In the presence of circulating succinylcholine, however, anticholinesterase drugs either will not affect or will enhance the succinylcholine-induced desensitizing block. Since no simple method for determining the succinylcholine level in plasma exists, these researchers suggest that anticholinesterase drugs should be avoided in the management of patients whose response to succinylcholine is prolonged.

As indicated above, we believe that attempts to antagonize a prolonged succinylcholine block may be appropriate in well-defined circumstances. To avoid the chance that neostigmine may prolong the block, we first use edrophonium as a diagnostic drug. If, following administration of edrophonium, tetanus becomes unequivocally sustained, post-tetanic facilitation disappears, and tidal volume, vital capacity, or inspiratory force increase for at least three to five minutes, it is reasonable to expect complete and prolonged antagonism of the succinylcholine blockade by neostigmine. Apparently, antagonism of a desensitizing neuromuscular block should not be attempted when the patient is apneic.[65] A review of reported cases of patients with low dibucaine numbers suggests that attempts to reverse succinylcholine desensitizing blocks before there was evidence of spontaneous muscle activity have resulted in more profound and prolonged neuromuscular blocks. Perhaps this indicates a high level of succinylcholine in the plasma. However, in those cases in which spontaneous muscle activity had begun to appear, there usually was an immediate and lasting antagonism of the neuromuscular block when an anticholinesterase was administered.[65]

DRUGS THAT PROLONG SUCCINYLCHOLINE BLOCK BY INHIBITION OF PSEUDOCHOLINESTERASE

Drugs that may prolong a succinylcholine neuromuscular blockade by inhibition of pseudocholinesterase (plasma cholinesterase) include: (1) echothiophate, (2) hexafluorenium, (3) phenelzine, (4) tetrahydroaminacrine (tacrine), and (5) cytotoxic drugs (alkylating agents) including nitrogen mustard and cyclophosphamide. Pseudocholinesterase breaks down succinylcholine by hydrolysis. If pseudocholinesterase is absent, a prolonged block may occur. The extent to which pseudocholinesterase must be reduced before a prolonged block occurs has not been defined, but it is estimated that a decrease of at least 20% is necessary. We discuss only those drugs that inhibit pseudocholinesterase sufficiently to bring about a clinically detectable effect.

Echothiophate iodide, which is used in the treatment of glaucoma, probably has received the most attention. It inhibits pseudocholinesterase from 15 to 40%.[68] It increases the duration of succinylcholine block by 10 to 20 minutes. More details can be found in the excellent review by Pantuck and Pantuck.[68]

Phenelzine, a monoamine oxidase inhibitor used for the treatment of mental depression, also increases the duration of a succinylcholine block by the inhibition of pseudocholinesterase. Apparently, pseudocholinesterase levels do not return to normal for 2 weeks after the discontinuance of phenelzine.[68] Even though phenelzine can dramatically reduce pseudocholinesterase levels in some patients, the reduction is unpredictable and sometimes nonexistent.[68] The reasons for this unpredictability are unclear.

It has been reported that cytotoxic or alkylating agents prolong succinylcholine neuromuscular block by the alkylation of pseudocholinesterase.[69,70] Recently Bennett et al. reported one case of prolonged pancuronium neuromuscular blockade in a patient who was receiving an alkylating drug, triethylenethiophosphoramide (thio-TEPA);[71] the interaction is unrelated to changes in pseudocholinesterase. This patient, however, was affected by myasthenia gravis; the presence of this condition casts some doubt on the mechanism of the interaction. Further studies are required to confirm this observation.[71]

HYPOTENSIVE DRUGS

Ganglionic blocking drugs, particularly trimethaphan (Arfonad), can affect neuromuscular blockade by several mechanisms, namely, changes in blood flow, inhibition of pseudocholinesterase, and decreased sensitivity of the postjunctional membrane. Drugs that are used to induce hypotension deliberately can affect the neuromuscular block because of changes in blood flow to the neuromuscular junction. In general, a reduction in muscle blood flow will delay the onset and will prolong the duration of neuromuscular blockade. A study by Goat et al. presents evidence that a reduction in muscle blood flow does not prolong a nondepolarizing blockade.[72] They reported that the times required to recover from the block by 25 to 75% were not prolonged, but the researchers did not actually report the duration of neuromuscular blockade. Hence it can be stated that the "slope" of recovery was not prolonged, but this study cannot provide conclusions on the duration of neuromuscular blockade on the basis of the reported data. For example, one might ask how long it would take to achieve 25% recovery. Furthermore, changes in blood flow were induced by a roller pump through a shunt, a system that probably does not approximate the low flow conditions caused by hypotensive drugs. Therefore, this study does not discredit the theory that a neuromuscular block may be prolonged by a decrease in muscle flow.

Can hypotensive drugs affect the neuromuscular junction directly, independently of changes in muscle blood flow? Apparently sodium nitroprusside has no direct effect.[73] Gergis et al. have proposed that trimethaphan (Arfonad) depresses the postjunctional membrane as evidenced by decreased sensitivity of the membrane to iontophoretically applied acetylcholine.[73]

This would explain a prolonged nondepolarizing blockade, but not the clinical observation that neostigmine may augment, rather than antagonize, the block.[74,75] Obviously the interaction among neostigmine, trimethaphan, and the nondepolarizing relaxants needs further study, and, until more information becomes available, we use an arbitrary and empiric approach to this type of drug interaction. If a prolonged nondepolarizing block occurs in a patient who has received trimethaphan, we administer neostigmine, 2.5 to 5.0 mg/70 kg, or pyridostigmine, 10 to 15 mg/70 kg. If the block is not antagonized, the patient's ventilation should be controlled until the block terminates spontaneously, since the administration of additional anticholinesterase may augment neuromuscular blockade.[73,75]

In addition to altering the effect of muscle relaxants by decreasing blood flow and by directly affecting the neuromuscular junction, trimethaphan inhibits pseudocholinesterase activity.[75] Sklar et al. have estimated that pseudocholinesterase activity is suppressed by trimethaphan to such an extent that the duration of action from succinylcholine is doubled.[76] However, sodium nitroprusside does not alter pseudocholinesterase activity.[76] In summary, trimethaphan alters the action of muscle relaxants in several ways, whereas sodium nitroprusside appears only to decrease muscle blood flow.

DRUG INTERACTIONS INVOLVING THE CARDIOVASCULAR EFFECTS OF d-TUBOCURARINE AND PANCURONIUM

CASE REPORT

A 69-year-old man was anesthetized with halothane and nitrous oxide (60%) for total hip arthroplasty. Halothane was maintained at an end-tidal concentration of 0.75 volume %. The patient's systolic blood pressure was 130 mm Hg. Three minutes after the administration of d-tubocurarine 12 mg/m^2 (21 mg total), his systolic blood pressure began to decrease. Ten minutes later, the systolic blood pressure was 70 mm Hg. Halothane was discontinued and ephedrine, 15 mg, was administered intravenously. The patient's systolic blood pressure promptly increased to 120 mm Hg. Halothane was gradually reinstituted without further difficulty with blood pressure.

Hypotension in this case appears to be related to the administration of d-tubocurarine. Although ephedrine administration was successful in reversing the hypotension, this approach can be dangerous. Ephedrine, which elicits both direct and indirect sympathetic responses, increases the incidence of dysrhythmias with halothane; this drug interaction is discussed in Chapter 6.

Hypotension from d-tubocurarine is probably due to histamine release and to ganglionic blockade.[77,78] The magnitude of hypotension probably depends on several factors, the most important of which are depth of anesthesia (Fig. 24–5), dose of d-tubocurarine administered, age, and intravascular volume.[79,80] The most likely situation in which hypotension might develop is in an elderly, bedridden patient who is deeply anesthetized, and who is receiving a large dose of d-tubocurarine. Hypotension can be rare when d-tubocurarine is used in doses of less than 9 mg/m^2 (15 mg/70 kg) (Fig. 24–5). Since doses larger than this are not necessary for adequate relaxation during halothane anesthesia, hypotension from d-tubocurarine should not be a problem.

Why is hypotension from d-tubocurarine more severe with higher concentrations of halothane? This may be because both drugs block ganglionic transmission in a dose-dependent manner and both may have an additive effect.[80,81] With deeper levels of halothane, the onset of d-tubocurarine ganglionic blockade occurs at lower doses; the opposite is also true. This situation probably applies to anesthetic agents other than halothane.

CASE REPORT

A 48-year-old 60-kg woman was scheduled for a radical mastectomy. She was anesthetized with halo-

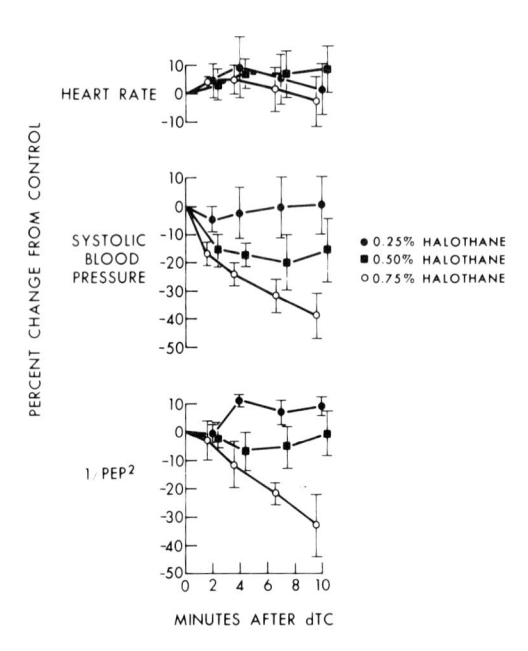

Fig. 24–5. Effects of alveolar halothane concentration on systolic blood pressure, heart rate, and myocardial inotropy (1/PEP^2) following administration of d-tubocurarine 12 mg/m^2, as an intravenous bolus. Each point represents the mean of values for five patients (± 1 SE). All patients also received nitrous oxide, 60%. (From Munger, W.L., Miller, R.D., and Stevens, W.C.: The dependence of d-tubocurarine hypotension on alveolar concentration of halothane, dose of d-tubocurarine, and nitrous oxide. Anesthesiology, 40:442, 1974.)

thane and nitrous oxide, 60%, after the administration of thiopental, 150 mg. After the induction of anesthesia, her systolic blood pressure was 130 mm Hg and her heart rate was 90 beats per minute. Pancuronium, 6 mg, was then administered intravenously. Within three minutes the patient's heart rate was approximately 180 beats per minute and her systolic blood pressure was 90 mm Hg. Administration of lidocaine, 100 mg, intravenously had no effect. Neostigmine, 1.5 mg, was administered intravenously. This resulted in a prompt decrease in heart rate to 80 beats per minute and in a systolic blood pressure to 120 mm Hg. The neuromuscular blockade was also antagonized. Anesthesia and the operation proceeded without any further difficulty. Postoperatively the patient was interviewed more thoroughly for possible drug intake information missed on the preoperative visit. It was then learned that she had been taking imipramine for over a year.

This case report represents a triple drug interaction—pancuronium, tricyclic antidepressants, and halothane. Pancuronium administration induces a transient tachycardia and slight hypertension.[82] The tachycardia is probably due to the vagolytic action of pancuronium, but the stimulation of the sympathetic nervous system has been suggested as a cause of tachycardia. Specifically, the negative chronotropic and inotropic actions of cholinergic drugs such as acetylcholine and carbachol are blocked by pancuronium. These actions support the theory of pancuronium's vagolytic mechanism of action.[83] Furthermore, the prior administration of atropine will attenuate the tachycardia from pancuronium (Fig. 24–6).[82] However, Seed and Chamberlain have found that pancuronium exerts a positive inotropic effect that is independent of an increase in heart rate.[84] Furthermore, reports of an increase in the plasma concentration of catecholamine following pancuronium and of a block of the reuptake of myocardial catecholamines suggest sympathetic activation.[85,86] The evidence supports a primarily vagolytic action. Even though Zsigmond et al. did not find an increase in plasma catecholamine concentrations, all other evidence points to a secondary stimulation of the sympathetic nervous system.[87]

A combined vagolytic and sympathomimetic effect is compatible with the observations in this case. It is well known that halothane "sensitizes" the myocardium to catecholamines. As a result, dysrhythmias such as ventricular extrasystoles or atrioventricular dissociation are more likely to occur with the administration of either atropine or vasopressors during halothane anesthesia.[82,88] Such dysrhythmias also are more likely when pancuronium is given during halothane anesthesia.[82] The propensity to cardiac dysrhythmias is further increased by tricyclic antidepressants, such as imipramine, which are known to block the reuptake of catecholamines.[89] Recent work in our laboratory indicates that such dysrhythmias are less likely to occur if one uses anesthetic agents that do not sensitize the myocardium to catecholamines, such

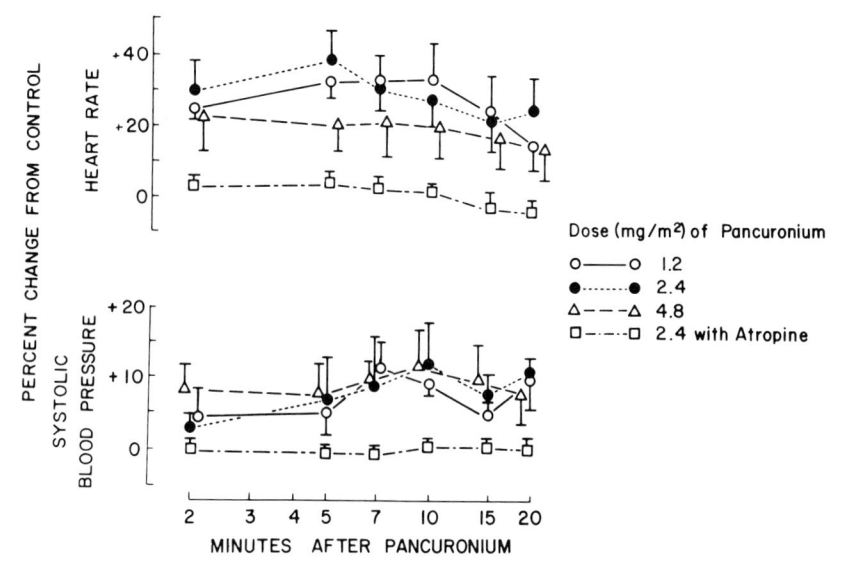

Fig. 24–6. Relationship between percentage increase in heart rate, systolic blood pressure, and time after pancuronium, 1.2, 2.4, or 4.8 mg/m². One group of patients received atropine, 0.33 mg/m², prior to pancuronium administration. Each symbol represents the mean ± 1 SE for five patients. (From Miller, R.D., et al.: Pancuronium-induced tachycardia in relation to alveolar halothane, dose of pancuronium, and prior atropine. Anesthesiology, 42:352, 1975.)

as enflurane or nitrous oxide-narcotic anesthesia.[89a]

Therefore, we use a muscle relaxant other than pancuronium or gallamine when a patient has taken tricyclic antidepressants. Conversely, if pancuronium is administered, we use anesthetics that do not sensitize the myocardium to catecholamines.

DRUGS THAT ALTER THE REQUIRED DOSES OF NEOSTIGMINE OR OF PYRIDOSTIGMINE

Several antibiotics increase the dose of neostigmine or of pyridostigmine required for antagonism, but these antibiotics also make it impossible for complete antagonism to occur no matter what dose of neostigmine is given. There are probably other drugs that act similarly, but they have not been identified. Those drugs that may interfere with the neostigmine-d-tubocurarine interaction are likely to intensify the neuromuscular blockade from nondepolarizing relaxants such as d-tubocurarine. Thus when a neuromuscular blockade cannot be antagonized it is difficult to know whether the block is too intense to be antagonized or whether a specific problem with the neostigmine-relaxant interaction exists.

Even though no other drugs are known to alter specifically the neostigmine-relaxant interaction, some drugs can create secondary conditions that interfere with the reversal of neuromuscular blockade. These conditions are: (1) neuromuscular blockade that is too intense (hypothermia and renal failure), (2) antibiotics, (3) respiratory acidosis, and (4) metabolic alkalosis (hypokalemia and hypocalcemia). In the case of the last three conditions, not only is more neostigmine required, but also it is impossible to antagonize the block completely unless the antibiotic is eliminated or unless the acid-base abnormality is corrected.

Narcotics have little or no effect on a nondepolarizing neuromuscular blockade as such. However, if respiratory acidosis ensues from their administration, complete antagonism by neostigmine is difficult and often impossible.[91,92] This is a spurious effect of the narcotic.

There are other drugs that may have little direct effect on neuromuscular transmission but that cause secondary changes that may have important consequences. Chronic diuretic therapy causes hypokalemia, which augments a nondepolarizing neuromuscular blockade and increases the dose of neostigmine required for neuromuscular blockade.[93] General anesthetic agents, particularly halothane and enflurane, decrease renal and liver function as well as the patient's ability to maintain normal body temperature. Diminished renal function and hypothermia delay the excretion of muscle relaxants (Figs. 24-3 and 24-7).[17,90,94-97] Administration of sodium bicarbonate sufficient to increase arterial pH above 7.5 creates a situation in which a d-tubocurarine or pancuronium neuromuscular blockade cannot be antagonized completely by neostigmine.[91,92] One may mistakenly conclude that the incomplete antagonism is due to the elevated pH; however, the administration of sodium bicarbonate also decreases plasma calcium and potassium levels. When plasma calcium and potassium levels are normal, an elevated pH has no effect on a nondepolarizing blockade or on its antagonism by neostigmine.[98]

Generally, neostigmine, 2.5 to 5.0 mg/70 kg, or pyridostigmine, 10 to 20 mg/70 kg, should antagonize a nondepolarizing neuromuscular blockade. What should be done if these doses fail? In this situation, additional antagonist should not be given unless certain questions have been answered:[99]

1. Has enough time been allowed for the neostigmine or pyridostigmine to act fully?
2. Is the neuromuscular blockade too intense to be antagonized?
3. What is the acid-base and electrolyte status of the patient?
4. What is the patient's temperature?
5. Is the patient receiving any drug that might interfere with reversal?

The answers to these questions may help to correct conditions that prevent prompt, complete reversal of neuromuscular blockade by either neostigmine or pyridostigmine.

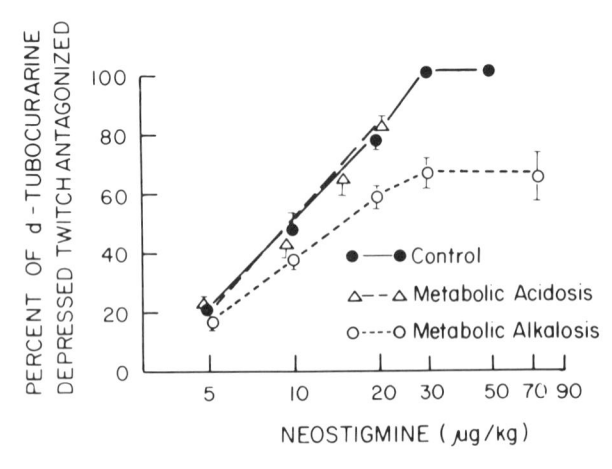

Fig. 24–7. Correlation by dose of neostigmine and percentage of dTC-depressed twitch antagonized. Each symbol represents the mean ±1 SE. (From Miller, R.D., et al.: The effect of acid-base balance on neostigmine antagonism of d-tubocurarine-induced neuromuscular blockade. Anesthesiology, 42:377, 1975.)

ATRACURIUM AND VECURONIUM

Vecuronium and atracurium are new nondepolarizing neuromuscular blocking drugs with durations of action between those of succinylcholine and pancuronium. To place them into perspective, we shall compare vecuronium and atracurium with three other neuromuscular blocking drugs discussed in this chapter: succinylcholine, pancuronium and d-tubocurarine.

Developmental Chemistry. Savage et al.[100] are responsible for the manipulation of the steroid nucleus that resulted in the development of many neuromuscular blocking drugs, the most successful to date being the bisquaternary, pancuronium. To achieve a nondepolarizing neuromuscular blocker with a more rapid onset of action and shorter duration of action than that of pancuronium, the monoquaternary vecuronium was developed. Although both vecuronium and pancuronium are hydrophilic, vecuronium is slightly more lipophilic because it is a monoquaternary rather than a bisquaternary compound. Because of this increased lipophilicity, vecuronium was predicted to have different pharmacokinetic and pharmacodynamic profiles from pancuronium,[100] as described in the pharmacokinetic section below. Increased lipophilicity should enhance penetration of membranes and could alter vecuronium's route of elimination as compared with pancuronium, as proved to be the case.

Stenlake et al.[101] used a different principle in developing a neuromuscular blocking drug having a short duration of action: a neuromuscular blocking drug spontaneously degraded to inactive breakdown products. Thus, atracurium was developed. This quaternary ammonium compound breaks down in the absence of plasma enzymes through Hofmann elimination and, to a lesser extent, ester hydrolysis. Hofmann elimination is a nonbiologic method of degradation that occurs at a physiologic temperature and pH. Lowering temperature or pH decreases the rate of this reaction. Ester hydrolysis does not require pseudocholinesterase and is facilitated by an acid pH. The major breakdown products are laudanosine and a related quaternary acid, neither of which has neuromuscular blocking effects.[102]

Potency. The potency of vecuronium is equal to or slightly greater than pancuronium; the ratios of their potencies range from 1.0 to 1.74.[103-110] Atracurium is less potent than pancuronium, the ratios of their potencies ranging from 0.25 to 0.33.[110-112]

Onset Time and Duration of Action. The onset time—from administration to peak effect—and duration of action—from administration to 90 or 95% recovery of control twitch tension—are similar for both vecuronium and atracurium.[103-108,110-112, 113-115,116-124] The doses of atracurium or vecuronium that depress twitch height less than 100% have onset times ranging from 4 to 8 minutes. Because larger doses depress twitch tension 100%, onset times appear to be shorter. For example, four times the ED_{95} of vecuronium has an onset time of 1.3 minutes.[118] When three times the ED_{95} of atracurium was given, onset times were 1.2[111] and 1.3[114] minutes. Even when large doses are given, neither vecuronium nor atracurium has an onset time as short as that of succinylcholine.[125] Not surprisingly, recovery time (time from 25 to 75% recovery of control twitch tension) was also shorter (30 to 50%[103,105,108-110,126]) for vecuronium and atracurium than for pancuronium. These times ranged from 9 to 12 minutes for both atracurium and vecuronium.[103-105,107,108, 112,115,120,126]

Cumulative Effect. Vecuronium and atracurium have little or no cumulative effect. Ali et al.[127] observed a slight cumulative effect with vecuronium and no cumulative effect with atracurium. Whether a neuromuscular blocking drug has a cumulative effect can be explained on a kinetic basis. With neuromuscular blockers that are not extensively metabolized (i.e., all blockers except succinylcholine and atracurium), recovery of neuromuscular function parallels the decrease in plasma concentration. Following a single dose of vecuronium or pancuronium, plasma concentration falls rapidly because of redistribution from the central to the peripheral compartment. With subsequent doses, the muscle relaxant in the peripheral compartment tends to limit this distribution phase, and the decrease in plasma concentration results from elimination or metabolism. Thus both pancuronium, and to a lesser extent, vecuronium can be demonstrated to have cumulative effects. For atracurium, pharmacokinetic analyses reveal that there is not a distinct distribution phase with a rapid decrease in plasma concentration. Thus, recovery from the effects of atracurium depends predominantly upon elimination (in this case metabolism by Hofmann elimination and ester hydrolysis) rather than redistribution. As a result, recovery from the neuromuscular effects of atracurium* is similar for the first and all subsequent doses.

Pharmacokinetics. Both vecuronium and atracurium have distinct pharmacokinetic properties as compared with currently used nondepolarizing muscle relaxants. For example, unlike pancuronium, metocurine, d-tubocurarine, or gallamine, neither vecuronium nor atracurium depends heavily on the kidney for elimination. Only 10 to 25% of an injected dose of vecuronium is excreted in the urine,[128–130] the predominant route of elimination probably being the bile.[128] Although vecuronium should be metabolized into compounds similar to those produced by the breakdown of pancuronium, only small amounts of these metabolites have been detected by methods such as thin-layer chromatography.[129] Although the precise extent to which vecuronium is metabolized has not been determined, apparently most of the drug excreted in the urine and bile is unchanged.[128]

Because atracurium is metabolized completely through Hofmann elimination and ester hydrolysis, it should only be excreted in the urine or bile in the form of a metabolite. Although urinary and biliary excretion has not been determined in humans, elimination half-life is about 20 to 30 minutes.[131,132]

Effects of Age. The potency of both vecuronium and atracurium are similar in pediatric and adult patients. On the other hand, d'Hollander et al.[133–135] found that a difference existed between vecuronium and atracurium in the elderly. Less vecuronium was required to sustain a steady state of paralysis, and recovery from neuromuscular blockade was longer in elderly patients (over 60 years) than in younger patients;[133] yet, these investigators observed no age-related changes associated with atracurium.[135] This is the only study with atracurium in the elderly. More study is required to better define the influence of age on the neuromuscular blockades produced by vecuronium or atracurium.

Cardiovascular Effects. The two major cardiovascular effects from older nondepolarizing blockers are tachycardia from vagal blockade (e.g., pancuronium and gallamine) and hypotension from histamine release (e.g., d-tubocurarine and metocurine). In contrast, vecuronium and, in large part, atracurium have little or no cardiovascular effects. For example, Booij et al.[136] gave 3 times the ED_{90} of vecuronium intravenously to dogs and observed no change in heart rate, blood pressure, or cardiac output. Marshall et al.[137] found that doses of vecuronium up to 20 times greater than those required for neuromuscular blockade produced no cardiovascular changes in cats and dogs. Although vecuronium does not release histamine, atracurium does, but in amounts less than those produced by metocurine or d-tubocurarine.[138] Doses of atracurium less than

---

*Further confirmation of rapid metabolism is the relatively prompt appearance of laudanosine in blood (within 5 to 20 minutes).[131]

0.6 mg/kg are rarely associated with cardiovascular changes.[139,113,114,115,140,141,142] Larger doses can cause a transient histamine response associated with hypotension, tachycardia, and flushing.[112] This response, however, is less than that associated with *d*-tubocurarine or metocurine.

Obstetrics. Because of their high degree of ionization and relatively low lipophilicity, there is no reason to believe that vecuronium or atracurium would cross the placental barrier in significant amounts. This prediction has been confirmed by several studies.[143–146]

Renal Disease. Since both vecuronium and atracurium rely little on the kidney for elimination, duration of neuromuscular blockade should not be prolonged in patients with renal failure. This conclusion has been confirmed with large doses of atracurium (0.5 to 2.3 mg/kg)[131,147] and vecuronium (0.28 mg/kg).[130] Thus, vecuronium and atracurium are the only two currently used, nondepolarizing blocking drugs whose neuromuscular blockades are not prolonged by renal failure.

Liver Disease. Because atracurium is metabolized through Hofmann elimination and ester hydrolysis, its pharmacokinetics and duration of neuromuscular blockade should not be altered by impaired hepatic function. On the other hand, vecuronium is significantly eliminated in the bile, and one might predict that the presence of liver disease would prolong a vecuronium-induced neuromuscular blockade. Indeed, the duration of neuromuscular blockade produced by vecuronium,[148] but not atracurium,[149] will be increased in patients with impaired hepatic function.

REFERENCES

1. Miller, R.D.: Antagonism of neuromuscular blockade. Anesthesiology, 44:293, 1976.
2. Foldes, F.F.: Factors which alter the effects of muscle relaxants. Anesthesiology, 20:464, 1959.
3. Miller, R.D.: Factors affecting the action of muscle relaxants. *In* Muscle Relaxants. Edited by R.L. Katz. Amsterdam, Excerpta Medica, North Holland Publishing Co., 1975.
4. Ali, H.H., and Savarese, J.J.: Monitoring of neuromuscular function. Anesthesiology, 45:216, 1976.
5. Dretchen, K.L., et al.: Azathioprine: effects on neuromuscular transmission. Anesthesiology, 45:604, 1976.
6. Standaert, F.G., Dretchen, K.L., and Skirboll, L.R.: A role of cyclic nucleotides in neuromuscular transmission. J. Pharmacol. Exp. Ther., 199:553, 1976.
7. Matteo, R.S., et al.: Urinary excretion of *d*-tubocurarine in man—effect of osmotic diuretic. *In* Abstracts of Scientific Papers, Chicago, American Society of Anesthesiology, 1975.
8. Miller, R.D., Sohn, Y.J., and Matteo, R.: Enhancement of *d*-tubocurarine neuromuscular blockade by diuretics in man. Anesthesiology, 45:442, 1976.
9. Scapaticci, K.A., et al.: Effects of furosemide on the motor nerve terminal. Fed. Proc. (In press.)
10. Ham, J., et al.: Effects of furosemide on neuromuscular transmission. (In press.)
11. Pittinger, C.B., and Adamson, R.: Antibiotic blockade of neuromuscular function. Annu. Rev. Pharmacol., 12:169, 1972.
11a. Foldes, F.F.: Personal communication.
12. Wright, J.M., and Collier, B.: The site of the neuromuscular block produced by polymyxin B and rolitetracycline. Can. J. Physiol. Pharmacol., 54:926, 1976.
13. Van Nyhuis, L.S., Miller, R.D., and Fogdall, R.P.: The interaction between *d*-tubocurarine, pancuronium, polymyxin B, and neostigmine on neuromuscular function. Anesth. Analg. (Cleve.), 55:237, 1976.
13a. Giesecke, A.H.: Personal communication.
14. Fogdall, R.P., and Miller, R.D.: Prolongation of a pancuronium-induced neuromuscular blockade by polymyxin B. Anesthesiology, 40:84, 1974.
15. Churchill-Davidson, H.C., Way, W.L., and de Jong, R.H.: The muscle relaxants and renal excretion. Anesthesiology, 28:540, 1967.
16. White, R.D., De Weerd, J.H., and Dawson, B.: Gallamine in anesthesia for patients with chronic renal failure undergoing bilateral nephrectomy. Anesth. Analg. (Cleve.), 50:11, 1971.
17. Miller, R.D., et al.: Influence of renal failure on the pharmacokinetics of *d*-tubocurarine in man. J. Pharmacol. Exp. Ther., 202:1, 1977.
18. Deutsch, S., et al.: Effects of halothane anesthesia on renal function in normal man. Anesthesiology, 27:793, 1966.
19. Meyers, E.F.: Partial recovery from pancuronium neuromuscular blockade following hydrocortisone administration. Anesthesiology, 46:148, 1977.
20. Miller, R.D., et al.: The dependence of pancuronium and *d*-tubocurarine induced neuromuscular blockades on alveolar concentrations of halothane and Forane. Anesthesiology, 37:573, 1972.
21. Miller, R.D., Criqui, M., and Eger, E.I., II: The

influence of duration of anesthesia on a d-tubocurarine neuromuscular blockade. Anesthesiology, 44:207, 1976.
22. Miller, R.D., et al.: Comparative neuromuscular effects of pancuronium, gallamine, and succinylcholine during Forane and halothane anesthesia in man. Anesthesiology, 35:509, 1971.
23. Fogdall, R.P., and Miller, R.D.: Neuromuscular effects of enflurane alone and in combination with d-tubocurarine, pancuronium, and succinylcholine in man. Anesthesiology, 42:173, 1975.
24. Vitez, T.S., Miller, R.D., and Eger, E.I., II: An in vitro comparison of halothane and isoflurane potentiation of neuromuscular blockade. Anesthesiology, 41:53, 1974.
25. Ngai, S.H., Hanks, E.C., and Farhie, S.E.: Effects of anesthetics on neuromuscular transmission and somatic reflexes. Anesthesiology, 26:162, 1965.
26. Gergis, S.D., et al.: Effect of anesthetics on acetylcholine release from the myoneural junction. Proc. Soc. Exp. Biol. Med., 141:629, 1972.
27. Waud, B.E., and Waud, D.R.: The effects of diethyl ether, enflurane, and isoflurane at the neuromuscular junction. Anesthesiology, 42:275, 1975.
28. Waud, B.E., and Waud, D.R.: Comparison of drug-receptor dissociation constants at the mammalian neuromuscular junction in the presence and absence of halothane. J. Pharmacol. Exp. Ther., 187:40, 1973.
29. Karis, J.H., Gissen, A.J., and Nastuk, W.L.: Mode of action of diethyl ether in blocking neuromuscular transmission. Anesthesiology, 27:42, 1966.
30. Gissen, A.J., Karis, J.H., and Nastuk, W.L.: Effect of halothane on neuromuscular transmission. J.A.M.A., 197:770, 1966.
31. Ngai, S.H.: Action of general anesthetics in producing muscle relaxation: interaction of anesthetics and relaxants. In Muscle Relaxants. Edited by R.L. Katz. Amsterdam, Excerpta Medica, North-Holland Publishing Co., 1975.
32. Telivuo, L., and Katz, R.L.: The effects of modern intravenous local analgetics on respiration during partial neuromuscular block in man. Anaesthesia, 25:30, 1970.
33. Usubiaga, J.E., et al.: Interaction of intravenously administered procaine, lidocaine, and succinylcholine in anesthetized subjects. Anesth. Analg. (Cleve.), 46:39, 1967.
34. Usubiaga, J.E., and Standaert, F.: The effects of local anesthetics on motor nerve terminals. J. Pharmacol. Exp. Ther., 159:353, 1968.
35. Steinback, A.B.: Alteration by xylocaine (lidocaine) and its derivatives on the time course of end plate potentials. J. Gen. Physiol., 52:144, 1968.
36. Kordas, M.: The effect of procaine on neuromuscular transmission. J. Physiol., 209:689, 1970.
37. Gesler, R.M., and Matsuba, M.: Neuromuscular blocking actions of local anesthetics. J. Pharmacol. Exp. Ther., 103:314, 1951.
38. Thorpe, W.R., and Seeman, P.: The site of action of caffeine and procaine in skeletal muscle. J. Pharmacol. Exp. Ther., 179:324, 1971.
39. Harrah, M.D., Way, W.L., and Katzung, B.G.: The interaction of d-tubocurarine with antiarrhythmic drugs. Anesthesiology, 33:406, 1970.
40. Grogono, A.W.: Anesthesia for atrial defibrillation. Effect of quinidine on muscle relaxation. Lancet, 2:1039, 1963.
41. Miller, R.D., Way, W.L., and Katzung, B.G.: The potentiation of neuromuscular blocking agents by quinidine. Anesthesiology, 28:1036, 1967.
42. Miller, R.D., Way, W.L., and Katzung, B.G.: The neuromuscular effects of quinidine. Proc. Soc. Exp. Biol. Med., 129:215, 1968.
43. Johnston, R.R., Miller, R.D., and Way, W.L.: The interaction of ketamine with neuromuscular blocking drugs. Anesth. Analg. (Cleve.), 53:496, 1974.
44. Cronnelly, R.: Interaction of ketamine HCl with neuromuscular agents. Fed. Proc., 31:535, 1972.
45. Del Castillo, J., and Engback, L.: The nature of the neuromuscular block produced by magnesium. J. Physiol., 124:370, 1954.
46. Giesecke, A.H., et al.: Of magnesium, muscle relaxants, toxemic parturients, and cats. Anesth. Analg. (Cleve.), 47:689, 1968.
47. Ghoneim, M.M., and Long, J.P.: The interaction between magnesium and other neuromuscular blocking agents. Anesthesiology, 32:23, 1970.
48. Borden, H., Clarke, M., and Katz, H.: The use of pancuronium bromide in patients receiving lithium carbonate. Can. Anaesth. Soc. J., 21:79, 1974.
49. Hill, G.E., Wong, K.C., and Hodges, M.R.: Potentiation of succinylcholine neuromuscular blockade by lithium carbonate. Anesthesiology, 44:439, 1976.
50. Walts, L.F., and Dillon, J.B.: Clinical studies of the interaction between d-tubocurarine and succinylcholine. Anesthesiology, 31:39, 1969.
51. Katz, R.L.: Modification of the action of pancuronium by succinylcholine and halothane. Anesthesiology, 35:602, 1971.
52. Ivankovich, A.D., et al.: Dual action of pancuronium on a succinylcholine block. Can. Anaesth. Soc. J., 24:228, 1977.
53. Miller, R.D.: The advantages of giving d-tubocurarine before succinylcholine. Anesthesiology, 37:569, 1972.
54. Miller, R.D., Way, W.L., and Hickey, R.L.: Inhibition of succinylcholine induced increased intraocular pressure by nondepolarizing muscle relaxants. Anesthesiology, 29:123, 1968.
55. Miller, R.D., and Way, W.L.: Inhibition of succinylcholine induced increased intragastric pressure by nondepolarizing muscle relaxants and lidocaine. Anesthesiology, 34:185, 1971.
56. Lamoreaux, L.F., and Urback, K.F.: Incidence and prevention of muscle pain following administration of succinylcholine. Anesthesiology, 21:394, 1960.
57. Birch, A.A.B., Mitchell, G.D., and Playford, G.A.: Changes in serum potassium response to succinylcholine following trauma. J.A.M.A., 210:490, 1969.

58. Miller, R.D., and Way, W.L.: The interaction between succinylcholine and subparalyzing doses of d-tubocurarine and gallamine in man. Anesthesiology, 35:567, 1971.
59. Cullen, D.J.: The effect of pretreatment with nondepolarizing muscle relaxants on the neuromuscular blocking action of succinylcholine. Anesthesiology, 35:572, 1971.
60. Dery, R.: The effects of precurarization with a protective dose of d-tubocurarine in the conscious patient. Can. Anaesth. Soc. J., 21:68, 1974.
60a. Miller, R.D., and Savarese, J.J.: Pharmacology of muscle relaxants, their antagonists, and monitoring of neuromuscular function. Anesthesia. Volume 1. Edited by Miller, R.D., New York, Churchill Livingstone, 1981, pp. 487–538.
60b. Miller, R.D., Eger, E.I. II, Way, W.L., et al.: Comparative neuromuscular effects of Forane and halothane alone and in combination with d-tubocurarine in man. Anesthesiology, 35:38, 1971.
60c. Rupp, S.M., Fahey, M.R., and Miller, R.D.: Neuromuscular and cardiovascular effects of atracurium during nitrous oxide-fentanyl and nitrous oxide-isoflurane anesthesia. Br. J. Anaesth., 55(Suppl.):67S, 1983.
60d. Duncalf, D., Nagashima, H., Hollinger, I., et al.: Relaxation with Org-NC45 during enflurane anesthesia. Anesthesiology. 55:A203, 1981.
60e. Rupp, S.M., Miller, R.D., and Gencarelli, P.J.: Vecuronium-induced neuromuscular blockade during enflurane, halothane and isoflurane in humans. Anesthesiology, 60:102, 1984.
60f. Foldes, F.F., Bencini, A., and Newton, D.: Influence of halothane and enflurane on the neuromuscular effects of Org NC 45 in man. Br. J. Anaesth., 52(Suppl 1):64S, 1980.
60g. Krieg, N., Rutten, J.M.J., Crul, J.F., et al.: Preliminary review of the interactions of Org NC 45 with anaesthetics and antibiotics in animals. Br. J. Anaesth., 52:33S, 1980.
60h. Foldes, F.F., Bencini, A., and Newton, D.: Influence of halothane and enflurane on the neuromuscular blocking effects of Org NC 45 in man. Br. J. Anaesth., 62:64S, 1980.
60i. Krieg, N., Crul, J.F., and Booij, L.H.D.J.: Relative potency of Org NC 45, pancuronium, alcuronium and tubocurarine in anaesthetized man. Br. J. Anaesth., 52:783, 1980.
60j. Stirt, J.A., Katz, R.L., Murray, A.L., et al.: Modification of atracurium blockade by halothane and by suxamethonium. A review of clinical experience. Br. J. Anaesth., 55(Suppl. 1):71S, 1983.
60k. Krieg, N., Hendricks, H.H.L., and Crul, J.F.: Influence of suxamethonium on the potency of Org NC 45 in anaesthetized patients. Br. J. Anaesth., 53:259, 1981.
60l. Walts, L.F., and Rusin, W.D.: The influence of succinylcholine on the duration of pancuronium neuromuscular blockade. Anesth. Analg., 56:22, 1977.
60m. Katz, R.L., Norman, J., Seed, R.F., et al.: A comparison of the effects of suxamethonium and tubocurarine in patients in London and New York. Br. J. Anaesth., 41:1041, 1969.
60n. d'Hollander, A.A., Agoston, S., De Ville, A., et al.: Clinical and pharmacological actions of a bolus injection of suxamethonium: Two phenomena of distinct duration. Br. J. Anaesth., 55:131, 1983.
60o. Fisher, D.M., and Miller, R.D.: Interaction of succinylcholine and vecuronium during N_2O-halothane anesthesia. Anesthesiology, 59:A278, 1983.
60p. Marshall, I.G., Agoston, S., Booij, L.H.D.J., et al.: Pharmacology of ORG NC 45 compared with other non-depolarizing neuromuscular blocking drugs. Br. J. Anaesth., 52:11S, 1980.
60q. Rutten, J.M., Booij, L.H., Rutten, C.L., et al.: The comparative neuromuscular blocking effects of some aminoglycoside antibiotics. Acta Anaesthesiol. Belg., 31:293, 1980.
60r. Basta, S.J., Ali, H.H., Savarese, J.J., et al.: Clinical pharmacology of atracurium besylate (BW 33A): A new nondepolarizing muscle relaxant. Anesth. Analg., 61:723, 1982.
60s. Fahey, M.R., Morris, R.B., Miller, R.D., et al.: Clinical pharmacology of ORG NC 45 (Norcuron™): A new nondepolarizing muscle relaxant. Anesthesiology, 55:6, 1981.
60t. Gencarelli, P.J., and Miller, R.D.: Antagonism of Org NC45 (vecuronium) and pancuronium neuromuscular blockade by neostigmine. Br. J. Anaesth., 54:53, 1982.
60u. Baird, W.L.M., Bowman, W.C., and Kerr, W.J.: Some actions of Org NC 45 and of edrophonium in the anaesthetized cat and in man. Br. J. Anaesth., 54:375, 1969.
60v. Katz, R.L., Stirt, J., Murray, A.L., et al.: Neuromuscular effects of atracurium in man. Anesth. Analg., 61:730, 1982.
60w. Durant, N.N., Houwertjes, and M.C., and Agoston, S.: Comparison of the neuromuscular blocking properties of Org NC 45 and pancuronium in the rat, cat and rhesus monkey. Br. J. Anaesth., 52:723, 1980.
60x. Marshall, I.G., Agoston, S., Booij, L.H.D.J., et al.: Pharmacology of ORG NC45 compared with other non-depolarizing neuromuscular blocking drugs. Br. J. Anaesth., 52:11S, 1980.
60y. Fahey, M.R., Morris, R.B., Miller, R.D., et al.: Clinical pharmacology of ORG 45 (Norcuron): A new nondepolarizing muscle relaxant. Anesthesiology, 55:6, 1981.
60z. Viby-Mogensen, J., Jørgensen, B.C., Engbaek, J., et al.: On Org NC 45 and halothane anaesthesia. Preliminary results. Br. J. Anaesth., 52:67S, 1980.
60aa. Krieg, N., Mazur, L., Booij, L.H.D.J., et al.: Intubation conditions and reversability of a new non-depolarizing neuromuscular blocking agent. Org-NC45. Acta. Anaesthesiol. Scand., 24:423, 1980.
60bb. Durant, N.N., and Marshall, I.G.: The effects of a 3,4-diaminopyridine on acetylcholine release at the frog neuromuscular junction. Eur. J. Pharmacol., 67:201, 1980. B31.
60cc. Molgo, J., Lemeignan, M., and Lechat, P.: Ef-

fects of 4-aminopyridine at the frog neuromuscular junction. J. Pharmacol. Exp. Ther., 203:653, 1977.
60dd. Durant, N.N., Lee, C., and Katz, R.L.: 4-Aminopyridine reversal of sympathetic ganglionic blockade in the anesthetized cat. Anesthesiology, 52:381, 1980.
60ee. Booij, L.H.D.J., Van der Pol, F., Crul, J.F., et al.: Antagonism of Org NC 45 neuromuscular block by neostigmine, pyridostigmine, and 4-aminopyridine. Anesth. Analg., 59:31. 1980.
60ff. Thesleff, S.: Aminopyridines and synaptic transmission. Neurosciences, 5:1413, 1980.
61. Baraka, A.: Suxamethonium-neostigmine interaction in patients with normal or atypical cholinesterase. Br. J. Anaesth., 49:479, 1977.
62. Nastuk, W.L., and Gissen, A.J.: Actions of acetylcholine and other quaternary ammonium compounds at the muscle postjunctional membrane. In Muscle. Edited by W.M. Paul and E.C. Daniel. Oxford, Pergamon Press, Ltd., 1967.
63. Miller, R.D., et al.: Comparative time to peak effect and duration of neostigmine and pyridostigmine. Anesthesiology, 41:27, 1974.
64. Churchill-Davidson, H.C., and Katz, R.L.: Dual, phase II, or desensitization block? Anesthesiology, 27:546, 1966.
65. Vickers, M.D.A.: The mismanagement of suxamethonium apnea. Br. J. Anaesth., 35:260, 1963, 1966.
66. Katz, R.L., and Katz, G.J.: Clinical use of muscle relaxants. In Advances in Anesthesiology: Muscle Relaxants. Edited by L.C. Clark and E.M. Papper. New York, Hoeber, 1967.
67. Gissen, A.J., Katz, R.L., and Karis, J.H.: Neuromuscular block in man during prolonged arterial infusion with succinylcholine. Anesthesiology, 27:242, 1966.
68. Pantuck, E.J., and Pantuck, C.B.: Cholinesterases and anticholinesterases. In Muscle Relaxants. Edited by R.L. Katz. Amsterdam, Excerpta Medica, North-Holland Publishing Co., 1975.
69. Zsigmond, E.K., and Robbins, G.: The effect of a series of anticancer drugs on plasma cholinesterase activity. Can. Anaesth. Soc. J., 19:75, 1972.
70. Wang, R.I.H., and Ross, C.A.: Prolonged apnea following succinylcholine in cancer patients receiving AB-132. Anesthesiology, 24:363, 1963.
71. Bennett, E.J., et al.: Muscle relaxants, myasthenia, and mustards? Anesthesiology, 46:220, 1977.
72. Goat, V.A., et al.: The effect of blood flow upon the activity of gallamine triethiodide. Br. J. Anaesth., 48:69, 1976.
73. Gergis, S.D., Sokoll, M.D., and Rubbo, J.T.: Effect of sodium nitroprusside and trimethaphan on neuromuscular transmission in the frog. Can. Anaesth. Soc. J., 24:220, 1977.
74. Wilson, S.L., et al.: Prolonged neuromuscular blockade associated with trimethaphan: a case report. Anesth. Analg. (Cleve.), 55:353, 1976.
75. Deacock, A.R., and Davis, T.D.W.: The influence of certain ganglionic blocking agents on neuromuscular transmission. Br. J. Anaesth., 30:217, 1958.
76. Sklar, G.S., and Lanks, K.W.: Effects of trimethaphan and sodium nitroprusside on hydrolysis of succinylcholine in vitro. Anesthesiology, 47:31, 1977.
77. Norman, N., and Lofstrom, B.: Interaction of d-tubocurarine, ether, cyclopropane, and thiopental on ganglionic transmission. J. Pharmacol. Exp. Ther., 114:231, 1955.
78. Westgate, H.D., and Van Bergen, F.H.: Changes in histamine blood levels following d-tubocurarine administration. Can. Anaesth. Soc. J., 9:497, 1962.
79. Stoelting, R.K., and Longnecker, D.E.: Influence of end-tidal halothane concentration on d-tubocurarine hypotension. Anesth. Analg. (Cleve.), 51:364, 1972.
80. Munger, W.L., Miller, R.D., and Stevens, W.C.: The dependence of d-tubocurarine hypotension on alveolar concentration of halothane, dose of d-tubocurarine, and nitrous oxide. Anesthesiology, 40:442, 1974.
81. Price, H.L., and Price, M.L.: Has halothane a predominant circulatory action? Anesthesiology, 27:764, 1966.
82. Miller, R.D., et al.: Pancuronium-induced tachycardia in relation to alveolar halothane, dose of pancuronium, and prior atropine. Anesthesiology, 42:352, 1975.
83. Saxena, P.R., and Bonta, I.L.: Specific blockade of cardiac muscarinic receptors by pancuronium bromide. Arch. Intern. Pharmacodyn., 189:410, 1971.
84. Seed, R.F., and Chamberlain, J.H.: Myocardial stimulation by pancuronium bromide. Br. J. Anaesth., 49:401, 1977.
85. Nana, S., Cardan, E., and Domokos, M.: Blood catecholamine changes after pancuronium. Acta Anaesthesiol. Scand., 17:83, 1973.
86. Domenech, J.S., et al.: Pancuronium bromide: an indirect sympathomimetic agent. Br. J. Anaesth., 48:1143, 1976.
87. Zsigmond, E., et al.: The effect of pancuronium bromide on plasma norepinephrine and cortisol concentrations during thiamylal induction. Can. Anaesth. Soc. J., 21:147, 1974.
88. Jones, R.E., Deutsch, S., and Turndorf, H.: Effects of atropine on cardiac rhythm in conscious and anesthetized man. Anesthesiology, 22:67, 1961.
89. Axelrod, J., Whitby, L.G., and Hertting, G.: Effect of psychotropic drugs on the uptake of H[3]-norepinephrine by tissues. Science, 133:383, 1961.
89a. Edwards, R., et al.: Unpublished data.
90. McLeod, K., Watson, M.J., and Rawlines, M.D.: Pharmacokinetics of pancuronium in patients with normal and impaired renal function. Br. J. Anaesth., 48:341, 1976.
91. Miller, R.D., and Roderick, L.: Acid-base and a pancuronium neuromuscular blockade and its antagonism by neostigmine. Br. J. Anaesth., 50:317, 1978.
92. Miller, R.D., et al.: The effect of acid-base bal-

ance on neostigmine antagonism of d-tubocurarine-induced neuromuscular blockade. Anesthesiology, 42:377, 1975.
93. Miller, R.D., and Roderick, L.: Diuretic-induced hypokalemia and a pancuronium neuromuscular blockade and its antagonism by neostigmine. Br. J. Anaesth., 50:541, 1978.
94. Miller, R.D., Van Nyhuis, L.S., and Eger, E.I., II: The effect of temperature on a d-tubocurarine neuromuscular blockade and its antagonism by neostigmine. J. Pharmacol. Exp. Ther., 195:237, 1975.
95. Miller, R.D., and Roderick, L.: Pancuronium-induced neuromuscular blockade and its antagonism by neostigmine at 29, 37, and 41°C. Anesthesiology, 46:333, 1977.
96. Ham, J., et al.: The effect of temperature on the pharmacodynamics and pharmacokinetics of d-tubocurarine. Anesthesiology, 49:324, 1978.
97. Miller, R.D., et al.: Hypothermia and the pharmacodynamics and pharmacokinetics of pancuronium in the cat. J. Pharmacol. Exp. Ther., 207:532, 1978.
98. Miller, R.D., Agoston, S., and Van der Pool, F.: Is the effect of metabolic alkalosis on a pancuronium neuromuscular blockade and its antagonism by neostigmine a pH effect? (In preparation).
99. Miller, R.D.: Reversal of neuromuscular blockade. Regional Refresher Courses in Anesthesiology, 5:134, 1977.
100. Savage, D.S., Sleigh, T., and Carlyle, I.: The emergence of Org NC 45, 1-[(2 beta, 3 alpha, 5 alpha, 16 beta, 17 beta-3, 17-bis(acetyloxy)-2-(1-piperidinyl)-androstan-16-yl]-1-methylpiperidinium bromide, from the pancuronium series. Br. J. Anaesth., 52(Suppl. 1):3S, 1980.
101. Stenlake, J.B., Waigh, R.D., Urwin, J., et al.: Atracurium: Conception and inception. Br. J. Anaesth., 55(Suppl. 1):3S, 1983.
102. Chapple, D.J., and Clark, J.S.: Pharmacological action of breakdown products of atracurium and related substances. Br. J. Anaesth., 55(Suppl. 1):11S, 1983.
103. Fahey, M.R., Morris, R.B., Miller, R.D., et al.: Clinical pharmacology of ORG NC45 (Norcuron™): A new nondepolarizing muscle relaxant. Anesthesiology, 55:6, 1981.
104. Agoston, S., Salt, P., Newton, D., et al.: The neuromuscular blocking action of Org NC 45, a new pancuronium derivative, in anaesthetized patients. A pilot study. Br. J. Anaesth., 52(Suppl. 1):53S, 1980.
105. Crul, J.F., and Booij, L.H.D.J.: First clinical experiences with Org NC 45. Br. J. Anaesth., 52(Suppl. 1):49S, 1980.
106. Baird, W.L.M., and Herd, D.: A new neuromuscular blocking drug, Org NC 45. A pilot study in man. Br. J. Anaesth., 52(Suppl. 1):61S, 1980.
107. Buzello, W., Bischoff, G., Kuhls, E., et al.: The new nondepolarizing muscle relaxant Org NC 45 in clinical anaesthesia: Preliminary results. Br. J. Anaesth., 52(Suppl.):62S, 1980.
108. Krieg, N., Crul, J.F., and Booij, L.H.D.J.: Relative potency of Org NC 45, pancuronium, alcuronium and tubocurarine in anaesthetized man. Br. J. Anaesth., 52:783, 1980.
109. Walts, L.F., Stirt, J.A., and Katz, R.L.: A comparison of neuromuscular blocking effects of Norcuron and pancuronium. Anesthesiology, 55:A210, 1981.
110. Gramstad, L., Lilleaasen, P., and Minsaas, B.: Comparative study of atracurium, vecuronium (Org NC 45) and pancuronium. Br. J. Anaesth., 55(Suppl. 1):95S, 1983.
111. Payne, J.P., and Hughes, R.: Evaluation of atracurium in anaesthetized man. Br. J. Anaesth., 53:45, 1981.
112. Basta, S.J., Ali, H.H., Savarese, J.J., et al.: Clinical pharmacology of atracurium besylate (BW 33A): A new nondepolarizing muscle relaxant. Anesth. Analg., 61:723, 1982.
113. Katz, R.L., Stirt, J., Murray, A.L., et al.: Neuromuscular effects of atracurium in man. Anesth. Analg., 61:730, 1982.
114. Savarese, J.J., Basta, S.J., Ali, H.H., et al.: Neuromuscular and cardiovascular effects of BW 33A (atracurium) in patients under halothane anesthesia. Anesthesiology, 57:A262, 1982.
115. Sokoll, M.D., Gergis, S.D., Mehta, M., et al.: Safety and efficacy of atracurium (BW33A) in surgical patients receiving balanced or isoflurane anesthesia. Anesthesiology, 58:450, 1983.
116. Ørding, H., Viby Mogensen, J.: Dose-response curves for OR NC 45 and pancuronium. Acta Anaesthesiol. Scand., 25(Suppl. 1):73, 1981.
117. Swen, J.: Org NC 45: Initial experiences. Br. J. Anaesth., 52(Suppl. 1):66S, 1980.
118. Viby-Mogensen, J., Jørgensen, B.C., Engback, J., et al.: On Org NC 45 and halothane anaesthesia. Preliminary results. Br. J. Anaesth., 52(Suppl. 1):67S, 1980.
119. Duncalf, D., Nagashima, H., Hollinger, I., et al.: Relaxation with Org-NC45 during enflurane anesthesia. Anesthesiology, 55:A203, 1981.
120. Fragen, R.J., Robertson, E.N., Booij, L.H.D.J., et al.: A comparison of vecuronium and atracurium in man. Anesthesiology, 57:A253, 1982.
121. Rupp, S.M., Miller, R.D., and Gencarelli, P.J.: Vecuronium-induced neuromuscular blockade during enflurane, halothane and isoflurane in humans. Anesthesiology, 60:102, 1984.
122. Nguyen, H.D., Nagashima, H., Kaplan, R., et al.: Relaxation with BW33A under neurolept and enflurane anesthesia. Anesthesiology, 57:A277, 1982.
123. Ramsey, F.M., White, P.A., Stullken, E.H., et al.: Enflurane potentiation of neuromuscular blockade by atracurium. Anesthesiology, 57:A255, 1982.
124. Foldes, F.F., Nagashima, H., Boros, M., et al.: Muscular relaxation with atracurium, vecuronium and Duador under balanced anaesthesia. Br. J. Anaesth., 55(Suppl. 1):97S, 1983.
125. Scott, R.P.F., and Goat, V.A.: Atracurium: Its speed of onset. A comparison with suxamethonium. Br. J. Anaesth., 54:909, 1982.
126. Bencini, A., Agoston, S., and Ket, J.: Use of the human "isolated arm" preparation to indicate

qualitative aspects of a new neuromuscular blocking agent, Org NC 45. Br. J. Anaesth., 52(Suppl. 1):43S, 1980.
127. Ali, H.H., Savarese, J.J., Basta, S.J., et al.: Evaluation of cumulative properties of three new non-depolarizing neuromuscular blocking drugs BW A444U, atracurium and vecuronium. Br. J. Anaesth., 55(Suppl. 1):107S, 1983.
128. Upton, R.A., Nguyen, T-L., Miller, R.D., et al.: Renal and biliary elimination of vecuronium (ORG NC 45) and pancuronium in rats. Anesth. Analg., 61:313, 1982.
129. Sohn, Y.J., Bencini, A., Scaf, A.H.J., et al.: Pharmacokinetics of vecuronium in man. Anesthesiology, 57:A256, 1982.
130. Fahey, M.R., Morris, R.B., Miller, R.D., et al.: Pharmacokinetics of Org NC 45 (Norcuron) in patients with and without renal failure. Br. J. Anaesth., 53:1049, 1981.
131. Fahey, M.R., Rupp, S.M., Fisher, D.M., et al.: The pharmacokinetics and pharmacodynamics of atracurium in patients with and without renal failure. Anesthesiology. 59:A263, 1983.
132. Ward, S., Neill, E.A.M., Weatherley, B.C., et al.: Pharmacokinetics of atracurium besylate in healthy patients (after a single i.v.) bolus dose. Br. J. Anaesth., 55(Suppl. 1):113, 1983.
133. d'Hollander, A., Massaux, F., Nevelsteen, M., et al.: Age-dependent dose-response relationship of Org NC 45 in anaesthetized patients. Br. J. Anaesth., 54:653, 1982.
134. d'Hollander, A.A., Nevelsteen, M., Barvais, L., et al.: Effect of age on the establishment of muscle paralysis induced in anaesthetized adult subjects by ORG NC45. Acta Anaesthesiol. Scand., 27:108, 1983.
135. d'Hollander, A.A., Luyckx, C., Barvais, L., et al.: Clinical evaluation of atracurium besylate requirement for a stable muscle relaxation during surgery: Lack of age-related effects. Anesthesiology, 59:237, 1983.
136. Booij, L.H.D.J., Edwards, R.P., Sohn, Y.J., et al.: Cardiovascular and neuromuscular effects of Org NC 45, pancuronium, metocurine, and d-tubocurarine in dogs. Anesth. Analg., 59:26, 1980.
137. Marshall, R.J., McGrath, J.C., Miller, R.D., et al.: Comparison of the cardiovascular actions of Org NC 45 with those produced by other non-depolarizing neuromuscular blocking agents in experimental animals. Br. J. Anaesth., 52(Suppl. 1):21S, 1980.
138. Basta, S.J., Savarese, J.J., Ali, H.H., et al.: Histamine-releasing potencies of atracurium besylate (BW 33A), metocurine, and D-tubocurarine. Anesthesiology, 57:A261, 1982.
139. Rupp, S.M., Fahey, M.R., and Miller, R.D.: Neuromuscular and cardiovascular effects of atracurium during nitrous oxide-gentanyl and nitrous oxide-isoflurane anaesthesia. Br. J. Anaesth., 55(Suppl. 1):67S, 1983.
140. Hilgenberg, J.C., Stoelting, R.K., and Harris, W.A.: Haemodynamic effects of atracurium during enflurane-nitrous oxide anaesthesia. Br. J. Anaesth., 55(Suppl. 1):81S, 1983.
141. Brandom, B.W., Woelfel, S.K., Cook, D.R., et al.: Clinical pharmacology of atracurium in infants. Anesth. Analg., (In press).
142. Goudsouzian, N.G., Liu, L.M.P., Cote, C.J., et al.: Safety and efficacy of atracurium in adolescents and children anesthetized with halothane. Anesthesiology, 59:459, 1983.
143. Baraka, A., Noueihed, R., Sinno, H., et al.: Succinylcholine-vecuronium (Org NC 45) sequency for cesarean section. Anesth. Analg., 62:909, 1983.
144. Dailey, P.A., Fisher, D.M., Shnider, S.M., et al.: Pharmacokinetics, placental transfer, and neonatal effects of vecuronium and pancuronium administered during cesarean section. Anesthesiology, 60:569, 1984.
145. Demetriou, M., Depoix, J-P., Diakite, B., et al.: Placental transfer of Org NC 45 in women undergoing cesarean section. Br. J. Anaesth., 54:643, 1982.
146. Frank, M., Flynn, P.J., and Hughes, R.: Atracurium in obstetric anaesthesia. A preliminary report. Br. J. Anaesth., 55(Suppl. 1):113S, 1983.
147. Hunter, J.M., Jones, R.S., and Utting, J.E.: Use of atracurium in patients with no renal function. Br. J. Anaesth., 54:1251, 1982.
148. Ward, S., and Neill, E.A.M.: Pharmacokinetics of atracurium in acute hepatic failure (with acute renal failure). Br. J. Anaesth., 55:1169, 1983.
149. Miller, R.D., Rupp, S.M., Fisher, D.M., et al.: Clinical pharmacology of vecuronium and atracurium. Anesthesiology, 61:444, 1984.

25

LOCAL ANESTHETICS

EDWIN S. MUNSON

A drug interaction occurs when the effects of one drug are modified by the prior or concurrent administration of another drug. Interactions arising from the administration of local anesthetic drugs may result from alterations in absorption, distribution, or elimination of one drug by another or from the combination of their actions on various organ systems. The mechanism of drug allergies, adverse reactions, and the problems arising from physical and chemical incompatibility, as well as the effects of excipients and preservatives, is beyond the scope of this chapter.

ABSORPTION

CASE REPORT

A healthy 36-year-old woman was admitted to the hospital for repair of a severely deviated nasal septum. Preoperatively she received meperidine 100 mg, pentobarbital 100 mg, and atropine 0.4 mg, intramuscularly. Anesthesia was induced with thiopental, 250 mg, and maintained with nitrous oxide, 60%, and halothane, 1%. Cocaine flakes, 100 mg, and 1 ml of 1:1,000 epinephrine (1,000 µg) were mixed and placed on three cotton pledgets, which were inserted into the nasal cavity for 3 minutes and were subsequently removed. During the 3 minutes, 20 ml of a 2% lidocaine solution, which contained 0.5 ml of 1:1,000 epinephrine (500 µg), was prepared; 3 ml of this solution was injected into the dorsum of the nose and infraorbital areas. When the skin incision was made, the blood was noted to be dark; after a few minutes the anesthetist reported an irregular pulse and hypotension. Cardiac asystole occurred and resuscitative efforts were unsuccessful.

This case report illustrates the risk of using large doses (>1,000 µg) of epinephrine in association with cocaine and an inhalation anesthetic agent that may induce such cardiac dysrhythmias. It is well known that cocaine and epinephrine associated with some inhalation anesthetic agents (particularly halothane and cyclopropane) can precipitate serious and life-threatening dysrhythmias.

Cocaine

If cocaine 10% is applied to the nasal mucosa in humans, absorption may be delayed because of concomitant vasoconstriction. Van Dyke et al. found that, although plasma levels of cocaine reached a peak (0.12 to 0.47 µg/ml) from 15 to 60 minutes after administration, the drug persisted in the plasma for 4 to 6 hours.[1] Since residual cocaine was detectable on the nasal mucosa for as long as 3 hours, absorption probably continued, resulting in persistent plasma levels. Also, plasma cocaine levels rise higher and last longer in dental patients with cardiovascular disease. The possibility of potentiating sympathomimetic amines administered during the course of anesthesia and surgical procedure should be anticipated. In addition, drugs such as cocaine that interfere with intraneural uptake of catecholamines can promote epinephrine-induced dysrhythmias during halothane anesthesia.[2]

391

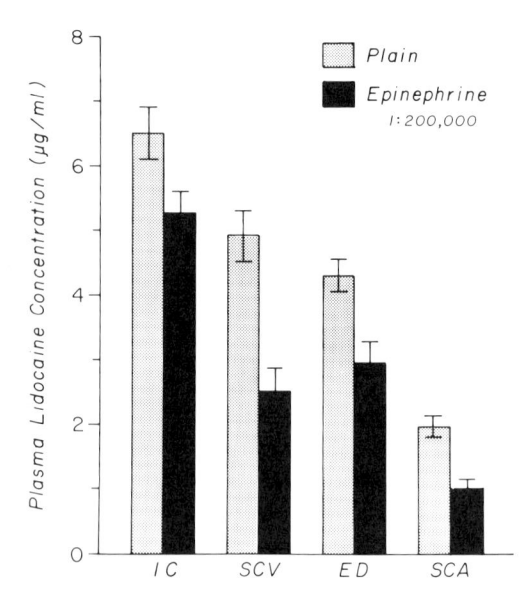

Fig. 25–1. Mean (± SE) maximum plasma concentrations following the injection of 400 mg lidocaine for intercostal (IC), subcutaneous vaginal (SCV), epidural (ED), and subcutaneous abdominal (SCA) block. The addition of epinephrine significantly ($P<0.01$) reduced lidocaine plasma levels in each instance. (Redrawn from Scott, D.B., et al.: Factors affecting plasma levels of lignocaine and prilocaine. Br. J. Anaesth. 44:1040, 1972.)

Epinephrine

The addition of epinephrine to local anesthetic solutions reduces plasma concentrations of local anesthetic, prolongs the block, and has little, if any, effect on the time of onset of analgesia. Scott et al. showed that the addition of 1:200,000 epinephrine to a 2% lidocaine solution lowered plasma levels when 400 mg of lidocaine was injected for various block procedures (Fig. 25–1).[3]

Whenever solutions containing epinephrine are administered in the presence of an inhalation anesthetic agent, the potential for dysrhythmias increases. The halothane-epinephrine interaction is well known (see Chap. 7, "Sympathomimetic Drugs"). The addition of a 0.5% lidocaine solution makes the use of epinephrine safer during halothane and enflurane anesthesia[4] (see "Inhalation Anesthetic Agents" section of this Chapter).

Sodium bisulfite, a reducing agent, is added to local anesthetic-epinephrine solutions by the manufacturer. Although oxidative decomposition of epinephrine is prevented, sodium bisulfite is strongly acidic and increases buffer demands in tissue.[5] Clinically, a greater initial concentration of local anesthetic is required to attain the same effect when a stabilizer has been added. When epinephrine is administered, ampules of local anesthetic-epinephrine solutions containing a single dose and no chemical stabilizers or freshly prepared epinephrine solutions should be employed.

Carbon Dioxide

Bromage et al. have shown that carbonated solutions of lidocaine and prilocaine (rather than the hydrochloride salts) increase the depth and shorten the onset of the block by some 20 to 40%.[6] The investigators suggest that the addition of carbon dioxide, a fast membrane penetrator and acidifying agent, improves the distribution of the anesthetic drug in the various components of nerve tissue. Carbon dioxide more readily converts the local anesthetic amide to the more active ammonium ion by lowering the pH *inside* the membrane. This effect of carbon dioxide is opposite to tissue acidosis, such as occurs from tissue infection or from the injection of sodium bisulfite, both of which increase *extramural* buffer demands.

Dextran

Adding low-molecular-weight dextran 40 to local anesthetic solutions prolongs the effectiveness of the anesthetic agent by decreasing its rate of absorption.[7–9] This technique offers particular advantage during intercostal nerve block for prolonged and postoperative analgesia. Kaplan et al. showed that the duration of nerve block with bupivacaine, 0.75%, and dextran 40 was 36 hours, as compared with 12 hours produced by bupivacaine and saline solutions in combination.[9]

DISTRIBUTION

CASE REPORT

A 27-year-old, 60-kg man with chronic glomerular nephritis and congestive heart failure was hospitalized for repair of an arteriovenous shunt previously established to facilitate long-term hemodialysis. A nerve block of the left brachial plexus was attempted by the axillary approach using 30 ml of lidocaine 1.5%, with 1:200,000 epinephrine. Since satisfactory anesthesia was not obtained, additional lidocaine was injected into the axillary space, which raised the initial dosage of 450 mg to a total of 1,400 mg within 1 hour. The patient developed twitching of the face and extremities, and oxygen was administered immediately by face mask. Seizure activity promptly subsided, but the patient remained drowsy and unresponsive. There were no appreciable changes in any of the vital signs during this episode. Small amounts of procaine were then administered locally for placement of a new shunt in the same arm. The patient's recovery was uneventful.[10]

This report describes the adverse reaction to an overdose of lidocaine in a patient whose cardiac and renal functions were compromised. A decrease in the volume of drug distribution and renal clearance as well as an excessive dose of the anesthetic may have contributed to the reaction.

Cardiac Failure

Lidocaine metabolism is decreased in patients with cardiac failure and cardiogenic shock after myocardial infarction.[11,12] In heart failure, both the volume of distribution and the plasma clearance of lidocaine are reduced. The plasma concentration of lidocaine during intravenous infusion is higher in patients with cardiac failure; the terminal plasma half-life may be prolonged as much as three- to sixfold. The administration of an amide-type local anesthetic for regional block procedures in these patients can produce potentially toxic levels of local anesthetics in the plasma, particularly if, in addition, lidocaine has been administered to control cardiac dysrhythmias. In patients with cardiovascular disease, levels of cocaine in the plasma after intranasal application are also higher, and their duration is more prolonged, than are cocaine levels in healthy dental patients.[1]

Hemorrhage

Lidocaine plasma levels are higher in animals during hemorrhage than in normovolemic animals.[13] An increased blood level reflects a decrease in both rate of clearance and volume of distribution. The elevated blood concentrations are similar to those observed in patients with congestive heart failure.

Vasopressors

The administration of sympathomimetic drugs during lidocaine infusion may influence lidocaine blood concentrations. Isoproterenol increases hepatic blood flow, while norepinephrine decreases it.[13] Steady-state lidocaine blood levels are directly related to changes in hepatic blood flow (Fig. 25–2). Alterations in the clearance of local anesthetic relate to change in hepatic blood flow rather than to an altered extraction ratio. Decreased lidocaine clearance after the administration of propranolol also has been described by Branch et al. in dogs.[14] Clinically, the administration of norepinephrine might induce lidocaine toxicity in patients with previously stable levels of local anesthetic drugs in plasma.

The use of vasopressor drugs for the treatment of arterial hypotension also may increase the toxicity of local anesthetics. Mather et al. found that, whereas intravenous ephedrine relieved cardiovascular depression after epidural block, lidocaine levels in plasma were elevated.[15] This increased systemic absorption from the epidural site would also curtail cardiovascular depression.

Protein Binding

Tucker and colleagues have described the following ranking of local anesthetics according to their ability to bind with plasma proteins: bupivacaine > mepivacaine > lidocaine.[16] This order correlates well with the blocking action (potency) of these drugs. Since the binding of drugs to plasma proteins is reversible and nonspe-

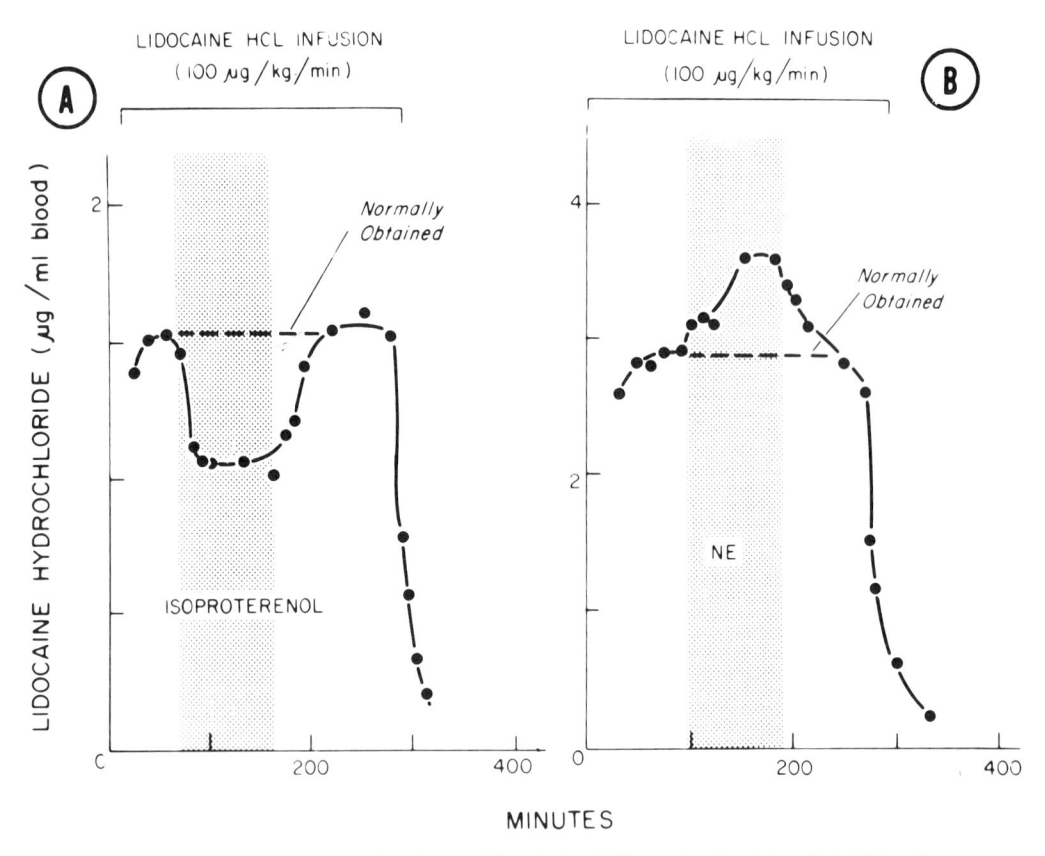

Fig. 25-2. The effects of isoproterenol and norephinephrine (NE) on steady-state arterial lidocaine concentrations in the rhesus monkey. The vasopressors were administered over the time period shown by the shaded area. Dashed lines indicate the lidocaine plasma levels normally obtained in the absence of vasopressors. (From Benowitz, N., et al.: Lidocaine disposition kinetics in monkey and man. II. Effects of hemorrhage and sympathomimetic drug administration. Clin. Pharmacol. Ther., 16:99, 1974.)

cific, drugs can compete with one another for binding sites (see "Pulmonary Extraction" section of this Chapter). Also, since protein binding influences drug distribution and elimination, changes in binding, either as the result of physiologic changes or from other drugs, may modify the action and duration of local anesthetics. For example, the addition of phenytoin (diphenylhydantoin), quinidine, meperidine, or desipramine to normal human plasma displaces bupivacaine.[17] If this effect occurs *in vivo*, patients receiving these drugs may have a four- to sixfold increase in unbound or active bupivacaine. Although drug interactions of this type have not been reported clinically, the possibility of increased toxicity of local anesthetics exists.

Feely et al. have reported that cimetidine increases toxicity and decreases clearance of lidocaine.[17A] Acute intravenous infusion of lidocaine, 1 mg/kg, in subjects receiving concomitant cimetidine, 300 mg 4 times daily, resulted in early signs and symptoms of lidocaine toxicity. Cimetidine pretreatment increased lidocaine plasma concentration and significantly decreased systemic clearance, volume at steady-state, and plasma protein binding. When administered acutely to patients receiving cimetidine, lidocaine should be infused slowly or given in repeated small doses.

Changes in the concentration of hydrogen ion may also alter the binding of local anesthetics to plasma proteins.[18] Lidocaine protein binding is decreased when plasma pH is decreased from 7.6 to 7.0, which suggests that a greater concentration of drug is available (active) in the presence of acidosis. Since acidosis usually accompanies central nervous system (CNS) and cardiovascular depressions, metabolic or respiratory acidosis should be corrected to lessen toxicity and to interrupt this self-perpetuating effect (see "Hydrogen Ion" section of this Chapter).

ELIMINATION

CASE REPORT

A 22-year-old woman was scheduled for dental extractions. A few minutes after the injection of procaine, she became weak and felt nauseated and dyspneic; she subsequently became cyanotic and lost consciousness. The patient was resuscitated successfully by ventilation with oxygen and by the administration of vasopressors. Seven years later, the same patient manifested prolonged apnea after the administration of succinylcholine. Subsequent examinations showed that she was an atypical homozygote with a dibucaine number of 18 and thus had reduced hydrolysis rates for benzylcholine and procaine. The family history revealed that the patient's sister had experienced cardiovascular collapse after the administration of 320 mg of procaine for pudendal nerve block anesthesia. Subsequent testing showed that her plasma cholinesterase activity and dibucaine number were also abnormally low.[19]

The occurrence of concomitant CNS and neuromuscular toxicity in the same patient is unusual. However, since ester-type local anesthetics and succinylcholine are each hydrolyzed by plasma pseudocholinesterase, a competitive phenomenon occurs whenever these drugs are administered together. Prolonged apnea after the use of succinylcholine should alert the clinician to the possibility of atypical plasma cholinesterase. Hence large amounts of ester-type local anesthetics may result in severe systemic toxicity in such patients. Many other drugs and diseases may also modify the elimination of local anesthetics.

Enzymatic Hydrolysis

Anticholinergic Drugs. Neostigmine and pyridostigmine are frequently used to reverse the neuromuscular blockade produced by nondepolarizing muscle relaxants. In addition to inhibiting acetylcholinesterase, neostigmine and pyridostigmine inhibit plasma cholinesterase.[20] The depression of plasma cholinesterase activity may last as long as two hours after the administration of pyridostigmine (Fig. 25–3). Patients who receive neostigmine or pyridostigmine should be given succinylcholine and ester-type local anesthetic agents in reduced amounts. In contrast, recent studies in rabbits show that a spinal block with tetracaine can be reversed by injecting cholinesterase into the subarachnoid space.[20a]

Echothiophate Iodide. Patients with glaucoma frequently are treated with echothiophate iodide eye drops. This organophosphorus compound is a long-acting inhibitor of both acetylcholinesterase and pseudocholinesterase. Although reported drug interactions involve increased neuromuscular blockade after the administration of succinylcholine, a potential inter-

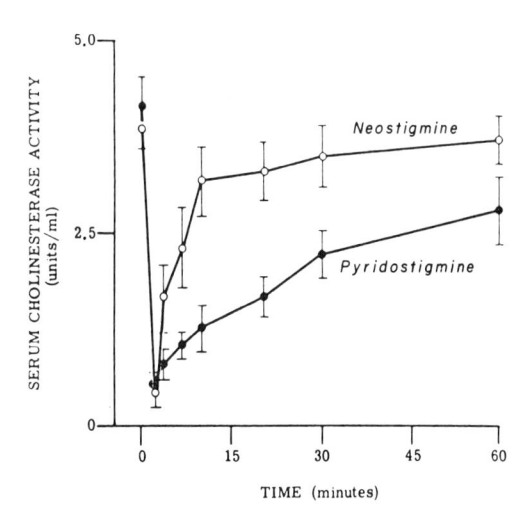

Fig. 25–3. Mean ($\pm$ SE) serum cholinesterase activity values were significantly ($P < 0.05$) reduced for five minutes after administration of neostigmine and for at least 120 minutes after pyridostigmine. (From Stoelting, R.K.: Serum cholinesterase activity following pancuronium and antagonism with neostigmine or pyridostigmine. Anesthesiology, 45:674, 1976.)

action with ester-type local anesthetics exists.[21]

Lanks and Sklar reported pseudocholinesterase levels that were 35 to 52% of normal in a group of patients receiving echothiophate iodide (phospholine) for treatment of glaucoma.[21a] With respect to a patient who showed normal response to chloroprocaine with a pseudocholinesterase level 43% of normal,[21b] these authors suggest that enzymatic activity would have to decrease to less than 15% of normal before the threshold to toxicity would decrease. Subsequently, a prolonged epidural block with chloroprocaine was described in a postpartum patient with abnormal pseudocholinesterase and an enzyme activity equivalent to 18.5% of normal for nonpregnant patients.[21c] Similar considerations should be given when patients are subjected to related alkylphosphate compounds, such as diisopropyl fluorophosphate (DFP). These compounds are still used in many insecticides.

Glucocorticoids. Foldes et al. reported that butylcholinesterase activity in plasma decreases about 50% in patients who receive large doses of prednisone.[22] Subsequent studies with dogs showed that both methylprednisolone and dexamethasone decrease cholinesterase activity (pseudocholinesterase) in plasma. The cholinesterase enzyme is responsible for the hydrolysis of both succinylcholine and the ester-type local anesthetics such as procaine and tetracaine. A decrease in cholinesterase by glucocorticoids, probably caused by inhibition of hepatic protein synthesis, also is expected to increase the systemic toxicity of procaine-related drugs.

Chemotherapeutic Drugs. Cholinesterase activity may be lower in patients suffering from certain types of cancer than in healthy persons.[23] In addition, prolonged apnea resulting from the use of succinylcholine in two patients receiving an antitumor drug was described by Wang and Ross.[24] The cancer chemotherapeutic agent, AB-132, that is, ethyl-N-(bis [2-2-diethylenimido]phosphoro) carbamate, has been shown to inhibit both plasma and erythrocyte cholinesterases. The warning that succinylcholine should be administered with caution to patients who receive this chemotherapeutic agent also applies to the ester-type local anesthetics. A similar drug interaction should be expected between hydrolyzable local anesthetics administered in the presence of other chemotherapeutic agents that inhibit cholinesterase activity in plasma.

Pregnancy. Cholinesterase activity in plasma decreases during pregnancy and the immediate postpartum period. Most reports of prolonged apnea during cesarean section have been attributed to a reduced rate of enzymatic hydrolysis. However, Blitt et al. found that cholinesterase activity in the plasma and the duration of paralysis from succinylcholine do not correlate.[25] Finster demonstrated that the rate of hydrolysis of chloroprocaine in parturient patients did not differ from that in either men or nonpregnant women.[26] The sensitivity of infants to ester local anesthetics may be increased, however, since Reidenberg has shown that newborn infants hydrolyze procaine much more slowly than do healthy adults.[27]

Enzyme Induction

Drugs that induce hepatic microsomal enzyme systems (for example, phenobarbital) may alter the rate of metabolism of amide local anesthetics and may increase the rate at which metabolites of lidocaine are formed. Pretreating dogs with phenobarbital increases the hepatic clearance of lidocaine from 25 to 50% (Fig. 25–4).[28] Plasma lidocaine levels in seven epileptic patients treated with phenobarbital were also lower than those in control subjects receiving the same intravenous dose of lidocaine (Fig. 25–5).[29] Although four of the seven patients had taken regular doses of some barbiturate for periods ranging from one to four years, almost all of them had also received phenytoin, as well as other

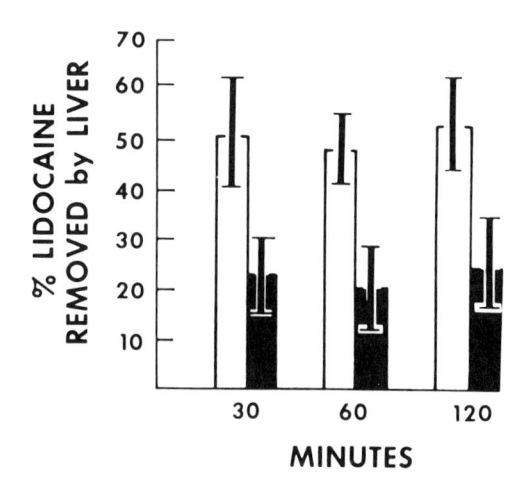

Fig. 25–4. Mean (± SD) hepatic extraction fractions of lidocaine in dogs pretreated with phenobarbital (open bars) were significantly greater than those in control animals (closed bars). (From DiFazio, C.A., and Brown, R.E.: Lidocaine metabolism in normal and phenobarbital-pretreated dogs. Anesthesiology, 36:238, 1972.)

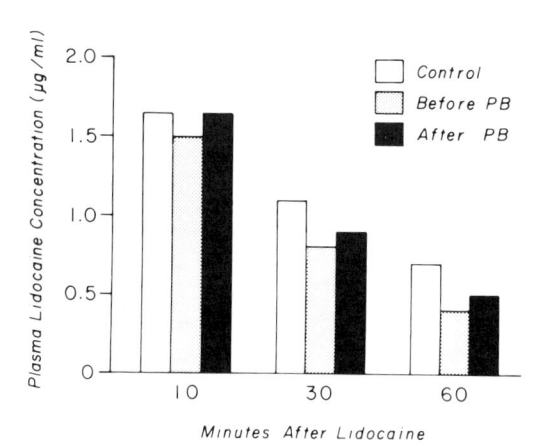

Fig. 25–5. Mean venous plasma lidocaine levels in untreated control subjects (open bars) before and after administration of phenobarbital (PB). Lidocaine plasma levels in both epileptic groups were significantly (P < 0.01) lower than in control subjects at 30 and 60 minutes. However, the addition of phenobarbital to other anticonvulsant medications taken before the experiment did not increase enzyme induction or lower lidocaine levels in the blood.[29]

drugs known to have enzyme-inducing properties. Patients who receive agents that induce drug-metabolizing enzymes may have a high tolerance to the systemic effects of repeated doses of lidocaine. However, this may not be apparent in patients with chronic liver disease because of their inability to respond to microsomal enzyme-inducing drugs.[30]

Hepatic Elimination

Liver Disease. Clearance of lidocaine from plasma is slow in patients with liver disease.[11,30] Central nervous system toxicity developed in a patient with liver disease after being given lidocaine at a rate usually well tolerated by patients with healthy livers.[31] Forrest et al. reported that lidocaine elimination is delayed in patients with chronic liver disease.[30] The mean (± SE) half-life of orally administered lidocaine in 19 of 21 patients with liver disease was 6.6 ± 1.1 hours, as compared with 1.4 ± 0.3 hours in healthy subjects.[30] Since lidocaine and other amide-type local anesthetics are eliminated primarily by hepatic metabolism, removal from plasma depends on blood flow through the liver. Impaired lidocaine elimination in patients with liver disease results from decreased hepatic blood flow secondary to cirrhosis and increased portosystemic shunting.[32]

The plasma half-lives of lidocaine, antipyrine, and paracetamol showed that significant correlations are related to serum albumin concentration. Of the three drugs studied, the prolonged half-life of lidocaine was the most sensitive indicator of hepatic dysfunction. In these patients who are known to have taken drugs that can cause microsomal enzyme induction, drug half-lives did not differ significantly from those in other patients with a similar degree of hepatic disease, as judged by routine liver function tests.[30] The severity of hepatic dysfunction should be taken into account when one considers lidocaine dosage for patients with chronic liver disease.

General Anesthesia. Decreased hepatic

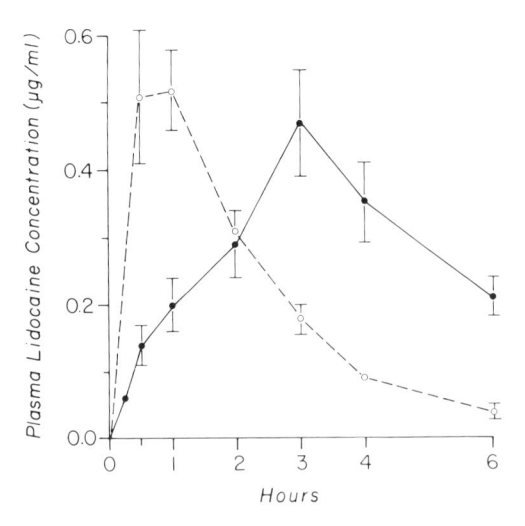

Fig. 25–6. Mean (± SE) plasma lidocaine concentration in seven awake subjects (open circles) and 12 anesthetized patients (closed circles) after ingestion of lidocaine, 400 mg. Note the marked delay in the rise of plasma lidocaine concentrations in the anesthetized patients, which indicates delayed absorption. The decreased rate of drug elimination from the plasma suggests impaired drug metabolism during anesthesia.[34]

removal of local anesthetics should be anticipated when patients are anesthetized with potent inhalation agents. The hepatic elimination of lidocaine in animals anesthetized with halothane was slower than in animals receiving nitrous oxide and curare.[28,33] Reduced elimination may be related to decreased hepatic blood flow and to depressed hepatic microsomes induced by halothane. Clinical studies in awake volunteers and patients anesthetized with a combination of nitrous oxide and gallamine, with or without halothane, have shown that general anesthesia delays the rise of lidocaine concentration in the plasma after oral administration of the drug.[34] This delay in absorption is accompanied by a delayed elimination of lidocaine from the plasma, which suggests that the metabolism of lidocaine is retarded during halothane anesthesia (Fig. 25–6).

Propranolol. The administration of propranolol to animals anesthetized with morphine and chloralose prolongs lidocaine plasma half-life by about 50% as compared with patients who have not had these drugs.[14] *Beta*-adrenergic blockade, in addition to decreasing both cardiac output and hepatic blood flow, reduces lidocaine clearance with little alteration in the rate of hepatic lidocaine extraction. This interaction results in higher plasma lidocaine levels than would be expected in patients not exposed to *beta*-adrenergic blocking drugs.

Pulmonary Extraction

The lung has been shown to function as a significant reservoir for lidocaine, mepivacaine, and bupivacaine.[34a] These lipophilic basic amines passively diffuse into pulmonary tissue from the pulmonary circulation, bind to saturation sites, and return unchanged to the circulating vascular compartment at a slow rate. It is reasonable to anticipate that patients treated with propranolol and having received amide local anesthetics may be more susceptible than normal to toxicity from altered pharmacokinetics. Jorfeldt et al. calculated that the peak arterial concentrations of lidocaine would have been three times higher had the pulmonary uptake of lidocaine not occurred.[34a] In this way, the lung serves as a capacitor to dampen the effect on the arterial concentration should a large dose of local anesthetic accidentally be injected intravenously. Rothstein and Pitt reported that the pulmonary extraction of bupivacaine was impeded both by the local anesthetic itself and by propranolol.[34b] Presumably, these drugs compete for common receptor sites.

Renal Excretion

The kidney is the major route of elimination of local anesthetic drugs and their metabolites. The ester-type drugs are hydrolyzed by plasma pseudocholinesterase, but the primary metabolite of procaine, para-aminobenzoic acid, is excreted by the kidney. Amide-type drugs, which have a small capacity for protein binding, such as prilocaine, demonstrate greater rates of renal clearance.[35] Renal clearance is inversely related to urine pH; hence any clinical situation that promotes renal acidification enhances the elimination of local anesthetics. Patients with impaired renal function hydrolyze procaine more slowly than do healthy adults.[27] Although the degree to which procaine hydrolysis slows in patients with renal disease is proportional to blood urea nitrogen levels, the mechanism is related to decreased levels of enzyme activity rather than to competitive enzyme inhibition. Ester local anesthetics should be administered in low dosage to patients who have kidney disease.

PHARMACOLOGIC INTERACTIONS

CASE REPORT

An 8-year-old boy weighing 25 kg was admitted to the hospital for an intravenous pyelogram and a renal biopsy. He received meperidine 50 mg, and pentobarbital 50 mg, intramuscularly 60 minutes before the placement of a catheter in a peripheral vein. Inadvertently, instead of radiopaque dye, mepivacaine, 300 mg (without epinephrine), was administered rapidly. Generalized seizures developed immediately and were terminated quickly by the administration of oxygen by mask and of intravenous diazepam 10 mg. Ventilation was supported, and one hour later the child was alert and conversing normally. Two days later diagnostic studies were performed without incident; the patient was discharged from the hospital the next day.[36]

This report of gross mepivacaine overdosage (12 mg/kg) in a child illustrates several points: (1) commonly used premedicant drugs offer little, if any, protection against CNS toxicity; (2) diazepam is a rapidly acting anticonvulsant agent that has minimal effects on circulation and ventilation; and (3) recovery from the administration of a single large dose of a local anesthetic is rapid, provided proper attention is given to the maintenance of the patient's ventilation and circulation.

The brain, the heart, and the neuromuscular system are particularly sensitive to the action of local anesthetics, which generally depress excitable membranes. Therefore, the use of other depressant drugs in clinical practice may result in significant drug interactions.

Anticonvulsant Drugs

Barbiturates have long been used to prevent and control local anesthetic toxicity. These agents enhance local anesthetic toxicity in mice and in dogs.[37,37a] When used before lidocaine-induced seizures, pentobarbital was detrimental, even when ventilation was supported.[37a] This suggests that a lidocaine-pentobarbital combination significantly depresses the cardiovascular system. Clinically, signs of central stimulation, behavioral changes, and seizures usually precede the circulatory depression that accompanies local anesthetic toxicity. Using drugs that suppress warning signs of impending toxicity deprives the clinician of valuable monitoring information.

In contrast to the barbiturates, pretreatment with the benzodiazepine derivative, diazepam, shows specific antagonism through its action on the limbic system of the brain. Clinically, compared with barbiturates, local anesthetic overdosage treated with diazepam appears to have less residual depression, and therefore, recovery is quicker. Pretreatment of animals with diazepam increases both the seizure dosage and the plasma concentration of lidocaine at which seizures occur.[38,39] Although diazepam elevates seizure threshold, it may also mask the signs of impending toxicity. When seizures develop in animals pretreated with diazepam, larger doses of the anticonvulsant drug are required to control seizures than are necessary when diazepam premedication is not given. Diazepam is recommended to control seizure activity, but seizures induced by the administration of local anesthetics can be treated effectively by other intravenous, as well as inhalation, anesthetic agents. Epileptic patients receiving long-term therapy with barbiturates, other anticonvulsant medication, or both may have a higher tolerance to local anesthetic drugs, since enzyme induction may be present (see the "Enzyme Induction" section of this chapter and Figure 25–5).

Blood Gases and Acid-Base Disturbances

Oxygen. The arterial oxygen tension level (>60 mm Hg) is not critical to the development of local anesthetic CNS toxicity. Although oxygen inhalation does not prevent CNS seizure activity, hyperemia after the onset of seizures may be beneficial.[40]

Carbon Dioxide. The seizure dosage for lidocaine has been demonstrated in anesthetized cats to be inversely related to the arterial carbon dioxide tension.[41] Other investigators have confirmed this relationship in dogs, but not in monkeys.[42,43] The effect of hypercapnia may be related to the role of carbon dioxide in increasing cerebral blood flow and therefore may increase the rate of delivery of the local anesthetic to the CNS.

Hydrogen Ion. Increased hydrogen ion concentration also increases cerebral toxicity.[42] Also, protein binding of lidocaine is reduced during acidosis, which increases the active portion of lidocaine and thereby augments toxicity.[18] The use of hyperventilation to reduce cerebral seizure threshold and to increase protein binding is recommended during the treatment of any seizure induced by local anesthetics. It should be noted that the cardiovascular responses to lidocaine in animals did not correlate with changes in arterial carbon dioxide tension (12 to 73 mm Hg) and in pH (7.69 to 7.11).[44]

Inhalation Anesthetic Agents

Local anesthetic toxicity may be modified by inhalation anesthetic agents. The administration of nitrous oxide or of low concentrations of more potent agents protects against seizures induced by lidocaine, procaine, or tetracaine.[45,46] De Jong et al. were able to increase the seizure threshold of lidocaine by 50% in cats breathing nitrous oxide, 70% (Fig. 25–7).[45] I have made

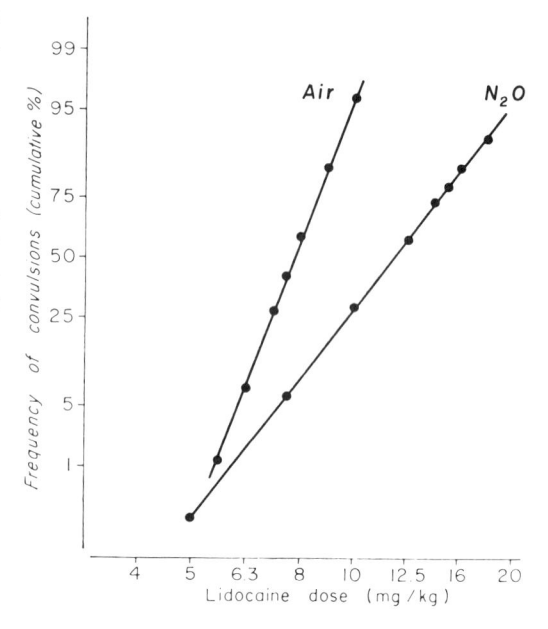

Fig. 25–7. Dose-response lines for awake cats (left) and those anesthetized with nitrous oxide, 70% (right) show that the lidocaine seizure threshold was elevated 50% in anesthetized animals. (From de Jong, R.H., Heavner, J.E., and de Oliveira, L.F.: Effects of nitrous oxide on the lidocaine seizure threshold and diazepam protection. Anesthesiology, 37:299, 1972.)

similar observations with nitrous oxide in rhesus monkeys. However, the inhalation of high concentrations of halothane, fluroxene, or methoxyflurane enhanced the lethal effects of both amide and ester-type drugs.[46] Increases in toxicity probably occur through an interaction of the depressive actions of these drugs on the cardiorespiratory system. The administration of lidocaine during diethyl ether anesthesia in man and during enflurane anesthesia in dogs results in ventilatory depression.[47,48] Since lidocaine also proportionally reduces anesthetic requirement (MAC), enhanced depression of ventilation can be avoided by reducing the concentration of the inhalation anesthetic.[48,49]

In dogs, equipotent, intravenously administered doses of lidocaine, bupivacaine, and etidocaine have equivalent antidysrhythmic effects in the presence of epinephrine during halothane anesthesia.[49a] Johnston, Eger, and Wilson studied this interaction in surgical patients anesthetized with halothane. They found that the addition of 250 to 400 mg lidocaine (0.5%) to an epinephrine solution for oronasal submucosal injection increased the dysrhythmogenic dose of epinephrine by about 75%.[49b] An even greater antidysrhythmic action of lidocaine subsequently was reported in similar clinical studies during enflurane anesthesia.[49c]

Local Anesthetic Mixtures

Local anesthetic drugs are frequently combined with one another to produce rapid onset and prolonged duration of anesthesia. Although the administration of large doses of multiple drugs is considered to be an important cause of local anesthetic toxicity, clinical reports indicate that local anesthetic solutions containing amide- and ester-type drugs can be used without an apparent increase in toxicity. However, mixtures of lidocaine-etidocaine and lidocaine-tetracaine in equipotent doses have approximately the same CNS toxicity in rhesus monkeys when given intravenously as either drug has when administered alone. That is, anesthetic toxicity is additive.[50]

Other reports indicate that repeated administration of local anesthetics cannot by itself alter seizure dosage or threshold.[39,51] The toxicity of mixtures of ester-type local anesthetics would be expected to be at least additive, since these drugs all depend on serum cholinesterase for their inactivation. However, the addition of tetracaine to procaine and to chloropropane has been shown to increase toxicity during constant-rate intravenous infusions in rats.[52]

In contrast to accidental rapid intravenous injections, the clinical tolerance for a mixture of local anesthetic drugs can be increased further after regional block procedures if the compounded drugs have different kinetic or metabolic characteristics. For example, the duration and high levels in the blood of ester derivatives such as procaine and tetracaine are limited by the activity of serum cholinesterase. In contrast, the decay of blood levels of amide derivatives such as lidocaine is subject to the slower processes of redistribution, hepatic metabolism, and elimination. Clinical studies with lidocaine-bupivacaine mixtures show that the pharmacokinetics of the individual drugs are unaffected.[52a]

Delirium induced by the combination of lidocaine and procaine amide has been reported, and bupivacaine and other amide local anesthetics (etidocaine) have also inhibited the hydrolysis of chloroprocaine by serum cholinesterase.[53,54] If these drugs are to be given concurrently, dosage should be reduced. Amide-ester mixtures containing chloroprocaine may also reduce the active (uncharged) amount of amide available in the solution. This phenomenon is related to the low pH (3.5) of chloroprocaine and may result in tachyphylaxis to the local anesthetic solution after repeated administrations to areas, such as the epidural space, with limited buffering capacities.[55] A prior injection of chloroprocaine has been reported to reduce the effectiveness of epidurally administered bupivacaine in parturients.[55a] It recently has been suggested that metabolism of chloroprocaine by cholinesterase in the nerve leaves behind a metabolite, i.e., 4-amino-2-chlorobenzoic acid, that interferes with the action of bupivacaine.[55b]

Muscle Relaxant Drugs

Combining local anesthetic agents with other drugs that share common metabolic pathways may cause significant drug interactions. Prolonged apnea, severe systemic toxicity, or both may occur if succinylcholine and the procaine-like ester drugs (including cocaine) are administered together, since serum cholinesterase is required for the hydrolysis and the inactivation of both types of compounds.[56] Other compounds known to possess anticholinesterase properties are pancuronium, hexafluorenium, and the hypotensive agent, trimethaphan.[57–59]

DeKornfeld and Steinhaus reported that the apneic period produced by a dose of succinylcholine ten minutes after the administration of lidocaine in dogs was almost twice as long as would have been anticipated if lidocaine had not been administered.[60] In addition, the administration of lidocaine after a subapneic dose of succinylcholine caused apnea in all animals studied. Whereas it is possible that this effect involves a drug interaction at the neuromuscular junction, these investigators suggested that the prolonged apnea is related to competition between the two drugs for plasma cholinesterase. A lidocaine dose of 10 mg/kg was employed in these animals anesthetized with pentobarbital. Although this dosage is greater than would be employed clinically, any combination of the two drugs should be used cautiously because the duration of the succinylcholine-induced apnea is likely to be longer in the presence of lidocaine.

The nondepolarizing muscle relaxants, gallamine and d-tubocurarine, elevate both the seizure dosage and the threshold of lidocaine in nonmedicated monkeys, whereas succinylcholine does not.[51] However, Acheson, Bull, and Glees found that the prior administration of succinylcholine (1 mg/kg) reduced the seizure dosage of lidocaine from 10 to 5 mg/kg in cats anesthetized with nitrous oxide.[61] In a related work, DeKornfeld and Steinhaus found that lidocaine (10 mg/kg) produced apnea in anesthetized dogs pretreated with subapneic doses of succinylcholine.[60] No explanation for these interactions has been proposed.

Local anesthetics may inhibit transmission at the neuromuscular junction by reducing either acetylcholine content or sensitivity of the postjunctional membrane by sodium channel blockade. Telivuo and Katz have shown that the intravenous administration of lidocaine, mepivacaine, prilocaine, or bupivacaine in man results in a small neuromuscular blocking action and depresses ventilation.[62] These studies and those using inhalation anesthetic agents suggest that the major cause of respiratory depression by local anesthetics, in the absence of muscle relaxants, is primarily related to a direct action on the CNS.

Matsuo et al., using the rat's phrenic nerve-hemidiaphragm, showed that neuromuscular blocking agents and local anesthetics increase the neuromuscular blocking effects of one another.[63] In clinical studies Zukaitis and Hoech have reported that lidocaine potentiates d-tubocurarine and, thus, allows more than a 50% reduction in the dosage of muscle relaxant when it is combined with lidocaine (2.5 mg/kg).[63a] This interaction should be considered when intravenous lidocaine is administered to surgical patients for the treatment of cardiac dysrhythmias when these patients have also received muscle relaxants.

Tricyclic Antidepressant Drugs

The seizure threshold of lidocaine appears to be indirectly related to levels of 5-hydroxytryptophan in the brain. Treatment of cats with 5-hydroxytryptophan decreases the seizure threshold of lidocaine and prolongs seizure activity.[64] In other studies, the increase of cerebral 5-hydroxytryptamine content induced by the administration of 5-hydroxytryptophan and the decrease of 5-hydroxytryptamine content induced by the administration of P-chloro-p-phenylalanine increase and decrease cerebral sensitivities to lidocaine, respectively.[65] This observation is interesting in regard to the sensitivity of the amygdala, a portion of the limbic system and an area of the brain known to have a high content of 5-hydroxytryptophan.

Local anesthetic solutions containing catecholamines may interact with tricyclic antidepressant drugs and, thus, cause hypertension and tachycardia. Lidocaine and mepivacaine solutions containing norepinephrine have produced severe headache in two dental patients who were given protriptyline.[66] A similar norepinephrine-desmethylimipramine interaction has been demonstrated in dogs.[67] The observed cardiovascular changes are related to the interaction of catecholamines and monoamine oxidase inhibitors. Other tricyclic agents that increase levels of norepinephrine at nerve terminals and the ester-type local anesthetic, cocaine, are likely to show a similar action.

An intravenous injection of amitriptyline has been shown to potentiate the anesthetic effects of lidocaine and procaine in animals. It is thought that this property relates to the sedative effect of amitriptyline. However, other tricyclic compounds (imipramine and protriptyline) have not been shown to interact with local anesthetics.[67a]

Local Anesthetic Drug Metabolites

Pharmacologically active metabolites of lidocaine may contribute to CNS toxicity in some patients. Strong et al. demonstrated that monoethylglycinexylidide and glycinexylidide are present in patients receiving lidocaine for the treatment of cardiac dysrhythmias.[68] Since some patients who showed signs of CNS toxicity had plasma concentrations of lidocaine within the accepted therapeutic range (less than 2.8 µg/ml), perhaps these metabolites are active and contribute to the observed toxicity. This speculation is supported by animal studies showing that lidocaine and monoethylglycinexylidide have equal potential for inducing convulsions.[69]

Monoethylglycinexylidide, the primary metabolite of lidocaine, is approximately 80% as potent as the parent compound in protecting against ouabain-induced dysrhythmias in guinea pig atria (Fig. 25–8). Glycinexylidide is only one-tenth as potent.[70] Plasma concentrations of these me-

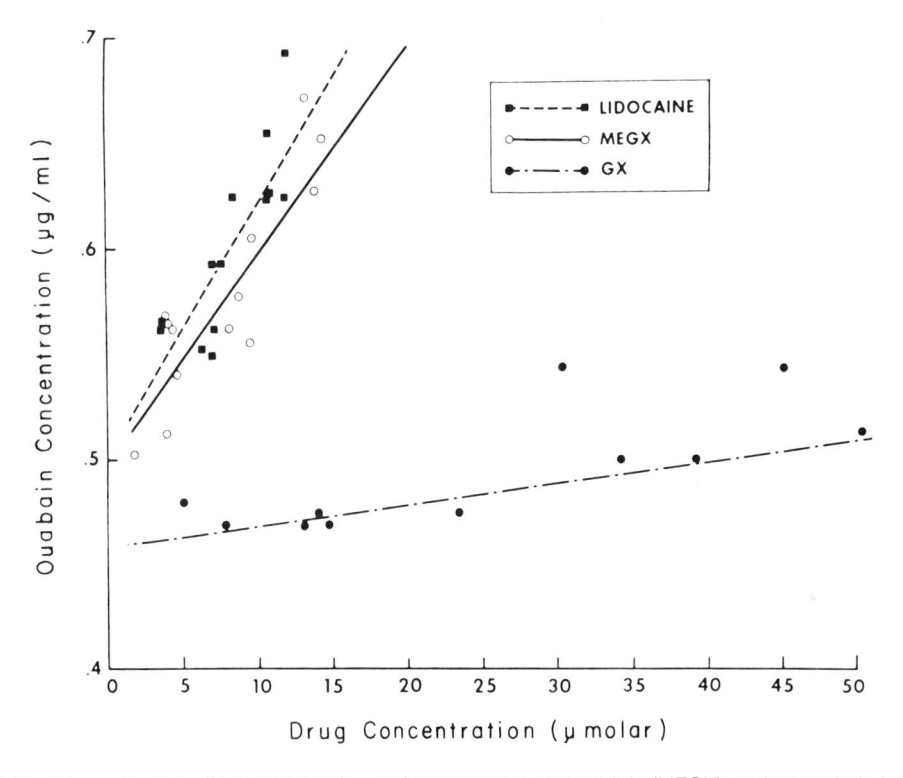

Fig. 25–8. The protective effects of lidocaine and monoethylglycinexylidide (MEGX) against ouabain-induced dysrhythmias in isolated guinea pig atria. Lidocaine and MEGX potency are nearly identical, whereas glycinexylidide (GX) potency is about one-tenth that of the parent compound. (From Burney, R.G., et al.: Antiarrhythmic effects of lidocaine metabolites. Am. Heart J., 88:765, 1974.)

tabolites, as well as those of lidocaine, should be considered when evaluating lidocaine therapy and local anesthetic toxicity. These principles might also apply when administering lidocaine or other amide-type local anesthetics to patients who have received prolonged lidocaine therapy.

The ability of para-aminobenzoic acid, the primary metabolite of procaine, to interfere with the therapeutic action of sulfonamides has long been recognized. Evidence also indicates that nontoxic doses of para-aminobenzoic acid, as well as sodium and ammonium benzoate, increase the lethal dosages of procaine and lidocaine in rats. Molgo et al. suggest that the mechanisms for these actions are directly related to cellular effects rather than to the inactivation of local anesthetic metabolism.[71]

Circadian Rhythm

Central nervous system responses of experimental animals to lidocaine may vary independently of drug dosage.[72] The responses are rhythmic and are closely related to the cyclic periods of light and darkness in the day. The importance and applicability of this phenomenon to clinical practice are unknown.

REFERENCES

1. Van Dyke, C., et al.: Cocaine: plasma concentrations after intranasal application in man. Science, 191:859, 1976.
2. Koehntop, D.E., Liao, J.C., and Van Bergen, F.H.: Effects of pharmacologic alterations of adrenergic mechanisms by cocaine, tropolone, aminophylline, and ketamine on epinephrine-induced arrhythmias during halothane-nitrous oxide anesthesia. Anesthesiology, 46:83, 1977.
3. Scott, D.B., et al.: Factors affecting plasma levels of lignocaine and prilocaine. Br. J. Anaesth., 44:1040, 1972.
4. Johnston, R.R., Eger, E.I., II, and Wilson, C.: A comparative interaction of epinephrine with enflurane, isoflurane, and halothane in man. Anesth. Analg. (Cleve.), 55:709, 1976.
5. De Jong, R.H., and Cullen, S.C.: Buffer-demand and pH of local anesthetic solutions containing epinephrine. Anesthesiology, 24:801, 1963.
6. Bromage, P.R., et al.: Quality of epidural blockade. III. Carbonated local anaesthetic solutions. Br. J. Anaesth., 39:197, 1967.
7. Loder, R.E.: A local anesthetic solution with longer action. Lancet, 2:346, 1960.
8. Rosenblatt, R.M., Lui, P., and Capener, C.: Dextran as a local anesthetic adjuvant. Anesthesiology, 53:S220, 1983.
9. Kaplan, J.A., Miller, E.D., Jr., and Gallagher, E.G., Jr.: Postoperative analgesia for thoracotomy patients. Anesth. Analg. (Cleve.), 54:773, 1975.
10. Marx, G.F., et al.: Drug overdose in axillary block of brachial plexus. N.Y. State J. Med., 68:304, 1968.
11. Thomson, P.D., et al.: Lidocaine pharmacokinetics in advanced heart failure, liver disease, and renal failure in humans. Ann. Intern. Med., 78:499, 1973.
12. Prescott, L.F., Adjepon-Yamoah, K.K., and Talbot, R.G.: Impaired lignocaine metabolism in patients with myocardial infarction and cardiac failure. Br. Med. J., 1:939, 1976.
13. Benowitz, N., et al.: Lidocaine disposition kinetics in monkey and man. II. Effects of hemorrhage and sympathomimetic drug administration. Clin. Pharmacol. Ther., 16:99, 1974.
14. Branch, R.A., et al.: The reduction of lidocaine clearance by dl-propranolol: An example of hemodynamic drug interaction. J. Pharmacol. Exp. Ther., 184:515, 1973.
15. Mather, L.E., et al.: Hemodynamic drug interaction: peridural lidocaine and intravenous ephedrine. Acta Anaesthesiol. Scand., 20:207, 1976.
16. Tucker, G.T., et al.: Binding of anilide-type local anesthetics in human plasma: 1. Relationships between binding, physiochemical properties, and anesthetic activity. Anesthesiology, 33:287, 1970.
17. Ghoneim, M.M., and Pandya, H.: Plasma protein binding of bupivacaine and its interaction with other drugs in man. Br. J. Anaesth., 46:435, 1974.
17a. Feely, J., et al.: Increased toxicity and reduced clearance of lidocaine by cimetidine. Ann. Intern. Med., 96:592, 1982.
18. Burney, R.G., DiFazio, C.A., and Foster, J.: Effects of pH on protein binding of lidocaine. Anesth. Analg. (Cleve.), 57:478, 1978.
19. Zsigmond, E.K., and Eilderton, T.E.: Abnormal reaction to procaine and succinylcholine in a patient with inherited atypical plasma cholinesterase: case report. Can. Anaesth. Soc. J., 15:498, 1968.
20. Stoelting, R.K.: Serum cholinesterase activity following pancuronium and antagonism with neostigmine or pyridostigmine. Anesthesiology, 45:647, 1976.
20a. Wang, B.C., et al.: Reversal of tetracaine spinal block by exogenous subarachnoid cholinesterase. Anesthesiology, 59:A209, 1983.
21. Pantuck, E.J.: Ecothiopate iodide eye drops and prolonged response to suxamethonium. A case report. Br. J. Anaesth., 38:406, 1966.
21a. Lanks, K.W., and Sklar, G.S.: Pseudocholinesterase levels and rates of chloroprocaine hydrolysis in patients receiving adequate doses of phospholine iodide. Anesthesiology, 52:434, 1980.
21b. Brodsky, J.B., and Campos, F.A.: Chloroprocaine analgesia in a patient receiving echothiophate iodide eye drops. Anesthesiology, 48:288, 1978.
21c. Kuhnert, B.R., et al.: A prolonged chloroprocaine

epidural block in a postpartum patient with abnormal pseudocholinesterase. Anesthesiology, 56:477, 1982.
22. Foldes, F.F., et al.: The influence of glucocorticoids on plasma cholinesterase (38219). Proc. Soc. Exp. Biol. Med., 146:918, 1974.
23. Kaniaris, P., et al.: Serum cholinesterase levels in patients with cancer. Anesth. Analg. (Cleve.), 58:82, 1979.
24. Wang, R.I.H., and Ross, C.A.: Prolonged apnea following succinylcholine in cancer patients receiving AB-132. Anesthesiology, 24:363, 1963.
25. Blitt, C.D., et al.: Correlation of plasma cholinesterase activity and duration of action of succinylcholine during pregnancy. Anesth. Analg. (Cleve.), 56:78, 1977.
26. Finster, M.: Toxicity of local anesthetics in the fetus and the newborn. Bull. N.Y. Acad. Med., 52:222, 1976.
27. Reidenberg, M.M., James, M., and Dring, L.G.: The rate of procaine hydrolysis in serum of normal subjects and diseased patients. Clin. Pharmacol. Ther., 13:279, 1972.
28. DiFazio, C.A., and Brown, R.E.: Lidocaine metabolism in normal and phenobarbital-pretreated dogs. Anesthesiology, 36:238, 1972.
29. Heinonen, J., Takki, S., and Jarho, L.: Plasma lidocaine levels in patients treated with potential inducers of microsomal enzymes. Acta Anaesthesiol. Scand., 14:89, 1970.
30. Forrest, J.A.H., et al.: Antipyrine, paracetamol, and lignocaine elimination in chronic liver disease. Br. Med. J., 1:1384, 1977.
31. Selden, R., and Sasahara, A.A.: Central nervous system toxicity induced by lidocaine. Report of a case in a patient with liver disease. J.A.M.A., 202:908, 1967.
32. Stenson, R.E., Constantino, R.T., and Harrison, D.C.: Inter-relationships of hepatic blood flow, cardiac output, and blood levels of lidocaine in man. Circulation, 43:205, 1971.
33. Burney, R.G., and DiFazio, C.A.: Hepatic clearance of lidocaine during N_2O anesthesia in dogs. Anesth. Analg. (Cleve.), 55:322, 1976.
34. Adjepon-Yamoah, K.K., Scott, D.B., and Prescott, L.F.: Impaired absorption and metabolism of oral lignocaine in patients undergoing laparoscopy. Br. J. Anaesth., 45:143, 1973.
34a. Jorfeldt, L., et al.: Lung uptake of lidocaine in man. Regional Anesth., 5:6, 1980.
34b. Rothstein, P., and Pitt, B.R.: Pulmonary extraction of bupivacaine and its modification by propranolol. Anesthesiology, 59:A189, 1983.
35. Eriksson, E., and Granberg, P.O.: Studies on the renal excretion of Citanest and Xylocaine. Acta Anesthesiol. Scand. (Suppl.), 16:79, 1965.
36. Mepivacaine overdosage in a child. (Discussion, E.S. Munson.) Anesth. Analg. (Cleve.), 52:422, 1973.
37. Richards, R.K., Smith, N.T., and Katz, J.: The effects of interaction between lidocaine and pentobarbital on toxicity in mice and guinea pig atria. Anesthesiology, 29:493, 1968.
37a. Caron, M., and LeLorier, J.: Potentiation of lidocaine toxicity by pentobarbital in the dog. Toxicol. Appl. Pharmacol., 51:537, 1979.
38. De Jong, R.H., and Heavner, J.E.: Diazepam prevents and aborts lidocaine convulsions in monkeys. Anesthesiology, 41:226, 1974.
39. Ausinsch, B., Malagodi, M.H., and Munson, E.S.: Diazepam in the prophylaxis of lignocaine seizures. Br. J. Anaesth., 48:309, 1976.
40. Munson, E.S., Pugno, P.A., and Wagman, I.H.: Does oxygen protect against local anesthetic toxicity? Anesth. Analg. (Cleve.), 51:422, 1972.
41. De Jong, R.H., Wagman, I.H., and Prince, D.A.: Effect of carbon dioxide on the cortical seizure threshold to lidocaine. Exp. Neurol., 17:221, 1967.
42. Englesson, S., and Grevsten, S.: The influence of acid-base changes on central nervous system toxicity of local anaesthetic agents II. Acta Anaesthesiol. Scand., 18:88, 1974.
43. Munson, E.S., and Wagman, I.H.: Acid-base changes during lidocaine induced seizures in Macaca mulatta. Arch. Neurol., 20:406, 1969.
44. Yakaitis, R.W., Thomas, J.D., and Mahaffey, J.E.: Cardiovascular effects of lidocaine during acid-base imbalance. Anesth. Analg. (Cleve.), 55:863, 1976.
45. De Jong, R.H., Heavner, J.E., and de Oliveira, L.F.: Effects of nitrous oxide on the lidocaine seizure threshold and diazepam protection. Anesthesiology, 37:299, 1972.
46. Staniweski, J.A., and Aldrete, J.A.: The effects of inhalation anaesthetic agents on convulsant (LD-50) doses of local anaesthetics in the rat. Can. Anaesth. Soc. J., 17:602, 1970.
47. Siebecker, K.L., et al.: Effect of lidocaine administered intravenously during ether anesthesia. Acta Anaesthesiol. Scand., 4:97, 1960.
48. Himes, R.S., Jr., Munson, E.S., and Embro, W.J.: Enflurane requirement and ventilatory response to carbon dioxide during lidocaine infusion in dogs. Anesthesiology, 51:131, 1979.
49. Himes, R.S., Jr., DiFazio, C.A., and Burney, R.G.: Effects of lidocaine on the anesthetic requirements for nitrous oxide and halothane. Anesthesiology, 47:437, 1977.
49a. Chapin, J.C., et al.: Lidocaine, bupivacaine, etidocaine, and epinephrine-induced arrhythmias during halothane anesthesia in dogs. Anesthesiology, 52:23, 1980.
49b. Johnston, R.R., Eger, E.I., and Wilson, C.: A comparative interaction of epinephrine with enflurane, isoflurane, and halothane in man. Anesth. Analg. (Cleve.), 55:709, 1976.
49c. Horrigan, R.W., Eger, E.I., and Wilson, C.: Epinephrine-induced arrhythmias during enflurane anesthesia in man: A nonlinear dose-response relationship and dose-dependent protection from lidocaine. Anesth. Analg. (Cleve.), 57:547, 1978.
50. Munson, E.S., Paul, W.L., and Embro, W.J.: Central-nervous-system toxicity of local anesthetic mixtures in monkeys. Anesthesiology, 46:179, 1977.
51. Munson, E.S., and Wagman, I.H.: Elevation of lidocaine seizure threshold by gallamine in rhesus monkeys. Arch. Neurol., 28:329, 1973.

52. Daos, F.G., Lopez, L., and Virtue, R.W.: Local anesthetic toxicity modified by oxygen and by combination of agents. Anesthesiology, 23:755, 1962.
52a. Seow, L.T., et al.: Lidocaine and bupivacaine mixtures for epidural blockade. Anesthesiology, 56:177, 1982.
53. Ilyas, M., Owens, D., and Kvasnicka, G.: Delirium induced by a combination of anti-arrhythmic drugs. Lancet, 2:1368, 1969.
54. Lalka, D., et al.: Bupivacaine and other amide local anesthetics inhibit the hydrolysis of chloroprocaine by human serum. Anesth. Analg. (Cleve.), 57:534, 1978.
55. Brodsky, J.B., and Brock-Utne, J.G.: Mixing local anaesthetics (Correspondence). Br. J. Anaesth., 50:1269, 1978.
55a. Hodgkinson, R., Husain, F.J., and Bluhm, C.: Reduced effectiveness of bupivacaine 0.5% to relieve labor pain after prior injection of chloroprocaine 2%. Anesthesiology, 57:A201, 1982.
55b. Corke, B.C., Carlson, C.G., and Dettbarn, W-D.: The influence of 2-chloroprocaine on the subsequent analgesic potency of bupivacaine. Anesthesiology, 60:25, 1984.
56. Jatlow, P., et al.: Cocaine and succinylcholine sensitivity: A new caution. Anesth. Analg. (Cleve.), 58:235, 1979.
57. Stovner, J., Oftedal, N., and Holmboe, J.: The inhibition of cholinesterase by pancuronium. Br. J. Anaesth., 47:949, 1975.
58. Bennett, E.J., et al.: Pancuronium and the fasciculations of succinylcholine. Anesth. Analg. (Cleve.), 52:892, 1973.
59. Poulton, T.J., James, F.M., and Lockridge, O.: Prolonged apnea following trimethaphan and succinylcholine. Anesthesiology, 50:54, 1979.
60. DeKornfeld, T.J., and Steinhaus, J.E.: The effect of intravenously administered lidocaine and succinylcholine on the respiratory activity of dogs. Anesth. Analg. (Cleve.), 38:173, 1959.
61. Acheson, F., Bull, A.B., and Glees, P.: Electroencephalogram of the cat after intravenous injection of lidocaine and succinylcholine. Anesthesiology, 17:802, 1956.
62. Telivuo, L., and Katz, R.L.: The effects of modern intravenous local analgesics on respiration during partial neuromuscular block in man. Anaesthesia, 25:30, 1970.
63. Matsuo, S., et al.: Interaction of muscle relaxants at the neuromuscular junction. Anesth. Analg. (Cleve.), 57:580, 1978.
63a. Zukaitis, M.G., and Hoech, G.P.: Train of 4 measurement of potentiation of curare by lidocaine. Anesthesiology, 51:S288, 1979.
64. de Oliveira, L.F., Heavner, J.E., and de Jong, R.H.: 5-hydroxytryptophan intensifies local anesthetic-induced convulsions. Arch. Int. Pharmacodyn. Ther., 207:333, 1974.
65. de Oliveira, L.F., and Bretas, A.D.: Effects of 5-hydroxytryptophan, iproniazid and p-chlorophenylalanine on lidocaine seizure threshold of mice. Eur. J. Pharmacol., 29:5, 1974.
66. Dornfest, F.D.: Drug interaction (Letter to the editor). S. Afr. Med. J., 46:1104, 1972.
67. Goldman, V., Astrom, A., and Evers, H.: The effect of a tricyclic antidepressant on the cardiovascular effects of local anaesthetic solutions containing different vasoconstrictors. Anaesthesia, 26:91, 1971 (abstract).
67a. Lechat, P., Fontagne, J., and Giroud, J-P.: Influence of a previous administration of tricyclic antidepressant compounds on the activity of local anesthetics. Therapie, 24:393, 1969.
68. Strong, J.M., Parker, M., and Atkinson, A.J., Jr.: Identification of glycinexylidide in patients treated with intravenous lidocaine. Clin. Pharmacol. Ther., 14:67, 1973.
69. Blumer, J., Strong, J.M., and Atkinson, A.J., Jr.: The convulsant potency of lidocaine and its N-dealkylated metabolites. J. Pharmacol. Exp. Ther., 186:31, 1973.
70. Burney, R.G., et al.: Anti-arrhythmic effects of lidocaine metabolites. Am. Heart J., 88:765, 1974.
71. Molgo, J., Montoya, G., and Guerrero, S.: Influencia del benzoato de sodio, benzoato de amonio y acido p-aminobenzoico sobre la dosis letal media de procaina y lidocaina en la rata macho. Arch. Biol. Med. Exp. (Santiago), 9:50, 1973.
72. Lutsch, E.F., and Morris, R.W.: Circadian periodicity in susceptibility to lidocaine hydrochloride. Science, 156:100, 1967.

This work was done while Dr. Munson was Professor of Anesthesiology at the University of Florida and Chief, Anesthesia Services at the Veterans Administration Medical Center at Gainesville, Florida.

26

DRUGS AND ANESTHETIC DEPTH

DAVID J. CULLEN

CASE REPORT

A 33-year-old white woman with a history of ulcerative colitis was admitted to the hospital, complaining of abdominal pain, bloody diarrhea, and anorexia. In 1971, she had undergone exploration for a possible toxic megacolon; her colon had not been removed although an appendectomy had been performed. Anesthesia, consisting of halothane, nitrous oxide, oxygen, and curare, had been uneventful at that time, as had been the patient's postoperative course. Medications included sulfadiazine, prednisone 30 mg/day, tincture of opium with belladonna, diazepam, iron, and Fiorinal.

On admission to the hospital, the patient's hematocrit was 35% and her white blood count was 8,900/mm.[3] An abdominal film showed large loops of distended colon and elevation of the left hemidiaphragm from a large dilated splenic flexure. She required meperidine 75 to 100 mg q3h to control pain from increasing distension and toxicity. Three days after hospital admission, the patient underwent surgical exploration for toxic megacolon and possible colonic perforation.

The patient was 5 ft. 4 in. tall and weighed 130 lbs. After 1.5 ml of Innovar intravenously, thiopental 250 mg and succinylcholine 100 mg were administered IV. The patient's trachea was intubated rapidly and easily. Anesthesia was maintained with nitrous oxide, 4 L in combination with oxygen, 2 L. Additional thiopental (50 mg) and Innovar (1.5 ml) were given followed by pancuronium (4 mg) prior to incision. Approximately 30 minutes after the incision, fentanyl was given incrementally to a total of 0.15 mg. Total medication prior to abdominal closure was thiopental, 300 mg, Innovar, 3 ml, fentanyl, 0.15 mg, and pancuronium, 6 mg.

Before the induction of anesthesia, her pulse was 140 and her blood pressure was 120/60. After induction, her pulse slowed to 120; her blood pressure remained between 100 and 120 systolic throughout the operation. Her temperature fell from 37.5° to 36°C during the three-hour procedure. Respiration was controlled. According to the anesthetist, pupillary movement or dilation, tearing, perspiration, grimacing, movement, hypertension, rise in heart rate, or any other signs of light anesthesia were not evident.

The patient's postoperative course, with two exceptions, was uncomplicated. She was discharged from the hospital three weeks later. Complications included

I. On the first postoperative day, the surgeon noted that "patient reports rather accurately the remembrance of sensations during the procedure, including the memory of hearing a 'four-letter word' that was used when the colon was entered at its place of perforation into the diaphragm." The anesthetist reported that the patient recalled conversation, abdominal discomfort, inability to move, and details of various manipulations. Although the patient was not unduly upset by her experience, her state of awareness during the procedure went unnoticed by the anesthetist and was not detected by the usual clinical signs.

II. On admission to the recovery room, a chest roentgenogram was obtained in order to determine the location of the central venous pressure (CVP) line. A total pneumothorax was seen, suggesting that the diaphragm had been entered inadvertently during the colonic dissection. The patient was awake and in no respiratory distress. She was neither hyperpneic nor cyanotic. After the insertion of a chest tube, the patient's lung was fully expanded. Prior to inserting the chest tube, her respiratory rate was 20 to 24 per minute, her CVP 7 to 9 cm H_2O, her blood pressure 120/70 mm Hg, and her apical pulse 100 per minute and regular. Following insertion of the chest tube, the patient's vital signs did not change. Blood gases were not obtained prior to the insertion of the chest tube. Pa_{O_2} (on room air five hours after the chest tube was placed) was 82 mm Hg, Pa_{CO_2} 39 mm Hg, pH 7.44.

One year later, the patient had an arthrodesis under enflurane-nitrous oxide and oxygen anesthesia. One month after the arthrodesis, she underwent total knee replacement under halothane, nitrous oxide, and oxygen anesthesia. Both anesthetic courses were uneventful. One year after the latter procedure, the patient

407

had a total knee replacement on the other side. Again, the anesthesia was uneventful, even though only 4 ml of Innovar, 7 mg of morphine, and 42 mg of curare were used. She had taken no narcotic during the previous 2 years.

The patient is a pleasant, intelligent, articulate person who has a realistic view of her illness and hospital experiences. During her hospitalization for colectomy, the events of which she recalled, she was interviewed by her anesthetist, who recorded the following conversation:

" 'Tell me how you felt when you first came down to the operating room.'

'I would say when I first came down to the operating room I was extremely apprehensive. I wasn't rested because I hadn't had any drugs in advance of the operation, and I was so tense, I didn't know what to expect quite. My spirits were good though, I won't say they weren't. I was quite optimistic. I wasn't in a worried state at all and I felt that I was looking forward to the surgery only insofar as I knew that it would be a tremendous relief to the pain that I was having.'

'Can you remember the skin incision at all from the start of the surgery?'

'I can remember the skin incision. Only in my words, I wouldn't have put it that way. As I said earlier, I felt as if somebody had a pair of hedgeclippers and was going to clip a little bit at a time and decided not enough grass had been mowed back and took the lawnmower and started pushing a bit harder from the right side to the left side. And they kept going through this process and they would get about half way across my stomach and the lawnmower would kind of sink a bit deeper and cause a tremendous amount of undue pressure and pain which I was trying to express but had no way of doing so. I wanted to move my arms or my legs or speak, and I literally had no power within me to do that.'

'What specific conversation can you recall while you were asleep?'

'One of the things I believe I remember during the course of the surgery, I remember two or three people saying, do you think the machinery is working properly? I don't know whether this was just something that was in my mind or whether I had heard somebody say it and I just projected upon it. I began to get nervous in a way, laying there thinking that the machinery wasn't working because I was feeling so much pain and I was wondering whether anyone else was aware of this or not.'

'Can you recall any of the surgeons speaking specifically?'

'I do from time to time remember comments between the various surgeons—not necessarily all business, but just comments about what they were doing as far as passing instruments and checking that my blood pressure was up to par and things along this line. I think at one point I remembered someone saying how much longer is it going to be, but I'm not quite sure about that.'

'Do you remember anything that I did to you at all, touching you or anything like that?'

'I do remember that quite well. I remember you were trying to open my eyes many times and they just wouldn't stay open. By opening my eyes, I wanted to tell you something, that I was in this tremendous pain, and yet I had no way of communicating with you really. I didn't know if you could understand how I felt or not. I wasn't sure if the monitor that you must have had attached to me showed this pain or not, but I was in pain and I wanted to say something all the time by either some eye movement or wrist movement. But, since my arms were spread apart so far, it was just a complete lack of coordination to get my message across. But I did almost feel at one period, almost in a state of panic because I felt that maybe you were losing your grip on me for some reason.'

'Can you describe the character of your pain, was it sharp, or was it dull, was it constant, did it come and go?'

'I would have to say that the pain came and went and it would start off slowly and then a tremendous pain wave would come. And then this (I use lawnmower for goodness knows why) as it got to going up hill again, the pain was released, and then as it came back down again, because of the area where obviously the incision must have been, the pain would intensify so much more again. But I was definitely in pain which I hadn't anticipated. I literally felt as though I lived through the whole operation. If I had known what I know now, I probably would have been too afraid to go under it and to undergo the operation, that is because of all the feeling of pain that I felt as I went under it, feeling that I would be out of my misery somehow. It didn't happen and when I woke up finally, I was absolutely exhausted and I felt, I didn't feel relaxed or relieved at all and in fact, I don't think I really slept very much after the operation. I was awake more than anything else.'

'Were things fuzzy at all during the operation?'

'They were quite fuzzy. One of the things that is rather peculiar to me is everybody sort of knows me as an organized person and I always have this little black book with me. It's like a little bible; somehow, everything important ends up in it. I can remember laying on the operating table and having one book in one hand and one in the other and trying to itemize everything that you were doing to me so that when I came around, I could discuss these things because I was interested in them. I wanted to form an objective point of view but after a while, so many things happened, one upon another, that the whole sequence became lost.'

'Would you be frightened to undergo another anesthesia procedure at all?'

'No, I would not. It hasn't destroyed my faith in so-called medicine, and because, in fact, I anticipate having another operation in a couple of months, I realize that it was just one of those freaks of nature that do happen. I have the feeling that one of the reasons that I didn't go under as deep is because, perhaps, I wasn't prepared early enough. So many patients are prepared hours before and given sedatives and I don't think I had that much time to relax and I think that may have had a bearing on it. But I definitely would say I wouldn't hesitate to have surgery again if I had to have it.' "

Anesthesia is defined as a state of general insensibility to pain and other sensations. In order for the anesthesiologist to realize that the patient perceives pain or other sensations, the patient must be able to respond to various noxious stimuli. This case illustrates that general anesthesia had not been achieved. Yet the patient was unable to communicate this to the anesthesiologist by either somatic or sympathetic responses. Only retrospectively was it established that the patient was not anesthetized.

The most likely explanation for this patient's state of awareness was the relatively small dose of narcotic administered with nitrous oxide to analgesia in the presence of a potent surgical stimulus. Additionally, the prior 3-day use of meperidine for the relief of pain from toxic megacolon probably increased the patient's tolerance to the narcotics received intraoperatively. Finally, muscle relaxants used to facilitate abdominal surgery rendered her unable to communicate with the anesthesiologist.

Anesthetic depth can be quantitated by using the concept of MAC. MAC is the Minimum Alveolar Concentration of anesthetic that produces immobility in 50% of those patients or animals exposed to a noxious stimulus. MAC was chosen to measure anesthesia because it is a reliable, reproducible, visible index of potency.[1] Its end point, the abolition of movement, is of clinical importance. MAC can be applied to all inhalation anesthetics and relates the observation of movement or nonmovement in response to a painful stimulus to the partial pressure of anesthetic at the anesthetic site of action in the brain (assuming that the alveolar partial pressure has equilibrated with brain concentration).

Once MAC was determined for various inhalation anesthetics, variables that alter MAC or depth or anesthesia were identified.[2] A drug that reduces MAC 30% indicates that the drug provides 30% of the anesthesia, even though that drug may not be an anesthetic in itself. Many of the currently known modifiers of anesthetic depth are drugs. Their effects on the depth of anesthesia are discussed in this chapter and are related to clinical management whenever possible. In addition, common pathophysiologic changes that may alter anesthetic depth are mentioned.

QUANTITATING DEPTH OF ANESTHESIA

In 1965, Eger et al. described MAC and began to outline factors that affect MAC in animals.[2] These investigators defined one point on a dose-response curve where the dose was alveolar anesthetic concentration and the response was the reaction of the patient to a surgical incision (Table 26–1).

Additional points on this dose-response curve have been described recently. One is the end-tidal halothane or enflurane concentration required for successful endotracheal intubation (MAC EI).[2a,2b] In children, MAC for successful intubation for both agents was approximately 30% higher than MAC for surgical incision. Another point was defined by Roizen et al.: the anesthetic concentration required to Block an Adrenergic Response—MAC-BAR. This dose was 1.45 MAC for halothane and 1.6 MAC for enflurane.[2c] Thus, it appears even more likely that the dose-response curves for inhalation anesthetics are roughly parallel to each other within the clinical range. De Jong and Eger have estimated a point toward the other end of the curve–the dose of anesthetic that anesthetizes not 50%, but 95% of the patient population (AD_{95}) (Fig. 26–1).[3] This criterion is important because

Table 26-1
Five well-defined end points describing alveolar anesthetic concentration and the response of the patient

	AWAKE MAC[39]		MAC[1-3]		ED$_{95}$[3]		MAC EI$_{50}$[2a,2b]	MAC-BAR[2c]
	(alveolar concentration)	(% of MAC)	(alveolar concentration)	(% of MAC)	(alveolar concentration)	(% of MAC)	(% of MAC corrected for age)	(% of MAC corrected for age)
Halothane	0.41%	55%	0.74%	100%	0.90%	122%	133%	145%
Methoxyflurane	0.081%	51%	0.16%	100%	0.22%	138%		
Ether	1.41%	73%	1.92%	100%	2.22%	116%		
Fluroxene	2.2%	65%	3.4%	100%	3.57%	105%		
Enflurane			1.68%	100%			139%	160%
Nitrous oxide*	65–86%	59–78%	104%	100%				

*Eger—personal communication

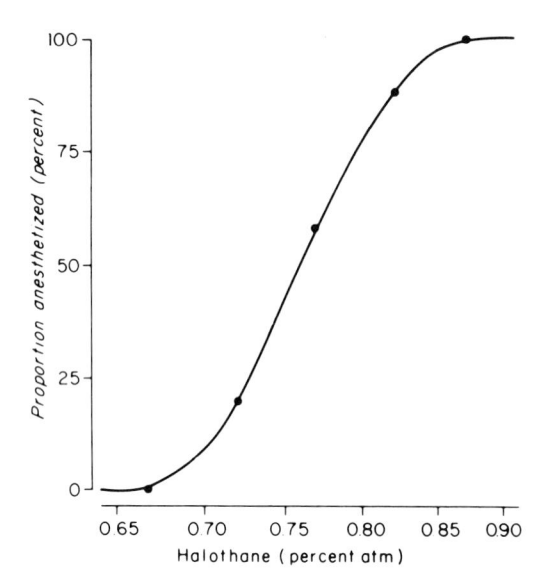

Fig. 26–1. Halothane log dose-response curve. Percentage of subjects anesthetized (i.e., not responding to skin incision) within each of five halothane dose ranges is on the vertical axis. The horizontal axis is scaled to the logarithm of the alveolar halothane concentration. Note the curve symmetry around the median (50% response) points. (From De Jong, R.H., and Eger, E.I., II: MAC expanded: AD_{50} and AD_{95} values of common inhalation anesthetics in man. Anesthesiology, 42:386, 1975.)

no clinician attempts to anesthetize patients with an anesthetic concentration that provides a 50% chance of movement during a skin incision—a much higher probability is clinically desirable. For some of the inhalation anesthetics, the AD_{95} is close to the AD_{50}, or MAC concentration, whereas for other anesthetics, the AD_{95} is farther from MAC (Table 26–1). Assessing anesthetic depth is difficult since a given increase in inspired concentration does not yield a comparable increase in alveolar concentration and anesthetic depth because of variations in uptake and distribution.[4]

De Jong et al. and Freund et al. suggest that anesthetic "depth" is also a function of the impact of anesthetics on the central nervous system (Fig. 26–2). They demonstrated an almost linear response of monosynaptic pathways and the susceptibility of the H-reflex to increasing concentrations of anesthetic agents. They also documented that anesthesia *is a continuum*, not an all or none response.[5,6]

Cullen and Larson have urged that anesthesiologists give serious attention to the assessment of "depth" of anesthesia because:

in any patient, only that level of anesthesia needed to meet the surgical requirements should be established. We hold the basic premise that the less the involvement of the patient's critical organs and system (i.e., the lower the concentration of the agent, or the less "deep" the anesthesia), the less will be the damage to the patient, whether this be temporary or perhaps permanent. We emphasize, however, that we firmly believe in providing sufficient anesthesia to meet the surgical requirements. We believe that anesthesia that is "light" enough so that response to surgical stimuli such as hypertension, tachycardia, recollection of stimuli and increased muscle tension may result in unnecessary harm. Consequently, it is essential that the anesthesiologist learn how to assess the various responses of the patient that give clues to the depth of anesthesia. All patients are not the same. In major surgical procedures, the condition of most patients is not the same during or at the end as at the beginning. Further, all surgeons are not the same, all surgical requirements are not the same, and all operating conditions are not the same. We submit that, if there are these many variables in an anesthetic situation, the anesthetist must learn to recognize and respond to those subtle as well as obvious changes that take place in the individual patient. Fortunately, many patients have responses that are peculiar to them. For example, some patients move a hand in response to a stimulus, other patients wrinkle an eyebrow, and other patients make more gross effort such as leg movement; other patients respond by elevation of blood pressure, increase or decrease in pulse rate, perspiration, tearing, and pupillary changes, while still others have characteristic respiratory patterns.[7]

Administration of anesthesia must be individualized, with the patient serving as his own control. Although Cullen and Larson have described clinical signs of light, moderate, and deep anesthesia, these signs vary greatly with the anesthetic agent and are not generally applicable.[8]

The clinical signs used to assess depth

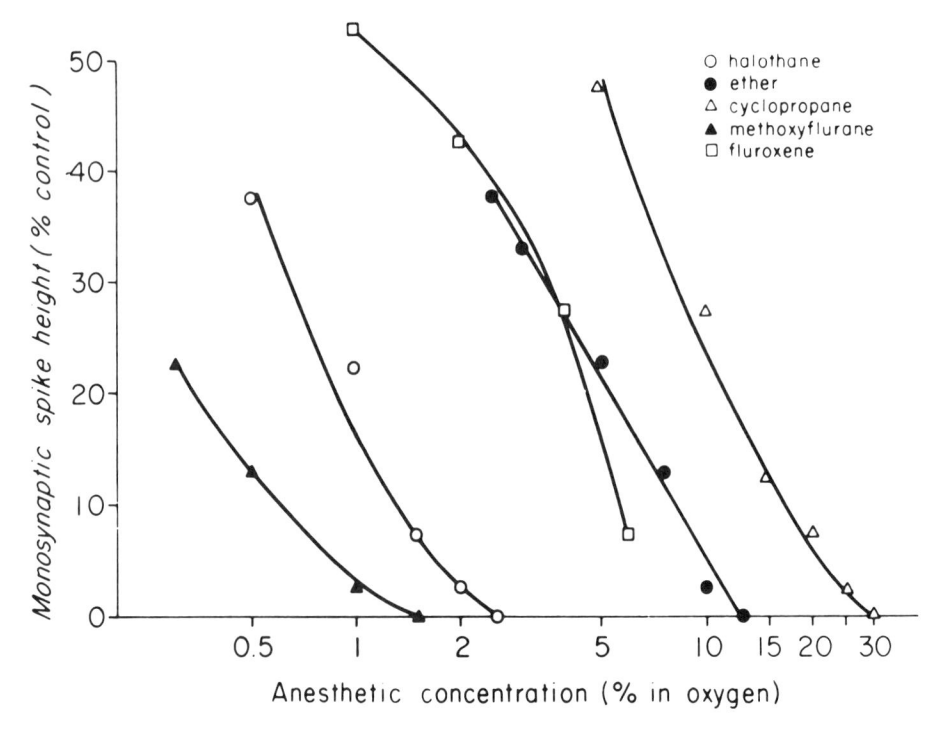

Fig. 26-2. Mean monosynaptic spike heights are plotted against inspired concentrations of five commonly used anesthetics on a semilog scale. As anesthetic concentration rose, the amplitude of the spike began to fall. Thus depression of synaptic transmission was inversely proportional to the log of the anesthetic concentration. (From De Jong, R.H., et al.: Anesthetic potency determined by depression of synaptic transmission. Anesthesiology, 29:1142, 1968.)

of anesthesia include: heart rate, blood pressure, pupil diameter, pupillary reactivity to light, tearing, eye movement, tidal volume, respiratory rate, and abdominal muscle tone. Most of these clinical signs define the depth of anesthesia for only specific inhalation anesthetics.[8] For example, falling blood pressure is characteristic of deepening halothane anesthesia whereas rising blood pressure indicates deepening fluroxene anesthesia (Fig. 26-3). Since similar examples abound, it is impossible to use blood pressure as the sole guide to anesthetic depth. To confuse matters further, many factors other than anesthetic depth alter the common signs of anesthesia. These factors include: preanesthetic medication; induction agents; a patient's illness, age, and general health; the site and extent of surgical stimulation; the use of muscle relaxants and/or controlled ventilation; patient's body temperature; Pa_{CO_2}; and the duration of anesthesia. Our data related the clinical signs of anesthesia to the concentration of several inhaled anesthetics in human volunteers in whom all of the variables mentioned were controlled.[8] Although guidelines emerged to evaluate anesthetic depth specific to each anesthetic drug, each clinical situation will undoubtedly modify many of the signs of anesthesia.

For clinical purposes, it is most important to assess depth of anesthesia just prior to incision, at the time of incision, and at various times during the surgical procedure as the level of painful stimulation is directly related to surgical manipulations (e.g., traction manipulation of viscera). *Anesthetic depth must always be considered in the context of the surgical stimulus.*

Clinical experience indicates that pre-

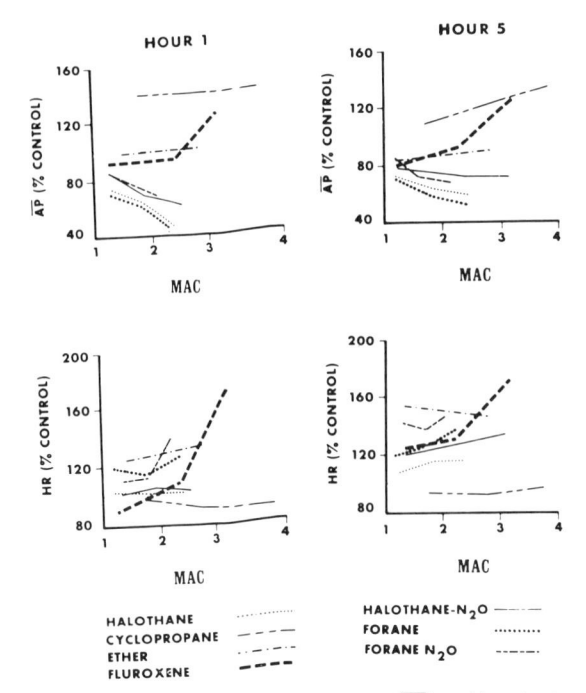

Fig. 26-3. Mean arterial pressure ($\overline{AP}$) and heart rate (HR) responses to several concentrations of seven anesthetics are shown. To permit comparison of anesthetic agents at equipotent concentrations, the horizontal axis represents multiples of MAC. On the ordinate, 100 represents the awake control value. Note that $\overline{AP}$ responses vary widely from one anesthetic to another and that for the same agent $\overline{AP}$ response changes with prolonged anesthesia.

dicting the level of the subsequent response to an operation is extremely difficult on the basis of clinical signs prior to surgical incision. It is more practical to use the response to surgical incision as the focal point for estimating anesthetic depth. Prior to incision, the anesthesiologist determines tidal volume and respiratory rate (if he allows the patient to breathe spontaneously), blood pressure and heart rate, eye position, pupillary diameter, presence or absence of tearing, perspiration, and, if possible, abdominal muscle tone. Three possible responses to a surgical incision can be described (known as the "Goldilocks" assessment): (1) if anesthesia is *too light*, the patient moves, coughs, and bucks on the endotracheal tube (a phenomenon common with enflurane) or shows a dramatic rise in blood pressure and heart rate; (2) if *too deep*, the patient does not move, but also, more important, has no autonomic reflex response to incision, that is, no tachycardia, blood pressure increase, pupillary dilatation, deepening tidal volume, or faster respiratory rate; and (3) when *"just right,"* the patient does not move in response to incision, but rather shows reflex awareness that a painful stimulus has been applied. The pupils may dilate, heart rate and blood pressure usually increase 10 to 20%, and the patient's respiratory rate may increase, whereas tidal volume definitely increases (Fig. 26-4). Interestingly, two minutes after skin incision, during an operation, the reflex changes in clinical signs abate and in most cases return to the preincision state, indicating the prognostic importance of skin incision as compared with other surgical stimuli. During the surgical procedure, it is helpful to reduce inspired anesthetic concentration gradually to evoke mild reflex responses in order to determine that anesthesia is indeed at the appropriate level. Since a constant inspired concentration results in a rising alveolar concentration, a patient will become more deeply anesthetized unless the inspired concentration is reduced.[4] Testing for the appearance of clinical responses will indicate when additional reduction of inspired concentration is unwise.

EFFECT OF DRUGS ON ANESTHETIC DEPTH (TABLE 26-2)

Aside from the expected potentiation of general anesthetics by sedatives and narcotics, only one other major drug group has been shown to interact with general anesthesia. These are drugs that alter central nervous system catecholamine function. Those drugs that increase central nervous system norepinephrine levels increase MAC; conversely, drugs that decrease central norepinephrine levels decrease MAC.

lends further support to the concept that anesthetic depth is influenced by central nervous system catecholamine concentration.[12]

Naloxone: Finck et al. reported that they had antagonized anesthesia with naloxone (10 mg/kg IV) in rats that were anesthetized with either halothane or enflurane.[13] Most recent studies demonstrate that naloxone has no significant effect on halothane,[13a] nitrous oxide,[13b,13c] or thiopental.[13d] One recent study, however, suggests that naloxone may reverse nitrous oxide analgesia in man.[13e] In any case, the mechanism for the phenomenon, if it exists, remains to be elucidated.

Hypernatremia: Although not drug-induced, changes in anesthetic depth may result from changes in electrolyte concentrations. Tanifuji and Eger showed that hypernatremia to a serum sodium of 179 mEq/L, sufficient to increase cerebrospinal fluid (CSF) sodium to 181 mEq/L, increased halothane MAC in dogs 43%. Mannitol, which increases osmolarity, increased MAC because dehydration raised CSF Na+ to 176 mEq/L. Hyperosmolarity not associated with increased CSF Na+ did not raise MAC. Potassium changes had no effect on MAC[14] (Table 26–3).

Hyperthermia: Steffey and Eger showed that halothane MAC in dogs increased as their temperatures rose from 37 to 42°C, after which MAC decreased (Fig. 26–5, Table 26–3). The rate of increase to 42°C was 8%/°C. This suggests that febrile patients may require a higher concentration of halothane to achieve an adequate anesthetic level.[15]

Potentiation of General Anesthesia

Depletion of brain norepinephrine and dopamine without change in brain serotonin concentration decreases halothane MAC by a small but significant amount.[16] Similarly, drugs that decrease brain serotonin without altering norepinephrine or dopamine concentrations also decrease halothane MAC to a small degree. However, this effect was not seen in rats exposed to cyclopropane. Mueller suggested that only anesthetics that progressively depress neuronal activity such as halothane are affected by central catecholamine levels, whereas a drug such as cyclopropane, which initially excites neurons, is not affected by this central level of catecholamines.[16]

Roizen et al. destroyed specific areas of brain that contain high concentrations of norepinephrine or of serotonin and achieved a maximal 40% reduction in halothane MAC.[17]

In a clinically applicable report, Miller, Way, and Eger observed that patients who received 1 to 6 g/day of *alpha*-methyldopa

Table 26–3
Pathophysiologic states that change anesthetic requirement

State	Anesthetic	MAC (% change)	Species	Reference #
Hypernatremia (Serum Na+ 179 mEq/L)	Halothane	↑ 43	Dogs	14
Hyperthermia (37° to 42°C)	Halothane	↑ 8/°C	Dogs	15
Hypoxia (Pa$_{O_2}$ 30 mm Hg)	Halothane	↓ Progressively towards 0	Dogs	32
Hypercapnia (Pa$_{CO_2}$ 95 to 245 mm Hg)	Halothane	↓ Progressively to 0	Dogs	34
Hypocapnia (Pa$_{CO_2}$ 10 mm Hg)	Halothane	No change	Dogs	35
Pregnancy	Halothane	↓ 25	Pregnant Ewes	37
Pregnancy	Methoxyflurane	↓ 32	Pregnant Ewes	35
Pregnancy	Isoflurane	↓ 40	Pregnant Ewes	37
Hypotension (mean AP 40 to 50 mm Hg)	Halothane	↓ 20	Dogs	41

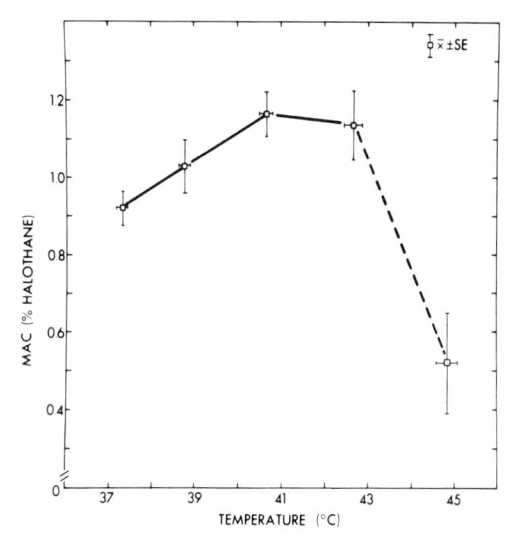

Fig. 26–5. The effect of hyperthermia on halothane MAC. Note the increase in halothane MAC until approximately 41°C. Death occurred at a mean temperature of 45.9°C. (From Steffey, E.P., and Eger, E.I., II: Hyperthermia and halothane MAC in the dog. Anesthesiology, 41:393, 1974.)

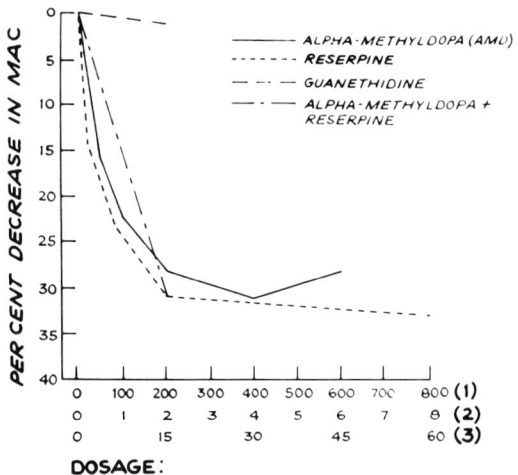

Fig. 26–6. Administration in dogs of *alpha*-methyldopa, reserpine, or *alpha*-methyldopa with reserpine decreased MAC in dose-related fashion. There was no change in halothane MAC with guanethidine. (From Miller, R.D., Way, W.L., and Eger, E.I., II: The effects of *alpha*-methyldopa, reserpine, guanethidine and iproniazide on minimum alveolar anesthetic concentration (MAC). Anesthesiology, 29:1156, 1968.)

(AMD) required lower concentrations of inhalation anesthesia to maintain adequate surgical anesthesia.[9] These investigators postulated that *alpha*-methyldopa displaces central nervous system norepinephrine thus potentiating anesthetic depth. In dogs, *alpha*-methyldopa and reserpine, which reduce central and peripheral norepinephrine levels, reduced MAC in dose-related fashion by approximately 30% (Fig. 26–6). Guanethidine, which only depletes peripheral catecholamines, did not affect MAC.

Clonidine, a potent central analgesic in animals whose effect is not reversed by naloxone, is also a potent centrally acting antihypertensive agent. Since it produces profound sedation when administered acutely IV, its effect on halothane MAC was studied by Bloor and Flacke.[17a] Clonidine 5 μg/kg decreased halothane MAC 42% within 2.3 hours while 20 μg/kg decreased halothane MAC 48% after 2.6 hrs. Tolazoline, an *alpha*-adrenergic antagonist, immediately reversed these effects upon injection, further demonstrating the role of central adrenergic neurotransmitters in modulating the depth of anesthesia.

Isoproterenol and Propranolol: Tanifuji and Eger reported that both isoproterenol, in doses sufficient to double the heart rate, and propranolol, 2 or 10 mg/kg IV, had no effect on halothane MAC in dogs.[18] Isoproterenol has not been reported to enter the CNS in significant amounts. Although propranolol crosses the blood-brain barrier, it does not alter brain norepinephrine.[19]

Levodopa: The authors suggested that lower doses of levodopa increase dopamine levels, thus inhibiting neurotransmission. The oral administration of levodopa increases CNS dopamine content in the basal ganglia, and this may in turn increase CNS catecholamine synthesis. Johnston et al. postulated that this agent may reduce MAC. Lower doses of L-dopa—5, 10, or 25 mg/kg IV—decreased halothane

MAC in dogs by as much as 52% (Fig. 26–7). However, L-dopa, 50 mg/kg, increased MAC by 41% for the first and second hour, but by the third and fourth hour, MAC decreased to 37% below control. Long-term administration of levodopa yielded variable results. The authors suggested that smaller doses of levodopa would increase dopamine levels, which, by inhibiting neurotransmission, could reduce MAC. However, larger doses of levodopa might displace norepinephrine from nerve terminals in the central nervous system. This suggestion is consistent with the researchers' previous findings; namely, that increased central norepinephrine levels increased MAC.[20]

Verapamil: Verapamil, 0.5 mg/kg, was infused over 10 minutes to achieve a pharmacologic depression of intracardiac conduction (40% increase in the PR interval). MAC decreased 25%, with no clinically significant neuromuscular blockade.[20a] Verapamil is supplied as a racemic mixture of both the d and l stereoisomers. The d form has local anesthetic effects owing to blockade of fast sodium channels, while the l form blocks slow calcium channels. Hence, the authors infer that the d isomer is responsible for reducing MAC. It would be prudent to decrease halothane concentration in the presence of verapamil, because of its effect on MAC as well as its negative chronotropic and inotropic effects on the myocardium.

Ketamine: Ketamine (50 mg/kg IM) produced a dose-dependent reduction in halothane MAC in rats (Fig. 26–8). MAC remained low for several hours, demonstrating ketamine's long-lasting effect.[21]

Phencyclidine: Phencyclidine, 2 mg/kg or 4 mg/kg, decreased cyclopropane MAC 32 and 42% respectively, a response which is unaltered by naloxone pretreatment.[21a]

Lidocaine: Lidocaine has been used as

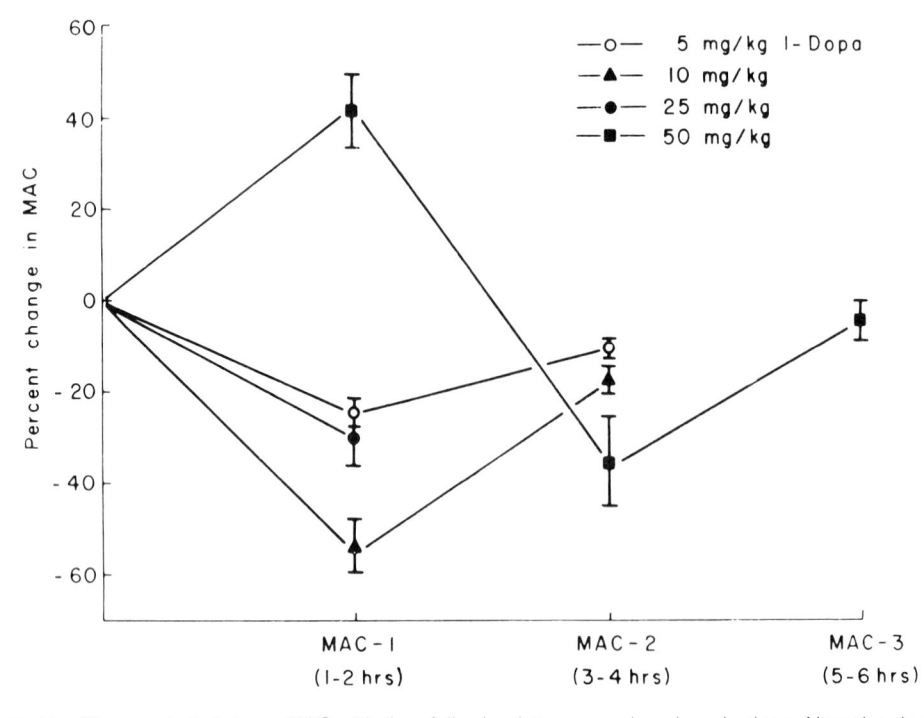

Fig. 26–7. Changes in halothane MAC with time following intravenous levodopa in dogs. Note the decrease in MAC with the lower doses of L-dopa and the 41% increase in MAC with the high dose L-dopa in the first two hours. All values are mean ±1 SE. (From Johnston, R.R., et al.: Effect of levodopa on halothane anesthetic requirement. Anesth. Analg. (Cleve.), 54:179, 1975.)

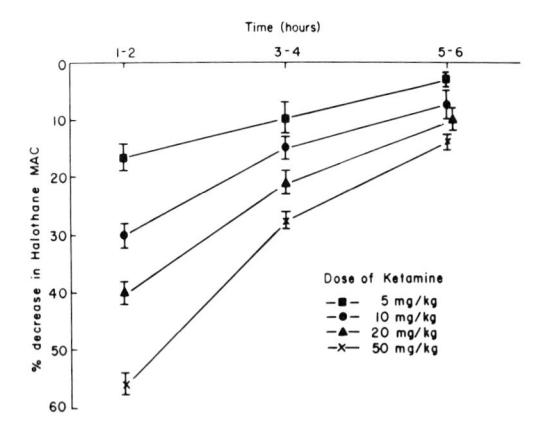

Fig. 26-8. Change in halothane MAC with time after intramuscular injection of ketamine. All values are mean ±1 SE. (From White, P.F., Johnston, R.R., and Pudwill, C.R.: Interaction of ketamine and halothane in rats. Anesthesiology, 42:183, 1975.)

an adjunct to general anesthesia.[22] Its effects, however, were not quantitated until DiFazio reported that lidocaine linearly reduced cyclopropane MAC up to 42% in rats as plasma concentrations rose to 1 μg/ml.[23] Himes et al. reported that plasma lidocaine concentrations of 2 to 6 μg/ml during nitrous oxide anesthesia in man contributed 0.13 to 0.28 of the anesthetic requirement.[24] The ED_{50} (median effective dose) in these studies was 3.2 μg/ml. In dogs anesthetized with halothane, MAC decreased up to 45% when plasma and CSF lidocaine were higher than 3 μg/ml (Figs. 26-9A & 26-9B). In view of this decrease, the anesthetist might reduce the concentration of depressant anesthetics such as halothane when lidocaine is used to suppress coughing in such procedures as bronchoscopy, pulmonary resection, and tracheal reconstruction.

Morphine: When administered as a preanesthetic medication, morphine slightly reduces MAC. Morphine sulfate, 8 to 15 mg subcutaneously, about 1.5 hours prior to surgery, reduced halothane MAC from 0.75% to 0.68% (Fig. 26-10).[25] Morphine sulfate, 10 to 12 mg IM, given approximately 1.5 hours prior to surgical incision reduced fluroxene MAC from 3.4% to 2.7% (Fig. 26-11).[26]

Fentanyl and Sufentanil: During a continuous infusion of fentanyl in dogs to provide steady-state conditions, enflurane MAC fell by a maximum of 65% at a fentanyl concentration of 30 ng/ml. Increasing the fentanyl concentration threefold led to a minimal additional reduction in MAC. This suggests the existence of a ceiling effect to this concentration-response relationship.[26a] Sufentanil, a drug 5 to 10 times more potent than fentanyl, reduced halothane MAC by 90% in rats.[26b] Naloxone completely reversed analgesia and respiratory depression induced by sufentanil. A plateau or ceiling effect was not observed until nearly complete anesthesia was obtained, a response that is quite different from that produced by fentanyl. Perhaps the difference rises from a species difference.

Diazepam: Diazepam, 0.2 mg/kg IV, 15 to 30 minutes prior to an operation reduced halothane MAC in man from 0.73% to 0.48%, a 35% reduction.[27] Diazepam, 0.4 mg/kg IV, further reduced halothane MAC, although that dose is too large for routine clinical use.

Nitrous Oxide: Nitrous oxide decreases MAC for halothane, fluroxene (Fig. 26-11), and isoflurane by approximately 1% for each percent of nitrous oxide administered.[25,26,28]

Pancuronium: The administration of pancuronium, 0.1 mg/kg, to 17 patients in whom a limb was isolated to prevent the total muscle relaxant effect of the drug decreased halothane MAC by 25% more than a control group receiving no pancuronium.[28a] The mechanism of action of this interesting phenomenon has not been elucidated. It is possible that small quantities of nondepolarizing muscle relaxants do, in fact, cross the blood-brain barrier and block CNS synaptic transmission, or that patients may be relatively deafferentated with far less muscle spindle afferent input to their reticular activating system. Per-

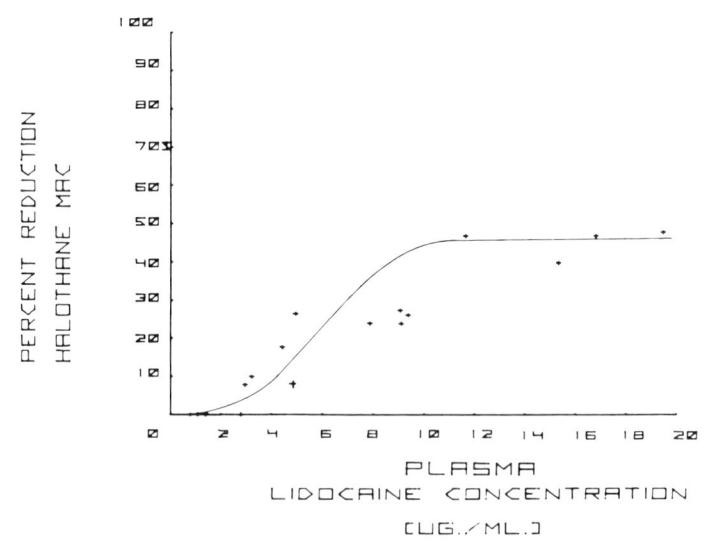

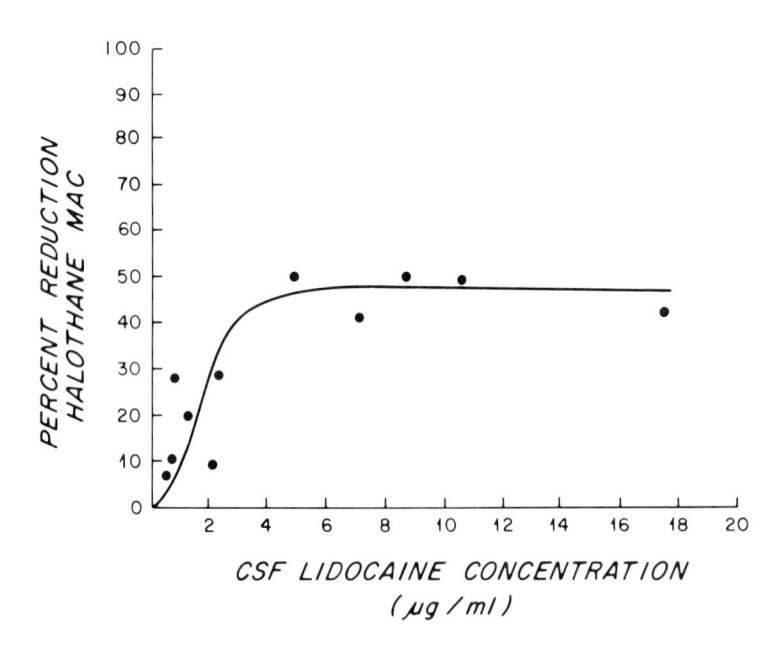

Fig. 26–9. A Plot of reduction in halothane MAC against increasing plasma lidocaine concentrations. B Plot of reduction in halothane MAC against increasing CSF lidocaine concentration. (From Himes, R.S., Di Fazio, C.A., Burney, R.G.: Effects of lidocaine on the anesthetic requirements for nitrous oxide and halothane. Anesthesiology, 47:437, 1977.)

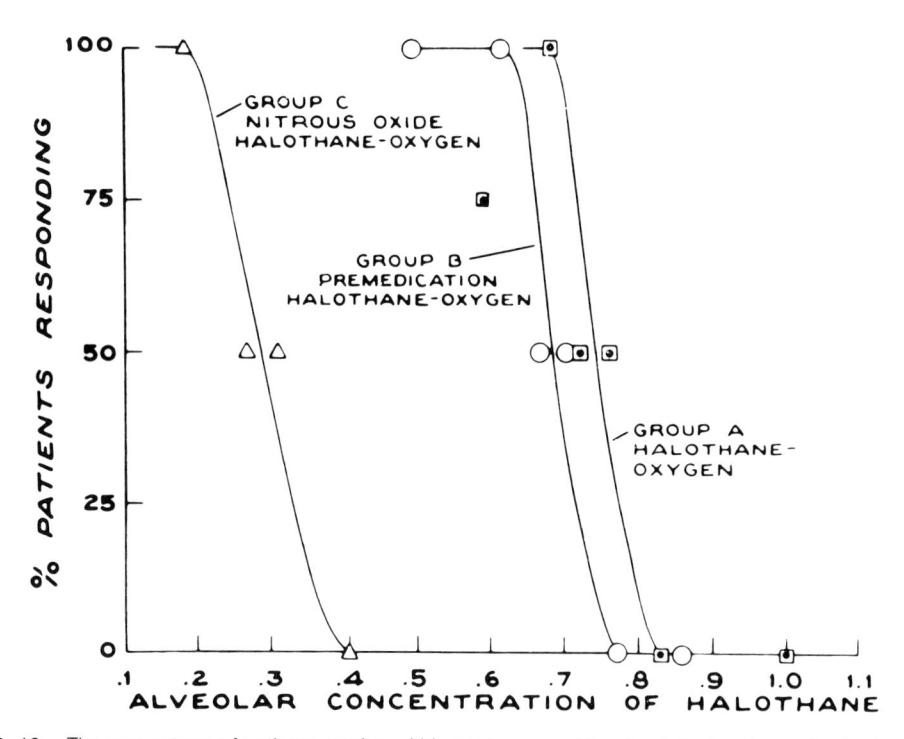

Fig. 26-10. The percentage of patients moving within each group of four is plotted on the vertical axis against the average alveolar concentration of the four which is plotted on the horizontal axis. Note that premedication with morphine sulfate, 8 to 15 mg subcutaneously, yielded a small reduction in MAC (Group B). Nitrous oxide administered with halothane resulted in a large reduction in MAC (Group C). (From Saidman, L.J., and Eger, E.I., II: Effect of nitrous oxide and of narcotic pre-medication on the alveolar concentration of halothane required for anesthesia. Anesthesiology, 25:304, 1964.)

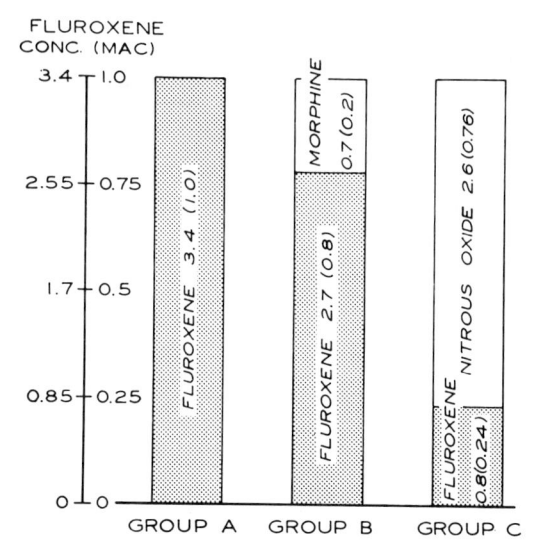

Fig. 26-11. Fluroxene concentration in volumes per cent with equivalent fractional MAC values are shown on the vertical axis. The concentration of fluroxene and MAC value are written within the bars. In group A, 3.4% fluroxene represents MAC 1.0. In group B, morphine is equivalent to 0.7% fluroxene (0.2 MAC). In group C, nitrous oxide (72% alveolar concentration) is equivalent to 2.6% fluroxene (0.76 MAC). (From Munson, E.S., Saidman, L.J., and Eger, E.I., II: Effect of nitrous oxide and morphine on the minimum anesthetic concentration of fluroxene. Anesthesiology, 26:137, 1965.)

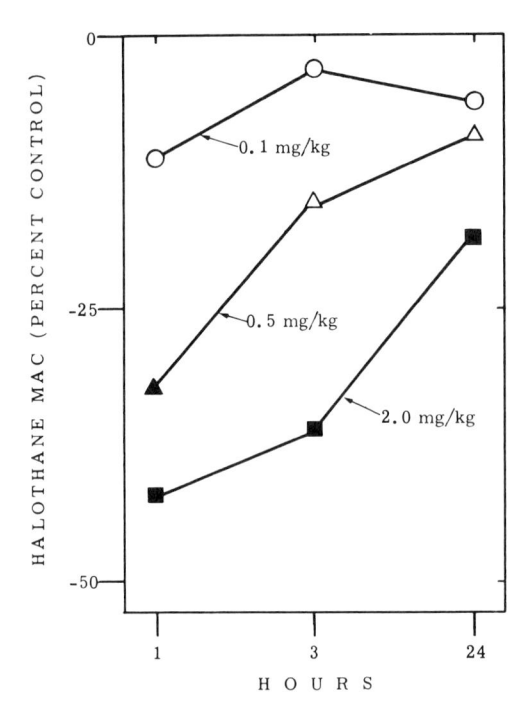

Fig. 26-12. Alterations in MAC after administration of tetrahydrocannabinol plotted as percentage of change from control. (From Stoelting, R.K., et al.: Effects of delta-9-tetrahydrocannabinol on halothane MAC in dogs. Anesthesiology, 38:523, 1973.)

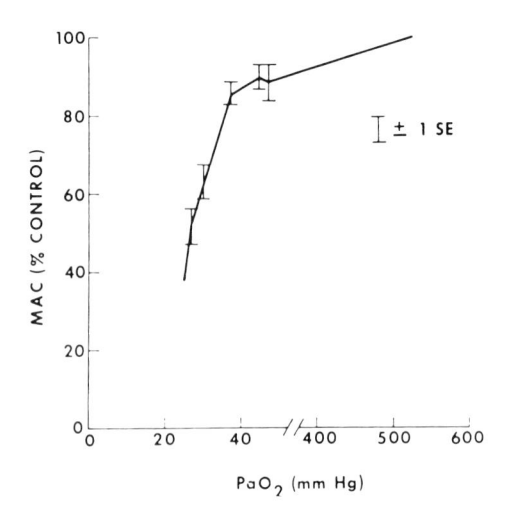

Fig. 26-13. MAC did not change significantly until arterial Pa_{O_2} decreased below 38 mm Hg. Thereafter, a precipitous decrease in MAC developed.

haps further studies with vecuronium, a more lipid soluble muscle relaxant which could penetrate the blood-brain barrier in greater amounts than pancuronium will shed further light on this interesting observation.

Atropine and Scopolamine: Although atropine has not been shown to affect MAC, large doses of scopolamine, 0.48 mg/kg, cause a maximal decrease in MAC of 14% in rats.[29] Clinical relevance is doubtful because much smaller doses of scopolamine are used for preanesthetic medication in man.

Tetrahydrocannabinol: Vitez et al. calculated that cyclopropane MAC fell by 15% and 25% in rats given tetrahydrocannabinol (THC), 1 or 2 mg/kg IP (intraperitoneally), respectively.[30] THC, 0.5 mg/kg, decreases MAC by 32% 1 hour after injection with a return to control after 3 hours in dogs (Fig. 26-12).[31] This short-lived effect is compatible with clinical observations that analgesia, sedation, and prolonged barbiturate sleeping time occur following THC injections. Whether these effects are clinically important to man, in whom 0.05 mg/kg of THC yields the desired euphoria, cannot be determined.

Alcohol: Chronic ingestion of ethyl alcohol increases isoflurane MAC 30 to 45%,[31a] and increases halothane MAC approximately 33%.[31b]

INTERACTION OF ANESTHETIC DEPTH AND PATHOPHYSIOLOGIC CHANGES (TABLE 26-3)

Hypoxia reduces halothane MAC in dogs rapidly and progressively, beginning at Pa_{O_2} 38 mm Hg (Fig. 26-13).[32] This Pa_{O_2} is close to the level of 35 mm Hg in man, at which level consciousness is lost as a result of acute hypoxia. MAC decreases as metabolic acidosis develops when Pa_{O_2} is held constant at 30 mm Hg.[32] To explore the mechanism responsible for the reduction of MAC, brain surface electrodes were applied to the cerebral cortex of dogs during hypoxia. Cerebral extracellular fluid

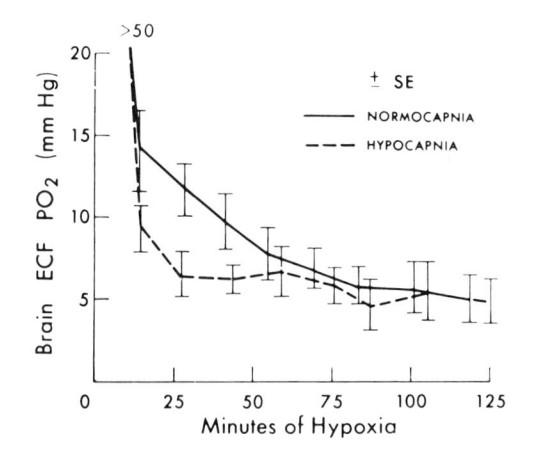

Fig. 26–14. Cerebral ECF P$_{O_2}$ decreased at Pa$_{O_2}$ 30 mm Hg and corresponded to a decrease in halothane MAC.

(ECF) Po_2 decreased to a range of 1 to 10 mm Hg when hypoxia to Pa$_{O_2}$ 30 mm Hg began (Fig. 26–14). After two hours of hypoxia, cerebral ECF pH decreased to 6.93 and cerebral ECF bicarbonate decreased to about 10 mEq/L (Fig. 26–15). Cerebral metabolic demand appears to exceed supply at this level of hypoxia, which in turn depresses MAC.[33]

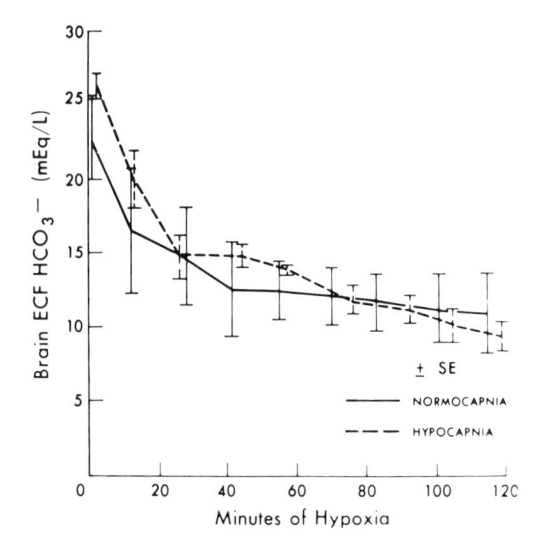

Fig. 26–15. Cerebral ECF bicarbonate values fell rapidly at Pa$_{O_2}$ 30 mm Hg in both hypocapnic and normocapnic dogs, and corresponded to a decrease in halothane MAC.

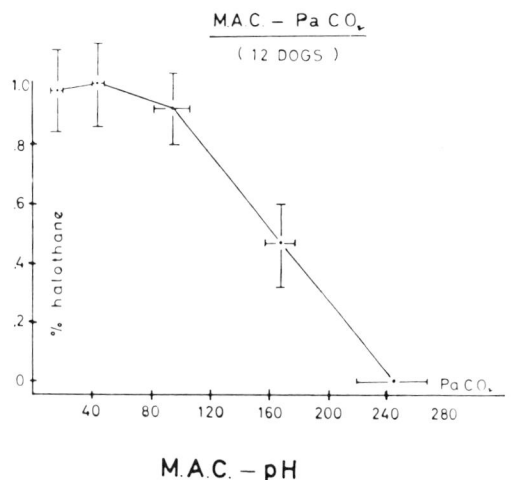

Fig. 26–16. Up to Pa$_{CO_2}$ 95 mm Hg, MAC is relatively constant. Above Pa$_{CO_2}$ 95 mm Hg, MAC declines progressively until CO$_2$ becomes fully anesthetic. (From Eisele, J.H., Eger, E.I., II, and Muallem, M.: Narcotic properties of carbon dioxide in the dog. Anesthesiology, 28:858, 1967.)

Carbon Dioxide

Within clinically relevant ranges, CO$_2$ has no effect on MAC. Until Pa$_{CO_2}$ levels above 95 mm Hg were achieved, MAC remained constant.[34] Above 95 mm Hg, Pa$_{CO_2}$ progressively reduced MAC and was completely anesthetic at 245 mm Hg (Fig. 26–16). When CSF pH fell below 7.1, MAC began to decrease; CO$_2$ became fully anesthetic at CSF pH of 6.8. The anesthetic potentiation by CO$_2$, however, is not pH dependent. Hypoxia studies showed that even when brain ECF pH was as low as 6.3, halothane MAC was above zero.[33] Perhaps CO$_2$ itself, or CO$_2$ plus decreased pH, is anesthetic at high concentrations. Despite the similarity of their physical properties, CO$_2$ is more potent than nitrous oxide, of which slightly more than one atmosphere is required for general anesthesia.

Hypocapnia to Pa$_{CO_2}$ 10 mm Hg, which maximally reduces cerebral blood flow, does not significantly reduce MAC,[35] despite the clinical impression that hyperventilated patients appear to be more deeply anesthetized than spontaneously breathing patients. Assuming equivalent alveolar anesthetic concentrations and time for cerebral equilibration, a possible mechanism for this observation is that hypocapnia abolishes spontaneous activity of the reticular formation, reducing afferent impulses to the cerebral cortex and to the phrenic nerve.[36]

Pregnancy

Although not a pathophysiologic disorder, pregnancy decreases the requirements for inhaled anesthetic agents.[37] Halothane MAC decreased 25%, methoxyflurane MAC 32%, and isoflurane MAC 40% in pregnant ewes. The decreased MAC may be related to the large increase in progesterone levels during late pregnancy. In addition to decreased MAC, uptake and distribution are more rapid in pregnant patients. If an anesthetic state is reached at a lower alveolar concentration, the dangers of aspiration and of airway obstruction are increased.

In summary, most drugs and clinical situations reduce the anesthetic requirement. Those few that increase the anesthetic requirement increase also CNS catecholamine levels. When all the variables that affect anesthetic requirement, such as age,[38] preoperative medication, anesthetic adjuvants, patient's illness, type of procedure, acid-base balance, oxygenation, temperature, and imprecise delivery systems, are taken into account, clinical signs of anesthesia must be closely observed to avoid anesthetic overdose or inadequate anesthesia. The time to test the depth of anesthesia is at the moment of surgical incision, when immediate responses are more evident, particularly in the nonparalyzed patient. Once an adequate anesthetic depth is assured, a relaxant can be given, if appropriate, and inspired anesthetic concentration can be gradually reduced until signs of light anesthesia appear. By observing the patient's clinical signs and by carefully manipulating the inspired concentration accordingly, the appropriate depth of anesthesia can be maintained despite the factors that affect MAC. These factors provide a frame of reference to guide the anesthetist, but the ultimate criterion is the patient's unique response to the balance between anesthetic depression and surgical stimulation.

REFERENCES

1. Eger, E.I., II: Anesthetic Uptake and Action. Baltimore, Williams & Wilkins, 1974, pp. 1–25.
2. Eger, E.I., II, Saidman, L.J., and Brandstater, B.: Minimum alveolar anesthetic concentration: A standard of anesthetic potency. Anesthesiology, 26:756, 1965.
2a. Yakaitis, R.W., Blitt, C.D., and Angiulo, J.P.: End-tidal halothane concentration for endotracheal intubation. Anesthesiology, 47:386, 1977.
2b. Yakaitis, R.W., Blitt, C.D., and Angiulo, J.P.: End-tidal enflurane concentration for endotracheal intubation. Anesthesiology, 50:59, 1979.
2c. Roizen, M.F., Horrigan, R.W., and Frazer, B.M.: Anesthetic doses blocking adrenergic (stress) and cardiovascular responses to incision—MAC BAR. Anesthesiology, 54:390, 1981.
3. De Jong, R.H., and Eger, E.I., II: MAC expanded: AD_{50} and AD_{95} values of common inhalation anesthetics in man. Anesthesiology, 42:384, 1975.
4. Eger, E.I., II: Anesthetic Uptake and Action. Baltimore, Williams & Wilkins, 1974, pp. 77–96.
5. De Jong, R.H., et al.: Anesthetic potency determined by depression of synaptic transmission. Anesthesiology, 29:1139, 1968.
6. Freund, F.G., Martin, W.E., and Hornbein, T.F.: The H reflex as a measure of anesthetic potency in man. Anesthesiology, 30:642, 1969.
7. Cullen, S.C., and Larson, C.P., Jr.: Essentials of Anesthetic Practice. Chicago, Yearbook Medical Publishers, 1974.
8. Cullen, D.J., et al.: Clinical signs of anesthesia. Anesthesiology, 36:21, 1972.
9. Miller, R.D., Way, W.L., and Eger, E.I., II: The effects of *alpha*-methyldopa, reserpine, guanethidine and iproniazide on minimum alveolar anesthetic requirement (MAC). Anesthesiology, 29:1153, 1968.
10. Johnston, R.R., Way, W.L., and Miller, R.D.: Alteration of anesthetic requirement by amphetamine. Anesthesiology, 36:357, 1972.
11. Johnston, R.R., Way, W.L., and Miller, R.D.: The effects of CNS catecholamine-depleting drugs on dextroamphetamine-induced elevation of halothane MAC. Anesthesiology, 41:57, 1974.
12. Stoelting, R.K., Creasser, C.W., and Martz, R.C.: Effect of cocaine administration on halothane MAC in dogs. Anesth. Analg. (Cleve.), 54:422, 1975.
13. Finck, A.D., Ngai, S.H., and Berkowitz, B.A.: Antagonism of general anesthesia by naloxone in the rat. Anesthesiology, 46:241, 1977.
13a. Harper, M.H., Winter, P.M., Johnson, B.H., et

al.: Naloxone does not antagonize general anesthesia in the rat. Anesthesiology, 49:3, 1978.
13b. Bennett, P.B.: Naloxone fails to antagonize the righting response in rats anesthetized with halothane. Anesthesiology, 49:9, 1978.
13c. Smith, R.A., Wilson, M., and Miller, K.W.: Naloxone has no effect on nitrous oxide anesthesia. Anesthesiology, 49:6, 1978.
13d. Duncalf, D., Nagashima, H., and Duncalf, R.M.: Naloxone fails to antagonize thiopental anesthesia. Anesth. Analg., 57:558, 1978.
13e. Chapman, C.R., and Benedetti, C.: Nitrous oxide effects of cerebral-evoked potential to pain: Partial reversal with a narcotic antagonist. Anesthesiology, 51:135, 1979.
14. Tanifuji, Y., and Eger, E.I., II: Brain sodium, potassium and osmolality. Effects on anesthetic requirements. In Abstracts of Scientific Papers. San Francisco, American Society of Anesthesiologists, 1976.
15. Steffey, E.P., and Eger, E.I., II: Hyperthermia and halothane MAC in the dog. Anesthesiology, 41:392, 1974.
16. Mueller, R.A., et al.: Central monaminergic neuronal effects on minimum alveolar concentrations (MAC) of halothane and cyclopropane in rats. Anesthesiology, 42:143, 1975.
17. Roizen, M.F., White, P.F., Eger, E.I., II, et al.: Effects of ablation of serotonin or norepinephrine brain-stem areas on halothane and cyclopropane MACs in rats. Anesthesiology, 49:252, 1978.
17a. Bloor, B.C., and Flacke, W.E.: Reduction in halothane anesthetic requirement by clonidine, an alpha-adrenergic agonist. Anesth. Analg., 61:741, 1982.
18. Tanifuji, Y., and Eger, E.I., II: Effect of isoproterenol and propranolol on halothane MAC in dogs. Anesth. Analg. (Cleve.), 55:383, 1976.
19. Laverty, R., and Taylor, K.M.: Propranolol uptake into the central nervous system and the effect on rat behavior and amine metabolism. J. Pharm. Pharmacol., 20:605, 1968.
20. Johnston, R.R., et al.: Effect of levodopa on halothane anesthetic requirement. Anesth. Analg. (Cleve.), 54:178, 1975.
20a. Maze, M., Mason, D.M., Jr., and Kates, R.E.: Verapamil decreases MAC for halothane in dogs. Anesthesiology, 59:327, 1983.
21. White, P.F., Johnston, R.R., and Pudwill, C.R.: Interaction of ketamine and halothane in rats. Anesthesiology, 42:179, 1975.
21a. Raja, S.N., Moscicki, J.C., and DiFazio, C.A.: Phencyclidine alters MAC: Possible mechanisms. Anesthesiology, 55:A223, 1981.
22. Blancata, L.S., Peng, A.T.C., and Alonsabe, D.: Intravenous lidocaine: adjunct to general anesthesia for endoscopy. N.Y. State J. Med., 70:1659, 1970.
23. DiFazio, C.A., Niederlehner, J.R., and Burney, R.G.: The anesthetic potency of lidocaine in the rat. Anesth. Analg. (Cleve.), 55:818, 1976.
24. Himes, R.S., DiFazio, C.A., Burney, R.G.: Effects of lidocaine on the anesthetic requirements for nitrous oxide and halothane. Anesthesiology, 47:437, 1977.
25. Saidman, L.J., and Eger, E.I., II: Effect of nitrous oxide and of narcotic pre-medication on the alveolar concentration of halothane required for anesthesia. Anesthesiology, 25:302, 1964.
26. Munson, E.S., Saidman, L.J., and Eger, E.I., II: Effect of nitrous oxide and morphine on the minimum anesthetic concentration of fluroxene. Anesthesiology, 26:134, 1965.
26a. Murphy, M.R., and Hug, C.C., Jr.: The anesthetic potency of fentanyl in terms of its reduction of enflurane MAC. Anesthesiology, 57:485, 1982.
26b. Hecker, B.R., Lake, C.L., DiFazio, C.A., et al.: The reduction in halothane MAC with sufentanil. Anesthesiology, 59:A341, 1983.
27. Perisho, J.A., Buechel, D.R., and Miller, R.D.: The effect of diazepam (Valium) on minimum alveolar anesthetic requirement (MAC) in man. Can. Anaesth. Soc. J., 18:536, 1971.
28. Stevens, W.C., et al.: Minimum alveolar concentrations (MAC) of isoflurane with and without nitrous oxide in patients of various ages. Anesthesiology, 42:197, 1975.
28a. Forbes, A.R., Cohen, N.J., and Eger, E.I., II: Pancuronium reduces halothane requirement in man. Anesth. Analg., 58:497, 1979.
29. Eger, E.I., II: Anesthetic Uptake and Action. Baltimore, Williams & Wilkins, 1974.
30. Vitez, T.S., et al.: Effects of delta-9-tetrahydrocannabinol on cyclopropane MAC in the rat. Anesthesiology, 38:525, 1973.
31. Stoelting, R.K., et al.: Effects of delta-9-tetrahydrocannabinol on halothane MAC in dogs. Anesthesiology, 38:521, 1973.
31a. Johnstone, R.E., Kulp, R.A., and Smith, T.C.: Effects of acute and chronic ethanol administration on isoflurane requirement in mice. Anesth. Analg., 54:277, 1975.
31b. Barber, R.E.: Anesthetic requirement in alcoholic patients. Abstracts of Scientific Papers, Annual Meeting of the American Society of Anesthesiologists, 1978, pp. 623–624.
32. Cullen, D.J., and Eger, E.I., II: Effects of hypoxia and isovolemic anemia on the halothane requirement (MAC) of dogs. I: The effect of hypoxia. Anesthesiology, 32:28, 1970.
33. Cullen, D.J., et al.: The effects of hypoxia and isovolemic anemia on the halothane requirement (MAC) of dogs. II: The effects of acute hypoxia on halothane requirement and cerebral-surface P_{O_2}, P_{CO_2}, pH, and bicarbonate. Anesthesiology, 32:35, 1970.
34. Eisele, J.H., Eger, E.I., II, and Muallem, M.: Narcotic properties of carbon dioxide in the dog. Anesthesiology, 28:856, 1967.
35. Cullen, D.J., and Eger, E.I., II: The effect of extreme hypocapnia on the anesthetic requirement (MAC) of dogs. Br. J. Anaesth., 43:339, 1971.
36. Bonvallet, M., Hugelin, A., and Dell, P.: Sensibilité comparée du système réticule activateur ascendant et du centre respiratoire aux gaz du sang et à l'adrenaline. J. Physiol. (Paris), 47:651, 1955.
37. Palahniuk, R.J., Shnider, S.M., and Eger, E.I., II: Pregnancy decreases the requirement for inhaled anesthetic agents. Anesthesiology, 41:82, 1974.
38. Gregory, G.A., Eger, E.I., II, and Munson, E.S.: The relationship between age and halothane requirement in man. Anesthesiology, 30:488, 1969.

39. Stoelting, R.K., Longnecker, D.E., and Eger, E.I., II: Minimum alveolar concentrations in man on awakening from methoxyflurane, halothane, ether, and fluroxene anesthesia. MAC awake. Anesthesiology, 33:5, 1970.
40. Viegas, O., and Stoelting, R.K.: Halothane MAC in dogs unchanged by phenobarbital. Anesth. Analg. (Cleve.), 55:677, 1976.
41. Tanifuji, Y., and Eger, E.I., II: Effect of arterial hypotension on anesthetic requirement in dogs. Br. J. Anaesth., 48:947, 1976.

|27|

AGENTS IN OBSTETRICS: MOTHER, FETUS, AND NEWBORN

MILTON H. ALPER and SANJAY DATTA

Perinatal pharmacology is basically complex, since it involves mother, fetus, placenta, labor, and neonatal adjustment to extrauterine life. Despite this complexity and the increased clinical concern, information on drug interactions in this area is limited. This is surprising because many factors in pregnancy and parturition may dispose a patient to untoward drug reactions and interactions. These factors include:

1. Multiplicity of drugs, both prescription and over-the-counter, consumed by pregnant patients. In one study, the mean number of drugs taken during pregnancy was 10.3, with a range of 3 to 29, excluding anesthetic agents, intravenous fluids, vitamins, iron, cigarette smoking, and exposure to pesticides, paint, or chemicals.[1] The drugs most frequently ingested included analgesics (chiefly salicylates), diuretics, antihistamines, antibiotics, antiemetics, antacids, and sedatives. That the unexpected may occur is exemplified by one patient who had been ingesting 25 five-grain tablets (7.5 g) of salicylate daily during pregnancy and who experienced respiratory arrest after receiving "a routine dose of sedative and analgesic agent" during labor. During the postpartum period profuse uterine bleeding necessitated a hysterectomy.

2. Physiologic changes in pregnancy, particularly in hormonal, cardiovascular, renal, and hepatic function, which may lead to alterations in drug disposition. Thus, drug effects during pregnancy may be different from those in nonpregnant patients.

3. Differences in fetal and neonatal drug sensitivity and pharmacokinetics in comparison with the mature organism.

Despite these factors, descriptions of drug interactions in pregnancy, in parturition, or in neonatal life are sparse. In this chapter, the physiologic and pharmacologic milieu of the perinatal period will not be reviewed in detail. Rather, we shall present several case reports of documented or suspected drug interactions that pertain specifically to the practice of obstetric analgesia and anesthesia. In each instance, the pharmacologic and physiologic background of the interaction will be reviewed.

OXYTOCICS, VASOPRESSORS, AND ANESTHESIA

Oxytocic agents are commonly used in obstetric patients for inducing or augmenting labor, for facilitating placental expulsion, and for enhancing contractions of the uterus post partum to reduce bleeding or to treat atony.[2-5] The clinically useful drugs are oxytocin and two ergot alkaloids, ergonovine and methylergonovine. The ergot alkaloids are less often used today because of the greater incidence of complications and because of insufficient evidence for their superiority to oxytocin.

Oxytocin (Pitocin) is a synthetic octapeptide, identical to the one normally present in and released from the posterior lobe of the pituitary gland, but free from contamination by other polypeptide hormones and proteins found in earlier natural preparations. Many of the complications described in the earlier literature were the result of the admixture of oxytocin with vasopressin (ADH), a potent octapeptide vasopressor and coronary artery vasoconstrictor. Pure synthetic oxytocin has some cardiovascular effects, but fewer than ADH, and is a specific stimulant of frequency and intensity of uterine contraction.

Ergonovine maleate (Ergotrate) and methylergonovine maleate (Methergine) differ from oxytocin in their effects on the uterus. Although the uterine effects of oxytocin closely resemble normal contractions, those induced by the ergot derivatives are of longer duration. Uterine tonus or baseline contractile tension is also increased. The use of ergot preparations therefore is limited to the postpartum period.

Oxytocin is more safely administered as an intravenous infusion, which can be prepared by diluting 10 IU (1.0 ml) in 1,000 ml of infusion fluid. During labor, infusion rates vary from 1 mU/min to 10 mU/min, administered with an infusion pump and with careful monitoring to detect signs of fetal distress. Postpartum rates of 20 mU to 100 mU/min may be used. Effects appear within 3 minutes, are maximal at about 20 minutes, and disappear within 15 to 20 minutes after discontinuing the infusion.

Ergot alkaloids are commonly given intramuscularly in a dose of 0.2 mg for the management of postpartum bleeding and uterine atony. Onset of activity occurs within 10 minutes, and increased uterine activity persists for 2 to 6 hours. The following report illustrates an interaction between oxytocics and a commonly administered vasopressor, ephedrine.

CASE REPORT

A 23-year-old woman received spinal anesthesia with tetracaine for an uncomplicated, low-forceps delivery. Prior to the administration of the anesthetic, she was given ephedrine, 25 mg, intramuscularly (IM) to prevent hypotension. Her blood pressure was stable during delivery at 110/70. Following the birth of a healthy child, she was given Methergine, 0.2 mg IM, in addition to a slow intravenous infusion of dilute oxytocin solution. Her blood pressure was 120/80 as she left the delivery room. Twenty minutes later, the patient complained of severe, throbbing fronto-occipital headache. Her systolic blood pressure was over 220 mm Hg. She was treated with serial injections of 2.5 mg of chlorpromazine intravenously to a total of 10 mg over 20 minutes. Her blood pressure decreased to 140/80, and her headache disappeared. She recovered uneventfully.

Cardiovascular Effects of Oxytocics

The cardiovascular side effects of oxytocic drugs in the obstetric patient have long been recognized. For example, in 1949 Greene and Barcham observed an increase in systolic blood pressure of 50 to 100 mm Hg in patients receiving both a vasopressor and an oxytocic agent.[6] In fact, one patient suffered hemiplegia. The most extensive report is that of Casady et al., who studied 741 women who received continuous caudal analgesia, prophylactic methoxamine when the block was initiated, and an oxytocic drug (either ergonovine or methylergonovine and/or oxytocin) at the time of delivery of the placenta.[7] Thirty-four of the 741 patients (4.6%) developed systolic blood pressures over 140 mm Hg post partum. One patient experienced a ruptured intracranial aneurysm. This incident led to the abandonment of the routine use of prophylactic vasopressor therapy.

Hypertension following the combined use of vasopressors and oxytocics is a serious drug interaction, although it is not totally predictable. All commonly used vasopressors, including ephedrine, presently the drug of choice in obstetrics with either the ergot or the posterior pituitary oxytocics, have been incriminated. Severe hypertension is particularly likely to occur in patients who are already mildly hypertensive and who receive an ergot alkaloid post partum. It is less frequently observed after the dilute intravenous infusion of oxytocin.

Most ergot alkaloids exert complex actions on the cardiovascular system; of chief concern is peripheral vasoconstriction by direct action on vascular smooth muscle. The ergot alkaloids display a spectrum of activity characteristic of partial agonists in that they may both stimulate and block *alpha*-adrenergic receptors. Ergonovine and methylergonovine are devoid of *alpha*-receptor blocking activity and are weak vasoconstrictors, but they are additive in their effects with the vasopressors, ephedrine and phenylephrine.[8]

Oxytocin also has complex cardiovascular effects, including vasoconstriction and thereby hypertension, which is more pronounced after surgical or chemical blockade of sympathetic pathways.[9] This block is an inevitable concomitant of major conduction anesthesia.

It is wise to avoid the routine use of vasopressors, particularly since they are rarely necessary. Hypotension may often be prevented by intravenous fluid therapy and by uterine displacement. Persistent hypotension can be treated with ephedrine, which will not decrease uterine blood flow. If any vasopressor has been used, ergot alkaloids are best avoided in favor of a slow intravenous infusion of dilute oxytocin with careful monitoring of blood pressure to detect the first sign of hypertension. If the use of ergot alkaloids is necessary, intramuscular rather than intravenous injection is advisable. If hypertension does occur, therapy should be promptly begun. Chlorpromazine has proved to be both safe and effective when given intravenously in a dose of 2.5 mg every 15 to 20 seconds until acceptable levels of blood pressure are reached; the total dose required is usually 10 to 15 mg. Nitroprusside should be effective, but it has not received the extensive clinical use that chlorpromazine has.

In addition to the well-defined hazards associated with their use with vasopressors, oxytocics may also interact dangerously with anesthetic agents. Lipton and co-workers in 1962 demonstrated the lack of significant cardiovascular effects when *dilute* synthetic oxytocin was administered during general anesthesia.[10] This observation has been confirmed in both animals and humans. In contrast, concentrated intravenous bolus injections of either natural or synthetic oxytocin may cause hypotension, tachycardia, and dysrhythmias, particularly with halothane.[11-15] These effects are transient, lasting five to ten minutes, and are due to peripheral vasodilation. Although usually well tolerated by healthy patients, these cardiovascular responses may be dangerous to patients with hypovolemia or with intrinsic heart disease.[13,14]

By contrast, the intravenous injection of ergonovine or of methylergonovine has been associated with more serious reactions from intense vasoconstriction, such as hypertension, convulsions, cerebrovascular accidents, and retinal detachment.[7,13,16,17] These drugs should not be used in patients with preeclampsia, hypertension, or cardiac disease.

Recently, Moodie and Moir could detect no difference in blood loss in parturient patients who were receiving either ergonovine or oxytocin during continuous lumbar epidural analgesia.[18] The incidence of nausea, vomiting, or retching was 46% after ergonovine and nil after oxytocin. These data combined with the cardiovascular side effects described suggest that oxytocin is most safely administered by dilute intravenous infusion by a pump rather than by intravenous bolus injection, and that the use of ergot alkaloids should be restricted, probably to the management of postpartum uterine atony.

Other Effects of Oxytocin

The possibility of a different type of interaction involving oxytocin has been suggested by Davies and his co-workers, who observed that total bilirubin levels were higher in two- and five-day-old infants whose mothers were subjected to artificially induced labor by amniotomy followed immediately by intravenous oxytocin infusion.[19] In contrast, infants born after spontaneous labor augmented by oxytocin and those born after spontaneous labor without oxytocin showed no evidence of hyperbilirubinemia. The researchers postulated that the elevated bilirubin levels were due to the higher incidence of drug administration during artificially induced labor and delivery. They were particularly concerned about nitrazepam, a benzodiazepine sedative, and bupivacaine, for epidural analgesia. Although no direct association between the use either of these drugs or of oxytocin and neonatal hyperbilirubinemia is known, labor of spontaneous onset is associated with higher umbilical cord cortisol levels than induced labor.[20] Epidural block in labor prevents the usual rise in maternal cortisol levels.[21] Perhaps the liver enzymes induced by corticosteroids are low also in artificially induced labor followed by epidural analgesia, which may leave the fetal liver at a metabolic disadvantage with respect to the action of hepatic enzymes required to cope with the early postnatal bilirubin load. This interesting and provocative hypothesis requires further study.

Finally, Hodges and his associates in 1959 observed prolonged neuromuscular blockade from succinylcholine in a group of patients who had received oxytocin infusions for from eight hours to five days.[22] They suggested that the effects of succinylcholine are enhanced in such patients, possibly as the result of oxytocin-induced redistribution of potassium at the neuromuscular junction. Experiments in animals and in man failed to confirm Hodges's observations, although slightly elevated potassium levels were measured in man.[23,24] It seems likely that the altered response to succinylcholine resulted from other changes associated with prolonged labor rather than from the use of oxytocin.

MAGNESIUM SULFATE AND ANESTHESIA

The hypertensive disorders of pregnancy are hazardous to both mother and fetus. Despite intensive investigation and detailed characterization of the pathophysiology of preeclampsia and eclampsia, their cause remains unknown and their treatment empirical.[25,26] Toxemia probably occurs in 6 to 7% of pregnancies and is responsible for about 20% of all maternal deaths and for a perinatal mortality rate of 15 to 30%.

The anesthetic management of patients with hypertensive disorders of pregnancy is controversial. Regional anesthesia, particularly lumbar epidural block, and general anesthesia have been recommended for both vaginal delivery and cesarean section. If general anesthesia is selected, endotracheal intubation should be performed and neuromuscular blocking drugs are likely to be used. In these patients, a common drug interaction occurs between magnesium and neuromuscular blocking drugs, as illustrated in the following case report from the literature.[27]

CASE REPORT

A 24-year-old woman with preeclampsia was treated with phenobarbital, hydralazine, and magnesium sulfate (60 g intramuscularly in divided doses over 14 hours). Three hours after the last injection of magnesium sulfate, anesthesia for cesarean section was induced with thiopental, succinylcholine (50 mg), nitrous oxide, and oxygen, followed by 30 mg of *d*-tubocurarine to control ventilation. At the end of the operation, despite the usual measures, the neuromuscular block could not be reversed. Ten milliliters of calcium gluconate, 10%, caused some improvement, but the patient required artificial ventilation for 8 hours.

Pharmacology of Magnesium Sulfate

Parenterally administered magnesium sulfate is still the mainstay for the management of the toxemic patient. A common approach is to inject 20 ml of magnesium sulfate, 20% (4 g), intravenously over 3 minutes, followed immediately by 10 ml of 50% solution (5 g) injected deeply intramuscularly into each buttock. The latter injection is administered every 4 hours thereafter if the patellar reflex is present, if urine flow has been at least 100 ml in the previous 4 hours, and if respiration is not depressed.[28] If convulsions persist, sodium amobarbital is administered, up to 0.25 g, in small intravenous increments. If the patient's diastolic blood pressure remains over 110 mm Hg, hydralazine is administered intravenously in divided doses up to a total of 5 to 20 mg until the diastolic pressure falls to about 100 mm Hg. No maternal deaths occurred in the 154 patients with eclampsia who were so treated. Seventy-seven percent of the patients delivered vaginally and 23% by cesarean section. All fetuses survived who were alive when treatment was started and who weighed at least 1,800 g (4 pounds) when delivered.

The magnesium ion is normally present in plasma in a concentration of 1.5 to 2.2 mEq/L. When its concentration exceeds 4 to 5 mEq/L, following parenteral administration, deep tendon reflexes diminish. They disappear at concentrations of approximately 10 mEq/L. At 12 to 15 mEq/L, respiratory paralysis may ensue as well as electrocardiographic changes such as heart block.

Magnesium salts were at one time thought to be central nervous system depressants capable of producing general anesthesia. In 1916, Peck and Meltzer described three operations in patients who received no drugs other than magnesium sulfate.[29] In 1966, Somjen and co-workers disproved this notion by administering magnesium sulfate to two human volunteers sufficient to achieve blood levels of 14.6 and 15.3 mEq/L.[30] Both subjects were profoundly paralyzed and appeared anesthetized but remained conscious, in contact with their surroundings, sensitive to painful stimuli, and showed no evidence of depression of the central nervous system. The observations of Peck and Meltzer remain unexplained.

The major effect of excess magnesium ion is the suppression of peripheral neuromuscular function by a decrease in the amount of acetylcholine released from motor nerve terminals in response to nerve impulses.[31] Magnesium also decreases the sensitivity of the end-plate to applied acetylcholine as well as the direct excitability of muscle fibers themselves. Experimentally increasing the concentration of calcium antagonizes the action of magnesium at nerve terminals and restores neuromuscular transmission. In addition, from the point of view of fetal well-being, studies in monkeys have shown that magnesium decreases mean arterial blood pressure and increases uterine blood flow.[32]

Neuromuscular Blockers and Magnesium

The anesthetic implications of magnesium therapy in the obstetric patient were first described by Morris and Giesecke in 1968. They noted a decreased requirement for succinylcholine in a group of patients undergoing cesarean section after magnesium sulfate therapy for toxemia.[33]

In a subsequent study in cats, Giesecke et al. reported that, although only 1/1,000 as potent as *d*-tubocurarine at the neuromuscular junction, magnesium sulfate enhanced the neuromuscular blockade from both *d*-tubocurarine and succinylcholine.[34] Ghoneim and Long reported similar findings in the rat, except that *d*-tubocurarine and decamethonium were enhanced approximately fourfold and succinylcholine only twofold.[27] The lesser degree of potentiation of succinylcholine may be the result of its more rapid destruction in the presence of elevated magnesium concentrations since cholinesterase activity is enhanced by magnesium.[35] (See Chapter 23.)

In spite of a possible prolonged block in patients treated with magnesium, muscle relaxants are too convenient to use to be simply omitted. We believe that the dangers of induction by inhalation anesthesia in these seriously ill obstetric patients outweigh the hazards posed by the potentiation of neuromuscular blockade. It is probably safer to avoid or to reduce the dose of the long-acting nondepolarizing relaxants. Certainly the 30 mg of *d*-tubocurarine described in the case report was excessive. Succinylcholine should be given at half the usual dose and with careful monitoring of neuromuscular function with a nerve stimulator. Although experimental magnesium-induced neuromuscular block can be antagonized by calcium, this is not so clinically.[31] The administration of calcium gluconate to two patients under these circumstances was ineffective.[27] The inability of calcium to antagonize completely a magnesium-induced neuromuscular block probably relates to the multiple actions of magnesium at the neuromuscular junction. At any rate, ventilatory support is required until the patient recovers spontaneously.

Other Effects of Magnesium

Magnesium, given intravenously, but not intramuscularly, may induce hypocalcemia in the mother and in the neonate.[36,37] In a study by Lipsitz, infants born after maternal intravenous therapy for 12 to 24 hours commonly showed signs associated with hypermagnesemia: flaccidity and hyporeflexia, respiratory depression, and a weak or absent cry.[38] The most severely affected infants required resuscitation and ventilatory support for 24 to 36 hours. In a large series of cases, Stone and Pritchard failed to find significant fetal or neonatal effects after the intramuscular regimen described above.[39] This probably means that central nervous system and blood levels were lower when magnesium was given intramuscularly instead of intravenously.

Magnesium sulfate is being used more frequently as a uterine muscle relaxant and labor suppressant. In a recent case report, an infant born to a magnesium-treated mother suffered from hypotonia and hyporeflexia. At 12 hours of age, she was treated with gentamicin and stopped breathing. Subsequent animal experiments demonstrated a marked potentiation of neuromuscular blockade by a combination of hypermagnesemia and aminoglycoside antibiotics.[39a]

Finally, Alexander and co-workers reported no cardiovascular problems in the anesthetic management of 14 eclamptic patients who underwent cesarean section after large doses of reserpine and/or hydralazine.[40] The interaction between antihypertensive agents and anesthesia is covered in detail elsewhere in this volume.

TOCOLYTIC AGENTS

Prematurity is the leading cause of perinatal mortality and morbidity. Tocolytic agents, used to stop premature labor, inhibit uterine contraction by (1) preventing myometrial response to internal or external stimuli, e.g., *beta*-sympathomimetics, methylxanthines, prostaglandin inhibitors or (2) decreasing stimulus input to the uterus, e.g., ethanol.

The *beta*-sympathomimetics have entered widespread use for this purpose. In particular, ritodrine and terbutaline, agents with predominantly beta 2-receptor effects, have been extensively applied in an attempt to control labor while minimizing maternal and fetal cardiovascular and metabolic side effects.[40a,b,c,d] Large doses of these drugs can cause severe maternal tachycardia with hypotension and presumably decreased cardiac output and placental perfusion.[40e] Of further concern to the anesthesiologist is the possible induction of hyperglycemia with an associated increase in plasma insulin levels which may result in hypokalemia.

An interesting interaction is illustrated in the following case report.

CASE REPORT

A 30-year-old woman, gravida 2, para 1, at 29 weeks gestation with a twin pregnancy was admitted to the hospital in active labor. The cervix was 3 cm dilated and 80% effaced. The patient received terbutaline, 0.25 mg, subcutaneously and betamethasone, 12 mg, intramuscularly. Over the next 60 hours, the patient received 8 more doses of terbutaline and 2 more doses of betamethasone. Sixty-four hours after admission, her contractions increased in frequency with progressive cervical dilatation. The patient suddenly developed shortness of breath with bilateral wheezing and basilar rales. Chest roentgenogram confirmed bilateral pulmonary infiltrates, and the diagnosis of pulmonary edema was made. Vaginal delivery was performed successfully under epidural anesthesia. The patient was treated with fluid restriction and oxygen with resolution of her pulmonary edema over the next several hours.

The occurrence of pulmonary edema following the use of *beta*-sympathomimetics with or without corticosteroids is now well documented.[40f,g,h] Its mechanism remains unclear.

INTERACTIONS IN THE FETUS AND NEONATE

Fetal pharmacology is a new area of investigation, especially in humans. Anesthesiologists have long recognized that most drugs used for obstetric analgesia and anesthesia cross the placental barrier. Despite a better understanding of the pharmacokinetics of maternal-fetal drug transfer and increased sophistication in the measurement of fetal drug effects, no instances of drug interaction have been noted. One expects that such interactions will be detected eventually.

In the past, more concern has been voiced over the effect of maternally administered drugs on the newborn, who must make the major homeostatic adjustments required for the transition from intrauterine to extrauterine life. At the same time, the neonate is deprived of the umbilical connection to his mother and must cope with whatever drug load he has "inherited" during parturition.

Transplacentally acquired drugs may influence the neonate's physiologic adaptations, particularly respiration, circulation, and thermoregulation; conversely, these major functional changes may themselves influence drug distribution and effects in the newborn. As pointed out in recent reviews,[41-48] our knowledge of drug disposition in the newborn is limited, but it suggests that there are profound differences from older children and adults, so much so that the neonate has been termed a "unique drug recipient."[47] Some of the factors that account for these differences are listed in Table 27–1.

All of the factors listed in Table 27–1 may account for drug effects that may be both quantitatively and qualitatively different in the neonate from those effects in older children and adults. Several drug interactions of interest to the anesthesiologist have been described in the neonate.

Of particular significance in the newborn is the ability to handle an important endogenous substrate, bilirubin.[49,50] Drugs may interfere with the disposition of bilirubin in two ways: either by competing for binding sites on neonatal plasma protein or by altering hepatic enzyme systems responsible for bilirubin metabolism.

Bilirubin is transported in neonatal blood in two forms, conjugated and unconjugated. Unconjugated, lipid-soluble bilirubin is 99% bound to plasma albumin, hence limiting its access to the brain. Unbound unconjugated bilirubin is able to penetrate the brain; if sufficient concentration is achieved in the brain, bilirubin encephalopathy or kernicterus results. Any factor that decreases the binding of unconjugated bilirubin to its albumin binding sites increases the risk of encephalopathy. Clinically, this is more likely to be important in infants who are premature or who are faced with abnormally high bilirubin loads after delivery.[50]

Some drugs compete with bilirubin for

Table 27-1
Factors affecting drug disposition in the neonate

1. Developmental age and state of maturation
   a. organ development
   b. sensitivity of drug receptors
2. Reduced esterase activity
3. Plasma protein binding
   a. reduced protein concentration
   b. qualitatively different albumin
   c. high concentrations of bilirubin and free fatty acids
   d. lower blood pH
   e. competition for binding sites by both endogenous and exogenous substrates
   f. increased apparent volume of drug distribution
4. Drug distribution
   a. changing pattern of regional blood flows
   b. relatively greater brain and liver mass
   c. lower myelin content of brain
   d. higher total body water and extra/intracellular water content ratio
   e. scanty adipose tissue
5. Biotransformation
   a. immaturity of certain hepatic enzyme systems
   b. enzyme induction or inhibition
6. Reduced renal function

plasma protein binding sites in the newborn.[51] Perhaps the best-known example is sulfisoxazole (Gantrisin), whose administration to the neonate is associated with an increased frequency of kernicterus in both animals and human beings. Of particular concern to the anesthesiologist is parenteral diazepam (Valium). Schiff and co-workers in 1971 demonstrated *in vitro* that injectable diazepam was a potent displacer of bilirubin from plasma proteins. However, sodium benzoate in the buffer preservative was found to be the displacer, not the diazepam.[52] This finding correlated well with previous observations of the displacing activity of caffeine sodium benzoate, an analeptic drug formerly used as a respiratory stimulant in the newborn with depressed ventilation. Recently, another component of drug mixtures, methylparaben, frequently used as a preservative in local anesthetic solutions, in injectable saline, and in bacteriostatic water, has also been shown to have similar displacing activity.[53]

Since injectable diazepam is frequently used as an adjunct during labor, concern was expressed about bilirubin displacement in both the fetus and the neonate. However, Adoni and co-workers in 1973 demonstrated no alterations in bilirubin binding capacity of blood in the umbilical cord from infants whose mothers received diazepam during labor.[54] Benzoate probably either is unable to cross the placenta or is so rapidly metabolized by the maternal liver that significant concentrations are not achieved in the fetus. However, injectable diazepam must be used with caution in the neonate with hyperbilirubinemia. The ability of other analgesics and anesthetics to modify bilirubin-albumin binding in the neonate has not been systematically studied.

A second area of concern is that of drug-induced alterations in fetal and neonatal metabolism of various substrates, including bilirubin. The best-known example is the prenatal administration of phenobarbital to the mother with resultant accelerated conjugation of bilirubin through induction of the hepatic enzyme, glucuronyltransferase. Under these conditions, lower bilirubin levels in the neonate have been demonstrated.[44] Since over 200 enzyme inducers have been identified, the metabolism of exogenous substrates and drugs may be affected.

Clinically, Morselli and his associates have documented the effects of both phenobarbital administration to the mother and maturity of the newborn on the latter's ability to clear diazepam from the bloodstream.[55] The plasma half-life of diazepam was 18 ± 3 (SE) hours in children aged 4 to 8 years and 75 ± 37 hours with a range of 38 to 120 hours in four prematurely born infants (28 to 34 weeks). In a group of full-term newborns whose mothers had received diazepam within 24 hours of delivery, the plasma half-life averaged 31 ± 2 hours. The most striking finding was an average half-life of diazepam of 16 ± 2.5 hours in three full-term newborns whose mothers received phenobarbital for at least eight days before delivery and diazepam within 24 hours of delivery. The researchers infer that the phenobarbital treatment of the mothers accelerated the disposition of diazepam in these full-term newborns to the level observed in the older children.

Treatment of pregnant rats and rabbits with phenobarbital during the last week of pregnancy results in accelerated metabolism of both pentobarbital and meperidine in the newborn.[56] Although not studied during pregnancy, the treatment of calves with phenobarbital resulted in a faster disappearance of thiopental from their bloodstream and a decrease in the duration of postanesthetic depression.[57] Further examples of enzyme induction of specific clinical significance to obstetric anesthesia will undoubtedly appear.

Finally, Drew and Kitchen reported the influence of some 20 different maternally administered drugs on total bilirubin levels in over 1,000 infants at 48 and 72 hours of age.[58] They found that maternal administration of meperidine was associated with lower bilirubin levels in the newborn. Maternal diazepam administration was associated with slightly higher levels; various phenothiazine derivatives, regional anesthesia, and general anesthesia had no effect. In general, the magnitude of the changes was not great and their clinical significance was doubtful, except perhaps in infants at risk for hyperbilirubinemia.

Despite the hypothetically fertile physiologic grounds for drug interactions in the fetus and neonate as the result of maternally administered analgesics and anesthetics, reactions of clinical significance have not been described. One may, however, infer that as perinatal pharmacology develops further, such interactions will most likely be identified, especially in infants at risk.

REFERENCES

1. Hill, R.M.: Drugs ingested by pregnant women. Clin. Pharmacol. Ther., *14*:654, 1973.
2. Munsick, R.A.: The pharmacology and clinical application of various oxytocic drugs. Am. J. Obstet. Gynecol., *93*:442, 1965.
3. Pauerstein, C.J.: Ecbolic agents. Clin. Anesth., *10*:299, 1973.
4. Rall, T.W., and Schliefer, L.S.: Oxytocin, prostaglandins and ergot alkaloids. *In* The Pharmacologic Basis of Therapeutics. 7th Ed. Edited by A.G. Gilman, L.S. Goodman, T.W. Rall, and F. Murod. New York, Macmillan, 1985, pp. 867–880.
5. Brenner, W.E.: The oxytocics: actions and clinical indications. Contemp. OB/GYN, *7*:125, 1976.
6. Greene, B.A., and Barcham, J.: Cerebral complications resulting from hypertension caused by vasopressor drugs in obstetrics. N.Y. State J. Med., *49*:1424, 1949.
7. Casady, G.N., Moore, D.C., and Bridenbaugh, D.L.: Postpartum hypertension after use of vasoconstrictor and oxytocic drugs. J.A.M.A., *172*:1011, 1960.
8. Munson, W.M.: The pressor effect of various vasopressor-oxytocic combinations: a laboratory study and a review. Anesth. Analg. (Cleve.), *44*:114, 1965.
9. Lloyd, S., and Pickford, M.: The action of posterior pituitary hormones and oestrogens on the vascular system of the rat. J. Physiol., *155*:161, 1961.
10. Lipton, B., Hershey, S.G., and Baez, S.: Compatibility of oxytocics with anesthetic agents. J.A.M.A., *179*:410, 1962.
11. Nakano, J., and Fisher, R.D.: Studies on the cardiovascular effects of synthetic oxytocin. J. Pharmacol., *142*:206, 1963.
12. Andersen, T.W., et al.: Cardiovascular effects of rapid intravenous injection of synthetic oxytocin during elective cesarean section. Clin. Pharmacol. Ther., *6*:345, 1965.

13. Hendricks, C.H., and Brenner, W.E.: Cardiovascular effects of oxytocic drugs used post partum. Am. J. Obstet. Gynecol., 108:751, 1970.
14. Weis, F.R., and Peak, J.: Effects of oxytocin on blood pressure during anesthesia. Anesthesiology, 40:189, 1974.
15. Weis, F.R., et al.: Cardiovascular effects of oxytocin. Obstet. Gynecol., 46:211, 1975.
16. Gombos, G.M., Howitt, D., and Chen, S.: Bilateral retinal detachment occurring in the immediate postpartum period after methylergonovine and oxytocin administration. Eye Ear Nose Throat Mon., 48:680, 1969.
17. Abouleish, E.: Postpartum hypertension and convulsion after oxytocic drugs. Anesth. Analg. (Cleve.), 55:813, 1976.
18. Moodie, J.E., and Moir, D.D.: Ergometrine, oxytocin and extradural analgesia. Br. J. Anaesth., 48:571, 1976.
19. Davies, D.P., et al.: Neonatal jaundice and maternal oxytocin infusion. Br. Med. J., 2:476, 1973.
20. Ohrlander, S., Gennser, G., and Eneroth, P.: Plasma cortisol levels in human fetus during parturition. Obstet. Gynecol., 48:381, 1976.
21. Buchan, P.C., Milne, M.K., and Browning, M.C.K.: The effect of continuous epidural blockade on plasma 11-hydroxycorticosteroid concentrations in labour. J. Obstet. Gynaecol. Br. Commonw., 80:974, 1973.
22. Hodges, R.J.H., et al.: Effects of oxytocin on the response to suxamethonium. Br. Med. J., 1:413, 1959.
23. Keil, A.M.: Effects of oxytocin on the response to suxamethonium in rabbits, sheep, and pigs. Br. J. Anaesth., 34:306, 1962.
24. Ichiyanagi, K., Ito, Y., and Aoki, E.: Effects of oxytocin on the response to suxamethonium and d-tubocurarine in man. Br. J. Anaesth., 35:611, 1963.
25. Pritchard, J.A., and MacDonald, P.C.: Williams Obstetrics. 15th Edition. New York, Appleton-Century-Crofts, 1976.
26. Speroff, L.: Toxemia of pregnancy: mechanism and therapeutic management. Am. J. Cardiol., 32:582, 1973.
27. Ghoneim, M.M., and Long, J.P.: The interaction between magnesium and other neuromuscular blocking agents. Anesthesiology, 32:23, 1970.
28. Pritchard, J.A., and Pritchard, S.A.: Standardized treatment of 154 consecutive cases of eclampsia. Am. J. Obstet. Gynecol., 123:543, 1975.
29. Peck, C.H., and Meltzer, S.J.: Anesthesia in human beings by intravenous injection of magnesium sulphate. J.A.M.A., 67:1131, 1916.
30. Somjen, G., Hilmy, M., and Stephen, C.R.: Failure to anesthetize human subjects by intravenous administration of magnesium sulfate. J. Pharmacol., 154:652, 1966.
31. del Castillo, J., and Engbaek, L.: The nature of the neuromuscular block produced by magnesium. J. Physiol., 124:370, 1954.
32. Harbert, G.M., Cornell, G.W., and Thornton, W.N.: Effect of toxemia therapy on uterine dynamics. Am. J. Obstet. Gynecol., 105:94, 1969.
33. Morris, R., and Giesecke, A.H.: Magnesium sulfate therapy in toxemia of pregnancy. South. Med. J., 61:25, 1968.
34. Giesecke, A.H., et al.: Of magnesium, muscle relaxants, toxemic parturients and cats. Anesth. Analg. (Cleve.), 47:689, 1968.
35. Nachmanson, D.: Action of ions on cholinesterase. Nature, 145:513, 1940.
36. Monif, G.R.G., and Savory, J.: Iatrogenic maternal hypocalcemia following magnesium sulfate therapy. J.A.M.A., 219:1469, 1972.
37. Savory, J., and Monif, G.R.G.: Serum calcium levels in cord sera of the progeny of mothers treated with magnesium sulfate for toxemia of pregnancy. Am. J. Obstet. Gynecol., 110:556, 1971.
38. Lipsitz, P.J.: The clinical and biochemical effects of excess magnesium in the newborn. Pediatrics, 47:501, 1971.
39. Stone, S.R., and Pritchard, J.A.: Effect of maternally administered magnesium sulfate on the neonate. Obstet. Gynecol., 35:574, 1970.
39a. L'Hommedieu, C.S., et al.: Potentiation of magnesium sulfate-induced neuromuscular weakness by gentamicin, tobramycin and amikacin. J. Pediatr., 102:629, 1983.
40. Alexander, J.A., et al.: Cesarean section in the eclamptic patient on antihypertensive therapy: a review of fourteen cases. South. Med. J., 57:1282, 1964.
40a. Barden, T.P., Peter, J.B., and Merkatz, I.R.: Ritodrine hydrochloride: a betamimetic agent for use in preterm labor. Obstet. Gynecol., 56:1, 1980.
40b. Spellacy, W.M., Crux, A.C., Bink, S.A., et al.: Treatment of premature labor with ritodrine: a randomized controlled study. Obstet. Gynecol., 54:220, 1979.
40c. Persson, H., and Olsson, T.: Some pharmacological properties of terbutaline (INN), 1-(3,5 dihydroxy phenyl)-2-(t-butylamino)-ethanol: a new sympathomimetic β receptor-stimulating agent. Acta Med Scand, 512(suppl):11, 1970.
40d. Andersson, K.E., Bengtsson, L.P.H., and Gustafson, I.: The relaxing effect of terbutaline on the human uterus during labor. Am. J. Obstet. Gynecol., 121:602, 1975.
40e. Knight, J.: Labour retarded with beta-agonist drugs. Anaesthesia 32:639, 1977.
40f. Stubblefield, P.G.: Pulmonary edema occurring after therapy with dexamethasone and terbutaline for premature labor: a case report. Am. J. Obstet. Gynecol., 132:321, 1978.
40g. Tinga, D.J., and Aaroudse, J.G.: Postpartum pulmonary edema associated with preventive therapy for premature labor. Lancet, 1:1026, 1979.
40h. Benedetti, T.J., Hargrove, J.C., and Rosene, K.A.: Maternal pulmonary edema during premature labor inhibition. Obstet. Gynecol., 59:33S, 1982.
41. Yaffe, S.J., ed.: Symposium on pediatric pharmacology. Pediatr. Clin. North Am., 19:1, 1972.
42. Ecobichon, D.J., and Stephens, D.S.: Perinatal development of human blood esterases. Clin. Pharmacol. Ther., 14:41, 1973.
43. Dancis, J., and Hwang, J.C.: Perinatal Pharmacology: Problems and Priorities. New York, Raven Press, 1974.

44. Eriksson, M., and Yaffe, S.J.: Drug metabolism in the newborn. Annu. Rev. Med., 24:29, 1973.
45. Yaffe, S.J., and Juchau, M.: Perinatal pharmacology. Annu. Rev. Pharmacol., 14:219, 1974.
46. Gillette, J.R., and Stripp, B.: Pre- and postnatal enzyme capacity for drug metabolite production. Fed. Proc., 34:172, 1975.
47. Morselli, P.L.: Clinical pharmacokinetics in the neonate. Clin. Pharmacokinetics, 1:81, 1976.
48. Yaffe, S.J.: Developmental factors influencing interactions of drugs. Ann. N.Y. Acad. Sci., 281:90, 1976.
49. Odell, G.B.: The distribution and toxicity of bilirubin. Pediatrics, 46:16, 1970.
50. Dodson, W.E.: Neonatal metabolic encephalopathies, hypoglycemia, hypocalcemia, hypomagnesemia, and hyperbilirubinemia. Clin. Perinatol., 4:131, 1977.
51. Stern, L.: Drug interactions—Part II. Drugs, the newborn infant, and the binding of bilirubin to albumin. Pediatrics, 49:916, 1972.
52. Schiff, D., Chan, G., and Stern, L.: Fixed drug combinations and the displacement of bilirubin from albumin. Pediatrics, 48:139, 1971.
53. Rasmussen, L.F., Ahlfors, C.E., and Wennberg, R.P.: The effect of paraben preservatives on albumin binding of bilirubin. J. Pediatr., 89:475, 1976.
54. Adoni, A., et al.: Effect of maternal administration of diazepam on the bilirubin-binding capacity of cord blood serum. Am. J. Obstet. Gynecol., 115:577, 1973.
55. Morselli, P.L., et al.: Drug interactions in the human fetus and newborn infant. In Drug Interactions. Edited by P.L. Morselli, S.N. Cohen, and S. Garattini. New York, Raven Press, 1974.
56. Pantuck, E., Conney, A.H., and Kuntzman, R.: Effect of phenobarbital on the metabolism of pentobarbital and meperidine in fetal rabbits and rats. Biochem. Pharmacol., 17:1441, 1968.
57. Sharma, R.P., Stowe, C.M., and Good, A.L.: Alteration of thiopental metabolism in phenobarbital-treated calves. Toxicol. Appl. Pharmacol., 17:400, 1970.
58. Drew, J.H., and Kitchen, W.H.: The effect of maternally administered drugs on bilirubin concentrations in the newborn infant. J. Pediatr., 89:657, 1976.

INDEX

Page numbers in *italic* indicate figures; page numbers followed by *t* indicate tables.

AB-132, 396
Abdominal surgery, inhalation anesthetic agents in, 353
Abortion, possible, in case report analysis, 14*t*
Absorption, of *beta*-adrenergic blocking agents, 118, 119*t*
   of local anesthetic agents, 391-392, *392*
Abstinence syndrome(s), acute. *See* Acute abstinence syndrome
   from buprenorphine, 329
Acetaldehyde, accumulation of, from disulfiram, 75
   as paraldehyde metabolite, 297-298
   production of, 75
   trichloroethanol and, 290
Acetazolamide, action of, antiepileptic, 253
   as carbonic anhydrase inhibitor, 213
   dosage of, antiepileptic, 247*t*, 253
   half-life of, 247*t*, 253
   indications for use of, 213
   pharmacokinetics of, 247*t*, 253
   renal effects of, 213
   side effects of, 213
   sites of action of, 213, *215*
Acetaminophen, biotransformation of, 64
   substitution of for aspirin, 9
Acetylcholine, actions of, 24
   as neurotransmitter, 170
   cardiac effects of, 161-162
     mechanism of, 227
   discovery of, 161
   duration of action of, 25
   effects of, 161-162
   hydrolysis of, 161-162
   in autonomic nervous system physiology, 148, *148*
   in drug interactions with magnesium, 205
   in hypermagnesemia, 204
   in interaction of furosemide and d-tubocurarine, 365
   interaction of, with diazepam, 296
     with inhalation anesthetic agents, 370
     with ketamine, 372
     with lithium carbonate, 276
     with local anesthetic agents, 402
     with magnesium sulfate, 372, 431
     with muscarinic cholinolytic agents, 165-166
     with pancuronium, 380
     with polymyxin B, 367
   muscarine and, 161
   nicotine and, 161
   release of, anticholinesterase agents and, 164
   response to, 24
   synthesis of, 161
Acetylcholine analog(s), 24
Acetylcholinesterase, interaction of, with anticholinergic agents, 395
   with echothiophate, 395
   with neostigmine, 377
Acid(s), 4-amino-2-chloroprocaine, 401
   carbamic, esters of, 164
   carbonic, dissociation of, 52
     formation of, 210
   dipropylacetic. *See* Valproic acid
   ethacrynic. *See* Ethacrynic acid
   folic, phenytoin and, 248
   gamma amino butyric. *See* Gamma amino butyric acid
   glucuronic, pentobarbital and, 64
   ionization of, 51-53
   lactic, epinephrine and, 87
   mandelic, monoamine oxidase and, 73
   para-aminobenzoic, 398, 404
   trichloroacetic, 297
   uric, 218
   valproic. *See* Valproic acid
   vanillylmandelic, 75*t*
Acid-base balance, barbiturates and, 285
   digitalis toxicity and, 190, 193
   local anesthetic agents and, 400
Acidemia, morphine in, 59
Acid-forming salt(s), 212-213
Acidification, renal, 399
Acidifying salt(s), 212-213
Acidosis, amphetamine metabolism in, 60
   effects in, of lidocaine, 394-395
     of local anesthetic agents, 394-395
   effects of, 395
     on epinephrine, 87
     on halothane, 422-423, *422*
     on neuromuscular blocking agents, 381
   from acetazolamide, 213
   from ammonium chloride, 212-213
   from hypoglycemic agents and ethyl alcohol, 290
   hyperventilation as treatment of, 56
   hypothermia-induced, 92
   interaction in, of neuromuscular blocking agents and narcotics, 381-382
   of d-tubocurarine and neostigmine, *382*
   potassium levels in, 220
   serum calcium concentration and, 200
Actin, calcium and, 198
Action potential(s), cardiac. *See* Cardiac action potential(s)
   nerve, in sympathetic neuroeffector junction, 114, *115*
Active transport, in nephron, *209*
   of sodium, renal tubular, 208, *209*, *210*
Activity, triggered, defined, 227
Acute abstinence syndrome, from nalbuphine, 330
   from naloxone, 326*t*, 328
   from pentazocine, 330
   in narcotic addiction, 321
Acute myocardial infarction, treatment of, nitroglycerin in, 143
   propranolol in, 119
AD$_{95}$, defined, 409, 411
Addiction, drug. *See* Drug addiction
   narcotic. *See* Narcotic addiction
Addition, defined, 3-4, 26
   dose, 3-4
   effect, 3-4
Adenosine, interaction of, with diazepam, 296
   with theophylline, 102
Adenosinemonophosphate, calcium and, 138, 140, 199
   inotropic effect of digitalis and, 184*t*
Adenosinetriphosphatase, in digitalis toxicity, 181
   in myocardial contractility, 198-199
   inotropic effect of digitalis and, 182-183, 184*t*
   interaction of with cardiac glycosides, 199
Adenosinetriphosphate, calcium transport and, 197
Adenyl cyclase, in sympathetic neuroeffector junction, 114
Adhesion, platelet, 142
Adjuvant anesthetic agent(s), purpose of, 16
Adrenalectomy, 369
Adrenalin. *See* Epinephrine
Adrenergic agent(s), 88*t*
Adrenergic amine(s), 86-87, 88*t*, 89-91

439

Adrenergic receptor(s), classification of, 115-116, *117*
  defined, 114
  in autonomic nervous system physiology, 147-148, *148*
  in sympathetic neuroeffector junction, 114-115, *115*
  stimulation of, causes of, 120
  subtype selectivity in, *beta*-adrenergic blocking agents and, 116-118, 118*t*
Adrenocorticotropic hormone, after adrenalectomy, 369
  after hypophysectomy, 369
  in myasthenia gravis, 369
  interaction of, with narcotic antagonists, 336
    with phenothiazines, 265
Adrenolytic agent(s), 348
Aerosol(s), bronchodilatory, 108-109
  dosage of, 109
  intraoperative, 109
Affinity, drug-receptor, defined, 24-25
  intensity of effect and, 40
Afterdepolarization(s), cardiac, 227-228
Afterpotential(s), cardiac, 184
Age, anesthetic regimen and, 13, 14*t*
  atracurium and, 384
  digitalis and, 186-188
  drug dosage and, 42-43
  thiopental dosage and, 46
  d-tubocurarine and, 379
  vecuronium and, 384
Agonism, defined, 24-25
Agonist(s), *beta*-adrenergic receptor, 114-115
  dose-response curves to, *25*
  duration of action of, 25
Agranulocytosis, from captopril, 157
  from carbamazepine, 250
  from phenytoin, 248
Akineton. *See* Biperiden
Albumin, binding by, of barbiturates, 284
  calcium binding to, 200
  hepatic dysfunction and, 397
  hypocalcemia and, 200
  in protein binding of drugs, 44-45
  osmotic pressure exerted by, 208
Albuterol, 108*t*
Alcohol, ethyl. *See* Ethyl alcohol
Alcoholism, anesthesia in, general, 291
  induction of, 349
  benzodiazepines in, 289
  disulfiram in treatment of, 75
  drug tolerance in, 288
    inhalation anesthetic, 349
  ethyl alcohol metabolism in, 288
Aldactone. *See* Spironolactone
Aldehyde, 290
Aldomet. *See Alpha*-methyldopa; Methyldopa
Aldosterone, in renal salt and water regulation, 211
  interaction of with spironolactone, 214
  secretion of, 211
  sodium restriction and, 211
Aldosterone antagonist(s), 24
Alfentanil, as induction agent, 350
  chest wall rigidity from, 322
  interaction of with midazolam, 317
Alkalemia, 59

Alkalinization of urine, in treatment of drug overdose, 58
Alkalinizer(s), 286
Alkaloid(s), belladonna. *See* Belladonna alkaloid(s); specific agents
Alkalosis, acid-forming salts in treatment of, 213
  amphetamine metabolism in, 60
  from diuretics, 213-214
  in hypokalemia, 219
  in shock, 92-94
  interaction in of d-tubocurarine and neostigmine, *382*
  neuromuscular blocking agents and, 381-382
  serum calcium concentration and, 200
Alkylating agent(s), 378
Alkylphosphate(s), interaction of, with chlorcyclizine, 44
  with local anesthetic agents, 396
  with phenobarbital, 44
  receptor binding of, 49
Allergic drug reaction(s), 32-34
  to theophylline, 103
Alpha-adrenergic blocking agent(s), 148*t*, 151*t*, 155-156
  dosage of, 148*t*
  indications for use of, 156
    in intraoperative hypertension, 342
  interaction of with antipsychotic agents, 264
    with guanethidine, 155
    with ketamine, 310
    with monoamine oxidase inhibitors, 272
    with morphine, 324
  interactions of, 24-27
  mechanism of action of, 27, 340-341
  pharmacology of, 155-156
Alpha-adrenergic receptor(s), actions and interactions of, 86
  calcium transport and, 198
  classification of, 86, 115-116
  in autonomic nervous system physiology, 147-148, *148*
Alpha-adrenergic stimulating agent(s), in treatment of myocardial depression, 346
  interaction of, with calcium-channel blocking agents, 346
    with phenothiazines, 79, 348
Alpha-adrenergic stimulation, causes of, 120
Alpha-methyldopa, actions of, 75-76
  hypotension from, 76
  in biosynthesis of catecholamines, 75*t*, 75-76
  indications for use of, 76
  interaction of, with halothane, 342, 415*t*, 416-417, *417*
    with norepinephrine, 73, 340-341, *417*
    with thiazide diuretics, 217
  mechanism of action of, 340-341
  pharmacology of, 152-153
  See also Methyldopa
Alpha-methyldopamine, 152
Alpha-methylnorepinephrine, 152, 341
Alpha-methyl-para-tyrosine, interaction of with halothane, 414
Alpha-methyl-p-tyrosine, in biosynthesis of catecholamines, 75*t*

Alphaxalone-alphadolone, interaction of with lithium carbonate, 276
Alprazolam, interaction of with cimetidine, 294
Aluminum hydroxide, digitalis toxicity and, 189
Aluminum silicate, inactivation of drugs by, 19
Alveolar gas, uptake of inhalation anesthetic agents and, 20
Amiloride, interaction of with digoxin, 217
  site of action of, 214, *215*
Amiloride-hydrochlorthiazide, interaction of with digitalis, 181
Amine(s), adrenergic, direct action of, 86-87, 88*t*, 89-91
  sympathomimetic. *See* Sympathomimetic amine(s)
4-Amino-2-chlorobenzoic acid, 401
Aminoglycoside antibiotic(s), effects of, toxic, 31
  interaction of, with diuretics, 221
    with ethacrynic acid, 218
    with neuromuscular blocking agents, 30-31
Aminophylline, cardiac effects of, 348
  composition of, 101-102, 102*t*
  dosage of, 103
  indications for use of, 348
  interaction of, with cephalothin, 19*t*
    with chloramphenicol, 19*t*
    with diazepam, 296
    with enflurane, 105, 349
    with erythromycin, 19*t*
    with halothane, 100-101, 105-106, 348-349
    with inhalation anesthetic agents, 348-349
    with isoflurane, 349
    with ketamine, 101, 106, 257
    with lithium carbonate, 277
    with pancuronium, 108
    with verapamil, 140
  intraoperative administration of, 107
  toxicity of, 349
  treatment of bronchospasm with, 34
4-Aminopyridine, interaction of, with antibiotics, 365
  with vecuronium, 376
Amiodarone, actions of, 239
  cardiac effects of, 231
  indications for use of, 239
  interaction of with digitalis, 188
  side effects of, 239
Amitriptyline, as agent with anticholinergic activity, 172*t*
  conversion to nortriptyline of, 47*t*
  indications for use of, 268
  interaction of, with atropine, 270
    with calcium, 202
    with clonidine, 269
    with enflurane, 270
    with ethyl alcohol, 287-288
    with ketamine, 269
    with lidocaine, 270
    with meperidine, 269
    with monoamine oxidase inhibitors, 80
    with morphine, 269
    with neostigmine, 270
    with procaine, 270

Ammonium, quaternary. *See* Quaternary ammonium
Ammonium benzoate, 404
Ammonium chloride, 212-213
Amoxapine, actions of, 270
Amphetamine, actions of, 81
  indirect, 87
  dissociation of, 56
  excretion of, pH and, 59, 60
  in opiate anesthesia, 2
  interaction of, with anesthetic agents, 81
    with barbiturates, 285
    with chlorpromazine, 81
    with halothane, 414, 415t
    with monoamine oxidase inhibitors, 80, 272
    with norepinephrine, 73, 414
    with reserpine, 266
  ionization of, 56
  overdosage of, 81
  toxicity of, 81
Amphotericin B, indications for use of, 189
  interaction of, with digitalis, 189
    with diphenhydramine, 19t
    with penicillin G, 19t
    with tetracyclines, 19t
Amtriptyline, interaction of, with lidocaine, 403
  with procaine, 403
Analgesia, from narcotics, 321
  in anesthesia, 16
  in wounded soldiers, 40
  quantitation of, 323
  reversal of, from interaction of narcotics and naloxone, 335-336
Analgesic(s), interaction of with monoamine oxidase inhibitors, 80
  narcotic. *See* Narcotic analgesic(s); specific agents
Analog(s), theophylline, 102
Anaphylaxis, characteristics of, 33
  drug antagonism in, 26-27
  epinephrine-resistant, calcium in treatment of, 201
  in anesthesia, 32-34
Anemia, aplastic, from carbamazepine, 250
  from phenytoin, 248
  hemolytic, from methyldopa, 152
  megaloblastic, from phenytoin, 248
Anesthesia, anticholinesterase agents in, 164
  antipsychotic agents in, history of, 262
  as continuum, 411
  "balanced," 1, 2
  beta-adrenergic blocking agents in, initial concerns regarding, 114
    preoperative discontinuance of, 128-132, 131-132, 132t
    rationale for caution with, 121-128, 120, 121t, 122-127, 126t, 127t, 129
  calcium in, 196-202
  cardiac dysrhythmia incidence in, 225
  cholinergic agents in, 166-170
  clinical signs of, anesthetic depth and, 412-413, 413-414
  components of, 16

conduction. *See* Conduction anesthesia
corticosteroids in, 110
defined, 409
depth of. *See* Anesthetic depth
digitalis in, influences on, 180-182
digitalis toxicity during, 179-182
dissociative. *See* Dissociative anesthesia
drug changes during, narcotics and, 330
drug interactions in, with digitalis, 179-193
effects of, on glomerular filtration rate, 203-204
epidural. *See* Conduction anesthesia
hepatic necrosis as sequela of, 67-68
historical background on, 255-256
hypermagnesemia in, 205
hypertension in, 149
hypotension during, causes of, 87, 91-92
  treatment of, 88t, 92-94
in asthmatics, 100-110, 102t, 104t, 108t
in drug-dependent patients, 29-30
in epilepsy, general, 255-257
  procedure for, 254-255
in hyperkalemia, 93-94
in hypertensive patients, procedure for, 342
in hypokalemia, 93
in obstetrics, toxemia and, 431-432
in patients receiving nitroglycerin, 143
in patients taking antihypertensive agents, 79
in patients taking diuretics, preoperative evaluation of, 218
induction of. *See* Induction of anesthesia
inorganic cations in, 196-205
magnesium in, 204-205
modern, basis of, 16
multiple-drug, rationale for, 16
opiate, principles of, 2
potassium in, 204
regional. *See* Regional anesthesia
shock during, causes of, 91-92
  treatment of, 92-94
single-agent, disadvantages of, 16
sodium in, 202-204
spinal. *See* Conduction anesthesia
Anesthesiologist(s), anesthetic depth assessment by, 411-413
  preoperative assessment by, 10, 12-15, 14t
  responsibilities of, drug interactions and, 9-11
  unique role of in medicine, 17-18
Anesthetic agent(s), cardiac effects of, 82-83, 83t, 169, 228
  classification of, by catecholamine release, 124-125
  effects of, in hypovolemia, 203
  fixed, hepatic interactions in, 66
    volatile versus, 68
  general. *See* General anesthetic agent(s)
  halogenated, in hyperkalemia, 204
  in ischemic heart disease, propranolol and, 125-126
  inhalation. *See* Inhalation anesthetic agent(s)

interaction of, with amphetamine, 81
  with anticholinergic agents, 167-172
  with antihypertensive agents, 6-7, 148-155, 151t
  with antipsychotic agents, 261t, 263-264
  with aspirin, 427
  with atropine, 171-172
  with *beta*-adrenergic blocking agents, 124-128, 129
  with bretylium, 225, 239
  with calcium-channel blocking agents, 140-142
  with clonidine, 7, 153
  with digitalis, 184, 188, 216
  with disulfiram, 75
  with diuretics, 216, 220
  with ergot alkaloids, 429
  with glycopyrrolate, 167
  with guanethidine, 151t, 154-155
  with hydralazine, 156
  with hydroxyzine, 167
  with magnesium sulfate, 430-432
  with methyldopa, 151t, 152-153
  with monoamine oxidase inhibitors, 80, 270t, 271-275
  with nitroglycerin, 143
  with oxytocic agents, 429-430
  with preanesthetic agents, 28, 283-284, 349
  with propranolol, 7, 78-79, 225, 236, 238
  with rauwolfia, 76-77
  with reserpine, 76-77, 151-152, 151t
  with scopolamine, 171
  with tricyclic antidepressants, 268-270
  with verapamil, 225
  intravenous. *See* Intravenous anesthetic agent(s)
  intravenous induction, 349-350
  local. *See* Local anesthesia
  multiple, single versus, 16
  potency of, cardiac effects and, 29
  physicochemical properties and, 28-29
  time sequence of administration of, drug interactions and, 29-30
  volatile, fixed versus, 68
Anesthetic depth, clinical signs of, 412-413
  drug interactions and, case report of, 407-409
  effects on, of carbon dioxide, 423-424, 423
  of pathophysiologic changes, 416t, 422-424, 422-423
  "Goldilocks" assessment of, 413
  hypotension and, from d-tubocurarine, 379, 380
  in pregnancy, 416t, 424
  interaction of general anesthetic agents and, 413-414, 415t, 416-419, 422, 417-422
  interpatient variations in, 411-413, 424
  manipulation of, 413, 424
  pain response and, 283, 409
  quantitation of, central nervous system effects and, 411, 412
  dose-response curve in, 409, 410t, 411, 411

Aspirin, interaction of *(cont.)*
  with diuretics, 220
  with indomethacin, 41
  with nifedipine, 139
  with spironolactone, 217
  with thiopental, 46
  with verapamil, 139
Asthma, anesthesia in, 13, 14*t*, 100-110, 102*t*, 104*t*, 108*t*
  corticosteroids in, 109-110
  inhalation anesthetic agents in, 106-107
  ketamine in, 105-106
  muscle relaxants in, 107-108
  premedication in, 104-105
  sympathomimetic bronchodilators in, 108-109, 108*t*
  theophylline in, 101-108, 102*t*, 104*t*
  atenolol indications in, 123
  beta-adrenergic blocking agents in, 123
  bronchospasm in, from endotracheal intubation, 348
  cardiac dysrhythmias in, 106-108
  catecholamines in, 108-109, 108*t*
  corticosteroids in, 109-110
  defined, 100
  incidence of, 110
  intraoperative, aminophylline in, 107
  preoperative evaluation in, 110
  seizures in, 106
  sympathomimetic bronchodilators in, 108-109, 108*t*
  treatment of, 100
    aminophylline in, 348
    anticholinergic agents in, 168
    common drugs in, 110
    corticosteroids in, 100, 109
    sympathomimetic agents in, 100, 108-109
    theophylline in, 100, 102
Asthma-Dor, as anticholinergic antimuscarinic agent, 171*t*
Atenolol, cardioselectivity of 117, 118*t*, 343
  dosage regimen of, 118
  indications for in asthmatics, 123
  pharmacology of, 118, 119*t*
Ativan. *See* Lorazepam
Atony, uterine, 428-429
Atracurium, age and, 384
  cardiac effects of, 384-385
  developmental chemistry of, 383
  dosage of, 383-384
  duration of action of, 383
  effects of, cumulative, 383-384
    reversibility of, 375-376
  elimination of, 383-385
  half-life of, 384
  in liver disease, 385
  in renal disease, 385
  interaction of, with anticholinesterase agents, 375-376
    with edrophonium, 376
    with histamine, 384
    with inhalation anesthetic agents, 354, 374-375
    with isoflurane, 374
    with lithium carbonate, 276
    with neostigmine, 375-376
    with nitrous oxide, 374
    with succinylcholine, 375
  metabolites of, 383, 384*n*

neuromuscular transmission blocked by, 163
  obstetric use of, 385
  pharmacokinetics of, 384
  potency of, 383
  side effects of, 165
Atrial fibrillation, digoxin in, verapamil and, 139
  from interaction, of digitalis and reserpine, 191
  treatment of, digitalis in, 179-180
    phenytoin in, 238
    procainamide in, 237
    quinidine in, 236
    verapamil in, 239
Atrial flutter, lidocaine in, 234
  treatment of, digitalis in, 179
    phenytoin in, 238
    quinidine in, 236
    verapamil in, 239
Atrioventricular conduction, digitalis and, 179, 183-185
  effect on, of amiodarone, 239
    of anticholinergic and cholinergic agents, 169-170
    of aprindine, 239-240
    of *beta*-adrenergic blocking agents, 343
    of calcium-channel blocking agents, 345
    of disopyramide, 238
    of mexiletine, 240
    of phenytoin, 238
    of procainamide, 237
    of propranolol, 238
    of quinidine, 236
    of verapamil, 239
Atropine, action of, on esophageal sphincter, 169
  agonist activity of, 25
  anesthetic premedication with, contraindications to, 166-169
  as belladonna alkaloid, 171*t*
  cardiac effects of, 27, 165-166
    during anesthesia, 168
  central anticholinergic syndrome from, 170-172
  cocaine and procaine compared with, 81, *81*
  effects of, acetylcholine and, 161
    central nervous system, 171
    delirium as, 172
    "sympathomimetic," 166
  fatal dose of, 171
  in "balanced" anesthesia, 2
  indications for use of, in intraoperative hypotension, 342
  in obstetric anesthesia, 169-170
  interaction of, with amitriptyline, 270
    with anesthetic agents, 171-172
    with anticholinesterases, 108
    with antiparkinsonian agents, 263
    with antipsychotic agents, 263
    with *beta*-adrenergic blocking agents, 27, 121, 123-125, 126*t*
    with chloroform, 166
    with cyclopropane, 415*t*, 422
    with diethyl ether, 166
    with digitalis, 187
    with dopamine, 86
    with halothane, 380
    with inhalation anesthetic agents, 415*t*, 422

with metoclopramide, 173
    with monoamine oxidase inhibitors, 274
    with morphine, 324
    with muscarinic cholinergic receptors, 24
    with nalbuphine, 332*t*
    with narcotic analgesics, 171, 324
    with narcotic antagonists, 336
    with neostigmine, 160, 169-171
    with neuromuscular blocking agents, 108
    with nitrous oxide, 168-169
    with norepinephrine, 166
    with other anticholinergic agents, 267-268
    with pancuronium, 367, 380, *381*
    with pharmacologic receptors, 24-25
    with physostigmine, 171-173, 295
    with propranolol, 27, 123-125, 126*t*, 344, 345
    with quaternary ammonium anticholinesterase agents, 171
    with reserpine, 266
    with succinylcholine, 168-169
    with *d*-tubocurarine, 364
    with vecuronium, 376
  physiologic antagonism and, 27
  preanesthetic, anesthetic depth and, 283
  psychiatric use of, 171
  response to, 24-25
  side effects of, problem secretions as, 167
  treatment of cardiac dysrhythmias with, 74
Autoimmune disease(s), drug reactions in, 32
Autonomic nervous system, divisions of, 147-148, *148*
  effects on, of calcium-channel blocking agents, 138-139, *140*
    of digitalis, 184-185
  function of, 148-150
  ganglion blocking agents in, 165
  nicotinic cholinolytic agents in, 165
  stability of, in anesthesia, 16
Availability, systemic, defined, 43
Azathioprine, indications for use of, 364
  interaction of, with neuromuscular blocking agents, 364-365, 371

"Balanced" anesthesia, 1-2
Banthine. *See* Methantheline
Barbiturate(s), abuses of, 284, 285
  biotransformation of, 64-65, 284-285
  distribution of, 284-285
  dosage of, lethal, 288-289
  drug tolerance from, 285
  effects of, antiepileptic, 246*t*, 248-249, 255-256
    central nervous system, 283, 285
    in hepatic disease, 284
    in hypovolemia, 203
  enzyme induction from, 67, 356
  historical background on, 255
  in multiple-drug therapy, 9
  interaction of, with alkalinizers, 286
    with alkylphosphates, 44
    with amphetamine, 285
    with anticholinergic agents, 268

INDEX 445

with anticoagulants, 43-44, 282, 285-286
with antihistamines, 298
with antipsychotic agents, 261t, 262-263
with aspirin, 284
with benzodiazepines, 289
with *beta*-adrenergic blocking agents, 285
with *beta*-carboline carboxylate esters, 293
with carbamazepine, 250
with central nervous system depressants, 286
with cephalothin, 19t
with chloramphenicol, 19t, 309
with chlorpromazine, 44, 262-263
with clonidine, 153
with contrast media, 309
with corticosteroids, 285
with coumarin, 285-286
with dicumarol, 44, 282
with digitalis, 44, 189, 286
with EPN, 44
with erythromycin, 19t
with ethyl alcohol, 287-289
with general anesthetic agents, 28
with halothane, 66
with inhalation anesthetic agents, 66, 349
with kanamycin, 19t
with ketamine, 257, 297
with lidocaine, 295
with lithium carbonate, 275t, 276-277, 309
with local anesthetic agents, 396-397, 397, 399-400
with malathion, 44
with monoamine oxidase inhibitors, 80, 157, 270t, 273, 347
with morphine, 323
with naloxone, 336
with narcotics, 323-324
with neuromuscular blocking agents, 370
with nortriptyline, 44
with opiates, 285
with oral contraceptives, 285
with parathion, 44
with phenothiazines, 286
with phenytoin, 248, 286
with picrotoxin, 292
with promethazine, 254
with quinidine, 286
with reserpine, 265t, 266
with scopolamine, 254
with sulfonamides, 284
with tetrohydrocannabinol, 298-299
with tricyclic antidepressants, 44, 268t, 269-270, 286
with trifluoperazine, 262-263
with valproic acid, 251
with warfarin, 44
pharmacokinetics of, 247t, 248-249
pharmacology of, 284-285
protein binding of, pH and, 59
routes of administration of, 284
substitution of other agents for, 9
tolerance to, in alcoholics, 288
un-ionized, actions of, 56
Baroreceptor(s), sensitization of, by digitalis, 184-185

Beclomethasone, indications for use of, 110
Belladonna alkaloid(s), anticholinergic antimuscarinic agents as, 171t
central anticholinergic syndrome from, 170-173
contraindications to, 166-167
preanesthetic, in epilepsy, 254
Benadryl. *See* Diphenhydramine
Benserazide, as decarboxylase inhibitor, 346
Benzocaine, toxicity of, pH and, 58-59
Benzodiazepine antagonist(s), 292-294
discovery of, 28
Benzodiazepines, antagonists of, 292-294
as central nervous system drugs, 28
binding sites of, 292-294
biotransformation of, 64
effects of, 312
central nervous system, 291-293
effects on, on muscle spasticity, 292
indications for use of, 291
interaction of, with anticoagulants, 286
with barbiturates, 289
with benzodiazepine antagonists, 293-294
with *beta*-carboline carboxylate esters, 293
with caffeine, 296-297
with digitalis, 182
with erganol, 289
with ethyl alcohol, 289-290
with gamma amino butyric acid, 292, 312-313
with general anesthetic agents, 28
with histamine H₂ blocking agent(s), 177
with inhalation anesthetic agents, 349
with ketamine, 257, 297
with lidocaine, 294-295
with meperidine, 295
with methylxanthines, 296-297
with muscarinic receptors, 24
with neuromuscular blocking agents, 297, 313
with normeperidine, 295
with pentobarbital, 292
with phenobarbital, 248
with phenytoin, 248
with physostigmine, 295-296
with picrotoxin, 292
with Ro 15-1788, 293-294
with valproic acid, 251, 296
with xanthines, 296-297
receptors to, 291-293
Benzothiadiazide(s), interaction of, with digitalis, 181, 189
Benztropine, as anticholinergic anti-Parkinson agent, 171t
indications for use of, 267
Benzylcholine, interaction of, with plasma cholinesterase, 395
Beta-adrenergic blocking agent(s), absorption of, 118, 119t
actions of, 77-78, 121, 122
administration of, intraoperative, 121-122, 124-126
anesthesia and, initial concerns regarding, 114
rationale for caution with, 121-128,

120, 121t, 122-127, 126t, 127t, 129
as antidysrhythmic agents, 230-231
available, 343
cardiac dysrhythmias with, reduced incidence of, 169
cardiac effects of, 78, 116-118, 118t, 343
calcium transport and, 200
in ischemic heart disease, 121, 121t, 122-123
catecholamine hypersensitivity induced by, 115, 116
classification of, 77-78
clinical applications of, 118-132, 119-120, 121t, 122-127, 126t, 127t, 129, 131-132, 132t
contraindications to, 123, 127
desensitization to, 42
digitalis toxicity treated with, 201
discontinuance of, rebound hypertension from, 342
dosage of, 118, 129, 131-132
drug interactions with, 78-79
effects of, in hyperkalemia, 204
local anesthetic, 231
elimination of, 78, 118, 119t
hypertension from, postoperative, 130-131
in asthma, 123
in cardiopulmonary bypass, 121-122
in heart failure, 123, 127
in ischemic heart disease, 121, 121t, 122-123
indications for use of, 78, 343
in asthma, 123
intraoperative, 121-122, 124-126
nonsurgical, 118-119
spurious, 118-119
interaction of, with anesthetic agents, 124-128, 129
with anticholinesterase, 27
with atropine, 27, 121, 123-125, 126t
with barbiturates, 285
with calcium, 201
with calcium chloride, 123, 126t
with calcium-channel blocking agents, 30, 139, 140
with catecholamines, 119-120, 120, 123, 127
with clonidine, 154
with cyclopropane, 125, 128, 129
with diazoxide, 158
with diethyl ether, 125, 128, 129
with digitalis, 124, 126t, 201, 345
with dobutamine, 124, 126t
with dopamine, 86, 124
with endotracheal intubation, 342, 344
with enflurane, 125-128, 129, 344
with epinephrine, 124, 126t
with gallamine, 121
with glucagon, 345
with halothane, 125-128, 129, 344
with hydralazine, 156
with inhalation anesthetic agents, 132, 342-345
with isoflurane, 125, 128, 129, 344
with isoproterenol, 124, 126t, 127t
with ketamine, 125, 310
with lidocaine, 398
with methoxyflurane, 125-128, 129, 343-344

Beta-adrenergic blocking agent(s), interaction of (cont.)
  with minoxidil, 157
  with monoamine oxidase inhibitors, 272, 348
  with morphine, 324
  with narcotics, 125-126, 128, 129
  with nifedipine, 139, 345
  with nitrous oxide, 125-126
  with opioids, 125
  with pancuronium, 121, 126
  with pharmacologic receptors, 24-26
  with potassium, 219, 220
  with prenalterol, 124, 126t
  with succinylcholine, 124, 125-126
  with thiopental, 125-126
  with trichloroethylene, 125, 128, 129, 344
  with verapamil, 139, 239, 345-346
 intrinsic sympathomimetic activity of, perioperative, 123, 132
 mechanism of action of, 341-343
 myocardial oxygen consumption and, 121, 121t
 overdosage of, calcium in treatment of, 201
 partial agonism by, 117, 118t
 postoperative inotropic support and, 130
 preoperative discontinuance of, 114, 128-132, 131-132, 132t
 properties of, 116-118, 118t
 prophylactic use of, 114, 129-130
 pure antagonism by, 117, 118t
 types of, 343
Beta-adrenergic receptor(s), actions of, 86, 115-116
 agonists of, 114-115
 antagonists of, 77-78, 114-115, 116
 calcium transport and, 198
 classification of, 86, 115-116, 342-343
 in autonomic nervous system, physiology of, 147-148, 148
 interaction of, with dopamine, 86
 mediators of, 114-115
 stimulation of, cardiac effects of, 115-116, 117
 effects of, 342-343
Beta-adrenergic stimulating agent(s), actions of, 108-109
 bronchodilatory effects of, 108-109, 108t
 indication for, 14t
 interaction of, with calcium-channel blocking agents, 138-139
  with corticosteroids, 110
  with halothane, 13
  with methylxanthines, 109
  with potassium, 219
Beta-carboline carboxylate ester(s), interactions of, 293
Beta-endorphin(s), opioid receptors and, 327t
Betamethasone, interaction of, terbutaline, 433
Beta-sympathomimetic agent(s), 432, 433
Bethanechol, clinical use of, 164
Bethanidine, interaction of, with tricyclic antidepressants, 27
Bicarbonate, cerebral extracellular fluid, 422-243, 423
 effect of, on phenobarbital distribution, 59
 loss of, 213

reabsorption of, furosemide and, 214
Biliary colic, from narcotics, 322
Bilirubin, interaction of, with caffeine sodium benzoate, 434
 with diazepam, 434-435
 with methylparaben, 434
 with phenobarbital, 434-435
 with sodium benzoate, 434
 with sulfisoxazole, 434
 neonatal, 433-435
 protein binding of, 41
Biotransformation, hepatic, 63-65, 66
 immune mechanisms in, 69
 in drug disposition, neonatal, 434t
 in pharmacokinetic drug interactions, 21-22
 of central nervous system drugs, 63
 of drugs, abnormal shunting of, 67
 of fixed drugs, 68
 of lipophilic drugs, chemical reactions in, 64-65
 of volatile drugs, 68
 oxidative, enzymes of, 65, 66
Biperiden, 171t
Bishydroxycoumarin, 297
Bittersweet, 171t
Block, celiac plexus. See Conduction anesthesia
Blood flow, cerebral, 142-144
 hepatic, histamine H$_2$ blocking agents and, 177
 pulmonary. See Pulmonary blood flow
 renal, 208
Blood pressure, anesthetic depth and, 412-413, 413
 effects on, of pancuronium, 380, 381
  of d-tubocurarine, 379, 380
 monitoring of, in shock, 92
 preoperative, in patients taking diuretics, 218
 antihypertensive therapy and, 342
 sympathetic nervous system and, 71
Bone marrow depression, from antiepileptic agents, 253
 from diuretics, 213
 from phenytoin, 248
 from trimethadione, 252
Bowman's capsule, plasma flow in, 208
Bradycardia, effects of, in anesthesia, 150
 from anticholinergic and anticholinesterase interaction, 169-170
 from anticholinesterase agents, 169-170
 from antihypertensive agents, 150, 341
 from cholinergic agents, 170
 from digitalis, 187
 from diltiazem, 138
 from guanethidine, 154
 from methoxamine, 90
 from methyldopa, 152
 from mexiletine, 240
 from muscarinic cholinolytic agents, 165
 from narcotics, 324, 350
 from nicotine, 163
 from phenylephrine, 90
 from propranolol, 120-121
 from succinylcholine, 168-169
 from timolol, 344

propranolol-associated, 123-124, 126t
 treatment of, 74
  anticholinergic agents in, 169
  pancuronium in, 324-325
Bretylium, actions of, 238-239
 dosage of, 239
 effects of, cardiac, 126, 230t, 231
  extracardiac, 230t
 indications for use of, 239
 interaction of, with anesthetic agents, 225, 239
  with digitalis, 239
  with neuromuscular blocking agents, 239
  with norepinephrine, 73, 238-239
  with vasopressors, 239
Bronchial obstruction, problem secretions and, 168
Bronchoconstriction, from beta-adrenergic blocking agents, 123
Bronchodilation, from beta-adrenergic stimulation, 148
 isoproterenol-induced, 89
 theophylline-induced, 102
Bronchodilator(s), interaction of, with inhalation anesthetic agents, 20
 sympathomimetic, 108-109, 108t
Bronchospasm, allergic, treatment of, 33-34
 anesthetic management of, 14t
 contraindication of propranolol in, 78
 corticosteroids in treatment of, 109-110
 from atropine and neostigmine interaction, 160
 from endotracheal intubation, in asthma, 348
 from neuromuscular blocking agent and anticholinesterase interaction, 108
 from timolol, 344
 inhibition of, by calcium-channel blocking agents, 142
 physiologic antagonism in, 27
Bumetanide, furosemide versus, 214
 interaction of, with digitalis, 181
Bupivacaine, effects of, neuromuscular, 402
 interaction of, with chloroprocaine, 401
  with desipramine, 394
  with dextran, 40, 392
  with epinephrine, 400
  with halothane, 400
  with lidocaine, 401
  with meperidine, 394
  with monoamine oxidase inhibitors, 274
  with nortoxiferine, 371
  with oxytocin, 430
  with phenytoin, 394
  with propranolol, 398
  with quinidine, 394
 protein binding of, 393-394
  diseases and, 46
 pulmonary extraction of, 398
 toxicity of, pH and, 58
Buprenorphine, 328-329, 330t
 as narcotic agonist-antagonist, 325t
 opioid receptors and, hypothetical interactions with, 327t
Burn(s), succinylcholine in, 204
Butorphanol, 329-331, 330t

as narcotic agonist-antagonist, 325t
opioid receptors and, hypothetical
   interactions with, 327t
Butoxamine, cardiac-sparing effects of,
   117
 interaction of, with norepinephrine,
   73
Butylcholinesterase, interaction of,
   with prednisone, 396
Butyrophenone(s), actions of, 18, 261-
   262
 contraindications to, 254
 indications for use of, 261
 interaction of, with anticholinergic
   agents, 261t, 263
  with clonidine, 153
  with dopamine, 347
  with inhalation anesthetic agents,
   349
  with methyldopa, 153
  with narcotic analgesics, 261t, 262
  with phenothiazines, 348
  with sympathomimetic agents,
   261t, 263
Butyrylcholinesterase, interaction of,
   with vecuronium, 375

Caffeine, effects of, anxiogenic, 296
 interaction of, with benzodiazepines,
   296-297
  with lorazepam, 296
  with procaine, 371
 theophylline compared to, 101
Caffeine sodium benzoate, 434
Calcium, binding to albumin of, 200
 blockade of, 135-139, 135t, 137
 cardiac effects of, 197-201
  therapeutic, 200-201
 channels of. See Calcium channel(s)
 concentration gradient of, 197
 in anesthesia, 196-202
  indications for use of, 196, 201
 intravenous preparations of, 202
 in cardiovascular cells, 135-139, 135t,
   137
 indications for use of, in citrate
   intoxication, 202
 in hyperkalemia, 202
 in treatment of myocardial
   depression, 346
 intraoperative, 196-197
 interaction of, with amitriptyline,
   202
  with antibiotics, 201, 365, 366t, 367
  with beta-adrenergic blocking
   agents, 201
  with calcium-channel blocking
   agents, 138-139, 346
  with catecholamines, 198
  with chlordiazepoxide, 296
  with curare, 205
  with decamethonium, 205
  with digitalis, 189, 201
  with diltiazem, 198
  with magnesium, 205, 431
  with methylxanthine, 198
  with monoamine oxidase
   inhibitors, 202
  with myocardial depressants, 201
  with neuromuscular blocking
   agents, 201, 205, 366t, 382
  with nifedipine, 198
  with pancuronium, 367

  with phenelzine, 202
  with phenytoin, 201
  with potassium, 201
  with procaine, 371
  with propranolol, 196-197, 345
  with succinylcholine, 205
  with sympathomimetic agents, 198
  with theophylline, 296
  with tranylcypromine, 202
  with tricyclic antidepressants, 202
  with d-tubocurarine, 366t
  with verapamil, 139, 198
 ions of, cardiac action potentials
   and, 226-227
  ethyl alcohol and, 287
  inotropic effect of digitalis and,
   182-183, 184t
 malignant hyperpyrexia and, 31
 metaraminol compared with, 201
 pharmacodynamic properties of,
   200-201
 physiologic role of, 197-201
 salts of, 202
 serum concentration of, 200
  in citrate intoxication, 202
 slow channel inhibition of, 135-139,
   135t, 137, 138t, 140
  mechanism of, 197-199
 treatment of hyperkalemia with, 204,
   220
Calcium channel(s), blockade of, 135-
   139, 135, 137
 defined, 198
 in ion transport, 197-201
Calcium chloride, interaction of, with
   beta-adrenergic blocking agents,
   123, 126t
  with propranolol, 123, 126t
Calcium gluconate, interaction of, with
   kanamycin, 19t
  with magnesium sulfate, 430-431
Calcium-channel blocking agent(s),
   action of, 30, 135-138, 135t, 137,
   138t
 reversal of, 138-139
 autonomic nervous system and, 138-
   139, 140
 available, 345
 cardiac effects of, 30, 137, 345-346
 cardiac pacemakers and, 139
 chelating agents versus, 135
 defined, 135
 discontinuance of, effects of, 142
 distribution of, drug interactions
   from, 139
 dosage titration of, 141
 hepatic dysfunction and, 139
 indications for use of, 136
 interaction of, with anesthetic
   agents, 140-142
  with beta-1 agonists, 138-139
  with beta-adrenergic blocking
   agents, 139, 140
  with calcium, 138-139
  with cardiac glycosides, 139-140
  with dantrolene, 142
  with dopamine, 138-139
  with endotracheal intubation, 346
  with epinephrine, 138
  with inhalation anesthetic agents,
   136, 141-142, 345-346
  with isoproterenol, 138
  with muscle relaxants, 142
  with narcotics, 141-142

  with potassium, 136, 140
  with propranolol, 78-79
  with theophylline, 140
 malignant hyperpyrexia treated
   with, 142
 mechanism of action of, 345
 metabolism of, drug interactions
   from, 139
 overdosage of, 139, 201
 physiologic effects of, 142
 potential interactions with, 30
 protein binding of, drug interactions
   from, 139
 Shy-Drager syndrome and, 139
 sick sinus syndrome and, 139
Calmodulin, defined, 197
 in calcium transport, 137, 197, 199
Cancer, cholinesterase levels in, 396
Cannabis, as enzyme inducer, 67
 extracts of, 299
 See also Tetrahydrocannabinol
Capillary(ies), in shock, 85
 peritubular, salt metabolism and,
   208
 schema of, 86
Capoten. See Captopril
Captopril, actions of, 157
 classification of, 148t
 dosage of, 148t
 indications for use of, 157
 interaction of, indomethacin, 157
  with potassium, 157
 mechanism of action of, 341
 pharmacology of, 157
 side effects of, 157
Carbachol, clinical use of, 164
 interaction of, with pancuronium,
   380
  with pharmacologic receptors, 24
Carbamate(s), organophosphates
   versus, 164
Carbamazepine, dosage of, 247t, 250
 indications for use of, 250
 interaction of, with anticoagulants,
   250
  with barbiturates, 250
  with epinephrine, 251
  with halothane, 251
  with propoxyphene, 251
 introduction of, 245, 246t
 pharmacokinetics of, 247t, 250-251
 side effects of, 250
 substitution of other agents for, 250
Carbamic acid, esters of, 164
Carbidopa, as decarboxylase inhibitor,
   346
Carbon dioxide, effects of, on
   anesthetic depth, 416t, 423-424,
   423
  on halothane, 416t, 423-424, 423
 epinephrine release induced by, 74
 in renal salt and water metabolism,
   210
 interaction of, with local anesthetic
   agents, 392, 400
  with prilocaine, 392
Carbon dioxide tension, lidocaine
   seizures and, 400
 nitrous oxide and, 351-352
Carbon tetrachloride, interaction of,
   with phenobarbital, 68
Carbonic acid, dissociation of, 52
 formation of, 210

Carbonic acid inhibitor(s), actions of, 213
Carbonic anhydrase, in renal salt and water metabolism, *209*, 210
  inhibitors of, 213
Cardiac action potential(s), defined, 225-226
  depolarization of, 225-227, *226*
  digitalis and, 182, 184
  physiology of, 199
Cardiac afterdepolarization(s), 227-228
Cardiac arrest, from anesthesia in renal failure, 220
  from interaction, of naloxone and narcotics, 336
    of potassium and digitalis, 191
Cardiac automaticity, abnormal, 227
  defined, 225-226
  normal, 226-227
Cardiac dysrhythmia(s), abnormal automaticity in, 227
  allergic, 33-34
  causes of, 31, 225
  conditions predisposing to, 168-169
  electrophysiology of, 225-228, *226*, *229*
  fatal, from digitalis and calcium, 189
  from abnormal automaticity, 227
  from anticholinergic agents, 169-170
  from atropine, 168
  from *beta*-adrenergic blocking agents, preoperative discontinuance of, 130, 132*t*
  from calcium-channel blocking agents, treatment of, 138-139
  from catecholamines, bronchodilatory, 108-109
  from cholinergic agents, 169-170
  from cocaine, epinephrine and, 82
  from conduction disturbances, 228
  from digitalis, 184-185, 187, 190, 192-193
  from disopyramide, 238
  from diuretics, potassium levels and, 215-217, 219-220
  from endotracheal intubation, 168, 342
  from epinephrine, 81-83, 83*t*
  from halothane, 71-72
  from hyperkalemia, 93-94, 204, 220
  from hypokalemia, 93, 204, 219-220
  from hypomagnesemia, 219-220
  from interaction, of antihypertensive agents and inhalation anesthetic agents, 341-342
    of atropine and neostigmine, 169
    of digitalis and calcium, 201
    of digitalis and diuretics, 215-216
    of digitalis and reserpine, 191
    of digitalis and succinylcholine, 191-192
    of halothane and aminophylline, 100-101, 348-349
    with tricyclic antidepressants, 269
  from levodopa, 346
  from maprotiline overdosage, 271
  from mercurial diuretics, 213
  from ouabain, lidocaine metabolites in treatment of, 403, *403*
  from phenothiazines, 264
  from physostigmine, 296
  from reserpine, electroconvulsive therapy and, 266
  from succinylcholine, in hyperkalemia and renal failure, 216-217
  from sympathomimetic agents, 82-83, 83*t*, 354-355
  from sympathomimetic amines, 354-355
  from theophylline, 103, 107
  from tricyclic antidepressants, 347
  in anesthesia, incidence of, 225
  in asthma, 106-108
  in thyroid disease, 192, 231
  incidence of, anesthetic regimen and, 169
    during sleep, 163
  induction of anesthesia and, 31-32
  intraoperative, 82
    beta-adrenergic blocking agents in, 121-122, *125*
  mechanisms of, 225-228
  paroxysmal, 231
  treatment of, 74
    amiodarone in, 239
    aprindine in, 239-240
    beta-adrenergic blocking agents in, 121-122, *125-126*
    bretylium in, 239
    cardioversion in, 236
    criteria for, 225
    digitalis in, 185
    disopyramide in, 238
    lidocaine in, 237
    mexiletine in, 240
    parasympathetic stimulation in, 162-163
    phenytoin in, 238
    procainamide in, 238
    propranolol in, 78, 119, 238
    quinidine in, 236
    tocainide in, 240
    verapamil in, 136, 239
  ventricular, 237-240
Cardiac effect(s), of acetylcholine, 161-162
  of acidosis, 395
  of aminophylline, 348
  of amiodarone, 239
  of amphetamine, 81
  of anesthetic depth, 412-413, *413*
  of anticholinergic agents, 168-170
  of anticholinesterase agents, 169-170
  of antihypertensive agents, 149-150
  of aprindine, 239-240
  of atenolol, 117, 118*t*
  of atracurium, 384-385
  of atropine, 27
  of balanced anesthesia, 83
  of *beta*-adrenergic blocking agents, 116-118, 118*t*, 343
    beneficial, 121-122, *124-126*
    in heart disease, 121, 121*t*, *122-123*
    in normal heart, 119-120, *120*
    intraoperative, 121-122, *124-126*
  of *beta*-adrenergic stimulation, 115-116, *117*
  of bretylium, 238-239
  of butoxamine, 117
  of calcium, 197-201
  of calcium-channel blocking agents, 30, 135-142, *137*, 138*t*, *140*, 345-346
  of captopril, 157
  of catecholamines, 75
  of chlorpromazine, 79
  of cholinergic agents, 169-170
  of clonidine, 153-154
  of cocaine, 27, 81-82
  of digitalis, 31
    autonomic, 184-185,
    electrophysiologic, 183-184
    inotropic, 182-183, 184*t*
    negative dromotropic, 179
    positive inotropic, 179, 182-183, 184*t*
    toxic, 187-188, 192-193
  of disopyramide, 238
  of dobutamine, 89
  of dopamine, 89
  of ephedrine, 90-91
  of epinephrine, 1, 3
  of ethyl alcohol, 290
  of etomidate, 317
  of general anesthetic agents, hypovolemia and, 76-77
  of guanabenz, 155
  of guanethidine, 77, 154-155
  of halothane, 379-380, *380*
  of hydralazine, 156
  of hyperkalemia, 204
    anesthesia and, 216
  of hypokalemia, 204
    anesthesia and, 216
  of hyponatremia, 203
  of isoproterenol, 89
    age and, 43
  of ketamine, 83-84, 105-106, 310
  of labetalol, 117, 156
  of lidocaine, 237
  of lithium, 277
  of magnesium sulfate, 431
  of mephentermine, 91
  of metaraminol, 91
  of methoxamine, 90
  of methyldopa, 152-153
  of metoprolol, 117, 118*t*
  of mexiletine, 240
  of minoxidil, 156-157
  of nadolol, 117, 118*t*
  of narcotics, 322, 335, 350
  of neuromuscular blocking agents, 384-385
  of nicotine overdose, 163
  of nitroglycerin, 142-143
  of nitrous oxide, 352-353
  of norepinephrine, 89
  of oxytocic agents, 428-429
  of pancuronium, 379-381, *381*
  of parasympathetic stimulation, 162-163
  of phenothiazines, 264-265
  of phenoxybenzamine, 155-156
  of phentolamine, 27, 155-156
  of phenylephrine, 90
  of phenytoin, 237-238
  of physiologic antagonism, 27
  of physostigmine, 296
  of pindolol, 117, 118*t*
  of practolol, 117-118, 118*t*
  of prazosin, 155
  of procainamide, 236-237
  of procaine toxicity, 395
  of propranolol, 78, 117, 118*t*, 238
    sudden withdrawal of, 78
  of quinidine, 236
  of reserpine, 76, 151-152
  of shock, 92-94
  of succinylcholine, 168-169
  of sympathetic nervous system, 71

INDEX 449

of sympathomimetic agents, 82-83, 83t
of terbutaline, 89
of theophylline, 103
of thiopental, 308
of timolol, 117, 118t
of tocainide, 240
of tricyclic antidepressants, 81, 347
of d-tubocurarine, drug interactions from, 379-380, 380
of vagal stimulation, 162-163
of vecuronium, 384-385
of verapamil, 239
anesthetic depth and, 418
Cardiac glycoside(s). See Digitalis; specific preparations
Cardiac pacemaker(s), abnormal activity of, dysrhythmias from, 228
calcium-channel blocking agents and, 139
Cardiac risk index score, 342
Cardiac surgery, 210, 312-313, 314-316
Cardiogenic shock, 85
dobutamine in treatment of, 89
from interaction, of propranolol and anesthetic agents, 121
renal blood flow in, 89
treatment of, mephentermine in, 91
Cardiopulmonary bypass, beta-adrenergic blocking agents in, 122, 156
calcium in, indications for, 201
cardiogenic shock in, propranolol and, 121
cardiovascular depression following, 343, 355
digitalis in, 232-233
drug interactions in, 78
interaction in, of diazepam and heparin, 312
of diazepam and opiates, 312, 324
methoxyflurane in, 128
nitroglycerin in, 143
propranolol in, 344
Cardioversion, digitalis toxicity and, 189
direct current, in treatment of intraoperative dysrhythmias, 236
Carfentanil, opioid receptors and, 327t
Catapres. See Clonidine
Catecholamine(s), actions of, direct, 86-87, 88t, 89-91
schematic view of, 73
active transport of, 72, 73
biosynthesis of, 75, 75t
bronchodilating, 108-109, 108t
cardiac effects of, 73-75, 94, 228, 380
disposition of, 72-73, 73
drug interactions with, tolerance to anesthesia and, 92
in aldosterone secretion, 211
in asthma, 108-109, 108t
in hypokalemia, 204
in hypotension, 88t
in shock, 88t
interaction of, with beta-adrenergic blocking agents, 115, 116t, 123, 127
with calcium, 198
with cocaine, 71-72, 81-82
with cyclopropane, 416
with digitalis, 184t, 192

with guanethidine, 154-155
with halothane, 71-72, 416
with inhalation anesthetic agents, 414, 416-418
with ketamine, 83-84
with methyldopa, 152-153
with monoamine oxidase, 73, 73
with monoamine oxidase inhibitors, 73
with phenoxybenzamine, 155-156
with phentolamine, 155-156
with propranolol, 119-120, 120
with reserpine, 151-152, 265
metabolism of, 75, 75t
pheochromocytoma and, 75
release of, anesthetic agents classified by, 124-125
by calcium injection, 200-201
by pheochromocytoma, 75
reuptake of, 72, 73
sensitivity to, sympathectomy and, 75
similarity of methyldopa to, 152-153
synthesis of, 72, 73
tachyphylaxis and, 42
thyroid hormone and, 75
Catechol-O-methyl transferase, actions of, 72-73, 73-74
Cation(s), inorganic. See Inorganic cation(s); specific agents
Celiac plexus block. See Conduction anesthesia
Celontin. See Methsuximide
Central anticholinergic syndrome, 170-173, 171t, 172t
anticholinergic agents in, 267, 269
condition of patient and, 171
manifestations of, 267
physostigmine in treatment of, 171-173
prevention of, 268
symptoms of, 170
types of, 172
Central nervous system, acetylcholine in, 161
anesthetic depth and, 411, 412
catecholamines in, 414, 416-418
depressants of. See Central nervous system depressant(s)
depression of, treatment of with physostigmine, 172
drugs acting on, cross-tolerance among, 28
time course of action of, 29-30
types of, 28-29
effects on, of acidosis, 395
of amphetamine, 81
of anticholinergic agents, 170-173
of anticholinesterase agents, 164
of barbiturates, 255, 288-289
of benzodiazepines, 291-293
of chloral hydrate, 297
of cocaine, 81
of digitalis, 185, 187-188
of dopamine, 346-347
of ethyl alcohol, 288-289
of general anesthetic agents, 255
of glutethimide, 298
of hypermagnesemia, 205
of inhalation anesthetic agents, 370
of levodopa, 346-347
of lidocaine, 294-295
of local anesthetic agents, 401, 404

of mepivacaine overdosage, 399
of meprobamate, 298
of methylxanthines, 296
of morphine, 326t
of nalorphine, 326t
of narcotics, 321-322, 335
of pesticides, 164
of physostigmine, 295-296
of procaine toxicity, 395
of sedative-hypnotic agents, 283-284, 299
of tetrahydrocannabinol, 299
of theophylline, 102-103
opiate receptors in, narcotic antagonists and, 334-335
Central nervous system depressant(s), interaction of, with antipsychotic agents, 261t, 262-263
with barbiturates, 286
with ethyl alcohol, 283, 291
with narcotics, 323-324, 337
with tricyclic antidepressants, 81
Cephalosporin, 218
Cephalothin, 19t
Cesarean section, 396
Charcoal, inactivation of drugs by, 19
Cheese, as tyramine source, 80
"Cheese reaction," tyramine and, 22
Chelating agent(s), calcium-channel blocking agents versus, 135
Chemoreceptor(s), carotid body, 163
Chemotherapeutic agent(s), 396
Child(ren), atropine in, fatal dosage of, 171
digitalis toxicity in, 188
diuretics in, preoperative evaluation of, 218
preanesthetic medication in, anesthetic depth and, 283
seizure control in, 248-249, 251-252, 254
theophylline metabolism in, 103, 104t
with heart disease, induction of anesthesia in, 310
Chloral hydrate, actions of, 297
as enzyme inducer, 67
indications for use of, 297
interaction of, with anticoagulants, 297
with ethyl alcohol, 289, 290
metabolites of, 290, 297
Chloralose, 398
Chloramphenicol, interaction of, with aminophylline, 19t
with barbiturates, 19t, 309
with cephalothin, 19t
with diphenhydramine, 19t
with erythromycin, 19t
with hydrocortisone, 19t
with phenytoin, 19t
with polymyxin B, 19t
with tetracyclines, 19t
with thiopental, 309
with vancomycin, 19t
Chlorcyclizine, 44
Chlordiazepoxide, enzyme induction from, 67, 356
indications for use of, 291
interaction of, with anticoagulants, 297
with calcium, 296
with cimetidine, 177, 294
with ethyl alcohol, 289, 290

Chlordiazepoxide, interaction of *(cont.)*
   with physostigmine, 172t
Chloride, 292
Chlorisondamine, 165
Chloroform, interaction of, with atropine, 166
   with epinephrine, 1
   with phenobarbital, 68
   with sympathomimetic agents, 82
Chloroprocaine, hydrolysis of, in pregnancy, 396
   interaction of, with bupivacaine, 401
   with echothiophate, 396
   with etidocaine, 401
   with pseudocholinesterase, 396
   metabolism of, 401
   tachyphylaxis to, 401
Chloropropane, interaction of, with tetracaine, 401
Chloroquine, 42
Chlorpheniramine, 19t, 172t
Chlorpromazine, actions of, 79, 172t, 261
   convulsive threshold with, 264
   enzyme induction from, 356
   in lytic cocktail, 262
   indications for use of, 79
   interaction of, with anticholinergic agents, 263
      with antiparkinsonian agents, 263
      with barbiturates, 44, 262-263
      with conduction anesthesia, 264-265
      with enflurane, 263
      with epinephrine, 263
      with general anesthetic agents, 79
      with inhalation anesthetic agents, 348
      with isoflurane, 263
      with ketamine, 310
      with meperidine, 324
      with methoxamine, 79
      with monoamine oxidase inhibitors, 80, 272
      with narcotic analgesics, 79, 323
      with norepinephrine, 73, 263-264
      with penicillin G, 19t
      with phenylephrine, 79, 264
      with sedatives, 79
      with thiopental, 262-263
      with tricyclic antidepressants, 269
      with vasopressors, 428-429
   respiratory depression from, 324
   side effects of, 261
      central anticholinergic syndrome as, 267
   volume of distribution of, 41
Chlorpropamide, interaction of, with ethyl alcohol, 290-291
   with thiazide diuretics, 217-218
Cholestyramine, interaction of, with digitalis, 19, 188-189
   with thiazide diuretics, 19
   with thyroid preparations, 19
   with warfarin, 19
Cholinergic agent(s), biochemistry of, 161-163
   cardiac effects of, 169-170
   clinical use of, in anesthesia, 166-170
   morphology of, 161-163
   muscarinic, defined, 161
   nicotinic, defined, 161
   pharmacology of mechanisms of, 163-165
   physiology of, 161-163

Cholinergic receptor(s), defined, 148
Cholinesterase(s), in hydrolysis, of local anesthetic agents, 396
   of acetylcholine, 161
   inhibition of, 162, 164, 166
   interaction of, with succinylcholine, 22, 164-165
      with tetracaine, 395
   plasma levels of, lithium carbonate and, 275
   phenelzine and, 273
Cholinoceptive receptor(s), defined, 148
Cholinolytic agent(s), classification of, 163
   muscarinic, 165-166
   nicotinic, 165
   pharmacology of mechanisms of, 163, 165-166
Cholinomimetic agent(s), classification of, 163
   gastrointestinal effects of, 19
   interaction of, with muscarinic cholinolytic agents, 165-166
   muscarinic, 163-165
   nicotinic, 163
   pharmacology of mechanisms of, 163-165
Cimetidine, actions of, 104, 176-177, 294
   indications for use of, 176, 324
   interaction of, with alprazolam, 294
      with benzodiazepines, 177
      with chlordiazepoxide, 177, 294
      with desmethyldiazepam, 294
      with diazepam, 177, 294, 312
      with fentanyl, 324
      with halothane, 177
      with lidocaine, 177, 394
      with lorazepam, 177, 294
      with morphine, 176-177
      with nalbuphine, 332t
      with naloxone, 176
      with narcotic analgesics, 176
      with opiates, 176
      with oxazepam, 177, 294
      with pantopon, 176
      with phenytoin, 177, 248
      with propranolol, 177
      with temazepam, 294
      with theophylline, 104-105, 177
      with triazolam, 294
      with warfarin, 177
   ranitidine versus, 177
   structure of, 176
Circadian rhythm, local anesthetic agents and, 404
   drug responses and, 17
Circulatory depression, from interaction of anesthetic and *beta*-adrenergic blocking agents, 125-128
   propranolol-associated, components of, 123
   reversal of, 123-124, 126t, 127t
   treatment of, 126t
Cirrhosis, acetazolamide in, 213
   effects in, of lidocaine, 397
Citrate toxicity, 201-202
Clindamycin, interaction of, with calcium, 366t
   with neostigmine, 366t
   with succinylcholine, 366t
   with d-tubocurarine, 366t

   with vecuronium, 375
Clonazepam, diazepam as substitute for, 253
   dosage of, 247t, 253
   indications for use of, 252, 291
   interaction of, with Ro 15-1788, 293
      with valproic acid, 251
   pharmacokinetics of, 247t, 252-253
   plasma levels of, 247t, 252-253
   side effects of, 253
Clonidine, actions of, 77, 153-154
   cardiac effects of, 153-154
   classification of, 148t
   discontinuance of, 153-154
      rebound hypertension from, 342
   dosage of, 148t
   indications for use of, 77, 153
   interaction of, with amitriptyline, 269
      with anesthetic agents, 7, 153
      with barbiturates, 153
      with *beta*-adrenergic blocking agents, 154
      with butyrophenones, 153
      with digitalis, 153
      with droperidol, 153
      with general anesthetic agents, 77
      with halothane, 415t, 417
      with naloxone, 336
      with norepinephrine, 341
      with opiates, 154
      with thiazide diuretics, 217
      with tricyclic antidepressants, 27-28, 153
   mechanism of action of, 340-341
   pharmacology of, 153-154
   side effects of, 151t, 153-154
Clonopin. *See* Clonazepam
Clorazepate, indications for use of, 253, 291
   interaction of, with ketamine, 297
   introduction of, 245, 246t
   pharmacokinetics of, 247t, 253
Cocaine, absorption of, 392
   actions of, 81-82
   atropine and procaine versus, 81, *81*
   cardiac effects of, 27, 71-72, 81-82
   duration of action of, 391
   effects of, in heart disease, 393
   fatal dose of, 82
   habitual use of, 82
   indications for use of, 81-82
   interaction of, with antihypertensive agents, 34
      with catecholamines, 71-72
      with cyclopropane, 391
      with epinephrine, 4, 81-82, 391
      with guanethidine, 155
      with halothane, 29, 34-35, 71-72, 82, 391, 414, 415t, 416
      with norepinephrine, 26, 73, 81
      with succinylcholine, 401
      with tricyclic antidepressants, 269, 403
   introduction of, 81
Codeine, conversion of, to morphine, 47t
   interaction of, with glutethimide, 298
   opioid receptors and, 327t
Coenzyme A, 161
Coenzyme P-450, 43
Cogentin. *See* Benztropine
Colestipol, 189

INDEX 451

Colistimethate, 19t
Colistin, 366t
Columbia group, 82
Coma, from benzodiazepines, treatment of, 293
　from interaction, of meperidine and phenelzine, 325
　　of monoamine oxidase inhibitors and narcotics, 273, 347
　therapy for, atropine in, 171
Competitive inhibition, *beta*-adrenergic receptors and, 114
Compoz, 171t
Conduction, atrioventricular. *See* Atrioventricular conduction
Conduction anesthesia, indications for, monoamine oxidase inhibitors and, 274
　interaction of, with antipsychotic agents, 264-265
Congestive heart failure, *beta*-adrenergic blocking agents contraindicated in, 123, *127*
　catecholamines in, 75
　digitalis clearance in, vasodilators and, 190
　diuretics in, potassium administration with, 219-220
　potassium transport in, 215-216
　treatment of, nicotinic cholinolytic agents in, 165
Conjugation, in biotransformation of drugs, 64
Contraceptive(s), oral, 285
Contrast medium(a), angiographic, osmotic diuresis from, 212
　interaction of, with barbiturates, 308-309
Converting enzyme inhibitor(s), dosage of, 148t
　pharmacology of, 157
Convulsion(s). *See* Seizure(s)
Coomb's test, methyldopa and, 152
Cor pulmonale, digitalis toxicity and, 190
　isoproterenol in treatment of, 89
Coronary artery disease, anticholinergic agents in, 168
　hazards of, 170
　beta-adrenergic blocking agents in, 121, *123*
　　preoperative discontinuance of, 130, *131*, 132, 132t
　interaction in, of inhalation anesthetic agents, 352
　　of narcotics and nitrous oxide, 350
　treatment of, nifedipine in, 345
Coronary artery(ies), *beta*-adrenergic stimulation and, 116, *117*
Coronary steal, 143
Coronary vasospasm, 141
Corticosteroid analog(s), 24
Corticosteroid(s), antiasthmatic, 109-110
　enzyme induction and, 356, 430
　in anesthesia, adverse effects of, 110
　interaction of, with barbiturates, 285
　　with *beta*-agonists, 110
　　with *beta*-sympathomimetic agents, 433
　　with neuromuscular blocking agents, 369
　　with phenobarbital, 285
　　with theophylline, 110

　metabolism of, mixed-function oxygenases and, 64
Cortisol, levels of, in pregnancy, 430
Cortisone, as enzyme inducer, 67
　effects of, after adrenalectomy, 369
　　after hypophysectomy, 369
　interaction of, with narcotic antagonists, 336
　　with pancuronium, 369
Coumadin. *See* Warfarin
Coumarin anticoagulant(s), as problem drugs, 10
　interaction of, with aspirin, 9
　　with barbiturates, 9, 285-286
　　with phenylbutazone, 9
　postoperative adjustment of, 10
Creatinine, sodium and, 202
　clearance of, 186
Cross-tolerance, among central nervous system drugs, 28
　to ethyl alcohol, 287, 290
　to sedative-hypnotic agents, 299
Crystalloid solution(s), in shock management, 92
Curare, agents similar to, 24-25
　effects of, parasympathetic, 161
　in "balanced" anesthesia, 2
　interaction of, with calcium, 205
　　with diazepam, 313
　　with ether, 2
　　with local anesthetic agents, 371, 398
　　with magnesium, 205
　　with quinidine, 372
　neuromuscular transmission blocked by, 163
Cyanide, 158
Cyclazocine, opioid receptors and, 327t
　effects of pH in, 59
Cyclopentolate, 171t
Cyclophosphamide, interaction of, with succinylcholine, 378
Cyclopropane, anesthetic depth and, cardiac signs of, 413
　central nervous signs of, 412
　catecholamine release and, 124-125
　interaction of, with anticholinergic agents, 168, 170
　　with antihypertensive agents, 341
　　with atropine, 169, 415t, 422
　　with *beta*-adrenergic blocking agents, 125, 128, *129*
　　with catecholamines, 416
　　with cocaine, 391
　　with digitalis, 184, 188
　　with epinephrine, 3, 82-83, 83t, 354, 391
　　with iproniazid, 414, 415t
　　with lidocaine, 419
　　with naloxone, 415t
　　with neostigmine, 169
　　with neuromuscular blocking agents, 370
　　with phencyclidine, 415t, 418
　　with propranolol, 78, 125, 128, *129*, 343
　　with reserpine, 266
　　with scopolamine, 415t, 422
　　with tetrohydrocannabinol, 299, 415t, 422
　　with thiopental, 309
　sensitivity of, to epinephrine-induced dysrhythmias, 82-83, 83t

Cytochrome P-450, binding of cimetidine to, 177, 312
　defined, 65
　genetic abnormalities in, 65, 68-69
　in biotransformation, 65, *66*
　in metabolism of inhalation anesthetic agents, 355
　inducers of, 67-68
Cytosol, 199
Cytotoxic agent(s), 378

Dalgan. *See* Dezocine
Dantrolene, effects of, 30
　interaction of, with calcium-channel blocking agents, 142
　　with verapamil, 142
Darvon. *See* Propoxyphene
Datura stramonium, 171t
DDT, as enzyme inducer, 67
　reason for banning of, 23
Deafness, from aminoglycside antibiotics and ethacrynic acid, 218
　from loop diuretics, 214
Dealkylation, in biotransformation, 64
Death, from alterations in plasma proteins, 45-46
　from atropine, 171
　from *beta*-adrenergic blocking agents, preoperative discontinuance of, 130, 132t
　from hyperkalemia, 93
　from interaction, of atropine and neostigmine, 169
　　of barbiturates and anticoagulants, 286
　　of barbiturates and ethyl alcohol, 289
　　of chloroform and epinephrine, 1
　　of cocaine and halothane, 34-35, 391
　　of codeine and glutethimide, 298
　　of digitalis and calcium, 189
　　of ethyl alcohol and other agents, 288-289, 291
　　of glutethimide and codeine, 298
　　of insulin and ethyl alcohol, 291
　　of methoxyflurane and practolol, 128
　　of naloxone and narcotics, 336
　　of narcotics and monoamine oxidase inhibitors, 325
　　of phenothiazines and ethyl alcohol, 289
　　of tricyclic antidepressants and sympathetic amines, 268
　from lithium toxicity, 276
　from mercurial diuretics, 213
　from morphine, in combat use, 40
　from narcotic overdose, 322
　from phenothiazines, 264
　from reserpine and electroconvulsive therapy, 266
　from toxemia of pregnancy, 430
　from valproic acid hepatotoxicity, 251
　postoperative, phenothiazines and, 264-265
Decamethonium, contraindications to, 368
　effects of, in renal failure, 368
　interaction of, with calcium, 205
　　with gallamine, 373

Decamethonium, interaction of *(cont.)*
  with lithium carbonate, 79, 275-276
  with magnesium, 205
  with pancuronium, 373
  with d-tubocurarine, 373
  neuromuscular transmission blocked by, 163
Decarboxylase, inhibitors of, 346
Dehalogenation, in biotransformation, 64
Delirium, from atropine, 172
  from interaction of lidocaine and procaine amide, 401
  from scopolamine, 171-172
  postoperative, from naloxone, 335
Demoxepam, interaction of, with ethyl alcohol, 289
Dental procedure(s), cocaine in, heart disease and, 391, 393
  interactions in, 235-236
    plasma cholinesterase and, 395
Depakene. *See* Valproic acid
Depakote. *See* Valproic acid
Depolarization, antidysrhythmic agents and, 229-231
  calcium in, 198
  of cardiac action potentials, 225-227, 226
  of cardiac cells, 182-184, 184t
Depolarizing block, examples of, 163
Depression, bone marrow. *See* Bone marrow depression
  central nervous system, physostigmine in treatment of, 172
  circulatory. *See* Circulatory depression
  of nerve function, 29
  psychic, from guanabenz, 155
    from hydralazine, 156
    from reserpine, 151, 151t
    lithium in treatment of, 275
    tricyclic antidepressants in treatment of, 268
  respiratory. *See* Respiratory depression
Dermatitis, from antipsychotic agents, 18
  from thiazide diuretics, 214
Desipramine, as agent with anticholinergic activity, 172t
  indications for use of, 268
  interaction of, with bupivacaine, 394
    with epinephrine, 268
    with ethyl alcohol, 287-288
    with norepinephrine, 268
    with phenylephrine, 268
Deslanoside, 181
Desmethyldiazepam, diazepam converted to, 47t
  interaction of, with cimetidine, 294
    with ethyl alcohol, 289
Desmethylimipramine, interaction of, with local anesthetic agents, 402-403
    with norepinephrine, 402-403
Detoxification, drug, defined, 21-22
Dexamethasone, interaction of, with narcotics, 323
    with penicillin G, 19t
    with pseudocholinesterase, 396
Dexamethonium, interaction of, with magnesium sulfate, 431
Dexoxadrol, actions of, 84

Dextran 40, interaction of, with local anesthetic agents, 392
Dextroamphetamine, interaction of, with halothane, 414
Dextromethorphan, interaction of, with phenelzine, 273
Dextrorphanol, opioid receptors and, 327t
Dezocine, as narcotic agonist-antagonist, 325t
  interaction of, with inhalation anesthetic agents, 333
  morphine versus, 330t
  nalorphine versus, 330t
  opioid receptors and, hypothetical interactions with, 327t
  potency of, 330t
Diabenzyline. *See* Phenoxybenzamine
Diabetes insipidus, from lithium, 277
  hypernatremia in, 203
Diabetes mellitus, corticosteroids in, coma and, 110
  diuretics in, 217-218
  in preoperative evaluation of patient taking diuretics, 220
  insulin receptors and, 42
Diaminopyridine, interaction of, with vecuronium, 376
Diamox. *See* Acetazolamide
Diazepam, actions of, 294, 312
  as clonazapam substitute, 253
  as valproic acid substitute, 251
  dosage of, preanesthetic, 254
  drug interactions with, 312-313, 314-316
  effects of, 312
    anticonvulsant, 294-295
    in heart disease, 313
    in neonates, 434-435
  indications for use of, 291
    as induction agent, 349
    in regional anesthesia in epilepsy, 254
    in seizure control, 252, 399
  interaction of, with acetylcholine, 296
    with adenosine, 296
    with aminophylline, 296
    with antihistamines, 312
    with bilirubin, 434-435
    with cimetidine, 177, 294, 312
    with curare, 313
    with digoxin, 181-182, 189
    with diltiazem, 139
    with ethyl alcohol, 289
    with etomidate, 317
    with fentanyl, 312-313, 314-316, 324
    with gallamine, 297
    with gamma amino butyric acid, 312-313
    with halothane, 284, 313, 415t, 419
    with heparin, 312
    with imidazodiapines, 293
    with inhalation anesthetic agents, 349-350
    with ketamine, 256-257, 285, 294, 297, 310, 311
    with lidocaine, 294-295, 399
    with lithium carbonate, 276
    with local anesthetic agents, 294-295, 399
    with morphine, 312, 324
    with nalbuphine, 332t

  with naloxone, 336
  with narcotics, 349
  with neuromuscular blocking agents, 297, 313
  with nifedipine, 139
  with nitrous oxide, 313, 314, 349
  with opiates, 312-313, 314-316
  with pancuronium, 313
  with phenobarbital, 435
  with physostigmine, 172, 172t, 295-296
  with reserpine, 266
  with Ro 15-1788, 293
  with succinylcholine, 297, 313
  with theophylline, 296
  with valproic acid, 296
  with verapamil, 139
  interactions with, cardiopulmonary, 312-313
  pharmacokinetic, 312
  introduction of, 245, 246t
  lorazepam versus, 252-253
  oxybarbital versus, 295
  pentobarbital versus, 295
  pharmacokinetics of, 247t, 252
  plasma levels of, antiepileptic, 247t, 252
  protein binding of, effects of alterations in, 43
Diazoxide, actions of, 158
  diabetogenic, 217-218
  contraindications to, 159
  dosage of, 158
  in hypoglycemia, 158
  in toxemia, 158
  indications for use of, 158
    in hypertensive crises, 158-159
  interaction of, with *beta*-adrenergic blocking agents, 158
    with oxytocin, 158
  nitroprusside versus, 158
  protein binding of, 158
Dibenamine, nonsurmountable antagonism of, 26
Dibucaine number(s), 371-372, 377
Dicumarol, interaction of, with barbiturates, 44, 282
    with phenobarbital, 282, 286
Diethyl ether, anesthetic depth and, cardiac signs of, 413
  central nervous signs of, 412
  catecholamine release and, 124-125
  effects of, neuronal, 255
  interaction of, with anticholinergic agents, 168
    with atropine, 166
    with *beta*-adrenergic blocking agents, 125, 128, 129
    with curare, 2
    with digitalis, 184, 188
    with epinephrine, 82, 83t
    with lidocaine, 400
    with neuromuscular blocking agents, 353
    with nitrous oxide, 72, 352, 353
    with propranolol, 78, 120-121, 125, 128, 129, 343
    with reserpine, 266
  minimum alveolar concentration of, anesthetic depth and, 410t
  sensitivity of, to epinephrine-induced dysrhythmias, 82, 83t
Digitalis, 179-193, 184t

INDEX

anesthetic considerations with, 180-182
cardiac effects of, 31
  autonomic, 184-185
  calcium transport and, 200
  dromotropic, 179, 183-184
  electrophysiologic, 183-184
  inotropic, 179, 182-183, 184t, 199
  toxic, 187-188
dosage of, gastrointestinal absorption and, 188
  intraoperative, 186
  loading, 185-186
  maintenance, 185-186
effects of, autonomic tone and, 179, 184-185
  in hypokalemia, 204
  on blood coagulability, 190
electrical countershock and, 187
indications for use of, 179, 192-193
interaction of, with amiloride-hydrochlorthiazide, 181
  with amiodarone, 188
  with amphotericin B, 189
  with anesthetic agents, 184, 188, 216
  with antacids, 189
  with antibiotics, 189
  with atropine, 187
  with barbiturates, 189
  with benzodiazepines, 182
  with benzothiadiazines, 181, 189
  with *beta*-adrenergic blocking agents, 124, 126t, 345
  with bretylium, 239
  with bumetanide, 181
  with calcium, 189, 201
  with calcium-channel blocking agents, 139-140
  with carbohydrates, 190
  with cholestyramine, 189
  with clonidine, 153
  with cyclopropane, 184, 188
  with diazepam, 189
  with diethyl ether, 184, 188
  with diuretics, 181, 189-190, 215-216
  with droperidol, 184, 188
  with enflurane, 184, 188
  with epinephrine, 192
  with erythromycin, 189
  with ethacrynic acid, 181, 189
  with fentanyl, 184, 188
  with fluroxene, 184, 188
  with furosemide, 181, 189
  with glucose, 190
  with halothane, 184, 188
  with heparin, 190
  with hydralazine, 190
  with insulin, 190
  with isoflurane, 184, 188
  with isoproterenol, 192
  with kaolin-pectin, 190
  with ketamine, 184, 188
  with lidocaine, 180, 182, 187, 190
  with magnesium, 181, 190
  with mephentermine, 91
  with methoxyflurane, 184, 188
  with nifedipine, 190
  with nitroprusside, 190
  with norepinephrine, 192
  with pentobarbital, 184, 188
  with phenylbutazone, 190

  with phenytoin, 180-182, 187, 190, 201
  with potassium, 180-181, 184, 187, 189-191, 199, 201, 215-216
  with procainamide, 191
  with propantheline, 191
  with propranolol, 78, 124, 126t, 187, 191
  with quinidine, 191, 236
  with reserpine, 191, 267
  with spironolactone, 181, 189, 217
  with succinylcholine, 191-192
  with sympathomimetic agents, 192
  with tetracycline, 189
  with tetracyclines, 192
  with triamterene, 181, 189
  with vasodilators, 181-182
  with verapamil, 192
pharmacology of, 182-188, 184t
preoperative considerations with, 192
preparations of, 179
prophylactic, in coronary artery bypass, 233
renal function and, 180-181, 185-187, 191
therapeutic index of, 179, 192
toxicity of. *See* Digitalis toxicity
toxicology of, 187-188
Digitalis leaf, renal function impairment and, 181
Digitalis toxicity, age and, 187-188
  anesthetic considerations in, 179-182
  causes of, 180-182, 192-193
  diagnosis of, 188
  effects of, cardiac, 184, 187-188
    central nervous, 187-188
    gastrointestinal, 187
    visual, 188
  following open heart surgery, 233
  hypokalemia and, 180-181, 190-191, 233
    from amphotericin B, 189
  incidence of, 179
  manifestations of, 192-193
  serum level measurement in, 188
  treatment of, drug dosages in, 182
    phenytoin in, 180-182, 190, 201
    potassium in, 180-181, 190-191, 201
Digitoxin, dosage of, 185
  excretion of, 189
    renal impairment and, 191
  half-life of, 179
  hepatic disease and, 190
  indications for use of, 179
  interaction of, with barbiturates, 286
    with cholestyramine, 19, 189
    with colestipol, 189
    with phenobarbital, 189
    with phenylbutazone, 190
    with phenytoin, 190
    with quinidine, 181, 191, 236
    with spironolactone, 217
  serum levels of, 185
    therapeutic, 192
Digoxin, antidysrhythmic effects of, experimental, 233
  clearance of, in heart failure, 182
    renal function and, 180, 185-187, 191
    vasodilators and, 181-182
  distribution of, tissue, 42, 188
  dosage of, intraoperative, 186

    loading, 185-186
    maintenance, 185-186
    obesity and, 190
  half-life of, 179, 185-186
  hepatic disease and, 190
  indications for use of, 179
  interaction of, with amiloride, 217
    with amiodarone, 188
    with antacids, 188, 189
    with barbiturates, 286
    with cholestyramine, 188, 189
    with diazepam, 181-182, 189
    with disopyramide, 181
    with erythromycin, 189
    with furosemide, 206, 217
    with halothane, 233
    with hydralazine, 182, 190
    with kaolin-pectin, 188
    with nifedipine, 190
    with nitroprusside, 182, 190
    with phenobarbital, 44
    with potassium, 216
    with procainamide, 181
    with propantheline, 191
    with quinidine, 180-182, 191, 236
    with quinine, 181
    with spironolactone, 215, 217
    with tetracycline, 189
    with triamterene, 216, 217
    with vasodilators, 182, 190
    with verapamil, 139-140, 181, 192
  pharmacokinetics of, 185-187
  serum levels of, in children, 188
    measurement of, 185-186
    muscle mass and, 187
    obesity and, 190
    route of administration and, 186
    therapeutic, 188, 192
    toxic, 188
  thyroid disease and, 192
  toxicity of, renal function impairment and, 181, 191
  volume of distribution of, 41
Diisopropyl fluorophosphate, 396
Diltiazem, actions of, 137-138
  cardiac effects of, 137-138, 138t, 345
  comparison of with other calcium-channel blocking agents, 138t
  effects of, platelet adhesion inhibition as, 142
  indications for use of, 136
  interaction of, with aspirin, 139
    with calcium, 198
    with diazepam, 139
    with lidocaine, 139
    with propranolol, 139
  mechanism of action of, 341, 345
  protein binding of, 139
Dimethadione, plasma levels of, 247t, 252
Dioxolane(s), 84
Diphenhydramine, as agent with anticholinergic activity, 172t
  enzyme induction from, 356
  interaction of, with amphotericin B, 19t
    with anticoagulants, 298
    with chloramphenicol, 19t
Diphenylhydantoin. *See* Phenytoin
Diphenylhydramine, as enzyme inducer, 67
Dipropylacetic acid. *See* Valproic acid
Dipyridamone, 46

Disease(s), autoimmune, drug
    reactions in, 32
  drug interactions enhanced by, 10
  hepatic. See Hepatic disease(s)
  neuromuscular, succinylcholine in,
    204
  protein binding of drugs and, 41, 45-
    46
  pulmonary. See Pulmonary disease(s)
  thyroid, digitalis toxicity and, 192
  underlying, drug responses and, 17
Disipal. See Orphenidrine
Disopyramide, actions of, 238
  effects of, extracardiac, 230t
  electrophysiologic actions of, 230t
  interaction of, with digoxin, 181
    with inhalation anesthetic agents,
      238
    with neuromusclar blocking
      agents, 238
  side effects of, 238
Dissociative anesthesia, defined, 47
  from ketamine, 47, 310
Disulfiram, actions of, 75
  effects of, 290-291
  in biosynthesis of catecholamines,
    75, 75t
  indications for use of, 75
  interaction of, with anesthetic
    agents, 75
    with paraldehyde, 297-298
Diuresis, osmotic, 211-212, 212
  treatment of drug overdose with, 58
Diuretic(s), 206-221, 207, 209, 212, 215
  acid-forming salts as, sites of action
    of, 212-213
  actions of, 365
    renal tubular, 208
  carbonic anhydrase inhibiting, sites
    of action of, 213
  cardiac effects of, 31
    potassium levels and, 215-217,
      219- 220
  drug interactions with, 214-218
    awareness of, 220
    beneficial, 217
    clinical implications with, 218-221
    toxic, 218
  hypokalemia from, digitalis toxicity
    and, 181, 189-190
  in treatment of hyponatremia, 203
  indications for use of, 206
  interaction of, with aminoglycoside
    antibiotics, 221
    with anesthetic agents, 216, 220
    with anticoagulants, 220
    with anticonvulsant agents, 220
    with antihypertensive agents, 217
    with anti-inflammatory agents, 220
    with aspirin, 220
    with digitalis, 181, 189-190, 215-
      216
    with hydralazine, 156
    with indomethacin, 220
    with labetalol, 156
    with lithium, 217, 276-277
    with neuromuscular blocking
      agents, 216-217, 221, 365, 382
    with potassium, 215-216
    with succinylcholine, 216-217
    with d-tubocurare, 216
    with d-tubocurarine, 364-365, 364
  intraoperative considerations in, 220-
    221

loop, 214. See also Ethacrynic acid;
    Furosemide
  mechanism of action of, 340
  mercurial, 213, 215
  osmotic, 211-212, 212
  potassium-sparing, actions of, 214
    interaction of, with beta-
      adrenergic blocking agents, 220
    preoperative considerations in, 218,
      220
  sites of action of, 211-214, 212, 215
  supplemental potassium in patients
    taking, 219-220
  thiazide. See Thiazide diuretic(s)
Dobutamine, actions of, direct, 89
  interaction of, with beta-adrenergic
    blocking agents, 124, 126t
Dobutrex. See Dobutamine
DOPA, 75t
Dopa decarboxylase, 346
Dopamine, action of, direct, 86, 88t,
    89-90
  biosynthesis of, 75t
  cardiac effects of, 90, 354
  central nervous system effects of,
    346-347
  in shock management, 93
  indications for use of, 90
  interaction of, with antihistamines,
    86
    with antipsychotic agents, 263
    with atropine, 86
    with beta-adrenergic blocking
      agents, 86, 124
    with butyrophenones, 347
    with calcium-channel blocking
      agents, 138-139
    with halothane, 208
    with inhalation anesthetic agents,
      346-347
    with ketamine, 84
    with levodopa, 417-418
    with monoamine oxidase
      inhibitors, 22, 272, 347
    with narcotics, 323
    with norepinephrine, 73, 346
    with propranolol, 124
    with reserpine, 265, 267
  levodopa as precursor of, 346
  metabolism of, 75t
Dopaminergic receptor(s), defined, 86
Doriden. See Glutethimide
Dosage, drug, principles of, 39
Dose ratio, defined, 42
Dose(s), median effective, 410t
  in therapeutic ratio, 40
  median lethal, in therapeutic ratio,
    40
Dose titration, rationale for, 17
Dose-effect relationship, principles of,
    39
  tissue receptors and, 40
Dose-response curve(s), in allergic
    drug reactions, 33
  of inhalation anesthetic agents, 409,
    410t, 411, 411
  to agonist drugs, 25
Doxepin, as agent with anticholinergic
    activity, 172t
  indications for use of, 268
Droperidol, as agent with
    anticholinergic activity, 172t
  fentanyl and, as induction agents,
    350

interaction of, with clonidine, 153
  with digitalis, 184, 188
  with fentanyl, 262, 324
  with ketamine, 310
  with levodopa, 347
  with methyldopa, 153
  with monoamine oxidase
    inhibitors, 274
  with nalbuphine, 332t
  with phenothiazines, 348
  preanesthetic, anesthetic depth and,
    283
Drug absorption, pH shifts and, 53,
    56, 57t
Drug addiction, interactions in, of
    opiates and ethyl alcohol, 291
  narcotic. See Narcotic addiction
Drug detoxification, defined, 21-22
Drug disposition, in neonates, 433,
    434t
  in pregnancy, 427
  route of administration and, 40
Drug distribution, neonatal, 433-435,
    434t
  pH shifts and, 56, 57, 58, 58-59
  tissue selectivity of, 42
  volume of. See Volume of
    distribution
Drug dosage, principles of, 39
Drug interaction(s), acute allergic, 32-
    34
  additive, 26
  altered drug metabolism in, 43-44
  among oral agents, 19
  anesthetic depth and, 413-414, 415t,
    416-419, 417-422, 422
  categories of, 18
  dangers of, 1-3, 9-10
  dysrhythmic, possible, 233-234
  generic drug formulation and, 18
  genetic factors in, 10
  hemodynamic, 44-46
  hepatic mediation of, 63-69, 66
  historical background on, 1-2
  hospital pharmacists as consultants
    on, 18
  in obstetrics, 427-435, 434t
  in vitro incompatibilities and, 18-19,
    19t
  incidence of, 5, 5t
  mechanisms of, general principles
    of, 16-35, 19t, 25
  MEDIPHOR classification of, 7-9
  pharmacodynamic, 23-32, 25
  pharmacokinetic, 19-23
  pharmacokinetics and, 39-49, 42t, 43,
    47t
  pharmacologic receptors and, 23-29,
    25
  potential, defined, 5
  procedure for minimizing, 9-10
  quantifying, 4-5
  recognition of, 17
  research into, 3-11, 5t, 8
  sources of information on, 5-9, 8
  time sequence and, 29-30
  types of, 18-35, 19t, 25
  useful, 1-2
  viscerotoxicity and, 67-69
  with antidysrhythmic agents, 231-
    236, 233
  with beta-adrenergic blocking agents,
    78-79

INDEX

with calcium-channel blocking agents, 139-142
with digitalis, 179-193
with diuretics, 214-221
with ethyl alcohol, 287-291
with intravenous anesthetic agents, 308-317, 311t, 314-316
with local anesthetic agents, 391-404, 392, 394-395, 397-398, 400, 403
with narcotic agonists, 323-325
opioid receptors and, 325-326, 327t, 328
with orpganophosphate eyedrops, 164-165
with sedative-hypnotic agents, 285-286, 287-291, 293-299
Drug Interactions Handbook, 6
Drug Interactions Index, 6
Drug Interactions Indexed, 6
Drug Interactions Newsletter, 6
Drug metabolism, alterations in, as drug interaction, 43-44
hepatic, 43-44, *43*
inhibition of, causes of, 21-22
pH shifts and, 60-61
stimulation of, causes of, 21-22
Drug metabolite(s), activity of, 64
reactive, in halothane interactions, 68-69
Drug overdosage, narcotic, 322, 325
of monoamine oxidase inhibitors, 80
treatment of, 41, 58, 81, 201
Drug reaction(s), adverse, types of, 18
allergic, 32-34
as type B reactions, 18
Drugs, absorption of, 53, 56, 57t
acidic, protein binding of, 44-46
additive, defined, 26
basic, protein binding of, 45-46
biotransformation of, abnormal shunting of, 67
hepatic, 63-65, *66*
distribution of. See Drug distribution
dose-effect relationship of, 39
fixed, 68
formulation of, allergic reactions and, 33
generic. See Generic drug(s)
half-life of, defined, 40
high-extraction, defined, 43
hit and run, defined, 49
ionization of, 51-53, 54-55t
ionized, un-ionized versus, 51-53
metabolism of. See Drug metabolism
oral, interactions among, 19
plasma concentration of, measurement of, 42
route of administration and, 40
slope of decline in, 40
potency of, defined, 40
problem, 10
protein binding of. See Protein binding
restriction of by anesthesiologist, 9
route of administration of, allergic reactions and, 33
drug disposition and, 40
plasma concentration and, 40
steady state of, measurement of, 49
"street," with anticholinergic muscarinic activity, 172
toxicity of, pH shifts and, 60-61
un-ionized, distribution of, 56-58, *57-59*

volatile, 68
Drug-metabolizing enzyme(s), 64-65
Dyskinesia(s), drug-induced, 265
Dysrhythmia(s). See Cardiac dysrhythmia(s)

Echothiophate, as pseudocholinesterase inhibitor, 378
enzymatic hydrolysis of, local anesthetic agents and, 395-396
in eyedrops, 164
indications for use of, 378, 395
interaction of, with acetylcholinesterase, 395
with chloroprocaine, 396
with pseudocholinesterase, 395-396
with succinylcholine, 377-378, 395
nonsurmountable antagonism of, 26
Eclampsia, treatment of, 431
magnesium sulfate in, 204, 372
paraldehyde in, 297
ED$_{95}$, anesthetic depth and, 410t
Edema, cellular, osmotic diuretics in, 212
pulmonary. See Pulmonary edema
treatment of, diuretics in, 213
Edrophonium, indication for use of, 233-234
interaction of, with atracurium, 376
with neuromuscular blocking agents, 372
with pancuronium, 367
with quinidine, 372
with succinylcholine, 377
with vecuronium, 376
mechanism of action of, 233-234
Elavil. See Amitriptyline
Electroconvulsive therapy, lithium carbonate and, 275-276
reserpine and, 266
succinylcholine and, 273, 275
Electroencephalogram(s), general anesthetic agents and, 255-256
manifestations on, of physostigmine, 295-296
phenobarbital in studies of, 255
Electrolyte(s), disturbances of, from loop diuretics, 214
from osmotic diuretics, 212
imbalance of, digitalis toxicity and, 193
measurement of, urinary, 218
renal regulation of, 208, *209*, 210-211
Elimination, drug, principles of, 40
Hofmann, 383-385
Embolism, possible, in case report analysis, 14t
pulmonary, isoproterenol in treatment of, 89
Emergence phenomenon(a), from ketamine, 310-311
Encephalopathy, anoxic, thiopental for prevention of, 46-47
from bilirubin, 433
Endoplasmic reticulum, defined, 64
in biotransformation of drugs, 64-65
Endotracheal intubation, anesthetic depth quantification and, 410t
bronchospasm from, in asthma, 348

cardiac dysrhythmias associated with, 168
complications of, 342
contraindication for, 14t
hypertension during, beta-adrenergic blocking agents and, 122, *124*
hypertension following, 71-72
hypertension from, propranolol in, 235-236
inhalation anesthetic agents in, minimum alveolar concentration and, 409, 410t
interaction of, with antihypertensive agents, 342
with beta-adrenergic blocking agents, 342, 344
with calcium-channel blocking agents, 346
lithium and, 277
midazolam and, 316
tachycardia following, 71-72
Enflurane, actions of, postjunctional membrane, 353
anesthetic depth and, 413
cardiac dysrhythmias with, 169
effects of, antiepileptic, 256
central nervous system, 255-256
hepatoxicity from, 356
interaction of, with aminophylline, 105, 349
with amitriptyline, 270
with anticholinergic agents, 167
with antihypertensive agents, 341
with antipsychotic agents, 263
with atracurium, 374
with beta-adrenergic blocking agents, 125-128, *129*, 344
with chlorpromazine, 263
with diazepam, 266
with digitalis, 184, 188
with epinephrine, 3, 83, 83t, 107, 355, 392
with etomidate, 256
with fentanyl, 351, 415t, 419
with hydralazine, 156
with ketamine, 310, 350
with lidocaine, 234, 237, 392, 401, 400
with maprotiline, 271
with monoamine oxidase inhibitors, 274
with nalbuphine, 332t
with naloxone, 415t, 416
with neuromuscular blocking agents, 2, 353-354, 370, 374, 382
with nitrous oxide, 72, 351-352, 353
with oxprenolol, 128, 130, *132*
with pancuronium, 354
with phenobarbital, 266
with phenothiazines, 264
with propranolol, 78, 125-128, *129*, 238, 343-344
with quinidine, 236
with reserpine, 266
with succinylcholine, 354
with theophylline, 105-107
with tranylcypromine, 80
with tricyclic antidepressants, 256
with d-tubocurarine, 354
with vecuronium, 374-375
with verapamil, 345-346

Gallamine (cont.)
  effects of, in renal failure, 368
  interaction of, with beta- adrenergic blocking agents, 121
    with decamethonium, 373
    with diazepam, 297
    with epinephrine, 83
    with lidocaine, 398, 402
    with lithium carbonate, 275-277
    with muscarinic receptors, 24
    with succinylcholine, 373-374
    with tricyclic antidepressants, 381
  vecuronium versus, 384
Gamma amino butyric acid, actions of, 292
  benzodiazepine binding sites and, 292-293
  interaction of, with benzodiazepines, 292, 312-313
    with diazepam, 312-313
    with pentobarbital, 292
Gammahydroxybutrate, 374
Ganglion(a), autonomic, 147-148, 162, 165
  cholinesterase inhibition and, 162
  stimulation of, as drug side effect, 163
Ganglionic blocking agent(s), interaction of, with monoamine oxidase inhibitors, 348
  with neuromuscular blocking agents, 378-379
Gantrisin. See Sulfisoxazole
Gastrointestinal effect(s), of anticholinergic drugs, 19
  of aspirin, 19
  of cholinomimetic drugs, 19
  of digitalis, 187, 189-190
  of guanethidine, 154
  of metoclopramide, 19, 173
  of narcotics, 19, 322
  of nicotine overdose, 163
  of physostigmine, 296
Gemonil. See Metharbital
General anesthesia, contraindications to, in toxemia, 432
  in alcoholism, 291
  in epilepsy, 255-257
General anesthetic agent(s), actions of, 28-29
  adjuvant drugs and, 16
  biotransformation of, 64
  cardiac effects of, 31
  in shock, 93
  interaction of, with chlorpromazine, 79
    with clonidine, 77
    with ethyl alcohol, 291
    with local anesthetic agents, 397-398, 398
    with narcotic analgesics, 28
    with oxytocic agents, 429
    with premedication, 28
    with sympathomimetic agents, 93
    with theophylline, 105-107
  interactions with, anesthetic depth and, 414, 415t, 416-419, 422, 417-422
    antagonistic, 414, 415t, 416
  malignant hyperpyrexia from, 31
  toxicity of, 16
Generic drug(s), variations in formulation of, drug interactions and, 18

Genetic factor(s), drug responses and, 17
  in drug interactions, 10
Gentamicin, interaction of, with calcium, 201, 366t
  with neostigmine, 366t
  with pancuronium, 375
  with succinylcholine, 366t
  with d-tubocurarine, 363-364, 364, 366t
  with vecuronium, 375
Glaucoma, anticholinesterase agents in treatment of, 164
  from interaction between atropine and muscarinic cholinergic receptors, 24
  treatment of, echothiophate in, 378, 395-396
    pilocarpine in, 164
    timolol in, 344
Glomerular filtration, in renal excretion, 22-23
  of neuromuscular blocking agents, 365
Glomerular filtration rate, digitalis toxicity and, 187-188
  effect on, of carbonic anhydrase inhibitors, 213
  of diuretics, 211, 213
  in anesthesia, 203-204
  prostaglandins and, 211
Glucagon, interaction of, with beta-adrenergic blocking agents, 345
Glucocorticoid(s), anti-asthmatic actions of, 109
  enzymatic hydrolysis in, local anesthetic agents and, 396
  in shock management, 93
  interaction of, with procaine, 396
Glucose, interaction of, with digitalis, 190
  osmotic diuresis with, 212
  treatment of hyperkalemia with, 204, 216, 220
Glucuronic acid, 64
Glucuronyltransferase, induction of, bilirubin and, 434-435
Glutethimide, actions of, 298
  as enzyme inducer, 67
  central nervous system effects of, 298
  indications for use of, 298
  interaction of, with anticoagulants, 298
    with codeine, 298
    with ethyl alcohol, 289
    with physostigmine, 172t
    with warfarin, 298
Glycerol, osmotic diuresis with, 212
Glycinexylidide, 403, 403
Glycopyrrolate, interaction of, with anesthetic agents, 167
  with antipsychotic agents, 263
  with other anticholinergic agents, 268
  with physostigmine, 173
Glycoside(s), cardiac. See Digitalis; specific preparations
"Goldilocks" assessment of anesthetic depth, 413
Gout, from diuretics and anesthesia, 218
  in preoperative evaluation of patient taking diuretics, 220

Guanabenz, actions of, 155
  classification of, 148t
  discontinuance of, hypertension from, 154
  dosage of, 148t
  mechanism of action of, 340-341
  pharmacology of, 155
Guanethidine, actions of, 77, 154-155, 290
  cardiac effects of, 77, 154-155
  classification of, 148t
  contraindications to, 154
  discontinuance of, hypertension from, 154
  dosage of, 148t
  hypotension from, 77
  indications for use of, 77
  interaction of, with alpha- adrenergic blocking agents, 155
    with catecholamines, 154-155
    with cocaine, 155
    with ephedrine, 151t, 155
    with ethyl alcohol, 290
    with halothane, 151t, 342, 415t, 417, 417
    with imipramine, 81
    with ketamine, 155
    with monoamine oxidase inhibitors, 272
    with norepinephrine, 73, 154-155, 341
    with pancuronium, 155
    with pargyline, 158
    with sympathomimetic agents, 154
    with thiazide diuretics, 217
    with tricyclic antidepressants, 27, 77, 81, 155
  mechanism of action of, 341
  pharmacology of, 154-155
  side effects of, 151t, 154

Half-life, drug, defined, 40
Hallucination(s), from interaction of oxymorphone and tetrahydrocannabinol, 299
  from ketamine, 310
  illusions versus, 311
Halogenated ether(s), interaction of, with epinephrine, 354-355
Haloperidol, actions of, 261-262
  as agent with anticholinergic activity, 172t
  interaction of, with methyldopa, 153
  side effects of, 261-262
Halothane, anesthetic depth and, 411, 412, 413-414
  biotransformation of, 66
  cardiac effects of, 71-72
  mechanism of, 227
  discontinuance of, during general anesthesia, 330
  effects of, antiepileptic, 255
    in hypovolemia, 203
    neuromuscular, 370
    neuronal, 255
  environmental effects on, 17
  hepatoxicity of, 67-69, 356
  hypercapnia and, 416t, 423, 423
  hypernatremia and, 416, 416t
  hyperosmolarity and, 416
  hypersensitivity to, 356
  hyperthermia and, 416, 416t, 417
  hypocapnia and, 416t, 422-424, 423

hypoxia and, 416t, 422-423, *422-423*
in asthmatics, 106-107
indication for, in asthma, 14t
interaction of, with *alpha*-methyldopa, 342, 415t, 416-417, *417*
　with *alpha*-methyl-para-tyrosine, 414
　with aminophylline, 100-101, 105-106, 348-349
　with amphetamine, 414, 415t
　with anticholinergic agents, 167-170
　with antihypertensive agents, 150, 341-342
　with antimuscarinic anticholinergic agents, 170
　with antipsychotic agents, 263
　with atracurium, 374
　with atropine, 380
　with barbiturates, 66
　with *beta*-adrenergic blocking agents, 125-128, *129*, 344
　with *beta*-adrenergic stimulating drugs, 13
　with bupivacaine, 400
　with calcium-channel blocking agents, 345-346
　with carbamazepine, 251
　with catecholamines, 71-72, 416
　with cimetidine, 177
　with clonidine, 415t, 417
　with cocaine, 29, 34-35, 71-72, 82, 391, 414, 415t, 416
　with dextroamphetamine, 414
　with diazepam, 284, 313, 415t, 419
　with digitalis, 184, 188
　with digoxin, 233
　with dopamine, 416
　with droperidol, 263
　with enzyme-inducing drugs, 68-69
　with ephedrine, 91, 355
　with epinephrine, 3, 34, 82-83, 83t, 106-107, 354-355, 391-392, 400-401
　with ethyl alcohol, 291, 349, 415t, 422
　with etidocaine, 400
　with etomidate, 317
　with guanethidine, 151t, 342, 415t, 417, *417*
　with hexobarbital, 66
　with hypnotics, 68-69
　with imipramine, 81
　with iproniazid, 347
　with isoproterenol, 415t, 417
　with ketamine, 47, 84, 310-311, 311t, 350, 415t, 418, *419*
　with levodopa, 347, 415t, 417-418, *418*
　with lidocaine, 66, 234, 237, 392, 400-401, 398, 415t, 418-419, *420*
　with lithium carbonate, 277
　with local anesthetic agents, 400-401
　with mannitol, 416
　with mephentermine, 91
　with metaraminol, 355
　with methyldopa, 151t
　with midazolam, 314, 316-317
　with monoamine oxidase inhibitors, 274, 347
　with morphine, 284, 350, 415t, 419, *421*
　with naloxone, 415t, 416
　with neuromuscular blocking agents, 2, 374-375, 382
　with nialamide, 274
　with nifedipine, 141
　with nitroglycerin, 144
　with nitrous oxide, 28, 71-72, 351-353, 419
　with norepinephrine, 416
　with oxprenolol, 122, 130, *132*
　with oxytocin, 429
　with pancuronium, 354, 369, 379-380, 415t, 419, 422
　with pargyline, 80
　with pentazocine, 66
　with pheniprazine, 274
　with phenobarbital, 68, 248, 415t
　with phenylephrine, 90
　with phenytoin, 248
　with polychlorobiphenyls, 68
　with potassium, 416, 416t
　with prazosin, 155
　with propranolol, 78-79, 125-128, *129*, 238, 343-344, 415t, 417
　with quinidine, 236
　with reserpine, 151t, 266, 342, 414, 415t, 417
　with sedatives, 68-69
　with serotonin, 416
　with succinylcholine, 168, 354
　with sufentanil, 415t, 419
　with tetrohydrocannabinol, 299, 415t, 422, *422*
　with theophylline, 101, 105-107
　with thiopental, 309
　with tolazoline, 417
　with tricyclic antidepressants, 269, 347, 379-380
　with d-tubocurarine, 369-371, *370*, 379, *380*
　with valproic acid, 251
　with vasopressors, 380
　with vecuronium, 374-375
　with verapamil, 139, 141, 142, 345-346, 415t, 418
metabolites of, 68-69
minimum alveolar concentration of, adrenergic responses and, 409, 410t
antihypertensive agents and, 342
diazepam and, 313
hypotension and, 416t
hypoxia and, 416t, 422-423, *422-423*
pregnancy and, 416t, 424
overdosage of, calcium in treatment of, 201
sensitivity of, to epinephrine-induced dysrhythmias, 82-83, 83t
Halothane hepatitis, as possible drug interaction, 68-69
Haptene(s), defined, 69
Heart, oxygen consumption in. See Myocardial oxygen consumption
"stone," defined, 122
Heart block, *beta*-adrenergic blocking agents contraindicated in, 123
from calcium-channel blocking agents, treatment of, 138-139
from digitalis, 187
from interaction, of digitalis and verapamil, 192
of potassium and digitalis, 191
from magnesium sulfate, 431
Heart disease(s), abnormal cardiac automaticity in, 227
beta-adrenergic blocking agents in, preoperative discontinuance of, 121-122, *123*, 128-132, *131-132*, 132t
calcium administration in, 201
cardiac dysrhythmias from, 187
congenital, ketamine in, 310
effects in, of cocaine, 391, 393
of ethyl alcohol, 290
ergot alkaloids in, 429
interaction in, of anesthetic agents and oxytocin, 429
of diazepam and fentanyl, 313, *314-316*
of diazepam and morphine, 312
of digitalis and propranolol, 191
of narcotics and nitrous oxide, 350
of nitrous oxide and other inhalation agents, 352
of propranolol and catecholamines, 119-120, *120*
of thiopental and inhalation anesthetic agents, 349
ischemic, thiopental in, 308
ketamine use in, 84
valvular. See Valvular heart disease(s)
vasopressors in, intraoperative hypotension and, 342
Heart failure, *beta*-adrenergic blocking agents contraindicated in, 123, *127*
congestive. See Congestive heart failure
effects in, of local anesthetic agents, 393
nephritis and, lidocaine in, 393
treatment of, digitalis in, 179-180
Heart rate, anesthetic depth and, 412-413, *413-414*
preoperative evaluation of in patients taking diuretics, 218
Hemodynamic drug interaction(s), 44-46
Hemorrhage, 344, 393
Hemorrhagic shock, characteristics of, 92
treatment of, 92-94
mephentermine in, 91
naloxone in, 336
Henderson's equation, 52-53
Henderson-Hasselbalch equation, 53, 56
Heparin, interaction of, with antibiotics, 19t
with diazepam, 312
with digitalis, 190
with propranolol, 35
possible indication for, 14t
Hepatic disease(s), atracurium in, 385
barbiturates in, 284
calcium-channel blocking agents in, 139
citrate intoxication in, 202
digitalis toxicity in, 190
effects of, on local anesthetic agents, 397

Hepatic disease(s) (cont.)
  from ethyl alcohol, anticoagulant therapy in, 288
  indicators of, drug half-lives as, 397
  methyldopa in, 152
  protein binding and, 41, 46
  vecuronium in, 385
Hepatic enzyme(s), ethyl alcohol and, 287-288
  monoamine oxidase inhibitors and, 271, 273
  phenobarbital and, 284
  sedative-hypnotic agents and, 284
Hepatic failure, ammonium chloride in, 213
Hepatic function, antiepileptic agents and, preoperative studies of, 253
  effects of, on atracurium, 385
    on vecuronium, 385
Hepatic necrosis, centrolobular, from inhalation anesthetic agents, 356
  postanesthetic, 67-68
Hepatic toxicity, from valproic acid, 251
Hepatitis, from halothane, 67-69, 356
  from hydralazine, 156
  from methyldopa, 152
  from phenytoin, 248
Hepatocyte(s), characteristics of, 63-64
  enzyme induction and, 65
Hexafluorenium, interaction of, with local anesthetic agents, 401-402
Hexamethonium, as nicotinic cholinolytic agent, 165
  effects of, parasympathetic, 161
  interaction of, with pharmacologic receptors, 24
Hexobarbital, interaction of, with halothane, 66
  with imipramine, 270
  with nalbuphine, 332t
High-extraction drug(s), defined, 43
Histamine, calcium channels and, 135
  in allergic drug reactions, 32, 34
  interaction of, with atracurium, 384
    with epinephrine, 26-27
    with metocurine, 384
    with d-tubocurarine, 379, 384
  release of, narcotics and, 322
  sensitivity to, 160
Histamine H$_2$ blocking agent(s), 176-177, 322
Hit and run drug(s), defined, 49
Hofmann elimination, defined, 383
  of atracurium, 383-385
Homatropine, as belladonna alkaloid, 171t
  cardiac effects of, 165
  interaction of, with other anticholinergic agents, 268
Hormone(s), antidiuretic. See Antidiuretic hormone
  interactions of, in renal salt and water regulation, 210-211
  thyroid, response to catecholamines potentiated by, 75
Hydralazine, actions of, 156
  classification of, 148t
  dosage of, 148t
  indications for use of, 156
    in toxemia, 431
  interaction of, with anesthetic agents, 156

  with beta-adrenergic blocking agents, 156
  with digitalis, 182, 190
  with diuretics, 156
  with enflurane, 156
  with magnesium sulfate, 432
  mechanism of action of, 341
  pharmacology of, 156
  side effects, 151t, 156
Hydrochlorothiazide, 216
  cardiac dysrhythmias from, 220
Hydrocortisone, indications for use of, 110
  interaction of, with chloramphenicol, 19t
    with colistimethate, 19t
    with pancuronium, 369
Hydrogen ion(s), drug ionization and, 51-53, 54-55t
  interaction of, with local anesthetic agents, 394-395, 400
  secretion of, renal tubular, 209, 210
Hydrolysis, enzymatic. See Enzymatic hydrolysis
  ester, of atracurium, 383-385
  in biotransformation of drugs, 64
Hydromorphone, interaction of, with nalbuphine, 332t
3-Hydroxy-methyl-beta-carboline, 293
4-Hydroxypropranolol, 47t, 78
5-Hydroxytryptamine, 151, 402
5-Hydroxytryptophan, 402
Hydroxyzine, contraindications to, 254
  interaction of, with anesthetic agents, 167
    with ketamine, 285, 311
    with pentobarbital, 283
Hyoscine. See Scopolamine
Hypercapnia, cardiac dysrhythmias and, 169
  effects of, on halothane, 416t, 423, 423
  epinephrine and, 74, 82
  local anesthetics and, 400
Hyperglycemia from tocolytic agents, 432
Hyperkalemia, anesthetic considerations in, 93-94, 204, 216, 220, 346
  beta-adrenergic blocking agents in, 204
  calcium in treatment of, 201-202
  calcium-channel blocking agents and, 140
  cardiac effects of, 204, 215-216
  catecholamine potentiation from, 93
  citrate intoxication and, 202
  defined, 204
  digitalis and, 188, 215-216
  fatal, 93
  from potassium-sparing diuretics, 214
  from succinylcholine, 374
  iatrogenic, 219
  in renal disease, 204
  intraoperative, causes of, 94
  manifestations of, 220
  neuromuscular blocking agents in, 204, 216-217
  renal failure and, 216-217, 220
  treatment of, 204, 220
Hypermagnesemia, antibiotics and, 432
  effects of, 204-205

  neuromuscular blocking agents in, 205
  neonatal, 432
Hypernatremia, anesthetic depth and, 416, 416t
  causes of, 203
  halothane and, 416, 416t
  treatment of, 203
Hyperosmolality, from osmotic diuretics, 212
Hyperosmolarity, halothane and, 416
Hyperpolarization, cardiac, 227
Hyperpyrexia, in hypertensive crisis, 272
  malignant. See Malignant hyperpyrexia
Hypersensitivity, drug, 32-34
Hypertension, anesthesia and, 149
  anesthesia in, procedure for, 342
  crises of. See Hypertensive crisis(es)
  ergot alkaloids in, 429
  essential. See Essential hypertension
  from beta-adrenergic blocking agents, preoperative discontinuance of, 130, 131
  from endotracheal intubation, 342
    propranolol in, 235-236
  from ketamine, 310
  from levodopa, 346
  from monoamine oxidase inhibitors, 271-275, 347
    treatment of, 80, 272, 348
  from naloxone, 336
  from nicotine overdose, 163
  from oxytocin, 429
  from succinylcholine, 163
  from tricyclic antidepressants, 268, 402
  from tyramine ingestion, 80
  hypovolemia in, 76-77
  in pregnancy, drug interactions in, 428-429
    treatment of, 430-431
  induction of anesthesia followed by, 71-72
  intraoperative, beta-adrenergic blocking agents in, 121-122, 124
    treatment of, 342
  intraoperative hypotension in patients with, 149
  ketamine use in, 310
  postoperative, from beta-adrenergic blocking agents, 130-131
  pulmonary. See Pulmonary hypertension
  rebound, 77, 153-154
    from discontinuance of antihypertensive agents, 77, 153, 342
  renal, beta-adrenergic blocking agents in, 131
  treatment of, 76-78, 156
Hypertensive crisis(es), avoidance of, 272
  from ethyl alcohol, 288
  monoamine oxidase inhibitors and, 157, 271-272, 274
  treatment of, 156, 158-159, 272
Hyperthermia, anesthetic depth and, 416, 416t, 417
  malignant. See Malignant hyperpyrexia
Hyperthyroid crisis, 122

INDEX

Hyperthyroidism, catecholamines and, 75, 82
  digitalis dosage in, 188
  digitalis toxicity and, 192
Hyperuricemia, from loop diuretics, 214
  from thiazide diuretics, 213
Hyperventilation, hypocalcemia from, 200
  hypokalemia from, 181
  in shock, 92-93
  ketamine and, 257
  pH shifts induced by, 56
  seizures and, 257, 400
Hypnotic agent(s), sedatives and, 282-300. *See also* Sedative-hypnotic agent(s); specific agents
Hypocalcemia, causes of, 200
  from magnesium sulfate, 432
  manifestations of, 200
  neuromuscular blocking agents in, 200, 381-382
Hypocapnia, citrate intoxication in, 202
  halothane and, 416t, 422-424, *423*
  hypokalemia from, 233
  in shock, 92-94
Hypoglycemic agent(s), as problem drugs, 10
  interaction of, with ethyl alcohol, 290-291
    with thiazide diuretics, 217-218
Hypokalemia, alkalosis in, 219
  anesthetic considerations in, 93, 216, 219
  cardiac effects of, 31, 93, 204
  catecholamines in, 204
  causes of, 181, 189-190
  citrate intoxication and, 202
  defined, 204
  digitalis and, 180-181, 188-191, 204, 233
  epinephrine-related, 93
  from tocolytic agents, 432
  in shock, 92-94
  neuromuscular blocking agents in, 216-217
  pancuronium in, 233
  skeletal muscle in, 216
  treatment of, 190-191
    preoperative, 219
Hypomagnesemia, cardiac dysrhythmias from, 219-220
  digitalis and, 188, 190
  effects of, 204
Hyponatremia, causes of, 202-203
  manifestations of, 202-203
Hypotension, causes of, 91-92, 149
  during anesthesia, 87, 91-92
    treatment of, 88t, 92-94
  effects of, on halothane, 416t
  from *alpha*-methyldopa, 76
  from anesthetic agent(s), 76-77
  from antihypertensive agents, 149
  from antipsychotic agents, 261, 263
  from bretylium, 239
  from calcium-channel blocking agents, 138-139
  from chlorpromazine, 79
  from epinephrine, 3
  from guanethidine, 77
  from hypokalemia, 204
  from hyponatremia, 202-203
  from levodopa, 346

from metaraminol, 91
from metocurine, 384-385
from mexiletine, 240
from monamine oxidase inhibitors, 80, 273-274, 325, 347
  treatment of, 348
from narcotics, 141, 262, 324, 350
from nicotine overdose, 163
from nitroglycerin, 143-144
from opiates, 322
from pargyline, 157
from phenothiazines, 348
from propranolol, 123-124
from quinidine, 236
from reserpine, 266
from theophylline, 103
from timolol, 344
from tocolytic agents, 432
from d-tubocurarine, 384-385
hypovolemic, 203
in pregnancy, treatment of, 429
intraoperative, causes of, 341
  in hypertensive patients, 149
  management of, 141, 342, 355
orthostatic, from antihypertensive agents, 149, 151t
treatment of, 90, 92-94, 201
  agents in, 88t
  phenylephrine in, 312
Hypothermia, effects of, on neuromuscular blocking agents, 381-382
  in shock, 92
Hypothyroidism, cardiac dysrhythmias in, 231
  digitalis toxicity and, 192
Hypovolemia, anesthetic agents in, 203
  barbiturates in, 203
  from diuretics, 218
  from sodium loss, 202-203
  in hypertension, 76-77
  in shock, treatment of, 92-94
  lidocaine in, 393
  neuromuscular blocking agents in, 203
  preoperative treatment of, 218
Hypovolemic shock, 85
Hypoxia, cardiac dysrhythmias and, 169
  digitalis and, 188, 190
  halothane and, 356, 416t, 422-423, *422-423*
  liver damage caused by, 69
  tissue, potassium transport in, 215-216

Imidazodiazepine(s), interaction of, with diazepam, 293
Imipramine, actions of, 80-81
  as agent with anticholinergic activity, 172t
  cardiac effects of, 81
  indications for use of, 268
  interaction of, with epinephrine, 81, 268
    with guanethidine, 81
    with halothane, 81
    with hexobarbital, 270
    with lidocaine, 270
    with local anesthetic agents, 403
    with meperidine, 269

    with monoamine oxidase inhibitors, 80-81
    with morphine, 269
    with norepinephrine, 73, 268
    with pancuronium, 81, 379-381
    with phenylephrine, 268
    with procaine, 270
    with thiopental, 270
Immune system, in biotransformation of drugs, 69
Immunosuppression, from azathioprine, 363-364
Index, therapeutic, defined, 28
Indomethacin, interaction of, with aspirin, 41
  with captopril, 157
  with diuretics, 220
  with ethacrynic acid, 214
  with furosemide, 214, 217
  with phenylbutazone, 41
  with prazosin, 155
  substitution of for phenylbutazone, 9
Induction of anesthesia, cardiac arrhythmias during, 31-32, 71-72
  hypertension following, 71-72
  hypotension during, 341-342
  in alcoholism, 349
  narcotic antagonists in, 331, 332t, 333
Infant(s), digitalis toxicity in, 188
  effects in, of local anesthetic agents, 396
  hypocalcemia in, 200
  preterm, treatment of apnea in, 102
  theophylline metabolism in, 103, 104t
Inhalation anesthetic agent(s), 340-357
  balanced anesthesia versus, 76
  biotransformation of, 64
  catecholamine release and, 124-125
  contraindications to, in toxemia, 432
  distribution of, cardiac output and, 20-21
  dose-response curve of, 409, 410t, 411, *411*
  effects of, antiepileptic, 255-256
    in hypernatremia, 416, 416t
    in hyperthermia, 416, 416t, 417
    neuromuscular, 353, 370
  elimination of, 63
  ganglionic blocking by, 165
  hepatic interactions of, 65-66
  hepatotoxicity of, 67-69
  in pregnancy, 416t, 424
  indications for use of, in abdominal surgery, 353
  in seizure control, 399
  interaction of, anesthetic depth and 414, 415t, 416-419, 422, *417-422*
    antagonistic, 414, 415t, 416
    with acetylcholine, 370
    with aminophylline, 348-349
    with amphetamine, 414, 415t
    with antibiotics, 9-10
    with antihypertensive agents, 150, 341-342
    with antipsychotic agents, 261t, 263
    with atracurium, 354, 374-375
    with atropine, 415t, 422
    with barbiturates, 66, 349
    with benzodiazepines, 349

Inhalation anesthetic agent(s), interaction of *(cont.)*
  with *beta*-adrenergic blocking agents, 132, 343-345
  with bronchodilators, 20
  with butorphanol, 331
  with butyrophenones, 349
  with calcium-channel blocking agents, 136, 141, 345-346
  with catecholamines, 414, 416-418
  with chlorpromazine, 348
  with cocaine, 391, 414, 415*t*, 416
  with dezocine, 332
  with diazepam, 349-350, 415*t*, 419
  with disopyramide, 238
  with dopamine, 346-347
  with enzyme-inducing drugs, 68-69
  with epinephrine, 2-3, 354-355, 391
  with ethyl alcohol, 349, 415*t*, 422
  with fentanyl, 415*t*, 419
  with hexobarbital, 66
  with intravenous induction agents, 349-350
  with iproniazid, 414, 415*t*
  with isoproterenol, 415*t*, 417
  with ketamine, 350, 415*t*, 418, *419*
  with levodopa, 346-347, 415*t*, 417-418, *418*
  with lidocaine, 66, 415*t*, 418-419, *420*
  with lithium carbonate, 276
  with local anesthetic agents, 397-398, *398*, 400-401, *400*
  with monoamine oxidase inhibitors, 274, 347-348
  with morphine, 415*t*, 419, *421*
  with nalbuphine, 331, 332*t*, 333
  with naloxone, 336, 415*t*, 416
  with naltrexone, 336
  with narcotics, 323-324, 331, 332*t*, 333, 336, 349, 350-351, 413, 415*t*
  with neuromuscular blocking agents, 2, 353-354, 369-371, *370*
  with nifedipine, 345
  with nitroprusside, 158
  with nitrous oxide, 351-353, 415*t*, 419, *421*
  with norepinephrine, 354-355, 413
  with oxyprenolol, 344
  with pancuronium, 354, 415*t*, 419, 422
  with pentazocine, 66, 331
  with phencyclidine, 415*t*, 418
  with phenothiazines, 348, 349
  with preanesthetic medication, 349
  with procainamide, 237
  with propranolol, 20-21, 343-345, 415*t*, 417
  with reserpine, 265*t*, 266, 341-342
  with scopolamine, 415*t*, 422
  with sedative-hypnotic agents, 283-284
  with sedatives, 349, 413, 415*t*
  with sufentanil, 415*t*, 419
  with sympathomimetic agents, 93
  with sympathomimetic amines, 354-355
  with tetrahydrocannibinol, 415*t*, 422, *422*
  with theophylline, 106-107
  with thiopental, 349
  with tricyclic antidepressants, 347
  with d-tubocurarine, 354
  with vasopressors, 263, 342
  with vecuronium, 354, 374-375
  with verapamil, 136, 239, 345-346, 415*t*, 418
  metabolism of, 355-356
  minimum alveolar concentration of, anesthetic depth and, 409, 410*t*, 411, *413*
  defined, 409
  endotracheal intubation and, 409, 410*t*
  prior drug therapy and, 340-349
  tolerance to, in alcoholism, 349
Inhibition, competitive, *beta*-adrenergic receptors and, 114
  postsynaptic, defined, 26
Innovar, components of, 262
  interaction of, with methyldopa, 153
  with metrizamide, 254
  with nalbuphine, 332*t*
Inorganic cation(s), 196-205
Insecticide(s), interaction of, with local anesthetic agents, 396
  organophosphate, nonsurmountable antagonism of, 26
Insulin, desensitization to, 42
  interaction of, with digitalis, 190
  with ethyl alcohol, 291
  treatment of hyperkalemia with, 204, 216, 220
Insulin receptor(s), diabetes and, 42
Insulin release, diazoxide and, 158
Interaction(s), drug. *See* Drug interaction(s); specific agents
Intravenous anesthetic agent(s), distribution of, 20-21
  interactions with, 308-317, 311*t*, 314-316
  potential for, 308
  pharmacokinetics of, 46-47
  time course of action of, 29-30
Intravenous induction agent(s), 349-350
  See also specific agents
Intropin. *See* Dopamine
Intubation, endotracheal. *See* Endotracheal intubation
Iodipamide, 309
Ion channel(s), calcium transport in, 197-201
  in sodium transport, 198-199
Ion(s), calcium, 196-202
  enzymatic, inotropic effect of digitalis and, 182-183, 184*t*
  magnesium, 204-205
  potassium, 204
  sodium, 202-204
Ion trapping, defined, 60
Ionization of drugs, 51-53, 54*t*, 55*t*
Iproniazid, interaction of, with cyclopropane, 414, 415*t*
  with monoamine oxidase inhibitors, 347
Ischemia, myocardial. *See* Myocardial ischemia
Ischemic heart disease, *beta*-adrenergic blocking agents in, 121, 121*t*, *122-123*
  propranolol in, 119, 125-126
  thiopental in, 308
Ismelin. *See* Guanethidine
Isocarboxazid, 325

Isoflurane, anesthetic depth and, cardiac signs of, *413*
  effects of, antiepileptic, 255
  neuromuscular, 370
  hepatotoxicity from, 356
  interaction of, with aminophylline, 349
  with antihypertensive agents, 341
  with antipsychotic agents, 263
  with atracurium, 374
  with *beta*-adrenergic blocking agents, 125, 128, *129*, 344
  with chlorpromazine, 263
  with digitalis, 184, 188
  with ephedrine, 355
  with epinephrine, 3, 83, 83*t*, 107, 355
  with ethyl alcohol, 349, 415*t*, 422
  with metaraminol, 355
  with neuromuscular blocking agents, 2, 370, 374
  with nitrous oxide, 351-352, 419
  with pancuronium, 354
  with propranolol, 125, 128, *129*, 344-345
  with succinylcholine, 353-354
  with theophylline, 106-107
  with vecuronium, 354, 374
  with verapamil, 345
  minimum alveolar concentration of, pregnancy and, 416*t*, 424
  seizures from, 255
  sensitivity of, to epinephrine-induced dysrhythmias, 83, 83*t*
Isoflurophate, in eyedrops, 164
  nonsurmountable antagonism of, 26
Isoniazid, enzyme induction from, 356
Isoproterenol, action of, *beta*-adrenergic stimulating, 116
  direct, 86, 88*t*, 89
  cardiac effects of, 89
  age and, 43
  comparison of, with other bronchodilators, 108, 108*t*
  in shock management, 93
  inactivation of *beta*-adrenergic receptors by, 114-115, *116*
  indications for use of, 89
  interaction of, with *alpha*-adrenergic antagonists, 27
  with *beta*-adrenergic blocking agents, 124, 126*t*, 127*t*
  with calcium-channel blocking agents, 138
  with digitalis, 192
  with halothane, 415*t*, 417
  with ketamine, 84
  with lidocaine, 44, 393, *394*
  with norepinephrine, 73
  with propranolol, *116*, 124, 126*t*, 127*t*, 345
Isosorbide dinitrate, 142
Isuprel. *See* Isoproterenol

Jaundice, from antipsychotic agents, 18
  from halothane interactions, 69

Kanamycin, interaction of, with barbiturates, 19*t*
  with calcium, 201, 365, 366*t*
  with calcium gluconate, 19*t*
  with cephalothin, 19*t*

with heparin, 19t
with methicillin, 19t
with neostigmine, 366t
with phenytoin, 19t
with succinylcholine, 366t
with d-tubocurarine, 366t
Kaolin, inactivation of drugs by, 19
Kaolin-pectin, interaction of, with digitalis, 190
  with digoxin, 188
Keflin. See Cephalothin
Kemadrin. See Procyclidine
Ketamine, actions of, 83-84, 105-106, 310
  cardiac effects of, 83-84
  characteristics of, 47
  comparison of, with dioxolanes, 84
  effects of, antiepileptic, 256
    central nervous system, 256
  excretion of, pH and, 59-60
  in asthmatics, 105-106
  in epilepsy, guidelines for, 256-257
  in heart disease, 84
  in hypertension, 84
  indications for use of, as induction agent, 350
  interaction of, with acetylcholine, 372
    with *alpha*-adrenergic blocking agents, 310
    with aminophylline, 106, 257
    with amitriptyline, 269
    with barbiturates, 257, 297
    with benzodiazepines, 257, 297
    with *beta*-adrenergic blocking agents, 125, 310
    with chlorpromazine, 310
    with clorazepate, 297
    with diazepam, 256, 285, 294, 297, 310, 311
    with digitalis, 184, 188
    with dopamine, 84
    with droperidol, 310
    with enflurane, 310, 350
    with epinephrine, 84
    with flunitrazepam, 310
    with guanethidine, 155
    with halothane, 47, 84, 310-311, 311t, 350, 415t, 418, *419*
    with hydroxyzine, 285, 311
    with inhalation anesthetic agents, 350
    with isoproterenol, 84
    with lithium carbonate, 276, 311
    with lorazepam, 256
    with maprotiline, 271
    with meperidine, 310
    with midazolam, 310, 314, 316
    with monoamine oxidase inhibitors, 269
    with naloxone, 336
    with naltrexone, 336
    with neuromuscular blocking agents, 372
    with nitrous oxide, 350
    with norepinephrine, 73, 84
    with pentobarbital, 310
    with phenobarbital, 266
    with phenothiazines, 264
    with phenoxybenzamine, 310
    with propranolol, 105, 310
    with reserpine, 266
    with scopolamine, 310
    with secobarbital, 285, 311

with succinylcholine, 372
with sympathomimetic agents, 257
with theophylline, 101, 105-106
with thyroxine, 84
with tranylcypromine, 269
with tricyclic antidepressants, 257, 269
with trimethaphan, 310
with d-tubocurarine, 372
with tyramine, 84
with vecuronium, 374
with verapamil, 310
pharmacokinetics of, 47
side effects of, 310
similarity of, to cocaine, 84
thiopental compared with, 105
Ketoconazole, gastric pH and, 176
Key-words system, 13, 14t, 15
Kidney, diseases of. See Renal disease(s)
  drug excretion in, 63
  effects on, of sodium, 202-203
  function of. See Renal function
  regulation of water and electrolytes by, 208, *209*, 210-211
  toxicity of. See Nephrotoxicity
Kinetics. See Pharmacokinetics

Labetalol, actions of, 156
  adrenergic blockade by, 117
  classification of, 148t
  dosage of, 148t
  indications for use of, 156
  interaction of, with diuretics, 156
  mechanism of action of, 341
  pharmacology of, 156
Labor, induction of, 428-429
  premature, 432-433
  suppression of, 432
Lactic acid, 87
Lanoxin, interaction of, with propantheline, 191
Laparoscopy, drug interactions in, 235-236
Laryngoscopy, cardiac arrhythmias during, 31-32
  myocardial ischemia during, *beta*-adrenergic blocking agents and, 121-122, *124*
Laudanosine, 383, 384n
L-dopa. See Levodopa
Levallorphan, as narcotic agonist-antagonist, 325t
  as partial agonist, 334
  structure of, 333-334, *334*
Levodopa, as dopamine precursor, 346
  cardiac effects of, 346
  effects of, central nervous system, 346-347
  interaction of, with dopamine, 417-418
    with droperidol, 347
    with halothane, 347, 415t, 417-418, *418*
    with inhalation anesthetic agents, 346-347
    with monoamine oxidase inhibitors, 272
    with narcotic antagonists, 336
    with narcotics, 323
    with norepinephrine, 418
  side effects of, 346
Levophed. See Norepinephrine

Levorphanol, levallorphan as derivative of, 333-334, *334*
  opioid receptors and, 327t
  structure of, *334*
Librium. See Chlordiazepoxide
Lidocaine, actions of, 237
  cardiac effects of, during atrial flutter, 234
    on pacemaker current, 227
    treatment failure with, *126*
  digitalis toxicity treated with, 182, 201
  dosage of, therapeutic, 234, 237
  effects of, circadian rhythm and, 404
    convulsant, 294-295
    extracardiac, 230t
    in acidosis, 394-395
    in heart failure, 393
    in hepatic disease, 397
    in renal impairment, 393
    neuromuscular, 402
  electrophysiologic actions of, 230t
  enzyme induction and, 44
  half-life of, hepatic dysfunction and, 397
  hepatic metabolism of, 44
  indications for use of, 234, 237
    in epilepsy, 254
  interaction of, with amitriptyline, 270, 403
    with ammonium benzoate, 404
    with barbiturates, 295
    with benzodiazepines, 294-295
    with *beta*-adrenergic blocking agents, 398
    with bupivacaine, 401
    with calcium, 201
    with carbon dioxide, 392, 400
    with cimetidine, 177, 394
    with cyclopropane, 419
    with diazepam, 294-295, 399
    with diethyl ether, 400
    with digitalis, 180, 182, 187, 190, 201
    with diltiazem, 139
    with enflurane, 234, 237, 400, 401
    with enzyme inducers, 396-397
    with ephedrine, 393
    with epinephrine, 3, 82, 87, 355, 392, *392*
    with etidocaine, 401
    with gallamine, 402
    with halothane, 66, 234, 237, 398, 415t, 418-419, *420*
    with histamine H$_2$ blocking agent, 177
    with hydrogen ion, 394-395, 400
    with 5-hydroxytryptamine, 402
    with 5-hydroxytryptophan, 402
    with imipramine, 270
    with inhalation anesthetic agents, 397-398, *398*
    with isoproterenol, 44, 393, *394*
    with lidocaine metabolites, 403-404, *403*
    with midazolam, 295
    with nalbuphine, 332t
    with neuromuscular blocking agents, 371
    with nifedipine, 139
    with nitrous oxide, 398, 400, *400*, 419
    with norepinephrine, 393, *394*
    with nortoxiferine, 371

Lidocaine, interaction of *(cont.)*
 with pancuronium, 371
 with para-aminobenzoic acid, 404
 with P-chloro-p-phenylalanine, 402
 with pentobarbital, 399
 with phenobarbital, 396, 397, *397*
 with propranolol, 44, 393, 398
 with protriptyline, 270, 402
 with quinidine, 234, 237
 with sodium benzoate, 404
 with succinylcholine, 371, 402
 with tetracaine, 401
 with thiopental, 295
 with tubocurarine, 235, 371, 402
 with vasopressors, 393, *394*
 with verapamil, 139
metabolism of, 397
metabolites of, interactions with, 403-404, *403*
mexiletine versus, 240
overdosage of, calcium in treatment of, 201
phenytoin versus, 190, 238
propranolol versus, 122
protein binding of, 393-395
 diseases and, 46
pulmonary extraction of, 398
seizures from, carbon dioxide tension and, 400
side effects of, 237
tocainide as analog of, 240
toxicity of, metabolites in, 403-404
pH and, 58
treatment of cardiac dysrhythmias with, 74
Lifescan, thiopental coma monitored with, 47
Lincomycin, interaction of, with calcium, 366*t*
 with neostigmine, 366*t*
 with penicillin G, 19*t*
 with succinylcholine, 366*t*
 with d-tubocurarine, 366*t*
Lindane, as enzyme inducer, 67
Lipid(s), drug excretion and, 63-64
Lithium carbonate, actions of, 79
 anesthetic considerations with, 277
 in pregnancy, 276
 indications for use of, 275
 interaction of, with acetylcholine, 276
 with alphaxalone-alphadolone, 276
 with aminophylline, 277
 with atracurium, 276
 with barbiturates, 275*t*, 276-277, 309
 with decamethonium, 79, 275-276
 with diazepam, 276
 with diuretics, 217, 276-277
 with ethacrynic acid, 217, 277
 with furosemide, 217, 277
 with gallamine, 275-277
 with halothane, 277
 with inhalation anesthetic agents, 276
 with ketamine, 276, 311
 with local anesthetic agents, 276
 with methohexital, 276
 with neuromuscular blocking agents, 275*t*, 275-276, 372-373
 with norepinephrine, 275
 with pancuronium, 79, 275-276
 with pentobarbital, 309
 with plasma cholinesterase, 275

 with propanidid, 276
 with serotonin, 275
 with spironolactone, 277
 with succinylcholine, 79, 275-276, 372-373
 with thiazide diuretics, 276-277
 with thiopental, 276
 with triamterene, 277
 with d-tubocurarine, 275-277
pharmacology of, 275
serum levels of, therapeutic, 276
 toxic, 276
side effects of, 276, 277
Liver, diseases of. *See* Hepatic disease(s)
 drug interactions mediated by, 63-69, 66
 drug metabolism in, 43-44, *43*
 dysfunction of, from loop diuretics, 214
 effects on, of antipsychotic agents, 18
 of halothane, 67-69
 failure of, effects on thiopental of, 46
Local anesthesia, from antipsychotic agents, 18
 absorption of, 391-392, *392*
 acid-base disturbances and, 400
 antidysrhythmic agents as, 229, 230*t*, 231
 beta-adrenergic blocking agents as, 231
 cardiac effects of, myocardial action potential and, 199
 circadian rhythm and, 404
 drug interactions with, 399-404, *400*, *403*
 effects of, central nervous system, 404
 hemorrhage and, 393
 in acidosis, 394-395
 in heart failure, 393
 neuromuscular, 371, 402
 on sodium channel, 137
 protein binding and, 393-395
 effects on, of hepatic disease, 397
 elimination of, 59, 395-399, *395*, *397-398*
 enzyme induction of, 396-397, *397*
 excretion of, pH and, 59
 hydrolysis of, cholinesterase in, 396
 enzymatic, 395-396, *395*
 plasma pseudocholinesterase in, 398
 in epilepsy, 254
 interaction of, with AB-132, 396
 with acetylcholine, 402
 with alkylphosphates, 396
 with anticonvulsant agents, 399-400
 with barbiturates, 396-397, *397*, 399-400
 with carbon dioxide, 392, 400
 with curare, 371
 with dextran, 392
 with diazepam, 294-295, 399
 with epinephrine, 2-3, 21, 392, *392*
 with fluroxene, 400
 with general anesthetic agents, 397-398, *398*
 with halothane, 400-401
 with hexafluorenium, 401-402
 with hydrogen, 400
 with hydrogen ion, 394-395

 with inhalation anesthetic agents, 397-398, *398*, 400-401, *400*
 with insecticides, 396
 with lithium carbonate, 276
 with methoxyflurane, 400
 with mixed local anesthetic agents, 401
 with neostigmine, 395
 with neuromuscular blocking agents, 371, 401-402
 with oxygen, 400
 with oxytocic agents, 430
 with pancuronium, 401-402
 with pentobarbital, 295
 with phenobarbital, 396, *397*
 with plasma cholinesterase, 395
 with propranolol, 398
 with pyridostigmine, 395
 with sodium bisulfite, 392
 with thiobarbiturates, 295
 with thiopental, 295
 with tricyclic antidepressants, 402-403
 with trimethaphan, 402
 with vasopressors, 393
ionization of, to reduce toxicity, 56
metabolites of, toxicity of, 403-404, *403*
peripheral effects of, 29
respiratory depression from, 402
seizures from, treatment of, 399-400
tachyphylaxis to, 401
tolerance to, in combination, 401
 in epilepsy, 399-400
toxicity of, combined, 401
pH and, 56-59
Loniten. *See* Minoxidil
Lorazepam, actions of, 294
 diazepam versus, 253
 dosage of, 247*t*, 253-254
 indications for use of, 253, 291, 294
 interaction of, with caffeine, 296
 with cimetidine, 177, 294
 with ethyl alcohol, 289
 with ketamine, 256-257
 with physostigmine, 172*t*, 295-296
 introduction of, 245, 246*t*
 pharmacokinetics of, 247*t*, 253
Lorfan. *See* Levallorphan
Lormetazepam, interaction of, with ethyl alcohol, 289
Loxapine, seizures from, 264
LSD, receptor binding of, 49
Luminal. *See* Phenobarbital
Lung(s). *See* Pulmonary entries
Lysine, in meperidine excretion, 273
Lytic cocktail, defined, 262

Ma huang, ephedrine from, 90
MAC, defined, 28
Magnesium, calcium transport and, 197
 derangements in, 204-205
 fetal effects of, 431
 indications for use of, 204
 interaction of, with calcium, 205, 431
 with curare, 205
 with decamethonium, 205
 with digitalis, 181, 189-190
 with succinylcholine, 205
 serum concentrations of, 204
Magnesium sulfate, actions of, 372
 cardiac effects of, 431

dosage of, 431
indications for use of, 372, 431-432
interaction of, with acetylcholine, 372, 431
  with anesthetic agents, 430-432
  with dexamethonium, 431
  with gentamicin, 432
  with hydralazine, 432
  with neuromuscular blocking agents, 372, 430-432
  with reserpine, 432
  with succinylcholine, 372, 431-432
  with d-tubocurarine, 372, 430-431
neuromuscular effects of, 431-432
pharmacology of, 431
side effects of, 432
Malathion, 44
Malignant hyperpyrexia, causes of, 31
  drug responses and, 17
  preanesthetic evaluation and, 12
  treatment of, 30, 142
Mandelic acid, 73
Mannitol, indications for use of, 212
  with halothane, 416
  with neuromuscular blocking agents, 364-365, 364, 371
  osmotic pressure exerted by, 208
  renal effects of, 211-212, 212
  sites of action of, 211-212, 215
Maprotiline, 270-271
Marijuana. See Tetrahydrocannabinol
Mebaral. See Methylphenobarbital
Median effective dose, anesthetic depth and, 410t
Medical Letter, 6
MEDIPHOR classification system, 7-9
MEDIPHOR Drug Interaction Facts, 6, 7-9, 8
Medisc, 6
Medium(a), contrast. See Contrast medium(a)
Mellaril. See Thiorizadine
Membrane potential, in calcium transport, 198
Membrane stabilizer(s), defined, 28
Meperidine, biotransformation of, 64
  contraindication to, 325
  conversion of to normeperidine, 67
  dissociation of, 56
  effects of pH in, 59
  excretion of, techniques for effecting, 273
  fentanyl versus, 48
  histamine release in, 322
  in lytic cocktail, 262
  in neonates, 435
  indications for use of, as induction agent, 350
  interaction of, with amitriptyline, 269
    with anticholinergic agents, 268
    with benzodiazepines, 295
    with bupivacaine, 394
    with chlorpromazine, 324
    with epinephrine, 83
    with etomidate, 317
    with imipramine, 269
    with ketamine, 310
    with methohexital, 309
    with monoamine oxidase inhibitors, 22, 67, 80, 157, 272-274, 295, 347
    with muscarinic receptors, 24
    with phenelzine, 325

  with phenobarbital, 435
  with phenothiazines, 262
  with promethazine, 262
ionization of, 56
protein binding of, 42t
respiratory depression from, 324
toxicity of, pH shifts and, 61
Mephentermine, action of, indirect, 87, 88t, 91
  cardiac effects of, 91, 354
  interaction of, with digitalis, 91
    with halothane, 91
    with monoamine oxidase inhibitors, 272, 274
    with reserpine, 266
  metaraminol versus, 91
Mephenytoin, 246t
Mephobarbital. See Methylphenobarbital
Mepivacaine, effects of, neuromuscular, 402
  enzyme induction and, 44
  interaction of, with diazepam, 399
    with nortoxiferine, 371
    with protriptyline, 402
  protein binding of, 393
  pulmonary extraction of, 398
  toxicity of, pH and, 58
Meprobamate, actions of, 298
  enzyme induction and, 44, 67, 356
  interaction of, with anticoagulants, 298
    with ethyl alcohol, 298
Mercaptopurine, 364
Mercury poisoning, from mercurial diuretics, 213
Mesantoin. See Mephenytoin
Metabolism, drug. See Drug metabolism
Metanephrine, biosynthesis of, 75t
Metaproterenol, 108t
Metaraminol, action of, indirect, 87, 88t, 91
  calcium compared with, 201
  cardiac effects of, 91
  interaction of, with halothane, 355
    with isoflurane, 355
    with monoamine oxidase inhibitors, 272
    with penicillin G, 19t
    with reserpine, 266
Methacholine, 162-164
Methadone, interaction of, with ethyl alcohol, 291, 323
  protein binding of, diseases and, 46
  substitution of other narcotics with, 30
Methamphetamine, interaction of, with monoamine oxidase inhibitors, 272
Methantheline, as quaternary anticholinergic agent, 171t
  interaction of, with physostigmine, 173
Metharbital, introduction of, 246t
  pharmacokinetics of, 247t, 249
Methergine. See Methylergonovine
Methicillin, interaction of, with kanamycin, 19t
Methloxazepam, diazepam converted to, 47t
Methohexital, actions of, 309
  effects of, antiepileptic, 255
  half-life of, 309

interaction of, with fentanyl, 309
  with hyoscine, 309
  with lithium carbonate, 276
  with meperidine, 309
  with promethazine, 309-310
side effects of, 309
Methotrimeprazine, interaction of, with morphine, 262, 284
Methoxamine, action of, *alpha*-adrenergic stimulating, 116
  direct, 86, 88t, 90
  cardiac effects of, 354
  indications for use of, 90, 342
  interaction of, with chlorpromazine, 79
    with nitroprusside, 4
    with oxytocic agents, 428
  treatment of drug-induced hypotension with, 75
Methoxyflurane, anesthetic depth and, central nervous signs of, 412
  biotransformation of, 68
  cardiac effects of, in cardiopulmonary bypass, 128
  contraindication for, 14t
  interaction of, with *beta*-adrenergic blocking agents, 125-128, 129, 343-344
    with digitalis, 184, 188
    with ephedrine, 91
    with epinephrine, 83, 83t, 355
    with local anesthetic agents, 400
    with nitrous oxide, 72, 351
    with phenobarbital, 13, 14t, 65
    with practolol, 128
    with propranolol, 78, 125-128, 129
    with reserpine, 266
  metabolism of, nephrotoxicity and, 356
  minimum alveolar concentration of, anesthetic depth and, 410t
  pregnancy and, 416t, 424
  nephrotoxicity from, drug metabolism and, 356
  sensitivity of, to epinephrine-induced dysrhythmias, 83, 83t
3-Methoxymorphine, 327t
Methscopolamine, interaction of, with antipsychotic agents, 263
  with other anticholinergic agents, 268
Methsuximide, 246t, 247t, 252
Methylamide-*beta*-carboline, 293
Methylatropine, 165
Methylbarbiturate(s), 309
Methyl-*beta*-carboline-3-carboxamide, 293
Methyl-*beta*-carboline-3-carboxylate, 293
3-Methylcholanthrene, 65
Methyldopa, actions of, 152-153
  cardiac effects of, 152-153
  classification of, 148t
  composition of, 152
  contraindications to, 152
  discontinuance of, hypertension from, 154
  indications for, 152
  dosage of, 148t
  indications for use of, 152
  interaction of, with anesthetic agents, 152
    with butyrophenones, 153
    with catecholamines, 152-153

Methyldopa, interaction of (cont.)
  with droperidol, 153
  with ephedrine, 151t, 152
  with haloperidol, 153
  with halothane, 151t
  with norepinephrine, 152
  with propranolol, 153
  pharmacology of, 152-153
  side effects of, 151t, 152-153
  See also Alpha-methyldopa
Methylene blue, 144
Methylergonovine, 428-429
Methylparaben, interaction of, with bilirubin, 434
Methylphenidate, interaction of, with anticholinergic agents, 268
  with monoamine oxidase inhibitors, 272
  with reserpine, 266
Methylphenobarbital, 247t, 249
Methylprednisolone, interaction of, with pseudocholinesterase, 396
Methylscopolamine, interaction of, with physostigmine, 173
Methylxanthine(s), effects of, central nervous system, 296
  interaction of, with benzodiazepines, 296-297
  with beta-agonists, 109
  with calcium, 198
Metoclopramide, actions of, 173
  gastrointestinal effects of, 19, 173
  indications for use of, 173
  interaction of, with anticholinergic agents, 19, 173
  with atropine, 173
  with narcotics, 173
Metocurine, cardiac effects of, 384-385
  indication for use of, 235
  interaction of, with histamine, 384
  with nalbuphine, 332t
  with neostigmine, 375
  with propranolol, 236
Metoprolol, bioavailability of, 119t
  cardioselectivity of, 117, 118t, 343
  discontinuance of, hypertension from, 154
  elimination half-life of, 118
  interaction of, with barbiturates, 285
  metabolism of, 119t
Metrizamide, interaction of, with Innovar, 254
Mexiletine, 230t, 240
Microcirculation, in shock, 85
  schema of, 86
Microsomal enzyme(s), chloral hydrate and, 297
  defined, 64
  ethyl alcohol and, 287-288
  in biotransformation of drugs, 64-65, 66
  induction of, 65, 67
  sedative-hypnotic agents and, 284
Microsome(s), defined, 64
Midazolam, actions of, 294, 314
  endotracheal intubation and, 316
  gastric pH and, 176
  interaction of, with alfentanil, 317
    with ethyl alcohol, 289
    with etomidate, 316
    with fentanyl, 317
    with halothane, 314, 316-317
    with ketamine, 310, 314, 316
    with lidocaine, 295

  with morphine, 314
  with neuromuscular blocking agents, 316
  with nitrous oxide, 314, 316
  with opiates, 317
  with pancuronium, 316
  with physostigmine, 296
  with scopolamine, 314
  with succinylcholine, 316
  side effects of, 317
Milontin. See Phensuximide
Minimum alveolar concentration, anesthetic depth quantified by, 409, 410t, 411, 413
  defined, 409
  of halothane, acidosis and, 422-423, 422
    antihypertensive agents and, 342
    diazepam and, 313
    ketamine and, 311, 311t
    levodopa and, 347
    midazolam and, 316-317
    monoamine oxidase inhibitors and, 347
    thiopental and, 309
  of inhalation anesthetic agents, narcotics and, 331, 333
    nitrous oxide and, 351-352
    tricyclic antidepressants and, 347
    sedative-hypnotic agents and, 283-284
Minipress. See Prazosin
Minoxidil, actions of, 156-157
  classification of, 148t
  dosage of, 148t
  indications for use of, 157
  interaction of, with beta-adrenergic blocking agents, 157
    with norepinephrine, 156-157
    with thiazide diuretics, 217
  mechanism of action of, 341
  side effects of, 157
Monoamine oxidase, 73, 73-74
Monoamine oxidase inhibitor(s), actions of, 157
  anesthetic considerations with, 9, 347-348
  catecholamine levels and, 79-80
  distribution of, 22
  dosage of, 148t
  indications for use of, 22, 157, 271, 347
  interaction of, with alpha- adrenergic blocking agents, 272
    with amitriptyline, 80
    with amphetamine, 80, 272
    with analgesics, 80
    with anesthetic agents, 80, 274-275
    with atropine, 274
    with balanced anesthesia, 274
    with barbiturates, 80, 157, 270t, 273, 347
    with beta-adrenergic blocking agents, 272
    with bupivacaine, 274
    with calcium, 202
    with chlorpromazine, 80, 272
    with dopamine, 22, 272, 347
    with droperidol, 274
    with enflurane, 274
    with ephedrine, 22, 80, 157, 272, 274
    with epinephrine, 272
    with ethanol, 80

  with fentanyl, 347-348
  with guanethidine, 272
  with halothane, 274, 347
  with imipramine, 80-81
  with inhalation anesthetic agents, 347-348
  with ketamine, 269
  with lithium carbonate, 272
  with meperidine, 22, 67, 80, 157, 272-274, 295, 325, 347
  with mephentermine, 272, 274
  with metaraminol, 272
  with methamphetamine, 272
  with methylphenidate, 272
  with monoamine oxidase inhibitors, 274
  with morphine, 80, 273, 274
  with narcotics, 157, 270t, 272-274, 323, 325, 337, 347, 352
  with neuromuscular blocking agents, 270t, 273-274
  with nitroprusside, 80, 272, 275
  with nitrous oxide, 347-348
  with norepinephrine, 22, 73, 157-158, 272, 347
  with pentazocine, 273
  with pentolinium, 80
  with phenazocine, 273
  with phentolamine, 80, 272
  with phenylephrine, 22, 272, 274
  with phenylpropanolamine, 272
  with prednisolone, 273
  with propranolol, 274
  with reserpine, 272
  with sedative-hypnotic agents, 273
  with sedatives, 347
  with serotonin, 347
  with succinylcholine, 378
  with sympathetic amines, 268, 271-272
  with sympathomimetic agents, 22, 157, 270t, 271-272
  with sympathomimetic amines, 7, 347
  with thiazide diuretics, 274
  with tricyclic antidepressants, 80-81, 271
  with trimethaphan, 80
  with d-tubocurarine, 274
  with tyramine, 22, 80, 157, 272, 288
  mechanism of action of, 271, 347
  nonsurmountable antagonism of, 26
  overdosage of, 80
  pharmacology of, 157-158
  preoperative discontinuance of, 80, 325, 347
  receptor binding of, 49
  side effects of, 157-158
Monoethylglycinexylidide, 403, 403
Morphine, as analgesic standard, 329, 330t
  as central nervous system drug, 28
  cardiac effects of, 350
  characteristics of, 47-48
  codeine converted to, 47t
  dose-effect curves of, 328-329
  duration of action of, 335
  effects of, central nervous system, 326t
    in renal failure, 48
    peripheral, 326t
  effects of pH in, 59
  histamine release in, 322

INDEX 467

indications for use of, as induction agent, 350
interaction of, with *alpha*- adrenergic blocking agents, 324
  with amitriptyline, 269
  with atropine, 324
  with barbiturates, 323
  with *beta*-adrenergic blocking agents, 324
  with butorphanol, 330
  with cimetidine, 176-177
  with diazepam, 312, 324
  with epinephrine, 83
  with ethyl alcohol, 291, 323
  with fluroxene, 415*t*, 419, *421*
  with halothane, 284, 350, 415*t*, 419, *421*
  with histamine H_2 blocking agent(s), 177
  with imipramine, 269
  with lidocaine, 398
  with methotrimeprazine, 262, 284
  with midazolam, 314
  with monoamine oxidase inhibitors, 80, 273
  with nalbuphine, 330, 332*t*
  with nalorphine, 326, 327*t*, 328, *328*, *329*
  with naloxone, 325-326, 326*t*, 327*t*, *328*, 333, 335-336
  with nifedipine, 141
  with nitrous oxide, 72, 322, 331, 350
  with pentazocine, 331
  with phenothiazines, 262
  with physostigmine, 324
  with propranolol, 78, 126
  with reserpine, 267
  with sleep, 324
  with sympathomimetic agents, 24
  with thiopental, 331
  with d-tubocurarine, 323
  with verapamil, 141-142
opioid receptors and, 325-326, 327*t*, 328
overdose of, treatment of, 325
rebound respiratory depression from, 21
seizures from, 254
structure of, *334*
Muscarine, 161
Muscarinic agent(s), interaction of, with norepinephrine, 163
Muscarinic cholinergic receptor(s), 24
Muscarinic receptor(s), defined, 148
Muscle relaxant(s). *See* Neuromuscular blocking agent(s)
Muscle(s), blood flow in, inhalation anesthetic agents and, 370
  neuromuscular blockade and, 378-379
contractility of, calcium and, 200
in hypokalemia, 204, 216
narcotic agonists and, 322-323
pain in, from succinylcholine, 374
relaxation of, anesthetic agents and, 16, 353
skeletal, in hypokalemia, 216
spasticity of, benzodiazepines in treatment of, 292
ventricular, action potentials from, 226-227, *226*
  in reentry of excitation, *229*

Muscle tone, abdominal, anesthetic depth and, 412-413
Myasthenia gravis, anticholinesterase agents in treatment of, 164
effects in, of adrenocorticotropic hormone, 369
Myocardial action potential(s), calcium-channel blocking agents and, 136-138, *137*
physiology of, 199
Myocardial contractility, *beta*-adrenergic stimulation and, 148
bretylium and, 239
calcium in, 198-201
calcium-channel blocking agents and, 137-138, 138*t*, 345-346
diazepam and, 313
etomidate and, 317
fentanyl and, 313
in citrate intoxication, 202
inotropic effect of digitalis and, 182-183
quinidine and, 236
Myocardial depression, calcium in treatment of, 201
following cardiopulmonary bypass, propranolol and, 343
from *beta*-adrenergic blocking agents, 125-128, 238, 343-344
from calcium-channel blocking agents, 345-346
from disopyramide, 238
from inhalation anesthetic agents, 343-346, 349
from procainamide, 236
from quinidine, 236
from tricyclic antidepressants, 347
from verapamil, 138
intraoperative, treatment of, 346
Myocardial infarction, abnormal cardiac automaticity in, 227
digitalis serum levels in, 188
drug interactions in, 67
effects in, of lidocaine, 393
Myocardial ischemia, intraoperative, *beta*-adrenergic blocking agents in, 121-122, *124-125*
mannitol in treatment of, 212
predisposition to dysrhythmias in, 74
treatment of, 135
Myocardial oxygen consumption, *beta*-adrenergic blocking agents and, 121, 121*t*, 343
determinants of, 121, 233
ketamine and, 310
nitroglycerin and, 143
Myosin, calcium and, 198
inotropic effect of digitalis and, 184*t*
Myosin-phosphorylase light chain(s), 199
Mysoline. *See* Primidone
Myxedema, 188

Nadolol, absorption of, 118, 119*t*
beta-adrenergic blockade by, 117, 118*t*
dosage regimen of, 118
lack of cardioselectivity of, 343
Nalbuphine, as naloxone alternative, 336
as narcotic agonist-antagonist, 325*t*

butorphanol versus, 329
drug interactions with, 330-331, 332*t*, 333
opioid receptors and, hypothetical interactions with, 327*t*
potency of, 329, 330*t*
Nalline. *See* Nalorphine
N-allylnorcodeine, 333
N-allylmorphine. *See* Nalorphine
Nalorphine, as antagonistic standard, 329, 330*t*
as naloxone alternative, 336
as narcotic agonist-antagonist, 325*t*
as partial agonist, 334
dose-effect curves of, *328-329*
effects of, 328
  central nervous system, 326*t*
  peripheral, 326*t*
effects of pH in, 59
history of, 333
interaction of, with morphine, 326, 327*t*, 328, *328-329*
  with naloxone, 326*t*, 328
opioid receptors and, 326, 327*t*, 328
potency of, 330*t*
structure of, 333, *334*
Naloxone, acute abstinence syndrome from, 328
alternatives to, 336
as antagonistic standard, 329
as narcotic antagonist, 321, 334
dosage of, 335-336
dose-effect curves of, *328*
drug addiction and, 30
duration of action of, 335, 337
effects of, 326
history of, 333
indications for use of, 337
in shock, 336
interaction of, with barbiturates, 336
  with buprenorphine, 328-329
  with cimetidine, 176
  with clonidine, 336
  with cyclopropane, 415*t*
  with diazepam, 336
  with enflurane, 415*t*, 416
  with ethyl alcohol, 336
  with fentanyl, 335, 336
  with halothane, 415*t*, 416
  with inhalation anesthetic agents, 336
  with ketamine, 336
  with morphine, 325-326, 326*t*, 327*t*, *328*, 333, 335, 336
  with nalorphine, 326*t*, 328
  with narcotic agonist-antagonists, 328-329, 330*t*
  with narcotics, 4, 273, 333-336
  with nitrous oxide, 335, 415*t*, 416
  with nonnarcotics, 336
  with opioid peptides, 254
  with pentobarbital, 336
  with pharmacologic receptors, 24
  with phencyclidine, 418
  with propoxyphene, 336
  with sufentanil, 419
  with thiopental, 415*t*, 416
opioid receptors and, 325-326, 327*t*
potency of, 330*t*
side effects of, 335-337
structure of, 334, *334*
Naltrexone, as narcotic antagonist, 321, 334

Naltrexone *(cont.)*
  interaction of, with inhalation anesthetic agents, 226
    with ketamine, 336
    with pentobarbital, 336
  opioid receptors and, hypothetical interactions with, 327t
Naproxen, interaction of, with thiopental, 46
Narcan. *See* Naloxone
Narcotic addiction, anesthesia and, 29-30
  interactions of opiates and ethyl alcohol in, 291
  narcotic anesthesia and, 331
  narcotic antagonists in, 321
  treatment of, buprenorphine in, 329
Narcotic agonist(s), drug interactions with, 323-325
  effects of, cardiovascular, 322
    central nervous system, 321-322
    gastrointestinal, 322
    muscular, 322-323
    respiratory, 322
  interaction of, with butorphanol, 330
    with central nervous system depressants, 323-324
    with inhalation anesthestic agents, 331
    with monoamine oxidase inhibitors, 325
    with nalbuphine, 330-331
    with narcotic agonist-antagonists, 325-326, 327t, 328-331, 330t
    with narcotic antagonists, 330
    with neuromuscular blocking agents, 333
    with pentazocine, 330-331
    with sodium, 334-335
  pharmacology of, 321-323
  potency of, morphine versus, 329, 330t
  narcotic antagonists versus, 334
  See also Narcotic(s); Narcotic analgesic(s); specific agents
Narcotic agonist-antagonist(s), actions of, 325
  available, 325t
  dose-response curves of, 333
  in anesthesia, 331, 333
  interaction of, with naloxone, 328-329
    with narcotic agonists, 325-326, 327t, 328, 329-331, 330t
    with neuromuscular blocking agents, 333
  opioid receptors and, 325-326, 327t, 328, *328-329*
  side effects of, 329-330
Narcotic analgesic(s), analgesia from, mechanism of, 321-322
  as central nervous system drugs, 28
  buprenorphine as, 329
  catecholamine release and, 124
  dependence on, anesthesia and, 29-30
  effects of, in hypovolemia, 203
    respiratory, 321
  in anesthesia, alternatives in, 330-331
    balanced, 83
  interaction of, with antimuscarinic anticholinergic agents, 170
    with antipsychotic agent(s), 261t, 262

  with atropine, 171
  with *beta*-adrenergic blocking agents, 125-126, 128, *129*
  with butyrophenones, 261t, 262
  with calcium-channel blocking agents, 141-142
  with chlorpromazine, 79
  with cimetidine, 176
  with diazepam, 324
  with epinephrine, 83
  with general anesthetic agents, 28
  with inhalation anesthetic agents, 331, 332t, 333, 349-351
  with metoclopramide, 173
  with monoamine oxidase inhibitors, 80, 157, 270t, 272-274
  with nalbuphine, 330-331, 332t
  with naloxone, 273
  with narcotic antagonists, 321, 327t
  with nitrous oxide, 314, 322
  with pentobarbital, 324
  with phenobarbital, 324
  with phenothiazines, 261t, 262
  with physostigmine, 172, 171t
  with propranolol, 125-126, 128, *129*
  with reserpine, 267
  with sympathomimetic agents, 93, 324
  with thiopental, 324
  with tricyclic antidepressants, 268t, 269
  with valproic acid, 251
  opioid receptors and, hypothetical interactions with, 327t
  physical addiction to, 28
  potency of, standard of, 329, 330t
  seizures from, 254
  sparing effect of, 28
  substitution among, 30
Narcotic antagonist(s), actions of, 335
  analgesic, in anesthesia, 331-332
  narcotic agonists versus, 331
  side effects of, 331
  classification of, 334
  drug addiction and, 30
  duration of action of, 335
  history of, 333
  in anesthesia, 321, 331, 332t, 333
  indications for use of, in shock, 336
  interaction of, with adrenocorticotropic hormone, 336
    with atropine, 336
    with cortisone, 336
    with L-dopa, 336
    with narcotics, 321, 327t, 330, 337
    with nonnarcotics, 336
    with physostigmine, 336
    with propranolol, 336
    with sodium, 334-335
  mechanism of action of, 334-335
  opioid receptors and, hypothetical interactions with, 327t
  partial, 334
  pharmacology of, 333-336, *334*
  potency of, 329, 330t
  pure, 334
  side effects of, 335-336
  similarity of, to benzodiazepine antagonists, 292-294
  structure of, 333-334, *334*
  use of, in narcotic addiction, 321

Narcotics, addiction to. *See* Narcotic addiction
  analogs of, 321
  biotransformation inhibited by, 66
  effects of, analgesic, 321-322
    cardiac, 335
    central nervous system, 335
    hypotension from, 322
  illicit use of, 321
  in anesthesia, physical dependence from, 331
  indications for use of, 321
  interaction of, with atracurium, 374
    with barbiturates, 322-324
    with central nervous system depressants, 337
    with chlorpromazine, 323
    with dexamethasone, 323
    with diazepam, 349
    with dopamine, 323
    with enzyme-inducing drugs, 67
    with halothane, 351-352
    with histamine receptor blocking agents, 322
    with inhalation anesthetic agents, 323-324, 336, 350-351, 413, 415t
    with levodopa, 323
    with monoamine oxidase inhibitors, 323, 325, 337, 347
    with nalbuphine, 332t
    with naloxone, 4, 333-336
    with narcotic antagonists, 321, 337
    with neostigmine, 381-382
    with neuromuscular blocking agents, 324-325, 370, 374-375, 381-382
    with nitrous oxide, 352-353
    with pancuronium, 324-325, 380-381
    with phenelzine, 325
    with phenoxybenzamine, 323
    with propranolol, 78
    with reserpine, 323
    with sedative-hypnotic agents, 334
    with sleep, 324
    with sympathomimetic agents, 324
    with vecuronium, 374-375
    with verapamil, 345
  opioid receptors and, 325-326, 327t, 328
  overdose of, fatal, 322
    treatment of, 325
  respiratory depression from, 322-323
  tolerance to, 331
National Institutes of Health, 6
Natriuresis, postoperative, 204
  pressure, cause of, 208, 210
Neomycin, in multiple-drug therapy, 9-10
  interaction of, with calcium, 201, 365, 366t
    with neostigmine, 366t
    with pancuronium, 375
    with succinylcholine, 366t
    with d-tubocurarine, 366t
    with vecuronium, 375
Neonate(s), bilirubin in, 433-435
  diazepam in, 434-435
  drug interactions in, 433-435, 434t
  hypermagnesemia in, 432
  hypocalcemia in, from magnesium sulfate, 432
  sulfisoxazole in, 434
Neostigmine, contraindication for, 14t

INDEX 469

dosage of, drug interactions and, 381-382, *382*
duration of action of, 377
in "balanced" anesthesia, 2
interaction of, with
  acetylcholinesterase, 377, 395
  with amitriptyline, 270
  with antibiotics, 365, 366*t*, 367-368, 381
  with atracurium, 375-376
  with atropine, 160, 169-171
  with diuretics, 382
  with lithium carbonate, 275
  with local anesthetic agents, 395
  with metocurine, 375
  with narcotics, 381-382
  with neuromuscular blocking agents, 108, 366*t*, 379, 381-382, *382*, 395, *395*
  with pancuronium, 367-368, 376, 380, 382
  with plasma anticholinesterase, 377
  with plasma cholinesterase, 395, *395*
  with polymyxin B, 366*t*, 367-368
  with reserpine, 267
  with succinylcholine, 376-377, 395
  with d-tubocurarine, 364, 366*t*, 381-382, *382*
  with vecuronium, 375-376
Neostigmine-glycopyrollate, interaction of, with nalbuphine, 332*t*
Neo-Synephrine. *See* Phenylephrine
Nephrotoxicity, fluoride levels in, inhalation anesthetic agents in, 356
  of antibiotics, 31
Nerve block. *See* Conduction anesthesia
Nerves, depression of function of, 29
  peripheral, stimulation of, acetylcholine and, 161
  sensory, stimulation of, in drug side effects, 163
  vagus. *See* Vagus nerve
Nervous system(s), central. *See* Central nervous system
  sympathetic. *See* Sympathetic nervous system
  parasympathetic. *See* Parasympathetic nervous system
Netimicin, 375
Neuroeffector junction(s), sympathetic, 114-115, *115-116*
Neurogenic shock, 85
Neurohumoral transmitter(s), acetylcholine as, 161-162
Neurolept anesthesia, cardiac dysrhythmias with, 169
  interaction of, with anticholinergic agents, 170
  with etomidate, 317
Neuroleptic agent(s), actions of, 18
  predisposition to drug interactions of, 18
Neuromuscular blocking agent(s), as problem drugs, 10
  cardiac effects of, 107-108
  depolarizing, nondepolarizing versus, 373-374
  development of, 383
  duration of action of, 25
    muscle blood flow and, 378-379

effects of, in hyperkalemia, 204
  in hypermagnesemia, 205
  in hypocalcemia, 200, 381-382
  in hypokalemia, 381-382
  in hypovolemia, 203
  in metabolic alkalosis, 381-382
  in renal failure, 368-369, *369*
  in respiratory acidosis, 381
  reversibility of, 375-376
excretion of, diuretics and, 365
ganglion blocking agents versus, 165
in "balanced" anesthesia, 1-2
interaction of, with antibiotics, 9-10, 365, 366*t*, 367-368, 381
  with anticholinergic agents, 395
  with anticholinesterase agents, 22, 108, 164, 166, 375-377
  with antidysrhythmic agents, 235-236, 371-372
  with antihypertensive agents, 378-379
  with aprindine, 240
  with atropine, 108
  with azathioprine, 364-365, 371
  with barbiturates, 370
  with benzodiazepines, 297, 313
  with bretylium, 239
  with calcium, 205
  with calcium-channel blocking agents, 142
  with corticosteroids, 369
  with cyclopropane, 370
  with diazepam, 297, 313
  with diethyl ether, 353
  with disopyramide, 238
  with diuretics, 216-217, 221, 365, 382
  with enflurane, 2, 353-354, 370, 374
  with fluroxene, 370
  with furosemide, 364-365, *364*
  with ganglionic blocking agents, 378-379
  with halothane, 2, 311*t*, 369-371, *370*, 374-375
  with inhalation anesthetic agents, 2, 353-354, 369-371, *370*
  with isoflurane, 2, 370, 374
  with ketamine, 311*t*, 372
  with lidocaine, 371
  with lithium carbonate, 275*t*, 275-276, 372-373
  with local anesthetic agents, 371, 401-402
  with magnesium, 205
  with magnesium sulfate, 372, 430-432, 431-432
  with mannitol, 364-365, *364*, 371
  with mexiletine, 240
  with midazolam, 316
  with monoamine oxidase inhibitors, 270*t*, 273-274
  with narcotic agonist-antagonists, 333
  with narcotics, 324-325, 333, 370, 381-382
  with neostigmine, 108, 381-382, *382*
  with nitroprusside, 378-379
  with nitrous oxide, 354, 370, 374-375
  with other neuromuscular blocking agents, 373-374
  with potassium, 220

  with prednisone, 369
  with pyridostigmine, 379, 381-382
  with quinidine, 371-372
  with renal failure, 368-369, *369*
  with reserpine, 265*t*, 267
  with succinylcholine, 373-374
  with theophylline, 107-108
  with tocainide, 240
  with trimethaphan, 158, 378-379
malignant hyperpyrexia from, 31
nondepolarizing, depolarizing versus, 373-374
Neuromuscular effect(s), of antibiotics, 365, 367-368
  of antihypertensive agents, 378-379
  of inhalation anesthetic agents, 370
  of local anesthetics, 371
  of magnesium sulfate, 372, 431-432
  of procaine toxicity, 395
Neuromuscular function, measurement of, train-of-four response in, 376
  twitch height in, 363, *364*, 367
Neuromuscular junction, 161-162
Nialamide, interaction of, with halothane, 274
  with narcotics, 325
  with norepinephrine, 73
Nicotinamide-adenine dinucleotide, in biotransformation, 65, *66*
Nicotine, 161, 163
Nicotinic receptor(s), defined, 148
Nifedipine, actions of, 137-138
  cardiac effects of, 137-138, 138*t*, 345
  contraindication to, 138
  effects of, antibronchospastic, 142
    on pulmonary blood flow, 142
    platelet adhesion inhibition as, 142
  indications for use of, 136, 345
  interaction of, with aspirin, 139
    with *beta*-adrenergic blocking agents, 139, 345
    with calcium, 198
    with diazepam, 139
    with digitalis, 190
    with fentanyl, 141
    with halothane, 141
    with inhalation anesthetic agents, 141, 345
    with lidocaine, 139
    with morphine, 141
    with nitrous oxide, 141
    with propranolol, 78-79, 139
  mechanism of action of, 341, 345
  photosensitivity of, 141
Nitrate(s), 342
Nitrazepam, interaction of, with oxytocin, 430
  substitution of for barbiturates, 9
Nitrogen mustard, interaction of, with succinylcholine, 378
Nitroglycerin compounds, 142-144
Nitroprusside, actions of, 158
  cardiac effects of, 143
  dosage of, 158
  effects of, neuromuscular, 378-379
  interaction of, with cyanide, 158
    with digitalis, 182, 190
    with inhalation anesthetic agents, 158
    with methoxamine, 4
    with monoamine oxidase inhibitors, 80, 272, 275
    with neuromuscular blocking agents, 378-379

pH *(cont.)*
  effect of, 51-61, 54-55t, 57t, 57-59
  gastric, histamine H₂ blocking agents and, 176
  shifts in, effect of, 51-61, 54-55t, 57t, 57-59
Pharmacodynamics, defined, 20, 39
Pharmacokinetics, defined, 19-20, 39
  drug interactions and, 39-49, 42t, 43, 47t
Pharmacologic antagonism, defined, 24
Pharmacologic receptor(s), interactions involving multiple, 26-28
  interactions involving single, 23-26, 25
  interactions not mediated by, 28-29
  list of, 23-24
Phenacetamide, introduction of, 246t
Phenazocine, interaction of, with monoamine oxidase inhibitors, 273
Phencyclidine, actions of, 83-84
  excretion of, pH and, 59
  interaction of, with cyclopropane, 415t, 418
  opioid receptors and, hypothetical interactions with, 327t
Phenelzine, actions of, 79-80
  as pseudocholinesterase inhibitor, 378
  indications for use of, 271, 378
  interaction of, with calcium, 202
    with dextromethorphan, 273
    with meperidine, 325
    with narcotic analgesics, 325
    with succinylcholine, 273, 378
  plasma cholinesterase levels with, 273
Phenergan. *See* Promethazine
Phenformin, interaction of, with ethyl alcohol, 290
Pheniprazine, interaction of, with halothane, 274
Phenobarbital, as carbamazepine substitute, 250
  biotransformation of, 65
  dissociation of, 51-52
  distribution of, pH shifts and, 56, 57, 58, 58-59
  dosage of, antiepileptic, 247t, 249
  effects of, neonatal, 434-435
    on hepatic enzymes, 284
  electroencephalographic manifestations of, 255
  interaction of, with alkalinizers, 286
    with alklyphosphates, 44
    with anticoagulants, 7
    with benzodiazepines, 248
    with bilirubin, 434-435
    with carbon tetrachloride, 68
    with chloroform, 68
    with corticosteroids, 285
    with diazepam, 435
    with dicumarol, 282, 286
    with digitoxin, 189
    with digoxin, 44
    with EPN, 44
    with ethyl alcohol, 287-289
    with furosemide, 217
    with halothane, 68, 248, 415t
    with lidocaine, 396-397, 397
    with local anesthetic agents, 396, 397
    with malathion, 44
    with meperidine, 435
    with methoxyflurane, 13, 14t, 65
    with narcotics, 324
    with parathion, 44
    with pentobarbital, 435
    with picrotoxin, 292
    with primidone, 249-250
    with quinidine, 236, 286
    with reserpine, 266
    with tetrohydrocannabinol, 299
    with theophylline, 105
    with thiopental, 435
    with timolol, 285
    with valproic acid, 249
    with warfarin, 67
  ionization of, 56
    equation for, 52-53
    pH shifts and, 53, 55t
  ionized, 51-52
  pharmacokinetics of, 247t, 248-249
  preanesthetic, 248
  protein binding of, 42t
  un-ionized, 51-52
Phenothiazine(s), actions of, 18, 261-262
  biotransformation of, 64
  cardiac effects of, 264
  contraindications to, 254
  convulsive threshold with, 264
  effects of, in neonates, 435
  indications for use of, 261, 348
  interaction of, with adrenocorticotropic hormone, 265
    with *alpha*-adrenergic agonists, 79, 348
    with anticholinergic agents, 261t, 263
    with barbiturates, 286
    with butyrophenones, 348
    with cephalothin, 19t
    with droperidol, 348
    with enflurane, 264
    with epinephrine, 348
    with ethyl alcohol, 289
    with general anesthetic agents, 79
    with inhalation anesthetic agents, 348, 349
    with ketamine, 264
    with meperidine, 262
    with methoxamine, 79
    with morphine, 262
    with muscarinic receptors, 24
    with narcotic analgesics, 79, 261t, 262
    with nitrous oxide, 348
    with phenylephrine, 79
    with physostigmine, 295
    with quinidine, 264
    with sympathomimetic agents, 261t, 263
    with vasopressors, 348
  postoperative mortality with, 264-265
  side effects of, 265
Phenoxybenzamine, actions of, 155-156
  indications for use of, 156
  interaction of, with *alpha*-adrenergic receptors, 86
    with catecholamines, 155-156
    with ketamine, 310
    with narcotics, 323
    with norepinephrine, 73
  nonsurmountable antagonism of, 26
  pharmacology of, 155-156
Phensuximide, introduction of, 246t

Phentolamine, actions of, 155-156
  cardiac effects of, 27, 155-156
  indications for use of, 156
  interaction of, with antipsychotic agents, 264
    with catecholamines, 155-156
    with monoamine oxidase inhibitors, 80, 272
    with norepinephrine, 89
    with tricyclic antidepressants, 269
  pharmacology of, 155-156
Phenurone. *See* Phenacetamide
Phenylalanine, metabolism of, 75t
Phenylbutazone, as enzyme inducer, 67
  interaction of, with anticoagulants, 41
    with digitalis, 190
    with indomethacin, 41
    with thiopental, 46
    with warfarin, 21
  protein binding of, 42t
  volume of distribution of, protein binding and, 45
Phenylephrine, action of, direct, 86-87, 88t, 90
  cardiac effects of, 354-355
  indications for use of, 90
  in intraoperative hypotension, 342
  interaction of, with antihypertensive agents, 150
    with antipsychotic agents, 263
    with chlorpromazine, 79, 264
    with desipramine, 268
    with ergonovine, 429
    with halothane, 90
    with imipramine, 268
    with inhalation anesthetic agents, 263, 354-355
    with methylergonovine, 429
    with monoamine oxidase inhibitors, 22, 272, 274
    with norepinephrine, 73
    with penicillin G, 19t
    with reserpine, 267
  treatment of drug-induced hypotension with, 75
Phenylpropanolamine, interaction of, with monoamine oxidase inhibitors, 272
  with reserpine, 266
Phenytoin, actions of, 237-238
  cardiac effects of, 230t
  treatment failure with, 126
  displacement of protein binding of, 21
  dosage of, antiepileptic, 247, 247t
    in digitalis toxicity, 182, 201
    therapeutic, 238
  effects of, extracardiac, 230t
  enzyme induction from, 67, 356
  indications for use of, 182, 238
    antiepileptic, 247
  interaction of, with barbiturates, 248, 286
    with benzodiazepines, 248
    with bupivacaine, 394
    with calcium, 201
    with cephalothin, 19t
    with chloramphenicol, 19t
    with cimetidine, 248
    with digitalis, 180-182, 187, 190, 201
    with erythromycin, 19t

with ethanol, 44
with fluroxene, 248
with furosemide, 217
with halothane, 248
with histamine H$_2$ blocking
   agent(s), 177
with kanamycin, 19*t*
with lidocaine, 396-397
with penicillin G, 19*t*
with quinidine, 236
with theophylline, 105
with tricyclic antidepressants, 248
with tubocurarine, 235
introduction of, 246*t*
pharmacokinetics of, 246-248, 247*t*
preanesthetic, 246-247
side effects of, 247-248
Pheochromocytoma(s), *alpha*-
   adrenergic blocking agents in,
   122, 156
catecholamine release from, 75
diazoxide in, 159
dysrhythmias from, propranolol in
   treatment of, 238
guanethidine and, 154
labetalol in, 156
tests for, methyldopa and, 153
trimethaphan in, 158
Phosphate(s), renal reabsorption of,
   210
Phosphaturia, from acetazolamide, 213
renal tubular inhibition indicated by,
   210
Phosphodiesterase, 102, 365
Phospholamban, 199
Pholine. *See* Echothiophate
Physeptone, preanesthetic, anesthetic
   depth and, 283
"Physiologic" antagonism, defined, 26
Physostigmine, cardiac effects of, 296
central anticholinergic syndrome
   treated with, 171-173
contraindications to, 173
dosage of, 173
effects of, central nervous system,
   295-296
indications for use of, 172-173
interaction of, with anticholinergic
   agents, 173, 295
with atropine, 171-173, 295
with benzodiazepines, 295-296
with chlordiazepoxide, 172*t*
with diazepam, 172, 172*t*, 295-296
with glutethimide, 172*t*
with glycopyrrolate, 173
with lorazepam, 172*t*, 295-296
with methantheline, 173
with methylscopolamine, 173
with midazolam, 296
with morphine, 324
with narcotic analgesics, 172, 172*t*
with narcotic antagonists, 336
with phenothiazines, 295
with propantheline, 173
with reserpine, 267
with scopolamine, 173, 295
with tricyclic antidepressants, 295
overdosage of, 173
side effects of, 296
Picrotoxin, 292
Pilocarpine, 164
Pindolol, actions of, membrane
   stabilizing, 343

beta-adrenergic blockade by,
   cardioselectivity of, 117, 118*t*
elimination half-life of, 118
metabolism of, 119*t*
Pitocin. *See* Oxytocin
Plasma cholinesterase, effects on, of
   pancuronium, 373
in hydrolysis, of cocaine, 401
   of succinylcholine, 401
in pregnancy, 396
interaction of, with local anesthetic
   agents, 395
with neostigmine, 377, 395, *395*
with procaine, 401
with pyridostigmine, 395, *395*
with tetracaine, 401
Plasma concentration, drug,
   measurement of, 42
route of administration and, 40
volume of distribution and, 41
Plasma pseudocholinesterase, in
   hydrolysis, of local anesthetic
   agents, 398
Platelet(s), abnormalities of, from
   valproic acid, 251
adhesion of, calcium-channel
   blocking agents and, 142
aggregation of, nitroglycerin and,
   144
Polychlorobiphenyl(s), as enzyme
   inducers, 67
interaction of, with halothane, 68
Polymyxin A, 366*t*
Polymyxin B, effects of, muscle
   relaxant, 365, 367
toxic, 31
interaction of, with acetylcholine,
   367
with calcium, 366*t*
with cephalothin, 19*t*
with chloramphenicol, 19*t*
with neostigmine, 366*t*, 367
with neuromuscular blocking
   agents, 30-31, 366*t*
Postsynaptic inhibition, defined, 26
Potassium, cardiac effects of,
   dysrhythmias and, 93-94
   mechanism of, 228
on refractory period, 201
derangements of, 204
effects of, on neuromuscular
   blocking agents, 382
ideal levels of, 93
in anesthesia, 204
interaction of, with *beta*-2-agonists,
   219
with *beta*-adrenergic blocking
   agents, 219
with calcium, 201
with calcium-channel blocking
   agents, 136, 140
with captopril, 157
with cardiac glycosides, 199
with digitalis, 180-181, 184, 187,
   189-191, 201, 216
with diuretics, 213, 215-216
with halothane, 416, 416*t*
with neuromuscular blocking
   agents, 220
with sympathomimetic amines,
   220
with triamterene, 216
with verapamil, 140
ionic alterations and, 31

loss of, from acetazolamide, 213
myocardial action potentials and,
   136-137
preoperative administration of, 219
salts of, in salt substitute, 215
secretion of, diuretics and, 213
serum levels of, accuracy of, 219
   in acidosis, 220
supplemental, in patients taking
   diuretics, 219-220
total body, measurement of, 219
transport of, in congestive heart
   failure, 215-216
urinary secretion of, 210-211
See also Hyperkalemia; Hypokalemia
Potassium chloride, indications for use
   of, 182
interaction of, with digitalis, 180-181,
   190-191
Potency, drug, defined, 40
of anesthetic agents, cardiac effects
   and, 29
physicochemical properties and,
   28-29
Potentiation, defined, 3-4, 26
Practolol, cardioselectivity of, 117-118,
   118*t*
interaction of, with methoxyflurane,
   128
with norepinephrine, 73
unavailability of, 118
Prazepam, indications for use of, 291
Prazosin, actions of, 155
classification of, 148*t*
dosage of, 148*t*
indications for use of, 155
interaction of, with epinephrine, 155
with halothane, 155
with indomethacin, 155
mechanism of action of, 341
pharmacology of, 155
side effects of, 151*t*, 155
Preanesthetic medication. *See*
   Anesthetic premedication
Prednisolone, 273
Prednisone, interaction of, with
   butylcholinesterase, 396
with neuromuscular blocking
   agents, 369
with pancuronium, 369
Preeclampsia, ergot alkaloids in, 429
treatment of, magnesium sulfate in,
   372
Pregnancy, anesthetic depth in, 416*t*,
   424
drug interactions in, 427-435
effects of, on inhalation anesthetic
   agents, 416*t*, 424
enzymatic hydrolysis in, local
   anesthetic agents and, 396
ethyl alcohol in, therapeutic use of,
   286
hypertension in, drug interactions
   with, 428-429
   treatment of, 430-431
hypotension in, treatment of, 429
lithium in, 276
magnesium administration in, 204
magnesium sulfate in, 372
plasma cholinesterase in, 396
possibility of, anesthetic
   management and, 13, 14*t*
sympathomimetic bronchodilators
   in, 109

Pregnancy (cont.)
  toxemia of. See Toxemia of
    pregnancy
Premedication, anesthetic. See
    Anesthetic premedication
Prenalterol, 124, 126t
Preoperative anesthetic assessment,
    12-15, 14t
Prilocaine, effects of, neuromuscular,
    402
  enzyme induction and, 44
  excretion of, 399
  interaction of, with carbon dioxide,
    392
    with nortoxiferine, 371
  toxicity of, pH and, 58
Primidone, dosage of, antiepileptic,
    247t, 249-250
  interaction of, with phenobarbital,
    249-250
  introduction of, 246t
  metabolites of, 249
  pharmacokinetics of, 247t, 249-250
  preanesthetic, 250
Priscoline. See Tolazoline
Probanthine. See Propantheline
Probenecid, interaction of, with
    thiazide diuretics, 213, 218
Procainamide, actions of, 236-237
  cardiac effects of, 199, 227, 230t
    treatment failure with, 126
  effects of, extracardiac, 230t
    peripheral and central nervous, 29
  excretion of, pH and, 59
  indications for use of, 237
  interaction of, with anticholinergic
      agents, 268
    with digitalis, 191, 237
    with digoxin, 181
    with inhalation anesthetic agents,
      237
    with lidocaine, 401
    with propranolol, 237
    with quinidine, 237
    with tubocurarine, 235
    with vasodilators, 237
    with verapamil, 237
Procaine, atropine and cocaine
    compared with, 81, 81
  excretion of, 398
    renal function and, 399
  hydrolysis of, 396
  in heart failure, 393
  interaction of, with amitriptyline,
    270, 403
    with ammonium benzoate, 404
    with caffeine, 371
    with calcium, 371
    with glucocorticoids, 396
    with imipramine, 270
    with nitrous oxide, 400
    with para-aminobenzoic acid, 404
    with plasma cholinesterase, 395,
      401
    with protriptyline, 270
    with sodium benzoate, 404
  metabolite of, 398, 404
  overdosage of, calcium in treatment
    of, 201
  toxicity of, pH and, 58
Prochlorperazine, effects of,
    gastrointestinal, 264
  interaction of, with narcotic
      analgesics, 262
Procyclidine, 171t

Prolactin, antipsychotic drugs and, 261
Promazine, interaction of, with
    succinylcholine, 264
Promethazine, as agent with
    anticholinergic activity, 172t
  interaction of, with antipsychotic
      agents, 264
    with barbiturates, 254
    with meperidine, 262
    with methohexital, 309-310
    with narcotic analgesics, 262
    with scopolamine, 254
  side effects of, 264
Propanidid, interaction of, with
    lithium carbonate, 276
Propantheline, as quaternary
    anticholinergic agent, 171t
  interaction of, with digitalis, 191
    with physostigmine, 173
Propoxyphene, hepatic metabolism of,
    44
  interaction of, with carbamazepine,
    251
    with naloxone, 336
Propranolol, absorption of, 119t
  actions of, 78, 238
    membrane stabilizing, 343
    as clonidine replacement, 77
    as high-extraction drug, 43
  beta-adrenergic blockade by,
      cardioselectivity of, 117, 118t
  bronchospasm and, 78
  cardiac effects of, 78, 230t, 234
    beneficial, 122, 126
    in normal heart, 119-120, 120, 121
    intraoperative, 121-122, 124-126
  circulatory depression from, 123-124,
    126t, 127t
    reversal of, 123-124, 126t, 127t
  disadvantages of, 118
  discontinuance of, beta-adrenergic
      receptors and, 116
    chronotropic versus inotropic
      blockade and, 115
    hypertension from, 154
  displacement of protein binding of,
    21
  distribution of, cardiac output and,
    20
  dosage of, 118, 238
    in renal hypertension, 131
    intraoperative, 122
    preoperative adjustment of, 131-
      132
  duration of action of, 25, 119
  effects of, extracardiac, 230t
  hepatic metabolism of, 44
  hypertension from, postoperative,
    130-131
  indications for use of, 78, 234, 238
    in endotracheal intubation, 235-
      236
    intraoperative, 121-122
    nonsurgical, 118-119
  interaction of, with anesthetic
      agents, 7, 78-79, 225, 235
    with antihypertensive agents, 217
    with antipsychotic agents, 263
    with atropine, 27, 123-125, 126t,
      344, 345
    with barbiturates, 285
    with bupivacaine, 398
    with calcium, 196-197, 345
    with calcium chloride, 123, 126t

    with calcium-channel antagonists,
      78-79
    with catecholamines, 119-120, 120
    with cimetidine, 177
    with cyclopropane, 78, 125, 128,
      129, 343
    with diethyl ether, 78, 120-121,
      125, 128, 129, 343
    with digitalis, 78, 124, 126t, 187,
      191
    with diltiazem, 139
    with dobutamine, 124, 126t
    with dopamine, 124
    with enflurane, 78, 125-128, 129,
      238, 343-344
    with epinephrine, 124, 126t
    with halothane, 78-79, 125-128,
      129, 238, 343-344, 415t, 417
    with heparin, 35
    with histamine H_2 blocking
      agent(s), 177
    with inhalation anesthetic agents,
      20-21, 132, 343-345
    with isoflurane, 125, 128, 129, 344-
      345
    with isoproterenol, 116, 124, 126t,
      127t, 345
    with ketamine, 105, 310
    with lidocaine, 44, 393
    with local anesthetic agents, 398
    with methoxyflurane, 78, 125-128,
      129
    with methyldopa, 153
    with metocurine, 236
    with monoamine oxidase
      inhibitors, 274
    with morphine, 78, 126
    with narcotic antagonists, 336
    with narcotics, 78, 125-126, 128,
      129
    with nifedipine, 78-79, 139
    with nitroprusside, 130-131
    with nitrous oxide, 125-126, 344
    with norepinephrine, 73
    with opioids, 125
    with pancuronium, 126, 236
    with prenalterol, 124, 126t
    with procainamide, 237
    with protamine, 35
    with quinidine, 236
    with succinylcholine, 125-126
    with theophylline, 105
    with thiazide diuretics, 217
    with thiopental, 125-126
    with trichloroethylene, 125, 128,
      129, 343-344
    with tricyclic antidepressants, 270
    with tubocurarine, 235-236
    with vasopressors, 345
    with verapamil, 78, 139
  intraoperative hypotension from,
    treatment of, 344-345
  long-term therapy with, cessation of,
    116
  metabolism of, 119t
  myocardial oxygen consumption
    and, 121, 121t
  nonsurmountable antagonism and,
    25-26
  plasma levels of, variations in, 118,
    119
  postoperative inotropic support and,
    130
  preoperative, prophylactic, 129-130

preoperative discontinuance of, 78, 343-344
pros and cons of, 128-129
protein binding of, diseases and, 46
effects of alterations in, 43
short-term therapy with, cessation of, *116*
side effects of, 238
surmountable antagonism and, 25-26
Prostaglandin(s), calcium channels and, 135
effect on, of sodium restriction, 211
in renal salt and water regulation, 211
renal, loop diuretics and, 214
Protamine, interaction of, with propranolol, 35
Protein binding, alterations in, clinical effects of, 43
competition for sites of, drug interactions and, 41
diseases and, 41, 45-46
displacement of, criteria for, 21
drug interactions caused by, 21
effect of pH in, 59
in drug disposition, neonatal, 434*t*
in hemodynamic drug interactions, 44-46
in pharmacokinetic drug interactions, 21
liver disease and, 46
mechanisms of, 41-42
of acidic drugs, 44-46
of basic drugs, 45-46
of long-acting drugs, 21
plasma protein changes and, 45-46
renal disease and, 46
Proteins, in ionic transport, 197
plasma, effects of changes in, 45-46
Protriptyline, indications for use of, 268
interaction of, with lidocaine, 270, 402
with local anesthetic agents, 403
with mepivacaine, 402
with norepinephrine, 402
with procaine, 270
Pseudocholinesterase, inhibition of, succinylcholine and, 377-378
interaction of, with antihypertensive agents, 379
with chloroprocaine, 396
with dexamethasone, 396
with echothiophate, 395-396
with methylprednisolone, 396
Pseudocholinesterase deficiency, drug interactions and, 10
interaction of, with succinylcholine, 17
Psychotropic agent(s), 261-277, 261*t*, 265*t*, 268*t*, 270*t*, 275*t*
Pulmonary disease(s), digitalis toxicity and, 190
treatment of, aminophylline in, 348
Pulmonary edema, from reduced sympathetic activity, 149
from sympathomimetic bronchodilators, 109
from tocolytic agents, 433
osmotic diuretics in, 212
theophylline and, 102-103, 104*t*
Pulmonary embolism, isoproterenol in treatment of, 89

Pulmonary hypertension, from minoxidil, 157
treatment of, calcium-channel blocking agents in, 142
Purkinje fiber(s), digitalis dosage and, 183
electrophysiology of, 226-228, *226*
in reentry of excitation, *229*
Pyridostigmine, dosage of, drug interactions and, 381-382
interaction of, with acetylcholinesterase, 395
with antibiotics, 365, 366*t*, 367-368, 381
with local anesthetic agents, 395
with neuromuscular blocking agents, 379, 381-382, 395, *395*
with pancuronium, 367
with plasma cholinesterase, 395, *395*
with d-tubocurarine, *364*
with vecuronium, 376
Pyrogallol, in biosynthesis of catecholamines, 75*t*
interaction of, with norepinephrine, 73

Quaternary ammonium, atropine and scopolamine versus, 166
central nervous system effects of, 164
Quaternary ammonium anticholinergic agent(s), interaction of, with physostigmine, 173
Quaternary ammonium anticholinesterase agent(s), interaction of, with atropine, 171
Quaternary ammonium compound(s), atracurium as, 383
renal excretion of, 22
Quaternary anticholinergic agent(s), antimuscarinic, 171*t*
Quinidine, actions of, 236
anesthetic considerations with, 236
cardiac effects of, 199, 227, 230*t*
displacement of protein binding of, 21
effects of, anticholinergic, 236
extracardiac, 230*t*
peripheral and central nervous, 29
indications for use of, 236
interaction of, with barbiturates, 286
with bupivacaine, 394
with curare, 372
with digitoxin, 181, 191, 236
with digoxin, 180-182, 191, 236
with edrophonium, 372
with enflurane, 236
with halothane, 236
with lidocaine, 234, 237
with neuromuscular blocking agents, 371-372
with pentobarbital, 286
with phenobarbital, 236, 286
with phenothiazines, 264
with phenytoin, 236
with procainamide, 237
with propranolol, 236
with succinylcholine, 372
with thioridazine, 264
with d-tubocurarine, 235, 371-372
with vasodilators, 236

protein binding of, 46
verapamil versus, 239
Quinine, interaction of, with digoxin, 181

Ranitidine, effects of, 176-177
interaction of, with theophylline, 105
Rate theory, of drug efficacy, 24-25
Ratio, dose, defined, 42
therapeutic, defined, 40
Rauwolfia, interaction of, with anesthetic agents, 76-77
Rauwolfia alkaloid(s), interaction of, with digitalis, 191
Reaction(s), anaphylactic, drug antagonism in, 26-27
drug. *See* Drug reaction(s)
excitatory, to anticholinergic agents, 171-172
transfusion, osmotic diuretics in, 212
Rebound hypertension, 77, 153-154
Receptor(s), adrenergic. *See* Adrenergic receptor(s); specific receptors
age of patient and, 42-43
benzodiazepine, 291-293
beta-adrenergic, *beta*-adrenergic blocking agents and, 77-78
catecholamine disposition and, 72-73, *73*
cholinergic, defined, 148
cholinoceptive, defined, 148
desensitization of, 42
dopaminergic, antipsychotic agents and, 261
defined, 86
intensity of drug effect and, 40
muscarinic, defined, 148
muscarinic cholinergic, 24
nicotinic, defined, 148
opioid, 325-326, 327*t*, 328, *328-329*
pharmacologic. *See* Pharmacologic receptor(s); specific receptors
sites of, drug concentration at, 42-49, *43*, 47*t*
"spare," defined, 42
tissue, dose-effect relationship and, 40
Reentry of excitation, causes of, 228, *229*
Reflex compensation, autonomic, calcium-channel blocking agents and, 139, *140*
Regional anesthesia, in epilepsy, rationale for, 254-255
indications for, monoaine oxidase inhibitors and, 274
Regitine. *See* Phentolamine
Reglan. *See* Metoclopramide
Rena, 46
vecuronium in, 385
Renal dialysis, in lithium toxicity, 277
Renal disease(s), atracurium in, 385
effects in, of local anesthetic agents, 399
of procaine, 399
hydralazine in, 156
hyperkalemia and, 201, 204
methyldopa in, 152
protein binding and, 41, 46
vecuronium in, 385
Renal effect(s), of acetazolamide, 213
of loop diuretics, 214
of mercurial diuretics, 213
of osmotic diuretics, 211-212, *212*
of thiazide diuretics, 213

Renal excretion, general principles of, 22-23
  pH shifts and, 58-60
Renal failure, anesthesia in, potassium levels and, 220
  digitalis serum levels in, 188
  diuretics in, neuromuscular blocking agents and, 221
  drug-induced deafness in, 218
  effects in, of neuromuscular blocking agents, 363-365, 368-369, *369*, 371, 381-382, 385
  from captopril, 157
  hyperkalemia and, 216-217
  interaction of, with antibiotics, 363-364, 371
    with furosemide, 364, 371
  morphine in patients with, 48
  prazosin in, 155
  prevention of, osmotic diuretics in, 212
Renal function, anesthesia and, 203-204
  digitalis and, 180-181, 185-187, 191
  effects on, of calcium-channel blocking agents, 142
  guanethidine and, 154
  impaired, acid-forming salts in, 213
  impairment, causes of, 181
  local anesthetic agents and, 393
  neonatal, drug disposition and, 434*t*
  normal, pancuronium in, 368, *369*
    d-tubocurarine in, 368, *369*
  salt metabolism and, 208, *209*, 210-211
  verapamil and, 142
Renal perfusion pressure, hydrostatic pressure and, 208, 210
Renal regulation, of water and electrolytes, 208, *209*, 210-211
Renal transplantation, immunosupression in, with azathioprine, 363-364
Renal tubule(s), effect on, of osmotic diuretics, 211-212, *212*
  salt and water reabsorption in, 208, *209*, 210-211
Renin, 211
Renin-angiotensin system, 211
Reserpine, actions of, 76-77, 150-152
  anesthetic implications with, 265
  cardiac effects of, 76, 151-152
  classification of, 148*t*
  discontinuance of, hypertension from, 154
  dosage of, 148*t*
  hypotension from, anesthetic agents and, 76-77
  indications for use of, 76, 150
    psychiatric, 265
  interaction of, with amphetamine, 266
    with anesthetic agents, 76-77
    with anticholinergic agents, 266
    with anticholinesterase, 27
    with atropine, 266
    with barbiturates, 265*t*, 266
    with catecholamines, 151-152
    with cyclopropane, 266
    with diazepam, 266
    with diethyl ether, 266
    with digitalis, 191, 267
    with dopamine, 265, 267

  with electroconvulsive therapy, 266
  with enflurane, 266
  with ephedrine, 151-152, 151*t*, 266
  with epinephrine, 267
  with halothane, 151*t*, 266, 342, 414, 415*t*, 417, *417*
  with inhalation anesthetic agents, 265*t*, 266, 341-342
  with ketamine, 266
  with magnesium sulfate, 432
  with mephentermine, 266
  with metaraminol, 266
  with methoxyflurane, 266
  with methylphenidate, 266
  with monoamine oxidase inhibitors, 272
  with morphine, 267
  with narcotics, 267, 323
  with neostigmine, 267
  with neuromuscular blocking agents, 265*t*, 267
  with norepinephrine, *73*, 151, 265, 267, 341
  with pargyline, 158
  with phenobarbital, 266
  with phenylephrine, 267
  with phenylpropanolamine, 266
  with physostigmine, 267
  with serotonin, 265
  with sympathomimetic agents, 265*t*, 266-267
  with thiazide diuretics, 217, 267
  with trichloroethylene, 266
  with tricyclic antidepressants, 27, 151
  with d-tubocurarine, 267
  with tyramine, 266
  mechanism of action of, 265, 341
  pharmacology of, 150-152
  preoperative discontinuance of, 76
  receptor binding of, 49
  side effects of, 151, 151*t*
Respiration, anesthetic depth and, 412-413, *414*
Respiratory alkalosis, digitalis toxicity and, 193
  hypokalemia from, digitalis toxicity and, 181
  in shock, 92-94
Respiratory depression, from barbiturates, 289
  from benzodiazepines, 289
  from chlorpromazine, 324
  from diazepam, 313, 349
  from ethyl alcohol, 289
  from local anesthetic agents, 402
  from meperidine, 324
  from midazolam, 317
  from monoamine oxidase inhibitors, 273, 325, 347
  from morphine in combat use, 40
  from narcotic antagonists, 334
  from narcotics, 321-323
    sleep and, 324
    treatment of, 330-331, 335
  nitrous oxide and, 351-353
  rebound, from morphine, 21
  treatment of, narcotic antagonists in, 321
Ritodine, indications for use of, 432
Ro 15-1788, 293-294
"Robin Hood" effect, of beta-

adrenergic blocking agents, 121, *122*

Salicylate(s), interaction of, with anticoagulants, 41
  protein binding of, 42*t*
Salt, metabolism of, renal function and, 208, *209*, 210-211
  water and, diuretic-drug interactions from derangements in, 215-217, 218-220
  loop diuretics in distribution of, 214
  thiazide diuretics in distribution of, 213
Salt(s), acid-forming, 212-213
Sarcolemma, defined, 197
  in calcium transport, 197-199
  inotropic effect of digitalis and, 184*t*
Sarcoplasmic reticulum, calcium transport in, 199
  ion transport in, 183, 184*t*
Schizophrenia, treatment of, 261, 265, 348
Scopolamine, as belladonna alkaloid, 171*t*
  cardiac effects of, 165-166
  effects of, 170-172
  interaction of, with anesthetic agents, 171-172
    with antiparkinsonian agents, 263
    with antipsychotic agents, 263
    with barbiturates, 254
    with cyclopropane, 415*t*, 422
    with inhalation anesthetic agents, 415*t*, 422
    with ketamine, 310
    with midazolam, 314
    with nalbuphine, 332*t*
    with other anticholinergic agents, 267-268
    with physostigmine, 173, 295
    with promethazine, 254
  quaternary ammonium versus, 166
  side effects of, problem secretions as, 167
Secobarbital, dosage of, preanesthetic, 254
  interaction of, with ethyl alcohol, 289
    with ketamine, 285, 311
Second-gas effect, 351
Secretion(s), salivary, from anticholinergic agents, 167-168
Sedation, from antihypertensive agents, 150-151, 151*t*
  from antipsychotic agents, 18, 261
  from clonidine, 153
  from guanabenz, 155
  from labetalol, 156
  from scopolamine, 170-171
Sedative(s), hypnotic agents and, 282-300
  interaction of, with chlorpromazine, 79
    with halothane, 68-69
    with inhalation anesthetic agents, 349, 413, 415*t*
    with monoamine oxidase inhibitors, 347
Sedative-hypnotic agent(s), anesthetic considerations with, 282, 299-300

INDEX

anesthetic depth and, 283-284
as central nervous system drugs, 28
cross-tolerance to, 299
dependence on, anesthesia and, 29-30
effects of, central nervous system, 283-284, 299
indications for use of, 283
interaction of, with antipsychotic agents, 262-263
  with ethyl alcohol, 289
  with inhalation anesthetic agents, 68-69, 283-284
  with monoamine oxidase inhibitors, 273
  with narcotics, 334
  with tricyclic antidepressants, 269-270
pharmacologic mechanisms of, 283-284
preanesthetic, 283-284
time course of action of, 29-30
types of, 282
Seizure disorder(s), agents in treatment 245-257, 246t, 247t
  anesthesia in, 245
    general, 255-257
    procedure for, 254-255
  incidence of, 24
  See also Epilepsy; Antiepileptic agent(s)
Seizure(s), barbiturates and, 283
  control of, acetazolamide in, 253
    barbiturates in, 249
    carbamazepine in, 250-251
    clonazepam in, 252-253
    clorazepate in, 253
    diazepam in, 252, 399
    ethosuximide in, 251-252
    lorazepam in, 253
    methsuximide in, 252
    phenobarbital in, 249
    phenytoin in, 247
    preanesthetic, 253-254
    primidone, 249-250
    trimethadione in, 252
    valproic acid in, 251
  from *beta*-carboline carboxylate esters, 293
  from enflurane, 256, 266
  from hyperventilation, 257
  from isoflurane, 255
  from ketamine, 256, 266
  from lidocaine, 237, 400, 402
    prevention of, 294
    treatment of, 294-295
  from local anesthetic agents, 399-400
  from narcotics, 254, 322
  from phenothiazines, 264
  from tricyclic antidepressants, 270
  in asthmatics, 106
  in toxemia of pregnancy, treatment of, 431
  sedative-hypnotic agents and, 283
  theophylline-induced, 102-103
  treatment of, oxygen in, 399-400
    paraldehyde in, 297
Selective antagonism, in opiate anesthesia, 2
Septic shock, 85
  treatment of, naloxone in, 336
Septicemic shock, renal blood flow in, 89
Serotonin, calcium channels and, 135

interaction of, with halothane, 416
  with lithium, 275
  with monoamine oxidase inhibitors, 347
  with parachlorophenylalanine, 414
  with reserpine, 265
Serpasil. *See* Reserpine
Sexual dysfunction, from antihypertensive agents, 151t
  from guanethidine, 154
  from labetalol, 156
Shock, alkalosis in, 92-93
  anaphylactic, characteristics of, 33
    treatment of, 33-34
  cardiogenic. *See* Cardiogenic shock
  causes of, 91-92
  combat, morphine and, 40
  defined, 85
  dopamine in treatment of, 90
  during anesthesia, causes of, 91-92
    treatment of, 92-94
  hemorrhagic. *See* Hemorrhagic shock
  hypovolemic, defined, 85
  microcirculation in, 85
  monitoring of, 92
  neurogenic, defined, 85
  septic, defined, 85
  septicemic, renal blood flow in, 89
  terminal-phase, 85
  treatment of, 92-94
    agents in, 88t
    naloxone in, 336
Shy-Drager syndrome, calcium-channel blocking agents and, 139
Sick cell syndrome, cause of, 203
Sick sinus syndrome, calcium-channel blocking agents and, 139
Sinequan. *See* Doxepin
Sisomicin, 375
SK-Pramine. *See* Imipramine
Sleep, benzodiazepine receptors in, 293
  incidence of cardiac dysrhythmias during, 163
  interaction of, with narcotics, 324
  mechanism of, barbiturates and, 255
Sleep Eze, as anticholinergic antimuscarinic agent, 171t
Slow-reacting substance, sensitivity to, 160
Smoking, nicotine overdose from, 163
Sodium, active transport of, renal tubular, 208, *209*, 210
  anesthetic considerations with, 203-204
  calcium-channel blocking agents and, 136
  fast channels of, inactivation of, 137
  imbalance of, water imbalance versus, 204
  interaction of, with cardiac glycosides, 199
    with narcotic agonists, 334-335
    with narcotic antagonists, 334-335
  ion transport of, inotropic effect of digitalis and, 182-183, 184t
  ions of, cardiac action potentials and, 226-227
    ethyl alcohol and, 287
  loss of, causes of, 202-203
  myocardial action potentials and, 136-137, *137*, 199
  osmotic pressure exerted by, 208

physiologic role of, 202-204
reabsorption of, aldosterone in, 211
  antidiuresis and, *212*
  loop diuretics and, 214
  osmotic diuresis and, 211-212, *212*
  renal tubular, 210
  restriction of, hormonal effects of, 211
retention of, causes of, 203
  from antihypertensive agents, 151t
  from pargyline, 157
  treatment of, 203
transport of, ion channels in, 198-199
water distribution and, 207
Sodium amobarbital, 431
Sodium benzoate, interaction of, with bilirubin, 434
  with lidocaine, 404
  with procaine, 404
Sodium bicarbonate, interaction of, with pancuronium, 382
  with d-tubocurarine, 382
  renal tubular reabsorption of, *209*, 210
  treatment of acidosis with, hyperkalemia and, 220
  treatment of hyperkalemia with, 204, 216
Sodium biphosphate, 273
Sodium bisulfite, 392
Sodium chloride, metabolism of, renal function and, 208, *209*, 210-211
  transport of, water distribution and, 207
Sodium pump, defined, 182
  inotropic effect of digitalis and, 182-183, 184t
Solanum dulcamara,, as source of anticholinergic alkaloids, 171t
Solanum tuberosum, as source of anticholinergic alkaloids, 171t
Sominex, as anticholinergic antimuscarinic agent, 171t
"Spare receptor(s)," defined, 42
Spinal anesthesia. *See* Conduction anesthesia
Spironolactone, actions of, 214
  interaction of, with aldosterone, 214
  with aspirin, 217
  with digitalis, 181, 189, 215, 217
  with lithium carbonate, 277
  with succinylcholine, 217
  site of action of, 214, *215*
Stadol. *See* Butorphanol
Status epilepticus, 253, 294, 297
"Stone heart," defined, 122
Streptomycin, in multiple-drug therapy, 9-10
  interaction of, with calcium, 201, 365, 366t
  with neostigmine, 366t
  with succinylcholine, 366t
  with d-tubocurarine, 366t
Succinylcholine, atracurium versus, 383-384
  cardiac effects of, 31-32, 168-169
  during anesthesia, 234-235
  effects of, apnea as, 395
  in hyperkalemia, 204
  ganglionic stimulation by, 163
  hydrolysis of, 396
  hyperkalemia from, 94

Succinylcholine (cont.)
  in pregnancy, cholinesterase and, 396
  indication for use of, 234-235
  interaction of, with AB-132, 396
    with alkylating agents, 378
    with antibiotics, 366t
    with anticholinesterase agents, 377
    with antimuscarinic anticholinergic agents, 170
    with atracurium, 375
    with atropine, 168-169
    with beta-adrenergic blocking agents, 124
    with calcium, 205
    with cholinesterase, 164-165
    with cocaine, 401
    with cyclophosphamide, 378
    with cytotoxic agents, 378
    with diazepam, 297, 313
    with digitalis, 191-192
    with diuretics, 216-217
    with echothiophate, 377-378, 395
    with edrophonium, 377
    with enflurane, 354
    with gallamine, 373-374
    with halothane, 168, 354
    with isoflurane, 353-354
    with ketamine, 372
    with lidocaine, 371, 402
    with lithium carbonate, 79, 275-276, 372-373
    with magnesium, 205
    with magnesium sulfate, 372, 430-431
    with midazolam, 316
    with nalbuphine, 332t
    with neostigmine, 376-377, 395
    with nitrogen mustard, 378
    with nitrous oxide, 168
    with organophosphate eyedrops, 164-165
    with oxytocin, 430
    with pancuronium, 235, 373-374
    with pharmacologic receptors, 24
    with phenelzine, 273, 378
    with plasma cholinesterase, 395
    with promazine, 264
    with propranolol, 125-126
    with pseudocholinesterase deficiency, 17
    with pyridostigmine, 395
    with quinidine, 372
    with spironolactone, 217
    with tacrine, 378
    with thiopental, 309
    with triamterene, 217
    with d-tubocurarine, 235, 373-374
    with vecuronium, 375
  interactions with, pseodocholinesterase inhibition and, 377-378
  neuromuscular transmission blocked by, 163
  possible indication for, 14t
  response to, 24-25
  side effects of, 373-374
    nerve stimulation in, 163
  toxicity of, plasma cholinesterase and, 395
  treatment of cardiac dysrhythmias with, 74
Succinyldicholine, interaction of, with plasma cholinesterase, 22

Sufentanil, indications for use of, as induction agent, 350
  interaction of, with halothane, 415t, 419
    with naloxone, 419
Sulfafursaol, interaction of, with thiopental, 309
Sulfamylon, as carbonic anhydrase inhibitor, 213
Sulfisoxazole, 434
Sulfonamide(s), interaction of, with barbiturates, 284
    with para-aminobenzoic acid, 404
    with thiopental, 6, 309
  protein binding of, 41
Sulfonylurea(s), interaction of, with ethyl alcohol, 290-291
Supraventricular tachycardia(s), 236-239
Surgical incision, anesthetic depth and, 409, 410t, 412-413
Suxamethonium. See Succinylcholine
Sympathetic amine(s), interaction of, with monoamine oxidase inhibitors, 268, 271-272
    with tricyclic antidepressants, 268-269
Sympathetic nervous system, activation of, by digitalis, 184-185
  activity of, agents decreasing, 75-79
    agents increasing, 79-82, 81
    nonpharmacologic inducers of, 74-75
  cardiac effects of, 71
  function of, measurement of, 149-150
  neuroeffector junction in, 114-115, 115-116
  role of, 71, 162
  stimulation of, 71
Sympathetic neuroeffector junction(s), 114-115, 115-116
Sympatholytic agent(s), antihypertensive, pharmacology of, 150-153
  classification of, 148t
  dosage of, 148t
Sympathomimetic agent(s), actions of, 115, 150
  cardiac effects of, 92-83, 83t
  in hypotension, 88t
    treatment of, 91-94
  in shock, 88t
    treatment of, 91-94
  interaction of, with anticholinergic agents, 268
    with antihypertensive agents, 150
    with antipsychotic agents, 261t, 263
    with butyrophenones, 261t, 263
    with calcium, 198
    with chloroform, 82
    with digitalis, 192
    with guanethidine, 154
    with inhalation anesthetic agents, 93
    with ketamine, 257
    with monoamine oxidase inhibitors, 22, 157, 270t
    with narcotics, 93, 324
    with parasympathomimetic agents, 26
    with pharmacologic receptors, 24

  with phenothiazines, 261t, 263
  with reserpine, 265t, 266-267
  with tricyclic antidepressants, 268t, 268
Sympathomimetic amine(s), actions of, 87, 88t, 89-91
  cardiac effects of, 354-355
  indications for use of, in anesthesia, 87, 355
  interaction of, with inhalation anesthetic agents, 354-355
    with monoamine oxidase inhibitors, 347
    with potassium, 220
    with tricyclic antidepressants, 81
Sympathomimetic bronchodilator(s), actions of, 108-109
  comparison of, 108t
  drug interactions with, 109
  indications for use of, 109
Sympathomimetic drug(s), adrenergic mechanisms of, 71-75, 73-74
  adrenergic mechanisms of, influences on normal, 75-82, 75t
  anesthetic, 83-84
  anesthetic influence on, 82-83, 83t
  in shock, 84-87, 86, 88, 89-94
    classification of, 85-87
    management of, 91-94
Synaptic gap(s), in sympathetic neuroeffector junction, 114, 115
  size of, 161-162
Syndrome(s), abstinence, from buprenorphine, 329
  acute abstinence. See Acute abstinence syndrome
  antihypertensive withdrawal, 151t, 153
  central anticholinergic, 170-173, 171t, 172t
  lupus-like, from hydralazine, 156
  nephrotic, from trimethadione, 252
  rapid transit, digitalis toxicity and, 189-190
  Shy-Drager, calcium-channel blocking agents and, 139
  sick cell, cause of, 203
  sick sinus, calcium-channel blocking agents and, 139
  Wolff-Parkinson-White, aprindine in, 240
Synergism, defined, 3-4

Tachycardia, abnormal automaticity in, 227
  catecholamine-induced, 73-74
  endotracheal intubation followed by, 71-72
  from atropine, 168
  from beta-adrenergic blocking agents, 132t
  from chlorpromazine, 79
  from cholinergic agents, 170
  from digitalis, 187
  from disopyramide, 238
  from epinephrine, 3
  from gallamine, 384
  from ketamine, 310
  from minoxidil, 157
  from naloxone, 336
  from nicotine overdose, 163
  from pancuronium, 380, 384
  from succinylcholine, 163

from thiopental, 308
from tocolytic agents, 432
from trimethaphan, 158
induction of anesthesia followed by, 71-72
intraoperative, *beta*-adrenergic blocking agents in, 121-122, *125*
treatment of, 342
mechanism of, 228
nifedipine-induced, 138
nitroprusside-induced, 143
reentrant, 230
treatment of, *beta*-adrenergic blocking agents in, 121-122, *125-126*
with antidysrhythmic agents, 232-235
supraventricular, 232-239
treatment of, 136, 185
ventricular, 345
Tachyphylaxis, catecholamines and, 42
to chloroprocaine, 401
Tacrine, interaction of, with succinylcholine, 378
Talwin. *See* Pentazocine
Tegretol. *See* Carbamazepine
Temazepam, interaction of, with cimetidine, 294
Temgesic. *See* Buprenorphine
Terbutaline, actions of, 89
comparison of with other bronchodilators, 108*t*
indications for use of, 89, 432
interaction of, with betamethasone, 433
Terminal-phase shock, 85
Tetanus, treatment of, paraldehyde in, 297
Tetany, from hypomagnesemia, 204
Tetracaine, hydrolysis of, 396
interaction of, with chloropropane, 401
with cholinesterase, 395
with lidocaine, 401
with nitrous oxide, 400
with plasma cholinesterase, 401
with procaine, 401
with tetracaine, 401
Tetracycline(s), distribution of, 42
interaction of, with amphotericin B, 19*t*
with antacids, 19
with calcium, 366*t*
with cephalothin, 19*t*
with chloramphenicol, 19*t*
with digitalis, 189, 192
with erythromycin, 19*t*
with neostigmine, 366*t*
with succinylcholine, 366*t*
with d-tubocurarine, 366*t*
Tetrahydroaminacrine. *See* Tacrine
Tetrodotoxin, 199, 227
Tetrohydrocannabinol, actions of, 298-299
anesthetic considerations with, 298-299
effects of, anesthetic depth and, 422
central nervous system, 299
dosage and, 299
interaction of, with barbiturates, 298-299
with cyclopropane, 299, 415*t*, 422
with ethyl alcohol, 299
with halothane, 299, 415*t*, 422

with oxymorphone, 299
with pentobarbital, 299
with phenobarbital, 299
Theobromine, theophylline compared to, 101
Theophylline, allergy to, 103
clearance of, 103-104, 104*t*
congeners of, 102
dosage of, 102-104
effects of, 102-108
indications for use of, 102
interaction of, with adenosine, 102
with antibiotics, 105
with calcium, 296
with calcium-channel blocking agents, 140
with cimetidine, 104-105
with corticosteroids, 110
with diazepam, 296
with enflurane, 105-107
with erythromycin, 105
with halothane, 101, 105-107
with histamine H_2 blocking agent(s), 177
with inhalation anesthetic agents, 105-107
with isoflurane, 106
with ketamine, 101, 105-106
with muscle relaxants, 107-108
with pancuronium, 107-108
with phenobarbital, 105
with phenytoin, 105
with propranolol, 105
with ranitidine, 105
with troleandomycin, 105
mechanism action of, 102
metabolites of, 103
pharmacokinetics of, 103-104, 104*t*
preoperative levels of, 104, 107
preparations of, 101-102, 102*t*
Therapeutic index, defined, 28
Therapeutic ratio, defined, 40
Thiazide diuretic(s), actions of, 213-214
diabetogenic, 217-218
indications for use of, 214
interaction of, with *alpha*-methyldopa, 217
with antihypertensive agents, 217
with chlorpropamide, 217-218
with cholestyramine, 19
with clonidine, 217
with guanethidine, 217
with hypoglycemic agents, 217-218
with lithium carbonate, 276-277
with minoxidil, 217
with monoamine oxidase inhibitors, 274
with probenecid, 213, 218
with propranolol, 217
with reserpine, 217, 267
side effects of, 213-214
sites of action of, 213-214, *215*
Thiobarbiturate(s), interaction of, with local anesthetic agents, 295
Thiopental, actions of, 308
alternatives to, 314, 316
anoxic encephalopathy prevented by, 46-47
biotransformation of, 63, 308
cardiac effects of, 169, 308
clearance of, 46
distribution of, cardiac output and, 20
tissue, 42

dosage of, 46
duration of action of, 46
effects of, anticonvulsant, 295
neuronal, 255
indications for use of, 308
as induction agent, 349
interaction of, with anticholinergic agents, 167, 169, 170
with aspirin, 46
with chloramphenicol, 309
with chlorpromazine, 262-263
with contrast media, 308-309
with cyclopropane, 309
with halothane, 309
with imipramine, 270
with inhalation anesthetic agents, 349
with lidocaine, 295
with lithium carbonate, 276
with local anesthetic agents, 295
with morphine, 331
with nalbuphine, 331, 332*t*
with naloxone, 415*t*, 416
with naproxen, 46
with narcotics, 324
with nitrous oxide, 352
with phenobarbital, 435
with phenylbutazone, 46
with preanesthetic medication, 283
with propranolol, 125-126
with quinidine, 372
with succinylcholine, 309, 372
with sulfafurasol, 309
with sulfonamides, 6, 309
liver failure and, 46
pharmacokinetics of, 46-47
protein binding of, 41, 42*t*, 46, 308
Thioridazine, actions of, 261
as agent with anticholinergic activity, 172*t*
interaction of, with anticholinergic agents, 263
with antiparkinsonian agents, 263
with quinidine, 264
side effects of, 261, 267
Thio-TEPA, interaction of, with pancuronium, 378
Thioxanthene(s), indications for use of, 261
Threshold potential(s), electrophysiology of, 226-227, *226*
Thrombocytopenia, from carbamazepine, 250
from valproic acid, 251
Thrombosis, possible, in case report analysis, 14*t*
Thyroid function, digitalis toxicity and, 192
Thyroid preparation(s), interaction of, with cholestyramine, 19
Thyrotoxicosis, cardiac dysrhythmias in, 231, 238
propranolol in treatment of, 78, 238
Thyroxine, interaction of, with ketamine, 84
Tidal volume, anesthetic depth and, 412-413, *414*
Timolol, *beta*-adrenergic blockade by, 117, 118*t*
dosage regimen of, 118
interaction of, with phenobarbital, 285
lack of cardioselectivity of, 343

Timolol (cont.)
  metabolism of, 119t
  topical use of, 344
Titration of drug dose, rationale for, 17
Tobacco, side effects of, 163
Tobramycin, 375
Tocainide, 230t, 240
Tocolytic agent(s), 432-433
Tofranyl. See Imipramine
Tolazoline, interaction of, with halothane, 417
  similarity of, to clonidine, 77
Tolbutamide, interaction of, with ethanol, 44
Tolerance, acute, to intravenous anesthetic agents, 29
  drug, anesthetic premedication and, 14t
    enzyme induction and, 67
  from barbiturates, 285
  to anesthetic agents, 128, 129
  to barbiturates, 288
  to beta-adrenergic blocking agents, 128, 129
  to ethyl alcohol, 287
  to fentanyl, 331
  to local anesthetic agents, 401
    in epilepsy, 399-400
  to narcotics, 331
  to sympathomimetic bronchodilators, 109
Toxemia, diazoxide in, 158
  incidence of, 430
  magnesium administration in, 204, 372, 431
Toxicity, aminophylline, 349
  amphetamine, 81
  citrate, 201-202
  cocaine, 82
  cyanide, 158
  digitalis. See Digitalis toxicity
  drug, cytochrome P450 and, 177
    pH shifts and, 60-61
    plasma cholinesterase and, 395
    from alterations in plasma proteins, 45-46
  lithium, diuretics and, 217
    symptoms of, 276
    treatment of, 277
  of general anesthetic agents, 16, 355-356
  of local anesthetic agents, combinations of, 401
    metabolites of, 403-404, 403
    pH and, 56, 58-59
    seizures from, 399-400
  of mercurial diuretics, 213
  theophylline, 102-103
  valproic acid, 251
Train-of-four response, 376
Trandate. See Labetalol
Tranquilizer(s), as central nervous system drugs, 28
  biotransformation inhibited by, 66
  time course of action of, 29-30
Transaminase(s), serum, methyldopa and, 152
Transfusion reaction(s), osmotic diuretics in, 212
Transmembrane potential(s), electrophysiology of, 226-227, 226
Transplantation, kidney, 363-364
Transport, active. See Active transport
  passive, 209

Tranxene. See Clorazepate
Tranylcypromine, actions of, 79-80
  indications for use of, 271
  interaction of, with calcium, 202
    with enflurane, 80
    with fentanyl, 80
    with ketamine, 269
    with narcotics, 325
    with norepinephrine, 73
Trauma, head, central anticholinergic syndrome and, 171
  spinal, succinylcholine in, 204
Trazodone, actions of, 271
Triameterene, actions of, 214
  interaction of, with digitalis, 181, 189
    with digoxin, 217
    with lithium carbonate, 277
    with succinylcholine, 217
  site of action of, 214, 215
Triazolam, interaction of, with cimetidine, 294
  with ethyl alcohol, 289
Trichloroacetate, as chloral hydrate metabolite, 290
Trichloroacetic acid, as chloral hydrate metabolite, 297
  interaction of, with warfarin, 297
Trichloroethanol, as chloral hydrate metabolite, 290, 297
Trichloroethylene, interaction of, with beta-adrenergic blocking agents, 125, 128, 129, 344
  with epinephrine, 354
  with propranolol, 125, 128, 129, 343-344
  with reserpine, 266
Tricyclic antidepressant(s), actions of, 80-81
  anesthetic considerations with, 269
  cardiac effects of, 81, 347
  catecholamine synthesis and, 80-81
  indications for use of, 268
  interaction of, with anticholinergic agents, 268t, 269
    with antihypertensive agents, 27-28, 34, 347
    with barbiturates, 44, 268t, 269-270, 286
    with bethanidine, 27
    with calcium, 202
    with central nervous system depressants, 81
    with clonidine, 27-28, 153
    with cocaine, 269, 403
    with enflurane, 256
    with epinephrine, 81, 268
    with ethyl alcohol, 287-288
    with felypressin, 269
    with gallamine, 381
    with guanethidine, 7, 27, 77, 81, 155
    with halothane, 81, 269, 347
    with inhalation anesthetic agents, 347
    with ketamine, 257, 269
    with local anesthetic agents, 402-403
    with monoamine oxidase inhibitors, 80-81, 271
    with muscarinic receptors, 24
    with narcotics, 268t, 269
    with norepinephrine, 268
    with pancuronium, 81, 269, 379-381

  with phenytoin, 248
  with physostigmine, 295
  with propranolol, 270
  with reserpine, 27, 151
  with sedative-hypnotic agents, 269-270
  with sympathetic amines, 268-269
  with sympathomimetic agents, 268t, 268-269
  with sympathomimetic amines, 81
  with vasopressors, 268-269, 347
  mechanism of action of, 268, 347
  monoamine oxidase inhibitors compared with, 80
  new, 270-271
  side effects of, 267, 347
    seizure threshold and, 270
    with anticholinergic activity, 172, 172t
Tridione. See Trimethadione
Triethylenethiophosphoramide, 378
Trifluoperazine, 261-262
Triggered activity, defined, 227
Trihexyphenidyl, as anticholinergic anti-Parkinson agent, 171t
  indications for use of, 267
Trilene. See Trichloroethylene
Trimeprazine, preanesthetic, anesthetic depth and, 283
Trimethadione, indications for use of, 252
  pharmacokinetics of, 247t, 252
  side effects of, 252
Trimethaphan, actions of, 158
  contraindications to, 158
  effects of, 378-379
  in hypertensive crises, 158
  interaction of, with ketamine, 310
    with local anesthetic agents, 402
    with monoamine oxidase inhibitors, 80
    with neuromuscular blocking agents, 158, 378-379
Troleandomycin, interaction of, with theophylline, 105
Tropin, calcium binding to, 198
Tropolone, in biosynthesis of catecholamines, 75t
Troponin, calcium transport and, 137, 199-200
  inotropic effect of digitalis and, 184t
Troponin-tropomyosin complex, calcium and, 198
d-Tubocurare, interaction of, with diuretics, 216
d-Tubocurarine, actions of, postjunctional membrane, 353
  cardiac effects of, 384-385
  drug interactions from, 379-380, 380
  components of, 216
  effects of, antibiotics as similar to, 365
  in renal failure, 368-369, 369, 371
  ganglionic blocking by, 165
  indication for use of, 235
  interaction of, with antibiotics, 366t, 371, 381
    with antidysrhythmic agents, 371-372
    with atropine, 364
    with calcium, 366t
    with clindamycin, 366t
    with colistin, 366t

INDEX

with decamethonium, 373
with digitalis, 192
with diuretics, 364-365, *364*
with enflurane, 354, 374
with epinephrine, 83
with furosemide, 217, 364-365, *364*, 371
with gentamicin, 363-364, *364*, 366*t*
with halothane, 369-371, *370*, 374, 379, *380*
with histamine, 379, 384
with inhalation anesthetic agents, 354
with isoflurane, 354, 374
with kanamycin, 366*t*
with ketamine, 372
with lidocaine, 235, 371, 402
with lincomycin, 366*t*
with lithium carbonate, 275-277
with magnesium sulfate, 372, 430-431
with mannitol, 364, *364*
with monoamine oxidase inhibitors, 274
with morphine, 323
with neomycin, 366*t*
with neostigmine, 364, 366*t*, 381-382, *382*
with paromomycin, 366*t*
with phenytoin, 235
with polymyxin A, 366*t*
with polymyxin B, 366*t*
with procainamide, 235
with propranolol, 235, 236
with pyridostigmine, *364*
with quinidine, 235, 371-372
with reserpine, 267
with streptomycin, 366*t*
with succinylcholine, 192, 235, 373-374
with tetracycline, 366*t*
with viomycin, 366*t*
opioid receptors and, hypothetical interactions with, 327*t*
Turnover number(s), of drug-metabolizing enzymes, 64-65
Twitch height, neuromuscular function measured by, 363, *364*, 367, *370*, 370-371, *382*
Type A drug reaction(s), 18
Type B drug reaction(s), 18
Tyramine, action of, 87
"cheese reaction" and, 22
food sources of, 80, 157
interaction of, with ketamine, 84
with monoamine oxidase inhibitors, 22, 80, 157, 272, 288
with norepinephrine, 73
with reserpine, 266
Tyrosine, biosynthesis of, 75*t*
interaction of, with norepinephrine, 73

United States Pharmacopeia Dispensing Information, 6
Urinary output, measurement of in shock, 92
Urine, acidification of, in monoamine oxidase inhibitor-narcotic interactions, 273
alkalinization of, in lithium toxicity, 277

in treatment of drug overdose, 58
formation of, 208, *209*, 210-211
pH shifts in, drug excretion and, 58-61
retention of, from narcotics, 322
from pargyline, 157

Vagus nerve, actions of digitalis on, 183-184
cardiac dysrhythmias and, anticholinergic agents and, 170
stimulation of, 161-163
Valium. *See* Diazepam
Valproate. *See* Valproic acid
Valproic acid, dosage of, antiepileptic, 247*t*, 251
indications for use of, 251
interaction of, with barbiturates, 251
with benzodiazepines, 251, 296
with clonazepam, 251
with diazepam, 296
with halothane, 251
with narcotics, 251
with phenobarbital, 249
with picrotoxin, 292
with thiopental, 249
pharmacokinetics of, 247*t*, 251
side effects of, 251
Vancomycin, interaction of, with cephalothin, 19*t*
with chloramphenicol, 19*t*
substitution of for neomycin, 9
Vanillylmandelic acid, 75*t*
Vasoconstriction, epinephrine-induced, 87
from *alpha*-adrenergic stimulation, 148
from calcium transport, 198
from cocaine, 391
from ergot alkaloids, 429
from oxytocin, 429
in shock, 92-93
norepinephrine-induced, 89
Vasodilation, from *beta*-adrenergic blocking agents, 121, *122*
from *beta*-adrenergic stimulation, 148
from calcium-channel blocking agents, 345
from ethyl alcohol, 290
from isoproterenol, 89
Vasodilator(s), in intraoperative hypertension, 342
interaction of, with digitalis, 181-182, 190
with monoamine oxidase inhibitors, 348
with procainamide, 237
with quinidine, 236
peripheral, dosage of, 148*t*
pharmacology of, 156-157
Vasopressin, interaction of, with oxytocin, 428
Vasopressor(s), contraindication to, 233
in intraoperative hypotension, 342
interaction of, with bretylium, 239
with halothane, 380
with inhalation anesthetic agents, 263, 342
with lidocaine, 393, *394*
with local anesthetic agents, 393
with monoamine oxidase inhibitors, 348

with oxytocic agents, 428-430
with phenothiazines, 348
with propranolol, 345
with tricyclic antidepressants, 268*t*, 268-269, 347
Vasospasm, coronary, 141
Vasoxyl. *See* Methoxamine
Vecuronium, age and, 384
cardiac effects of, 384-385
developmental chemistry of, 383
dosage of, 383
effects of, cumulative, 383-384
reversibility of, 375-376
in liver disease, 385
in renal disease, 385
interaction of, with 4-aminopyridine, 376
with antibiotics, 375, 375
with anticholinesterase agents, 375-376
with atropine, 376
with butyrylcholinesterase, 375
with diaminopyridine, 376
with edrophonium, 376
with enflurane, 374-375
with etomidate, 374
with fentanyl, 374-375
with gammahydroxybutrate, 374
with halothane, 374-375
with inhalation anesthetic agents, 354, 374-375, 422
with isoflurane, 354, 374
with ketamine, 374
with neostigmine, 375-376
with pyridostigmine, 376
with succinylcholine, 375
neuromuscular transmission blocked by, 163
obstetric use of, 385
potency of, 383
side effects of, 165
Ventricular fibrillation, causes of, 85
from digitalis, 187
prevention of, methacholine in, 162
treatment of, in shock, 84-85
prior to epinephrine infusion, 87
Venule(s), in shock, 85
schema of, *86*
Verapamil, actions of, 137-138, 239
cardiac effects of, 137-138, 138*t*, 139, 228, 230*t*, 345
anesthetic depth and, 418
experimental, 231
comparison of with other calcium-channel blocking agents, 138*t*
dosage of, 239
effects of, antibronchospastic, 142
extracardiac, 230*t*
in hepatic dysfunction, 139
on renal function, 142
plasma levels and, 138
forms of, 418
indications for use of, 136, 138, 234, 239, 345
interaction of, with aminophylline, 140
with anesthetic agents, 225
with anticholinesterase, 142
with aspirin, 139
with *beta*-adrenergic blocking agents, 139, *140*, 239, 345-346
with calcium, 139, 198
with dantrolene, 142
with diazepam, 139

Verapamil, interaction of *(cont.)*
  with digoxin, 139-140, 181, 192
  with enflurane, 345
  with fentanyl, 141-142
  with halothane, 139, 141-142, 345-346, 415t, 418
  with inhalation anesthetic agents, 136, 141, 239, 345-346
  with isoflurane, 345
  with ketamine, 310
  with lidocaine, 139
  with morphine, 141-142
  with narcotics, 345
  with nitrous oxide, 141, 345
  with pancuronium, 142
  with potassium, 140
  with procainamide, 237
  with propranolol, 78, 139
 intraoperative dysrhythmias treated with, 122
 mechanism of action of, 345
 overdosage of, calcium in treatment of, 201
 protein binding of, 139
 structure of, 345
Veterans Administration Hospital(s), 10
Viomycin, 366t

Vitamin B, interaction of, with erythromycin, 19t
Vitamin K, in treatment of gastric bleeding, 282
Volume of distribution, defined, 40-41
 protein binding and, 45
 tissue binding and, 45

Warfarin, biotransformation of, drug interactions and, 67
 interaction of, with antihistamines, 298
  with barbiturates, 44
  with chloral hydrate, 297
  with cholestyramine, 19
  with ethacrynic acid, 217
  with ethyl alcohol, 44, 288
  with glutethimide, 298
  with histamine H$_2$ blocking agents, 177
  with phenobarbital, 67
  with phenylbutazone, 21
  with trichloroacetic acid, 297
 protein binding and, 43, 45
Water, body, sodium concentration and, 202-204
 dissociation of, 52

 distribution of, osmotic pressure and, 206-208, *207*
 in treatment of hypernatremia, 203
 osmotic diuretics and, 211-212, *212*
 salt and, diuretic-drug interactions from derangements in, 215-217, 218-220
  loop diuretics in distribution of, 214
  renal metabolism of, 208, *209*, 210-211
  thiazide diuretics in distribution of, 213
Water-soluble drug(s), 64-65, *66*
Wolff-Parkinson-White syndrome, treatment of, aprindine in, 240
Wyamine. *See* Mephentermine
Wytensin. *See* Guanabenz

Xanthine(s), inotropic effect of digitalis and, 184t
 interaction of, with benzodiazepines, 296-297
Xenobiotic(s), 63-64
Xerostomia, from captopril, 157
 from clonidine, 153
 from guanabenz, 155

Zarontin. *See* Ethosuximide